OXFORD MEDICAL PUBLICATIONS

Improving the Health of
Older People: a World View

Improving the Health
of
Older People: a World View

Edited by

ROBERT L. KANE
Dean of Public Health,
University of Minnesota

J. GRIMLEY EVANS
Professor of Geriatric Medicine,
University of Oxford

and
DAVID MACFADYEN
Chief, Global Programme for Health of the Elderly,
World Health Organization

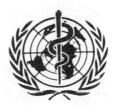

PUBLISHED ON BEHALF OF
THE WORLD HEALTH ORGANIZATION
BY
OXFORD UNIVERSITY PRESS
OXFORD   NEW YORK   TOKYO
1990

Oxford University Press, Walton Street, Oxford OX2 6DP
Oxford New York Toronto
Delhi Bombay Calcutta Madras Karachi
Petaling Jaya Singapore Hong Kong Tokyo
Nairobi Dar es Salaam Cape Town
Melbourne Auckland

and associated companies in
Berlin Ibadan

Oxford is a trade mark of Oxford University Press

Published in the United States
by Oxford University Press, New York

British Library Cataloguing in Publication Data
Improving the health of older people.
I. Kane, Robert L. (Robert Lewis, 1940–) II.
Evans, J. Grimley (John Grimley) III. Macfadyen,
David, 1931 –
613'.0438
ISBN 0–19–261792–3

Library of Congress Cataloging-in-Publication Data
Improving the health of older people: a world view/edited by Robert
L. Kane, J. Grimley Evans, and David Macfadyen.
(Oxford medical publications)
Rev. papers from the second meeting in Nov. 1987 of a WHO expert
committee.
Includes index.
1. Aged—Health and hygiene—Congresses. 2. Aged—Health and
hygiene—Government policy—Congresses. I. Kane, Robert L., 1940– .
II. Evans, J. Grimley. III. Macfadyen, David, 1935– .
IV. World Health Organization. V. Series.
RA564.8.I48 1990   362.1'9897—dc20   90-32316
ISBN 0–19–261792–3

Set by Graphicraft, Hong Kong
Printed and bound in Great Britain by
Courier International Ltd
Tiptree Essex

Foreword

For forty years, the World Health Organization has employed the mechanism of the Expert Committee to promote the provision of effective health care and to make practical recommendations on health programmes for the people of the world. Two such committees have prepared concise reports on aging. The first, in 1973, made recommendations on the planning and organization of services for older people. The second, in November 1987, made recommendations on the health of older people. For the second meeting, authorities on the many topics considered by the committee were invited to provide review articles summarizing current knowledge, highlighting progress in their field and identifying significant issues for the future. These papers were revised and co-ordinated, in consultation with the editors, and now appear in this book.

The book is a product of the programme for older persons which the World Health Organization established in 1982—the year in which the Vienna International Plan of Action focused global attention on the health and social consequences of population aging. Every month, the net balance of the world population aged 55 years or over increases by 1.2 million persons. More than 80 per cent of the monthly increase, a gain of nearly one million persons, occurs in developing countries. Thus aging is emerging as a public health issue for developing as well as for developed countries. This is one of the few texts which presents the health of older persons in a global context.

A preparatory step to preparing the most recent Expert Committee Report, and to producing this companion volume, was to assess, by a modified Delphi study, the progress made in various fields during the decade and a half between the two meetings. These perceptions influenced the content and structure of this book.

The initial emphasis on health and function stems, first, from the forty-year-old WHO constitution, the preamble of which defines health as a 'complete state of physical, mental and social well-being' and, secondly, from the 'Health for All' goal, which encompasses the Organization's aspirations for the elderly people of the world.

The text examines the world-wide growth of elderly populations and its consequence for future care, and the associated costs for this sector of the population. Living a longer life does not necessarily imply an improvement in its quality. Important issues about the overall quality of additional years gained through increases in life expectancy are addressed in the book.

Progress in specific dimensions of well-being are described. There is a perception that impressive gains in knowledge have been made in biology, and these are reviewed together with advances in our understanding of falls, sensory disorders, mental health in old age, osteoporosis, incontinence, drug therapy, and iatrogenic disorders. In many areas, for example in health promotion, disease prevention, and disability postponement, the search for effective interventions continues.

However, this is not a book which is narrowly focused on medical care. It extends to the family, which is the key issue for developing countries, community care, and nursing home and hospice care, as well as to the architectural design of facilities for older people. Health care services that are particularly appreciated by older persons are described, particularly with regard to people living in different sociocultural settings.

At all levels, countries lack staff who are skilled in providing support to elderly people and their families. With the year 2000 on the horizon, the target year for the World Health Organization's Health for All attainments, prominence is given to the production of adequately trained staff.

For all countries, but developing countries in particular, a prime need is to educate those who provide the majority of care—the informal network of carers comprising family, friends, and neighbours. Well-designed professional education is a priority for developed countries, where estimated personnel needs project great deficits in teaching, service, and research staff. The book provides guidance to those responsible for educational programmes for all categories of personnel.

What are the determinants of well-being in old age? Social and economic factors and pensions are at least as important as health care, and a section of the book deals with these issues. Social policies have therefore great potential impact on the future well-being of elderly people, although future scenarios of technology development provide prospects for maintaining autonomy in old age.

This book is a contribution, by the authors, to the World Health Organization's efforts to develop policies and programmes that will advance the well-being of the elderly people of the world. Such policies need to be rationally based, scientifically sound, socially acceptable, and technologically relevant. The book attempts to provide readers with a knowledge base for developing such policies and programmes.

D. Macfadyen
Chief, WHO Global Programme for the Elderly

Contents

List of contributors   xi

1. Perceived progress in aging: the results of a Delphi survey
   of international experts   1
   R. L. KANE

PART I: HEALTH AND FUNCTION

2. Introduction   15
   R. L. KANE

3. International demographic trends   19
   D. MACFADYEN

4. Compression of morbidity: issues and irrelevancies   30
   R. L. KANE, D. M. RADOSEVICH, AND J. W. VAUPEL

5. How are the elderly different?   50
   J. GRIMLEY EVANS

6. Assessment of health and functional status: an international
   comparison   69
   G. G. FILLENBAUM

7. Aging, quantitative health status assessment and the
   effectiveness of medical care   91
   R. B. WALLACE AND J. E. ROHRER

8. Social factors affecting the health of the elderly   107
   M. S. GORE

PART II: PROGRESS IN SPECIFIC AREAS

9. Introduction   127
   J. GRIMLEY EVANS

10. Progress in the biology of aging   128
    C. E. FINCH

11. Osteoporosis: 143

     Introduction   143
     J. GRIMLEY EVANS

     Scope for the prevention and treatment of osteoporosis   145
     B. E. C. NORDIN

12. Stroke: 172

     Introduction
     J. GRIMLEY EVANS

     Care of the patient with acute stroke   178
     T. YAMAGUCHI AND T. OMAE

     Stroke prevention and the population control of hypertension   187
     C. J. BULPITT

13. Drugs and old people: recent advances in geriatric pharmacology   211
     L. OFFERHAUS

14. Iatrogenic disorders   231
     F. I. CAIRD

15. Hearing disorders of aging: identification and management   237
     D. NOFFSINGER, J. P. MARTIN, AND S. H. LEWIS

16. The effectiveness of intervention for the mental health of the elderly   262
     B. J. GURLAND, R. MAYEUX, AND B. S. MEYERS

17. The efficacy of continence treatment   273
     J. G. OUSLANDER

18. Falls in later life   296
     M. J. GIBSON

19. Prevention in the aging   316
     A. M. DAVIES

PART III: HEALTH CARE

20. Introduction   341
     R. L. KANE

21. Role of primary health care for the elderly   346
     G. ANDREWS

22. The role of the family in the care of the elderly in developing countries 362
    N. A. APT

23. The role of the family in developed countries 381
    D. MAEDA

24. Case management and assessment of the elderly 398
    R. A. KANE

25. The efficacy of geriatric assessment programmes 417
    L. Z. RUBENSTEIN

26. The role of geriatric medicine 440
    R. A. BARKER

27. Home care and day care for the elderly 452
    B. HAVENS

28. Nursing home care for the elderly 473
    M. J. HIRSCHFELD AND R. FLEISHMAN

29. Hospice care for the elderly 491
    D. S. GREER

30. Housing for older people: the North American approach 502
    N. BLACKIE

31. Technology development and use for elderly people 528
    K. MASLOW

32. Assessing the impact of introducing new technologies and interventions for the elderly 544
    H. BECKER

PART IV: EDUCATION AND PERSONNEL NEEDS

33. Introduction 559
    D. MACFADYEN

34. Educating lay persons about the care of the elderly 561
    E. C. de LEHR

35. Educating health professionals in the care of the elderly 576
    C. EWAN

36. Planning for health personnel needed to serve elderly persons 596
    D. I. ZWICK and T. F. WILLIAMS

PART V: HEALTH AND SOCIAL POLICY ISSUES IN AGING

37. Introduction   617
    D. MACFADYEN

38. Planning more suitable environments for the elderly   621
    B. VELLAS, P. VELLAS, AND J. L. ALBAREDE

39. Economic factors affecting the health of the elderly   627
    N. OGAWA

40. The role of aging in establishing social priorities: an
    economic perspective   647
    K. WRIGHT

41. Contribution of social security to the well-being of the
    elderly   659
    J. ILIOVICI

42. Ethical issues and the care of the elderly   667
    A. L. CAPLAN

Appendix: Diagnosis and classification of dementias in the
elderly with special reference to the tenth revision of the
International classification of diseases (ICD-10)   683
A. JABLENSKY

Index   695

Contributors

Jean-Louis Albarede MD, Professor of Clinical Gerontology, Chief of Old Age Service, Centre Hospitalier Regional, Toulouse, France.

Gary Andrews MD, Chairman, Primary Care and Community Medicine, The Flinders University of South Australia, Bedford Park, South Australia.

Nana Araba Apt, Senior Lecturer and Co-ordinator, Social Administration Unit, Sociology Department, University of Ghana, Legon, Ghana.

Ronald A. Barker CBE FRCP FRACP, Formerly Director-General of Health, New Zealand, Waimauku, New Zealand.

Henk Becker Ph.D., Professor of Sociology, Utrecht University, The Netherlands.

Norman Blackie Arch D, Executive Director, Canadian Association on Gerontology, Winnipeg, Manitoba, Canada.

C. J. Bulpitt MD MSc FRCP, Division of Geriatric Medicine, Royal Postgraduate Medical School, Hammersmith Hospital, London, England.

F. I. Caird DM FRCP, David Cargill Professor of Geriatric Medicine, University of Glasgow, Scotland.

Arthur L. Caplan Ph.D., Director, Center for Biomedical Ethics, University of Minnesota, Minneapolis, MN, USA.

A. Michael Davies MD FFCM, Professor, School of Public Health and Community Medicine, The Hebrew University of Jerusalem, Israel.

Esther C. de Lehr, Director, Casa Hogar para Ancianos 'Arturo Mundet', Mexico.

J. Grimley Evans MD FRCP FFCM, Professor of Geriatric Medicine, University of Oxford, England.

Christine Ewan MB Ph.D., Associate Professor, School of Health Sciences, University of Wollongong, Australia.

Gerda G. Fillenbaum Ph.D., Associate Medical Research Professor, Duke University Medical Center, Durham, NC, USA.

Caleb E. Finch Ph.D., Professor, Ethel Percy Andrus Gerontology Center, University of Southern California, Los Angeles, CA, USA.

Rachel Fleishman MA, Brookdale Institute of Gerontology and Adult Human Development, Israel.

Mary Jo Gibson, International Federation on Aging, Washington DC, USA.

M. S. Gore Ph.D., Tata Institute of Social Sciences, Bombay, India.

David S. Greer MD, Dean of Medicine, Brown University, Providence, RI, USA.

Barry J. Gurland F.R.C. Psych, F.R.C.P., John E. Borne Professor of Clinical Psychiatry, Director of Center for Geriatrics and Gerontology, Columbia University, New York, NY, USA.

Betty Havens M.A., Provincial Gerontologist, Department of Health, Government of Manitoba, Winnipeg, Manitoba, Canada.

Miriam J. Hirschfeld RN DNSc, Senior Lecturer, Department of Nursing, Tel-Aviv University, Tel Aviv, Israel.

J. Iliovici Ph.D, Advisor to the General Secretariat, International Social Security Association, Geneva.

Assen Jablensky MD DMSc, Professor of Psychiatry, WHO Collaborating Centre for Research and Training in Mental Health, Sofia, Bulgaria.

Robert L. Kane MD, Dean, School of Public Health, University of Minnesota, Minneapolis, MN, USA.

Rosalie A. Kane DSW, Professor, School of Public Health and School of Social Work, University of Minnesota, Minneapolis, MN, USA.

Sheralyn Head Lewis MA, Co-ordinator of Aural Rehabilitation, VA Medical Center, West Los Angeles, CA, USA.

David Macfadyen MSc FRCPE FFCM, Chief, Global Programme for Health of the Elderly, WHO, Copenhagen, Denmark.

Daisaku Maeda, Director, Department of Sociology, Tokyo Metropolitan Institute of Gerontology, Tokyo, Japan.

James P. Martin MA, Co-ordinator of Employee Hearing Conservation, VA Medical Center, West Los Angeles, CA, USA.

Katie Maslow, Analyst, US Office of Technology Assessment, Washington DC, USA.

Richard Mayeux MD, Associate Professor, Clinical Neurology and Psychiatry, Columbia Presbyterian Neurological Institute, New York, NY, USA.

Barnett S. Meyers MD, Associate Professor of Clinical Psychiatry, New York Hospital, Cornell Medical Center, New York, NY, USA.

Douglas Noffsinger Ph.D., Chief, Audiology and Speech Pathology Service, VA Medical Center, West Los Angeles, CA, USA.

B.E.C. Nordin MD DSc FRCP FRACP, Senior Specialist, Institute of Medical and Veterinary Science, Visiting Professor, University of Adelaide, South Australia.

L. Offerhaus MD Ph.D., Directorate General for Public Health, Ministry of Welfare, Public Health and Cultural Affairs, Rijswijk, The Netherlands.

Naohiro Ogawa Ph.D., Professor and Deputy Director, Population Research Institute, Nihon University, Tokyo, Japan.

Teruo Omae MD, Director of Hospital, National Cardiovascular Centre, Osaka, Japan.

Joseph G. Ouslander MD, Assistant Professor of Medicine, UCLA School of Medicine, Los Angeles, CA, USA.

David M. Radosevich MSPH RNC, Research Assistant, School of Public Health, University of Minnesota, Minneapolis, MN, USA.

James E. Rohrer Ph.D., Program in Hospital and Health Administration, University of Iowa College of Medicine, Iowa City, IA, USA.

Laurence Z. Rubenstein MD MPH, Associate Professor, UCLA School of Medicine, Clinical Director, Geriatric Research, Education and Clinical Center, VA Medical Center, Sepulveda, CA, USA.

James W. Vaupel Ph.D., Professor, Hubert H. Humphrey Institute of Public Affairs, University of Minnesota, Minneapolis, MN, USA.

Bruno Vellas MD, Chief of Clinic, Old Age Service, Centre Hospitalier Regional, Toulouse, France.

Patrick Vellas, Director of Research Group on Aging and Architecture, University of Social Sciences, Toulouse, France.

Robert B. Wallace MD, Professor and Head, Department of Preventive Medicine and Environmental Health, The University of Iowa, Iowa City, IA, USA.

T. Franklin Williams MD, Director, National Institute on Aging, National Institutes of Health, Department of Health and Human Services, Bethesda, MD, USA.

Kenneth G. Wright, Senior Research Fellow, Centre for Health Economics, University of York, England.

Takenori Yamaguchi MD, Chairman, Cerebrovascular Division, Cardiovascular Centre, Osaka, Japan.

Daniel I. Zwick MA, Consultant, National Institute on Aging, National Institutes of Health, Department of Health and Human Services, Bethesda, MD, USA.

1

Perceived progress in aging: the results of a Delphi survey of international experts

ROBERT L. KANE

As part of the preparation of the report for the WHO Expert Committee on Aging, a survey of experts in different countries was undertaken to ascertain perceptions of the most significant advances in biology, care of the elderly, and social policies toward the elderly since the first Expert Committee report in 1974. A modified Delphi technique was employed.

A roster of experts was prepared (see Appendix). Each person was asked to list the most significant advances in each category. From the 56 experts consulted, 21 responses were received. Not all respondents addressed each area. Several indicated that they felt comfortable in only one or two areas. The responses in each area were then compiled, categorized, and rank ordered. These lists were again mailed to the expert panel, including both those who had and those who had not responded to the first invitation. The second mailing presented the lists and asked the respondents to rank the items in order of importance. Respondents were also invited to suggest additional topics for the list. The 35 responses were again tabulated and distributed to the entire panel, including those who had not responded to previous requests, for a final round. The additional suggestions from the second round were included to see whether they provoked new support. The third round produced 37 respondents.

As shown in Tables 1.1–1.3., the mean ratings changed very little between rounds two and three. In only one case did the relative rankings change—care for dementia and depression—in Table 1.2. The ratings are presented as the mean rank for each item; however, in some cases not everyone rated every item. In general there were only one or two abstainers for a given item. These were considered to be low ranks and given the bottom ranking.

Table 1.1 addresses the major advances in the biology of aging. The leading area of progress has been in the area of Alzheimer's disease. Indeed, the last decade has marked a distinct shift in our thinking about this process with a major emphasis on addressing it as a pathological process for which both prevention and cure are appropriate. The second area of progress has been in the development of better research around the mechanisms of aging. Although we have not yet uncovered these

Table 1.1 Most important advances since 1974 in our knowledge about the biology of aging (ranked in order of importance, when 1 = most important)

	Group mean (round two) (*n* = 35)	Group mean (round three) (*n* = 37)
The neuroanatomy and biochemistry of Alzheimer's disease, especially neurotransmitters	1.67	1.78
Theories of mechanisms involved in the aging process and strategies to intervene, especially genetics and biotechnology	2.29	2.64
The immune system as it relates to aging	3.06	3.15
The differences between age-related decline and pathological change, especially in the area of cardiac function	3.94	3.51
Application of new technologies for cerebral imaging (eg. CAT, PET, NMI)	4.45	3.92
Other issues raised:[a] Bio-epidemiology of aging		
Importance of social and behavioural interventions for maintaining health and functioning in the middle and latter years		
Improved understanding of psychological change with age as a result of information gained from longitudinal studies		

[a] (An insufficient number of responses were received on the additional three items to include them in the final ratings.)

mechanisms, much has been learned about the processes, especially in relation to our understanding of genetics. In a similar manner, the tremendous growth in our understanding of the immune mechanisms has been reflected in the appreciation of the role such systems play in the aging process.

The decade has also seen great changes in the way we view changes in organ system function with age. The early cross-sectional data from longitudinal studies has been supplanted by new longitudinal studies which suggest that there is much inter-organ system variation in the rate and extent of age-related changes. This is particularly true with regard to the cardiac system and measures of cognitive performance. At the same time, we have been privy to studies that show remarkable changes across different cohorts separated by only a few years. If these indications hold up, they suggest a potential for improvement that will challenge many of our cherished concepts about the inevitability of age-related changes. They raise a special flag of caution about any extrapolations based on present rates of disease or disability.

Another exciting area of marked development in the recent decade has come from advances in technologies that can be harnessed for the study and treatment of age-related diseases, especially the dementias. The major advances in computer-assisted tomography (CAT) to newer systems of metabolically active scanning have made available techniques for non-invasive study of the brain that allow better visualization of processes and anatomical changes that were not well understood before.

The listing of advances in care of the elderly, shown in Table 1.2, reflects a rather dramatic shift in emphasis over the decade. The greatest advance has occurred in the shift from institutional to community-based care. This is an especially important step because during the last momentous decade the balance of aging world wide has shifted from the developed to the developing countries. A model based on institutional care is not likely to prove feasible in much of the developing world where the majority of older persons now reside.

At the same time we have witnessed a growing appreciation of the multidimensional nature of care for the elderly and the consequent need to harness the talents of different disciplines. Such an approach threatens to be very expensive, just at the point when the people needing care are increasingly found in less affluent countries. The challenge will be to find ways of harnessing the skills of diverse disciplines without requiring their representation in most patient care encounters. This step poses great opportunities for those planning primary care training programmes in those countries.

The next three items on the list form a cluster conceptually. There is a growing body of expertise around the care of the elderly in terms of both medical and psychiatric care. In both cases, the emphasis is on the potential for improvement. Perhaps one of the greatest advances in geriatric care has come with the appreciation that much of what was formerly considered the inevitable decline of aging is now being addressed as remediable.

The ranking suggests that this change in philosophy and concentration of expertise has not been matched yet by parallel developments in better provision of primary care services for the elderly or by the infusion of these concepts into the training of the next generation of health professionals. These remain the challenges for the next decade, with particular urgency for the developing countries who are just beginning to confront the challenges of an aging society.

Table 1.2 Most important advances since 1974 in techniques for the care of the elderly (ranked in order of importance, when 1 = most important)

	Group mean (round two) ($n = 35$)	Group mean (round three) ($n = 37$)
The emphasis on home support services/ home care as an alternative to institutional care	1.62	1.61
Development of multidimensional approaches to assessment and care of the elderly	2.57	2.54
Increased attention to rehabilitation therapies and techniques	4.33	3.80
Improved psychogeriatric care for dementia and depression	5.37	4.35
Expansion/development of specialized geriatric medical care services	4.39	4.36
Improved primary care of the elderly	5.31	5.53
Better curricula for health professionals in the care of the elderly	5.68	5.76
Other issues raised[a]: Development of a range of housing alternatives as a component of the long term care system		
Scenario technique for planning health services for the future		
Improved standards of care quality assurance and improved techniques for evaluation		

[a] (An insufficient number of responses were received on the additional three items to include them in the final ratings.)

Other items of note in this regard include the centrality of housing. With the changing role of institutional care, issues of housing will become more salient. Many of the solutions for long-term care in the future will encompass mergers of housing and supportive services. The other major challenge will be to find ways of assuring and improving the quality of care. Especially since care is increasingly delivered outside of institutions, new ways of monitoring care will be required.

Table 1.3's list of advances in social policies reflects the advances in the

Table 1.3 Most important advances since 1974 in social policies towards the elderly (ranked in order of importance, when 1 = most important)

	Group mean (round two) ($n = 35$)	Group mean (round three) ($n = 37$)
Implementation of policies with respect to pensions and income security, transportation, retirement age, retirement planning and increased elderly participation in developing these policies	1.61	1.86
Shift in emphasis from institutional to non-institutional long-term care (e.g. day care, sheltered housing, home care, visiting services)	3.00	2.61
Generally improved awareness of the demographics of aging and their social implications	3.18	3.27
Special housing for the elderly	3.76	3.92
More emphasis on preventive health care and health promotion	4.59	4.97
Increased support for family care-givers to the elderly	6.16	5.16
Efforts to measure and improve quality of care, especially in nursing homes	6.50	6.01

other two areas and the related impact of demographic shifts. The most pressing issue is the development of income security for the growing numbers of persons entering old age. In some quarters, the gains made by the elderly and their rise as a political force have led to backlash and a belief that they have been disproportionately advantaged. The potential for intergenerational competition must be recognized and addressed.

The press for more community-based services to displace the heavy reliance on institutional care represents a call for creativity in both service structure and financing. It is part of a larger shift in the demographics of aging that must be reckoned with in almost every country in the world. Basic information on the growth of the elderly population and the effects of social phenomena like rural to urban migration is essential for even the most basic planning of services.

Among those services will be development of adequate and supportive housing for the elderly and the increased efforts to prevent disease. Much is said about health promotion among the elderly but little is clarified about precisely what is meant. Efforts to improve functioning by appropriate modifications of both health and environment seem much more feasible than the broader strategies for health promotion through behavioural change usually indicated by that phrase. At the same time, recent data on the benefits of preventive activities such as exercise or stopping smoking among the elderly suggest caution in dismissing such approaches without more careful testing in those age groups.

Discussion

This report suggests that there have been considerable activity and growth in knowledge over the period since 1974. About 5 years before the present study small panels of national experts were asked to forecast the future of gerontological issues up to the year 2000.[1] That report produced a rather more pessimistic scenario than the one laid out here. The energy that has been directed towards addressing the problems raised in responding to the challenges of an aging population provides a basis for optimism about the potential for achieving both social and scientific breakthroughs.

It is not at all clear that we want to eliminate aging, but we can learn to deal better with many of its untoward consequences. We must certainly learn to address the implications of demographic change and its social implications.

We can take some solace from the observation that several countries have already gone through their second major demographic revolution (in aging) and survived nicely. Those who see such a shift in population still well in the distance have the opportunity to learn from both the successes and the failures of those who have gone before. However, we cannot afford simply to close our eyes to the changes that seem to lie inevitably before us.

References

1. Selby, P. and Schecter, M. (1982). *Aging 2000: a challenge for society*, MTP Press, Hingham, MA.

APPENDIX A

Roster of Experts

	Responded to rounds 1, 2, or 3
Dr G. R. Andrews, Department of Primary Care and Community Medicine, Flinders University of South Australia, Australia	2, 3
Professor M. F. Antoninni, Institute of Geriatrics and Gerontology, University of Florence, Italy	
Ms Nana Araba Apt, Sociology Department, University of Ghana, Ghana	2, 3
Professor Edit Beregi, Gerontology Center, University of Budapest, Hungary	1, 2, 3
Dr Simon Bergman, School of Social Work, Tel Aviv University, Israel	2, 3
Dr Klaus Bergmann, The Maudsley Hospital, London, United Kingdom	1, 2, 3
Dr Eva Beverfelt, Gerontological Institute, Oslo, Norway	1, 3
Dr Jacob Brody, School of Public Health, University of Illinois at Chicago, United States	2, 3
Professor G. A. Broe, Department of Geriatric Medicine, Concorde Repartiation Hospital, Australia	2
Professor Robert H. Brook, The Rand Corporation, Santa Monica, United States	
Dr Robert Butler, Department of Geriatrics, Mount Sinai Medical Center, New York, United States	
Dr Ronald D. T. Cape, WHO Collaborating Centre for Research on Health of the Elderly, National Research Institute of Gerontology and Geriatrics, Australia	1, 2, 3

	Responded to rounds 1, 2, or 3
Dr Arthur Caplan, Biomedical Ethics Center, University of Minnesota, Minneapolis, United States	2, 3
Professor D. F. Chebotarev, WHO Collaborating Centre for Research on Aging, Institute of Gerontology of the Academy of Medical Sciences, USSR	1, 2
Dr Dennis Coakley, St James Hospital, Dublin, Ireland	
Professor Brian Cooper, Central Institute for Mental Health, Federal Republic of Germany	
Professor Ester Contreras de Lehr, Mexican Gerontological Society, Mexico	
Dr Caleb Finch, Andrus Gerontology Center, University of Southern California, Los Angeles, United States	2, 3
Dr Francoise Forrette, Foundation National Hopital Broca, Paris, France	1, 2
Dr David Greer, Center for Health Care Research, Brown University, Providence, United States	2, 3
Mr Jack Habib, Brookdale Institute for Gerontology and Adult Human Development, Israel	1, 2, 3
Dr R. Langton Hewer, Department of Neurology, Frenchay Health Authority, United Kingdom	
Ms Miriam J. Hirschfeld, Department of Nursing, Tel-Aviv University, Israel	2
Dr Malcolm Hodkinson, St Pancras Hospital, London, United Kingdom	2, 3
Dr Carl Hollander, Laboratories Merck Sharp & Dohme, Chibret, France	1, 2, 3
Dr Bernard Isaacs, Geriatric Medicine, University of Birmingham, United Kingdom	3
Dr A. V. Jablensky, WHO Collaborating Centre, Medical Academy, Bulgaria	
Professor S. Kanowski, Free University of Berlin, Germany	1, 3

	Responded to rounds 1, 2, or 3
Dr D. Kozarevic, Institute of Chronic Diseases and Gerontology, Yugoslavia	1, 2, 3
Profelssor G. Lambert, Centre International de Gerontologie Sociale, Paris, France	
Dr Peter Laslett, Cambridge Group for the History of Population and Social Structure, United Kingdom	
Dr M. Powell Lawton, Director of Research, Philadelphia Geriatric Center, United States	2, 3
Dr Leslie Libow, Department of Geriatrics and Adult Development, The Mount Sinai Medical Center, New York, United States	1
Professor Michael Lye, University Department of Geriatric Medicine, Royal Liverpool Hospital, United Kingdom	1, 3
Professor W. J. Maclennan, Department of Geriatric Medicine, City Hospital, Edinburgh, United Kingdom	1, 2, 3
Dr George Maddox, Council of Aging and Human Development, Duke University Medical Center, Durham, United States	3
Dr T. Omae, Director of Hospital, National Cardiovascular Center, Osaka, Japan	2, 3
Dr Paul Paillat, Department of Social Demography, National Institute for Demographic Sciences, Paris, France	
Professor Michael Philibert, Centre Pluridisciplinaire de Gerontologie, Universite d'Etudes Politiques, Grenoble, France	
Dr Colin Powell, Department of Geriatric Medicine, St Boniface Hospital, Winnipeg, Canada	2, 3
Dr Mathilda Riley, National Institute on Aging, National Institutes of Health, Bethesda, United States	2

	Responded to rounds 1, 2, or 3
Dr Duncan Robertson, Geriatric Rehabilitation, University of British Columbia, Canada	2
Sir Martin Roth, Department of Psychiatry, Addenbrookes Hospital, Cambridge, United Kingdom	2, 3
Dr John W. Rowe, Gerontology Division, Harvard Medical School, Beth Israel Hospital, Boston, United States	2, 3
Dr Laurence Rubenstein, GRECC, Veterans Administration, Los Angeles, United States	2, 3
Dr Sydney Sax, Department of Health, Canberra, Australia	1, 2, 3
Dr James Schultz, Florence Heller Graduate School, Brandeis University, Waltham, United States	1, 3
Dr Knight Steel, Division of Geriatrics, Boston University School of Medicine, United States	1, 2, 3
Professor I. H. Stevenson, Department of Pharmacology and Therapeutics, University of Dundee, Ninewells Hospital, United Kingdom	1, 2, 3
Dr Toru Tsumita, WHO Collaborating Centre for Health of the Elderly, Tokyo Metropolitan Institute of Gerontology, Japan	3
Professor W. van Eimeren, GSF-medis, Federal Republic of Germany	2, 3
Dr Robert J. Van Zonneveld, Laan Van Oud Poelgeest, Netherlands	2, 3
Dr Norman Vetter, College of Medicine, University of Wales, United Kingdom	1, 3
Dr T. Franklin Williams, WHO Collaborating Centre for Research on Care of the Aged, National Institute of Aging, National Institutes of Health, Bethesda, United States	1, 2, 3
Mr K. G. Wright, Center for Health Economics, University of York, England	1, 2, 3

Responded to rounds 1, 2, or 3

Dr Ng Yau Yung, Geriatrics Unit,
  Princess Margaret Hospital, Hong Kong   1, 2, 3

Part I

Health and function

2

Introduction

R. L. KANE

The last decade has seen incredible changes in the rate of mortality in older age groups. The numbers of elderly persons are increasing rapidly in both the developed and developing worlds. Within the latter, although the proportion of older persons is still generally quite modest, the overall number is remarkable. We have recently reached the point where the numbers of older persons in the developing countries exceed those in the developed world. While this shift reflects a triumph for health and medical care, some view it as mixed blessing, and express great concern about the rising cost of health care associated with an aging society. Some have called for drastic measures, including age-based rationing as way of controlling the rapidly rising cost of care. For those just beginning to encounter the growing numbers of elderly, the experience of geriatricians in parts of Europe and the United States can be especially relevant.

For purposes of both practice and policy, it is important to distinguish between those age-related differences that can be truly attributed to aging. Differences between old and young include both intrinsic (genetic) and extrinsic (environmental) true aging effects, but they also include differences derived from selective survival, cohort effects, and even differential challenges. Especially in the case of comparisons between different age groups at a point in time, it is important to realize that those who constitute the older group represent persons who lived during a different period and survived the experience. The observed differences may reflect the differences in both exposure and survival.

Function is the common language of gerontology. As the world becomes increasingly aware of the implications of an aging society, with its increasing burden of dependency, pressures from both clinical and financial quarters will urge efforts to control the distribution of services. One of the first tasks of gerontologists is to address the distinction between events associated with aging and those occurring as result of aging. For socially determined events, the distinction often disappears. To the extent that we adopt policies based on chronological age, we re-enforce age-based distinctions.

Age is an attractive measure for policy use. It is a universal device, and usually easy to determine. Its ease of use makes it a deceptively practical tool. The more we study aging, the more we appreciate the increasing variation that accompanies old age. In the simplest terms, chronological age is a good predictor of things for groups of persons but a very bad one for use with a given individual. Whether we look at physiology or activity, the older the group being studied the greater is the variation among them. Thus, age *per se* may be an easy measure to apply, but it may not be the best designator of need for service. Indeed age as a basis for eligibility is often used in social programmes such as retirement, but we must not equate getting old with necessarily becoming dependent.

The language of age-related performance better relies on function as the final common pathway to distinguish the need for levels of service. Whereas age may be grossly correlated with service needs, it is by no means inevitable that old age automatically implies major service requirements. In general, service needs increase as death approaches. In affluent societies, the cost of care in the last year of life represents a disproportionate share of the total life expenditures. The difficult task is, of course, to assess with reasonable certainty when that final chapter is about to begin. As one moves from chronological measures to functional ones, there is better predictability about such utilization.

The identification of functioning as the central focus of gerontology may inadvertently create some misunderstanding. Function as a goal does not imply a lack of concern about medical care. Quite the reverse. Improving function is the result of three combined activities. The first task is to remedy those conditions that are remediable. (One might correctly insert a caution that an even earlier task would be to prevent the condition from arising in the first place.) No amount of compassion will displace the failure of not attending to that which could have been corrected.

However, a key lesson of geriatrics is that traditional medical attention is necessary but not sufficient. Rendering good care is not enough. Having corrected that which is correctable, the next step is to address the environment to assure that it supports maximal functioning. In this context, environment refers to both the physical and the social milieu. It is often easier to see the physical barriers to function than the more subtle social ones. Poorly designed housing, which requires those with respiratory distress to climb stairs or walk long distances, is a easy example of a design problem. Indeed, there have evolved a number of very creative programmes to minimize the environmental barriers that keep impaired older persons from functioning as well as possible.

Changing the social environment requires a different approach. Here the difficulties are created by custom and anxiety. One of the social environmental problems to be addressed is the issue of risk aversion. Caregivers, whether family members or paid staff, may be reluctant to allow disabled elderly persons to do as much as possible for themselves for fear that they may get into difficulties. For example, family may fear leaving demented persons alone lest they neglect an open fire. Institutional personnel may have even greater anxieties about encouraging independence for fear of legal action attributed to neglect.

Another contributor to enforced dependency is pressure for greater productivity. When we measure productivity in a narrow sense, there is a real danger of encouraging personnel to do things for dependent elderly persons rather than working with them to help them do things independently. Everyone recognizes that it takes more time to work with clients to encourage automony than to take over the task and do it. Indeed, that is the fundamental principle of rehabilitation. If efficiency is improperly measured by short-term task performance, it is easy to see how such an essential rehabilitative approach might be undermined.

The final component of function is motivation. Here the caregiver, especially the professional, can play a vital role. If the client is encouraged to believe that improvement is possible, there will be greater efforts made to perform toward that goal. If, in contrast, the prognosis is bleak, it may become a self-fulfilling prophecy. It may well be that some of the effectiveness attributed to geriatric treatment programmes is related to this enthusiasm factor, the belief that clients can be improved in the face of general pessimism.[1]

Moreover, the attitude of the caregiver about his or her ability to help the client may affect the way he or she feels about that client. There is evidence to suggest that people feel hostile toward those they believe themselves impotent to help.[2]

Function, then, can be viewed as the final common pathway for assessing the effectiveness of geriatric care. It is especially useful as a way of comparing the status of persons in different situations and different cultures. At the same time, in such cross-cultural comparisons it is essential to recall that function, even when measured on the basis of performance, may be responding to environmental and attitudinal forces. The same level of performance may involve quite different levels of achievement in different settings.

Nonetheless function is the best available common language of aging. It provides a better way to discuss the distribution of care than chronological age. It is the result of a number of different, sometimes competing, forces.

One perennial and important question is the relationship between mortality and morbidity. Conceptual arguments can lead to quite different conclusions. On the one hand, if those who formerly perished are assisted to survive, the prevalence of morbidity should increase. But if the conditions that produce disease can be eliminated or reduced, then it should be possible to reduce both the rate of death and the level of disability in the population.

References

1. Kane, R. L. (1988). Beyond caring: the challenge to geriatrics. *Journal of the American Geriatrics Society,* **36**.
2. Lerner, M. J. and Simmons, C, H. (1966). Observer's reaction to the 'innocent victim': compassion or rejection. *Journal of Personality and Social Psychology*, **4**, 203–10.

3

International demographic trends

DAVID MACFADYEN

THE CENTURY OF HUMAN SURVIVAL

The twentieth century is the century of survival. For the first time men, and especially women, are beginning to live out their lifespans. National efforts and international action to advance health and reduce fertility have produced a world population which, for the first time, includes large numbers of elderly people. Already, the majority of the world's elderly people are living in developing regions (Fig. 3.1). And when we enter the twenty-first century, the third age will have emerged in the third world.

POPULATION GROWTH OF ELDERS IS FASTER IN DEVELOPING COUNTRIES

Every month, the net balance of the world population aged 55 years or over increases by 1.2 million persons. More than 80 per cent of the monthly increase, a gain of nearly one million persons, occurs in developing countries. The percentage annual growth rate in developing countries for this age group is 3.1, which is three times as high as in developed countries. Thus aging is becoming a public health issue for developing as well as for developed countries.[*]

Currently, some 23 countries have two million or more people aged 65 years or more, the age group which is traditionally used in presenting international comparisons. Before the year 2000, China will have more than eighty million citizens in this age group and India will reach this mark around 2015.

THE SPEED OF POPULATION AGING IS BREATHTAKING

While in developing countries the annual percentage growth rates of the older segment of the population are high, elderly people currently constitute only a small proportion of the total population.

[*] Developed countries comprise all nations in Europe (including the USSR) and North America plus Japan, Australia, and New Zealand. The remaining nations are classified as developing by the United Nations.

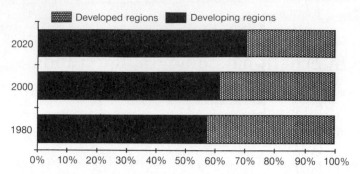

Fig. 3.1 Distribution of the world population aged 60 years and over between developed and developing regions.

By the year 2000, the proportion of aging people† in the total population will amount to about one in ten and the corresponding prediction for the year 2020 is one in eight (Fig. 3.2).

However, in some parts of the globe, countries are outpacing the historical and predicted trends in the rising proportion of elderly people. Japan, for example, has a high percentage annual growth rate of older people (2.7 per cent among those aged 65 to 74), and this will bring the proportion of its citizens who are aged 65 years and over to 14 per cent of the total population by the year 1996—double the proportion of 1970. The speed of aging in Europe and North America has been much slower (Fig. 3.3).

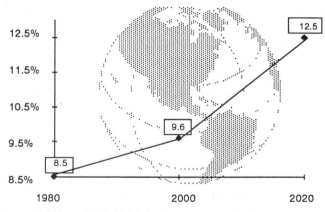

Fig. 3.2 World population aged 60 or more (as percentage of total population). Source: United Nations Population Division.

† In 1980, the United Nations defined 60 years as the age of transition of people to the aging segment of the population.

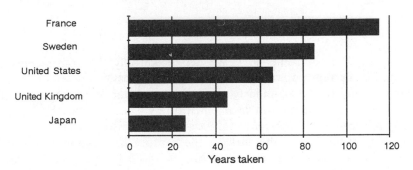

Fig. 3.3 Span of years required for the populatioin aged 65 years or more to transit from 7% to 14% of the total population.[1]

In Sweden, it took over 80 years to attain the corresponding transition, and in France it took over 100 years for its population aged 65 years and above to go from 7 to 14 percent of the total population, the level to which Japan jumped in only 26 years.

FERTILITY SHAPES POPULATION AGING

Population aging is an evolving process in which older persons appear in increasing proportions within the overall population. This demographic transition is brought about by declining fertility rates and falling death rates. Populations with high fertility have low proportions of older people. By contrast, countries which have sustained falls in fertility and which have made progressive reductions in mortality have growing proportions of older citizens. This is dramatically illustrated by the experience of China. A very large and growing population led China to adopt, in the 1970s, a policy of reducing fertility by encouraging married couples to restrict their families to one child. Effective implementation of this policy would result in 40 per cent of the population being over the age of 65 years by the middle of the next century. This would be almost double the level which Sweden, currently the world's oldest country, expects to attain by 2025. By that year, 22 per cent of Swedes will be in this age group and the corresponding proportions for the rest of Europe and the United States will be just a few percentage points behind.

Fertility reduction narrows the base of the population pyramid and, combined with mortality reduction, the effect is that the numbers in each quinquennial group become approximately equal. The projected United States population for 2025 approximates to such a shape rather than a pyramid.

OLDER AGE GROUPS GROW OLDER

Fertility patterns of some 60 years ago powerfully determine the age structure of current populations. Thus, many countries are experiencing a surge in the transit of elderly people through the upper age ranges. Persons of age 80 years and over constitute 14 per cent of the world's elderly population (19 per cent in the developed world and 11 per cent in developing regions). By the turn of the century the United States will have the oldest elderly population: one in three (31 per cent) elderly Americans will be aged 80 years or more in the year 2005. The need for health services is instensified by the growth in the proportion of older persons in the population and by the aging of the older population itself: that is, the growing proportion of older persons who are of extreme age.

Annual population growth rates are statistics which are frequently invoked by those involved in formulating pulblic policy. The high annual grwoth rates of very old people have largely escaped such scrutiny. Fig. 3.4 shows that several countries have annual rates of growth of the population aged 75 years and above that are 10- or 15-fold higher than that of the United Kingdom. The faster-growing older populations are in southern Europe (Italy, Greece, and Bulgaria), in Asia (China and Japan), and in Latin America (Brazil).

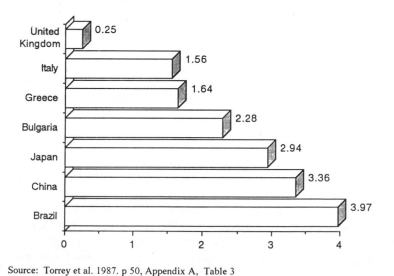

Source: Torrey et al. 1987. p 50, Appendix A, Table 3

Fig. 3.4 Average annual growth rate, 1985–2005; population aged 75 and over.[1]

URBANIZATION DOMINATES WORLD DEMOGRAPHIC CHANGE

Perhaps the most significant demographic trend in the second half of the twentieth century is urbanization. Elderly persons are not exempt from this population movement. Throughout the world, the older population became more concentrated in urban areas in the 1970s and early 1980s. However, in the developing countries, where the population as a whole is predominantly rural, only one in three (30 per cent) people aged 60 years or more live in urban areas. Even by the year 2000, the majority of aging people will be living in rural areas. Thus any programme which is centered only in urban areas will not reach the majority of elders. Latin America is unusual among developing regions in that the population as a whole lives predominantly in urban settings. Thus older Latin Americans tend to reside in urban areas.

Within urban populations, the proportion of older women tends to be higher than that of older men, which is attributable in part to sex differentials in mortality. This may also be related to the movement of widows from countryside to city for reasons of proximity to children after the loss of a spouse. This trend toward more urbanized societies raises questions as to whether traditional support systems for aged parents will be sustained.

HEALTH CONCERNS ARE LARGELY FOCUSED ON ELDERLY WOMEN

Elderly women outnumber elderly men in most countries of the world, greatly so at advanced age, especially in the industrialized countries (Fig. 3.5).

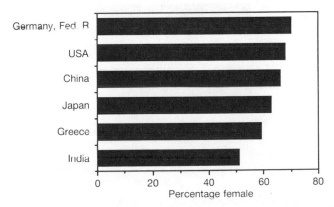

Fig. 3.5 Percentage of population female at age 80 years and above in 1985.[1]

There are nearly 6 million elderly women in the Federal Republic of Germany, compared with 3 million men in the age group of 65 years or more. However, the high ratio of German women to men is expected to decrease somewhat between 1985 and 2025—based largely on the assumption that male longevity will increase at a faster rate than that of women.

GLOBAL GOAL OF LIFE EXPECTANCY AT BIRTH OF 60 YEARS IS BEING REALIZED

With the exception of Africa, the developing regions of the globe are expected to achieve the World Health Organization's objective of attaining, by the year 2000, a life expectancy at birth of 60 years. Current levels of life expectancy in the developing world stand in striking contrast to those of developed countries. Average life expectancy at birth in 1988 in the developing world is 59 years, 19 per cent lower than the average of 73 years in developed countries. However there is considerable heterogeneity within the developing world. Some countries, such as Costa Rica and Jamaica, have life expectancies at birth which surpass levels found in France, the United States, and other industrialized countries. Thus, in comparing the figures which follow, the reader is reminded that averages mask wide variation among regions and countries. On an average regional basis, life expectancy at birth is highest in Latin America (67 years) and in the Caribbean (66 years). The Asian average, excluding Japan, is 6 years lower and that in the African region is lowest of all, at only 53 years (Fig. 3.6).

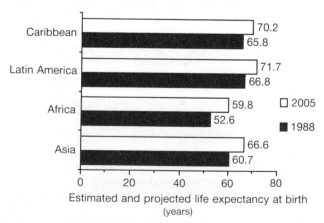

Fig. 3.6 Life expectancy at birth in developing regions.[2]

By the year 2005, considerable advances are predicted in life expectancy. In the Caribbean and in the Americas, life expectancies will reach into the seventh decade and Asians will look forward to life expectancy at birth of almost 67 years.

JAPAN HAS HIGHEST LIFE EXPECTANCY AT BIRTH, AND TRENDS ARE UPWARD

Japan's life expectancy (77 years in 1985) is the highest of the world's major countries. And there are further gains ahead. In a short work on the polemic of rectangularization of the survival curve and the compression of morbidity, it was noted that there is evidence that life expectancy is increasing and is projected to continue beyond the ninth decade, if current trends persists.[3]

The controversy on the rectangularization of the survival curve has had the welcome effect of focusing public discussion on the life-table and the various measures derived from it. As birth cohorts survive and transit through the lifespan with low exit frequency, decrements are delayed until late in life, with the effect that the survival curve takes a rectangular shape. Evolution of the survival curve may be observed in historical life-tables provided for Canadian provinces.[3] The 1925/1927 abridged life-table curve for Quebec women, for example, shows a stepwise decrement decade by decade over the lifespan. By 1980/1982 the corresponding survival curve took the form of a straight line until the sixth decade. This horizontal survival line together with the vertical terminal descent is the phenomenon referred to as the rectangularization of the life-table. In numerical terms, rectangularization is expressed as increasing life expectancy at birth or at higher ages, and as older median ages of the population.

INCREASE IN LIFE EXPECTANCY AT 65 OUTPACES THAT AT BIRTH

While expectation of life at birth increased by 12 per cent in Japan between 1960 and 1980, the average number of years remaining at 65 years increased by 26 per cent from 14.1 to 17.7 years (Fig. 3.7). The corresponding figures for the United States are a 6 per cent rise in life expectancy at birth and 15 per cent gain in life expectancy at age 65. Life expectancy of United States women at age 65 rose from 15.8 years in 1960 to 18.3 years in 1980, which exceeded the level attained by Australia and indeed by all other countries assessed.

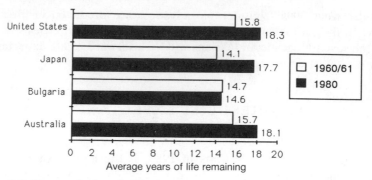

Fig. 3.7 Changes in female life expectancy at age 65 from 1960 to 1980.[1]

Although most countries show similar gains, some countries have experienced stagnation or decline in life expectancy at older ages. Elderly Bulgarian women, whose life expectancy at age 65 was 14.7 years in 1961, had a similar level (14.6 years) in 1979, and the expectation for Bulgarian men actually declined (not tabulated). Similar trends were observed in other East European countries. In countries with such patterns, more years can clearly be gained and the indications are that greater longevity at 65 is achievable through a life of healthy habits, avoiding risk factors such as smoking, excessive caloric and fat intake, physical inactivity, and alcohol abuse.

THE KILLERS—CANCER, HEART DISEASE, AND STROKE

The contribution to overall mortality of five major causes is presented in Fig. 3.8.

In developed countries, cancer claims one-quarter (26.5 per cent) of all deaths in men aged 65 to 74. A further quarter of total deaths in men in this age group is accounted for by ischaemic heart disease, which contri-

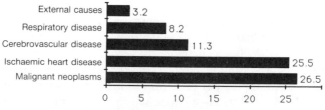

Fig. 3.8 Average percentage contribution to overall mortality: men, aged 65–74, developed countries, 1980–84.[5]

Table 3.1 Proportionate distribution of mortality by cause, at ages 65–74 for men

Cause of death	Range of proportionate contribution to overall deaths (%)		
Malignant neoplasms	16.2 (Romania)	to	35.5 (Netherlands)
Ischaemic heart disease	8.0 (Japan)	to	42.9 (Sweden)
Cerebrovascular disease	6.1 (USA)	to	26.7 (Portugal)
Respiratory disease	5.2 (Austria)	to	13.1 (Ireland)
External causes	1.5 (England & Wales)	to	5.4 (France)

Cause of death and ICD codes
(A refers to A list of ICD 8; B codes to the corresponding items on the Basic Tabulation list of ICD 9): malignant neoplasms A 45-A 60/B 08-14; cardiovascular disease A 80-88/B 25-30; ischaemic heart disease A 83/B 27; cerebrovascular disease A 85/B 85; respiratory disease A 89-A 96/B 31, B 32; external causes AE 138-Ae 150/Be 47-56.

butes 25.5 per cent to overall mortality; this is followed by cerebrovascular disease which contributes 11.3 per cent.

The relative importance of these five principal causes of death varies from country to country. In the period 1980 to 1984, the proportionate contribution of various causes to total mortality in men aged 65 to 74 ranged widely, and countries which feature in the lowest and highest ranges are given in Table 3.1.

Ischaemic heart disease, for example, is a leading cause of death in Sweden but is relatively less important in Japan. On the other hand, cerebrovascular disease is more important in Portugal (and in other countries of southern Europe as well as in Japan). The observed pattern is broadly consistent with known risk factors and indicates a potential for mortality reduction.

Variation is also observed in mortality attributed to respiratory disease (which is responsible for 8 per cent of deaths on average), and to external causes (which constitute 3 per cent of deaths on average). Although the ranges are smaller, these variations also indicate that there is potential for mortality reduction.

DRAMATIC FALLS IN MORTALITY

The best evidence of the potential for further gain in survival is obtained from analysis of trends since the 1970s in mortality at upper ages. In several developed countries, mortality rates have declined dramatically (Fig. 3.9).

From around 1970 to 1980/82, death rates plummeted in Australian,

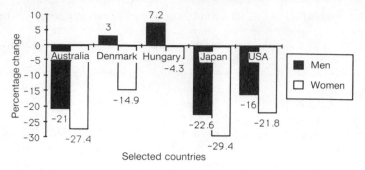

Fig. 3.9 Percentage change in death rates 1970–1974 to 1980–1982, ages 75–9 men and women.[5]

Danish, Japanese, and United States women aged 75 to 79. Australian, Japanese, and United States men in the same age group enjoyed percentage declines that are a few points below their female compatriots. However, in Danish and Hungarian men, mortality actually increased over the same period.

The dramatic declines are due primarily to falling death rates from ischaemic heart disease (Fig. 3.10) and stroke (Fig. 3.11).

The age-specific ischaemic heart disease mortality for Australian and United States men aged 65 to 74 years dropped markedly between the late 1960s and the early 1980s, in the case of the former from 23.4 per 1000 to 15.6 per 1000. Declines achieved in cerebrovascular disease are most striking in Japan. For both men and women in the age group 65 to 74 years, age-specific mortality from cerebrovascular disease fell in 1980–1984 to one third the level they had been two decades previously.

In contrast, little progress has been made in lowering cancer mortality, and the mortality challenge for the remaining years of the twentieth

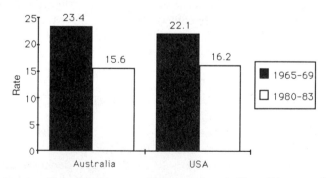

Fig. 3.10 Age-specific mortality per 1000 men aged 65 to 74 years from heart disease.[5]

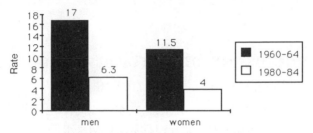

Fig. 3.11 Age-specific mortality per 1000 men aged 65 to 74 years from cerebrovascular disease, Japan.[5]

century is to find ways to achieve the same declines in cancer death rates that have been achieved in ischaemic heart and cerebrovascular disease.

Chapter 4 furnishes an appreciation of the personal and social impact of the years being added to overall life expectancy.

References

1. Torrey, B. B., Kinsella, K., and Taeuber, C. M. (1987). *An aging world*, International Population Report Series P 95, No. 78, pp. 7, 15, 21, 50. United States Department of Commerce, Bureau of Census, Washington DC.
2. Kinsella, K. G. (1988). *Aging in the Third World*. International Population Report Series P-95, No. 79, p. 14. United States Department of Commerce, Bureau of Census, Washington DC.
3. Schneider, E. L. and Brody, J. A. (1983). Aging, natural death and the compression of morbidity: another view. *New England Journal of Medicine*, **309**, 854–5.
4. Nagnur, D. (1986). *Longevity and historical life tables*. Ministry of Supply and Services, Canada.
5. Lopez, A. D. (1987). Demographic aspects of population aging in developed countries. *Revue Epidémologique et Santé Publique*, **35**, 195–205.

4

Compression of morbidity: issues and irrelevancies

ROBERT L. KANE, DAVID M. RADOSEVICH,
and JAMES W. VAUPEL

In Western countries, living a longer life does not necessarily imply an improvement in the quality of life. For example, Katz and his colleagues have shown that much of the advantage American women enjoy in additional years of life expectancy is lived in a dependent state.[1] (Fig. 4.1 shows this pattern with averages for 5-year age groups based on a small study in Massachusetts.)

Important questions have been raised about the overall quality of additional years gained through increases in life expectancy. On one side are those who see positive results from general and specific preventive efforts that have increased the health status of older persons. The incidence of serious diseases has been reduced and everyday observations suggest that many of the elderly are more vital than ever before. At the other pole are those who cite the 'failures of success' of medical advances,[2] and warn of a 'rising pandemic' of chronic diseases.[3] The truth may encompass both camps. We may be witnessing an improvement in the health of one group of elderly people while we also see some surviving into older age who would have perished in earlier times. Although the health status of the latter group has improved over the alternative of death, the overall effect is a worsening of the mean values of health status. For an appreciation of the personal and social impact of years added to overall life expectancy, an understanding of the inextricable relationship between mortality and morbidity is essential.

POLICY IMPLICATIONS OF TRENDS IN MORTALITY AND MORBIDITY

The growth in the elderly population has stimulated much discussion about the future of care and associated costs for this sector of the population. If life expectancy among the old continues to rise, the general fear is that the increased period of survival will occur in the context of dysfunctions that will require expensive care. An important ongoing debate, still unresolved, is whether the increase in older persons results

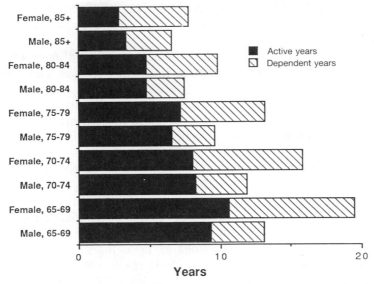

Fig. 4.1 Active vs dependent life expectancy, Massachusetts elderly, 1974.

from survival of those who would formerly have died from disease or whether there is a general improvement in the quality of persons surviving into old age. In the absence of better-informed data, current planning generally employs direct extrapolation of current age-specific rates, multiplied by expected numbers of elders in some future population. If the true numbers of disabled elderly in an age group are substantially different in future years, this can have profound implications for planning. Thus better forecasting of expected changes in disability rates will be very useful.

As part of the discussion about changes in morbidity among the elderly, James Fries[4-7] has emerged as a spokesman for a line of argument that proposes a compression in the number of years older persons will spend in a disabled state of ill health. This forecast is based on several assumptions:

—— the increase in life expectancy will be less than the postponed onset of disability;

—— disability can be postponed or avoided by appropriate preventive activities;

—— the increase in survival from formerly life-threatening conditions will not offset any gains achieved by such prevention.

The compression of morbidity concept is attractive to both planners and the elderly. It pictures the years gained as essentially disease free. At the same time, each of its assumptions has been challenged by one or more groups, while the evidence to support the theory is weak or non-existent.

Independent of the philosophical arguments on which much of Fries' proposals rest, there remain important health policy implications of the changing patterns of mortality and morbidity. As one of the most prominent sources of health care expenditures, institutionalization and physician services increase or decrease depending upon the scenario of mortality and morbidity to which one subscribes. Contrasting optimistic and pessimistic scenarios lead to dramatically different projections about the needs for services and their costs. For the former scenario, postponing the onset of disabling conditions resultant from chronic diseases will reduce the burden of disability in the population while adding quality to the years of life. The declining burden of years added implies a reduction in health service needs and proportionally lower costs in the future.

For the latter, more pessimistic scenario, living longer without delaying the onset of disabling conditions arising from chronic diseases gives rise to poor quality of years added through gains in life expectancy. The implication is that additional resources will need to be devoted to the care of the infirm, and that increasing resources in the form of institutionalization and physician services are to be expected in the course of providing care.

THE COMPRESSION OF MORBIDITY PARADIGM

The compression of morbidity paradigm is best presented in the form of a syllogism.[7] The logical argument is as follows: (1) if morbidity is defined as the time between onset of irreversible chronic disease and death; (2) if the age of onset of the chronic disease can be delayed until later ages (expected age of chronic disease onset); and (3) if the rate of change (increase) of chronic disease onset exceeds the rate of change (increase) in average life expectancy; then (4) morbidity is compressed into a shorter period of time.

Fries has argued that we can postpone the onset of morbidity by more active preventive actions aimed at risk factors. Many of these are the result of health behaviours, which can be altered once the individual assumes personal responsibility for his behaviour. He points to reductions in the incidence of chronic diseases such as heart disease, but the present evidence for these improvements is debatable. Moreover, to fulfil his paradigm, these reductions in incidence cannot increase lifespan. Thus the effects must be quite specific. At present, the data on delayed mortality seem stronger than those on morbidity.

Fries' argument in support of a fixed lifespan derives from a general theory of mortality and aging and the Hayflick limit.[8-10] As evidence that we are approaching a cap on life expectancy, Fries presents an overlay of survival curves for consecutive years. The resulting survival curves, laid one upon the other, project upward and to the right. This phenomena is referred to as the rectangularization of the survival curve and forms the basis for much of Fries' argument.

On inspection, the survival curves for successive years appear to terminate at a common upper age value, suggesting a cap on life expectancy. Fries concludes that future gains in life expectancy will be minimal, thereby creating a fixed upper limit against which the years free of disease may be compressed. However, little evidence for a compression of morbidity against this upper bound is proffered. As a whole, Fries' argument emerges as more of philosophical assertion than a case built on empirical evidence.

A fundamental policy shift is suggested in Fries' paradigm; that is, health resources should be shifted from the extension of life to the compression of morbidity. Chronic diseases, as the principal infirmity of aging, may be either postponed or prevented through a policy directed toward the modification of risk factors. Risk factors, such as cigarette smoking, obesity, saturated fat intake, hypertension, diet low in natural fibre, lack of exercise, and environmental exposures, act either to accelerate or to decelerate the development of chronic diseases. Improvements in lifestyle, or healthy habits will delay the onset of age-dependent diseases.[11] However, it remains to be shown whether risk factor changes carry the same attributable risk for disability at older ages as they do for death. To achieve the goals of compression of morbidity, the aggregate effect must be to shorten the period of time between the clinical manifestations of chronic disease and death. The existing evidence leaves this question unresolved.

VAGUE CONCEPTS

Despite considerable debate in the literature, there is a great deal of confusion surrounding the compression of morbidity paradigm and its concepts. There has been a general failure to discriminate between the interrelationship of key constructs in the paradigm, and a lack of understanding of the frequency measures which provide the supportive evidence.

Life expectancy and lifespan

Some of the confusion in the debate about the compression of morbidity stems from misunderstandings about the definitions of basic concepts. In particular, various measures of life expectancy and lifespan are often confounded.

The life expectancy of a group of people at a specific age is the average number of years of life an individual in the group can expect to live under existing mortality conditions. As a demographic measure, it is often expressed as life expectancy at birth; however, it may be expressed as life expectancy from any age. The assumption underlying its calculation and interpretation is that the current age-specific mortality rates will remain unchanged for the age cohort of interest.

The life expectancy of an individual is the life expectancy of the reference group in which the individual is assumed to belong. The same individual may belong to different groups, such as the population of US white males and the population of college graduates in Minnesota, and thus have different life expectancies depending on the reference group used.

The maximum life expectancy that a group of people could obtain is defined as the group's life expectancy under optimal conditions, that is, if mortality rates at all ages were as low as possible. Fries contends that major breakthroughs that are unlikely to be made for at least a century or two, if at all, are required before maximum human life expectancy can rise above about 85 years.

The maximum lifespan of an individual is the number of years the individual would live under optimal mortality conditions. The maximum of the lifespan of a population, usually an entire species, is the maximum of the lifespans of the individuals that comprise the population. Confusingly, this concept is sometimes simply called lifespan or specific lifespan, where specific is the adjectival form of species.

The notion of a maximum lifespan of a species can be operationalized in several ways. Usually it is measured as the longest observed lifespan. Sometimes it is defined as the expected lifespan of the longest-lived members of a population. Finally, in parallel with the usage of maximum life expectancy, it is sometimes conceived of as the maximum lifespan of a species under optimal mortality conditions.

The maximum lifespan for humans is frequently estimated at about 115 years, under all of these definitions. However, whether the maximum human lifespan under optimal mortality conditions is actually 115 depends on Fries' hypothesis that mortality rates at advanced ages cannot be reduced.

Morbidity

The term 'morbidity' has been used imprecisely in the literature. Fries himself has contributed to the confusion through his use of a variety of terms as synonyms for morbidity (e.g. disorder, infirmity, and disease). The concepts are never defined, nor are they consistently operationalized for purposes of research.

Kovar points to a failure to account for the difficulties of measuring morbidity as a major flaw evident in nearly all papers dealing with the compression of morbidity.[12] In addition to inadequately translating morbidity into a construct susceptible to study, the existing studies fail to provide adequate measures of irreversible morbidity.

Fries has argued that the limited scope of the medical model fails to reflect the emerging understanding of health. The World Health Organization raises concerns about limitations of the medical model and its failure to account for the range of problems that bring people into contact with the health care system.[13] The WHO conceptualization provides useful insights into the construct of morbidity. The medical model is incomplete, in the sense that it stops short of the consequences of disease, and it is these consequences that have greatest impact on health policy.

The concept of disease can be represented as a sequence of constructs from aetiology to manifestation to disease. First, something abnormal occurs within the individual. The aetiology, or the causative factors, gives rise to changes in the structure or functioning of the body, taking the form of pathology. If the pathological changes make themselves evident, they are described in terms of manifestations. The manifestations are clinically interpreted as symptoms and signs and constitute the principal components of the medical model of disease.

The WHO classification extends these illness-related phenomena; its progression from disease to impairment to disability to handicap represents a different plane of personal/social experience. In the WHO model, the morbid condition interferes with the individual's ability to carry out those functions and obligations that are expected of him. It is these consequences that intrude upon everyday life, accounting for the vast majority of calls on the health care system. As the burden of disease alters, the consequences assume greater importance. This is especially true for chronic and progressive or irreversible disorders.

In clinical disease, the manifestations may be either identified or unidentified. This distinction essentially differentiates the clinical from the subclinical case. Some symptoms cannot be linked to a single underlying disease process.

Impairment is broadly defined as any loss or abnormality of psychological, physiological, or anatomical structure or function. It represents any deviation from some norm in the individual's biomedical status; however, it does not necessarily imply that a disease is present. Impairment ensues only after a reaction is initiated which leads to the development of the pathological processes.

When the performance or behaviour of the individual is altered, and the impairment becomes objectified, common activities may become restricted. The consequences of impairment in terms of limiting functional performance and activity be the individual represent a disability. These involve integrated activities expected of the person (e.g. tasks, skills and behaviours). A disability is a person-level disturbance—any restriction or lack of ability to perform an activity in the manner considered normal for that person.

If the altered behaviour places the individual at a disadvantage relative to others, the experience then becomes socialized. This final plane reflects the response of society to the individual's experience and often takes the form of an expression of attitudes, or a behaviour. This consequence is referred to as a handicap. By definition, the handicap limits the fulfilment of a role that is normal for that individual. It is a social phenomenon since it is defined relative to other people.

In the search for the definition of morbidity, the concept most useful to research must be operationalizable and have direct implications for health policy. The construct of disability best meets this requisite criterion. Impairment is concerned with departures from the norms of structure and function. While they may be operationalized, only under narrowly defined conditions do they have immediate consequences for health care utilization; sensory impairments may represent a case in point. Handicap is heavily dependent upon cultural norms. As a consequence, a person may be handicapped in one group but not in another. Across time periods, there may be significant variance in how a handicap is defined. As such, it is susceptible to the effects of the period, making valid comparisons across time difficult. Disability can be objectified, and it carries consequences which have immediate impact upon health care resources.

Interrelationship of frequency measures of disease

There is a functional interrelationship between frequency measures of morbidity and mortality. Studies of morbidity and disability commonly use 'prevalence' as a frequency measure of disease. Prevalence is the probability of being afflicted with the disease at a particular point in time. It is measured through cross-sectional survey studies. 'Incidence' refers to the development of previously unrecognized disease during a specified observation period, which is usually a year in length. The measure of occurrence of 'new' disease is expressed as an incidence rate, and is directly measured through longitudinal, or prospective, studies.

While conceptually distinct, the notions of incidence and prevalence are interrelated. They differentiate both the time frame for measuring disease occurrence and how cases of disease are enumerated. Under certain conditions, the prevalence of a disease is a function of both the incidence rate of the disease and the duration of the disease. In the form of a simple mathematical relationship:

prevalence of disease = incidence rate of disease × duration of disease

As illustrated in Fig. 4.2, adapted from Kleinbaum *et al.*[14] prevalence is affected by a number of factors including both the incidence of disease and the rate of recovery from it. Thus, lower prevalence may result from preventing the onset of disease or from reduced survival after an episode.

'Risk factors' are the attributes of the environment or individuals that increase the likelihood of developing disease. For example, elevated serum cholesterol is a risk factor cardiovascular disease. Improved medical care usually acts to limit the serious consequences of disease and prolongs life while afflicted with the disease. 'Prognostic factors' refer to the attributes of the environment or individuals that affect the outcome of disease and the length of time the individual is afflicted with the particular disease. Once the disease has developed, its course may lead to recovery, continued affliction, or termination in death. The recovery rate measures recovery from the specific disease; the case fatality rate measures death from the specific disease.

Prevalence measures are confounded by survival, or a variety of factors which could yield measures that do not accurately reflect the true burden of disability in the population. First, the new occurrences of chronic disabling conditions may change. Over time, the incidence of diseases, such as musculoskeletal disorders and cardiovascular diseases, which have disability as a consequence, may change. There may be a decline in the

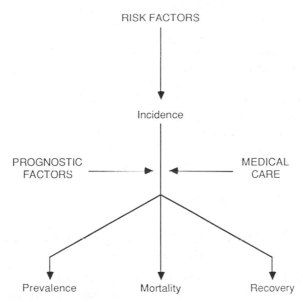

Fig. 4.2 Functional relationships among frequency measures.

onset of disability due to a modification of risk factors. Conversely, disability may increase as a result of unidentified risk factors. Second, rates of institutionalization may have changed over time. Increased rates of institutionalization would tend to remove the disabled from the community, thereby reducing the observed prevalence of disability among the population sampled. Changes in the threshold for institutionalization may change over time. For a period in which there is a relative scarcity of long-term care resources, only the more severe cases will find their way into the available institutions. Additionally, the relative case mix, or severity of disabled, within the population may change over time. This effect may be likened to a variation in the relative health of cohorts over time. Succeeding generations of the aged may prove to be more or less healthy. Improvements in medical care act to change the prognosis of chronic disabling conditions. Reduced case fatality or increased survival could have opposite effects. If the recovery is incomplete, they may expand morbidity rather than compress it. Improvements in mortality leave survivors. These survivors may be more susceptible to new illness by adding years of susceptibility for the development of chronic conditions or new illness. On the other hand, better care could lead to full recovery with a subsequent reduction in prevalence. Unfortunately, this more optimistic scenario is not often seen with chronic diseases.

Cases may be less severe than they were in the past because of improvements in medical care. Prognostic factors lead to additional individuals recovering from the disability.

Changes in disability-free life expectancy depend on two independent factors: the time of onset of morbidity and the life expectancy of the population.[15] Essentially, three scenarios are possible: stable population morbidity, increased population morbidity, and decreased population morbidity. Stable population morbidity, created by an increase in life expectancy equal to the increase in disability-free life expectancy, implies a societal burden unchanged over time. If the increase in life expectancy exceeds the onset of disability, increased population morbidity follows. Conversely, compression of morbidity results when the increase in disability-free life expectancy exceeds the increase in life expectancy. There should be an increase in active (functionally independent) years and a decrease in disabled years.

EVIDENCE TO SUPPORT COMPRESSION OF MORBIDITY

The empirical evidence to support or refute a compression of morbidity is not yet available. The literature both supports and opposes elements affecting the compression of morbidity. Better information is needed on each of the components and their combined effects, specifically the incidence of disability, its prevalence, and changes in life expectancy.

EVIDENCE OF A CAP ON LIFE EXPECTANCY

Although Fries advances several plausible theoretical arguments for a cap on human life expectancy, there is little empirical evidence either for or against such a cap.[16–19] If it exists at all, the cap on human life expectancy may well occur at some age substantially greater than age 85.

There remains a lack of accurate, carefully analysed data on the level of mortality rates, and on changes over time in these levels, at ages 85 and above. Accounts of very long-lived individuals and populations are probably myths. Furthermore, analysis of current demographic data sets for developed countries, such as age-specific mortality and population counts for the United States, is bedeviled by age exaggeration and misreporting: in the US the number of centenarians recorded in the 1980 census may have been twice the actual number.[20]

The available evidence on mortality patterns and trends at advanced ages is so sparse and questionable that it cannot judiciously be used to determine whether or not there is a cap on maximum life expectancy at any age, let alone at age 85. Some ways of looking at the data seem to suggest a possible cap somewhere around 85; other vantage points suggest a much higher limit. The available evidence does show progress in recent years in reducing mortality rates even after age 85 and some shift in the survival distribution out to more advanced ages. Furthermore, life expectancy continues to increase even among populations with life expectancies above 80 years, such as Swedish and Japanese women.[18]

Verbrugge identifies several factors that can increase the prevalence of disability.[25] First, there may actually be a higher incidence of chronic disease. Second, chronic diseases may be diagnosed earlier. This 'lead time bias' may result in increased reporting of diseases on survey, but it should not directly affect the consequences of the disease. Statistical survival is increased, but the true natural history of the disease is unchanged. Third, with earlier knowledge about a disease an individual may make earlier accommodations in his daily activities to the manifestations of the disease, for instance he may change jobs or cut down on usual activities faster when symptoms flare up.

Questionnaire changes can influence disability measures. Using the 1984 National Health Interview Survey (NHIS) and the 1984 Supplement on Aging (SOA), Kovar describes how different measures or different definitions of disability can yield markedly different levels of disability within the same interview.[12]

Aggregating reported statistics into broad age groups may obscure true changes in disability due to structural changes in the population. The effects of disproportionate increases among the older age groups may be misinterpreted as an increase in the crude prevalence of disability.

EVIDENCE OF REDUCED DISABILITY

Empirical evidence for reduced disability in the face of increasing life expectancy is difficult to find. Confirming trends requires comparable measures over a series of points in time. For this reason, a number of researchers have turned to the NHIS as a potential data source. These surveys are conducted annually by the US National Center for Health Statistics (NCHS). This continuous record of population health provides measures of acute and chronic morbidity, restricted activity and bed disability, and long-term limitations from chronic conditions on the non-institutionalized population of the United States since 1965.

Six major studies have used either the NHIS or a separate National Survey of the Aged to determine whether age-specific indices of disability have improved over time. Table 4.1, which builds on the work of Guralnik and Schneider,[15] summarizes these studies. Authors have used a core set of questionnaire items as indices of disability. In the NHIS, activity restriction is proffered as a measure for disability. Short-term disability is reflected in bed disability days and other restricted activity days, whereas a person's ability to carry on his main activity is used to assess chronic disability. This latter measure most closely approximates the irreversible disability premissed by Fries.

While not formally attempting to provide empirical evidence for or against a compression of morbidity, Kovar used NHIS for the years 1965–1977 to explore limitations in usual activity among US adults 65 years of age and older.[21] Her analysis disaggregated the disability measure by sex, age, and geographical region. She found that over these years there was increased prevalence of limitations in usual activities, but further noted that the age-specific prevalences were unchanged. She concluded that the changes observed were a consequence of changes in the population structure—specifically, increased proportions of aged in the population. For the single years 1966 and 1972, she observed no changes in limitations in mobility. No concomitant evaluation of institutionalization was noted, nor was there an evaluation of the levels of disability among the institutionalized.

Colvez and Blanchet used the NHIS surveys between the years 1966

Table 4.1 The evidence for compression of morbidity: principal studies of the United States and Canadian population

Reference	Population	Disability measure	Findings
Kovar[21] NHIS 1965–1977	US population 65 years of age and over	Prevalence of limitations in usual activity	Increased due to aging of the population; age specific rates unchanged
	65+ years	Limitations in mobility due to chronic conditions for 1966 and 1972 only	No change
Colvez and Blanchet[22] NHIS 1966–1974	US population 65 years of age and over	Prevalence main activity	Increased for men impossible
	< 45 years 45–64 years 65+ years	Prevalence main activity restricted	Decreased for men
		Prevalence other activity restricted	No change
Shanas[24] National Survey of the Aged 1962, 1975	US population 65 years of age and over	Degree of mobility: bedfast housebound Ambulatory	No change No change No change
	65–69 years 70–74 years 75–79 years 80+ years	Index of incapacity for self-care: goes outdoors walking stairs walks about house bathes self desses self cuts toenails	No change Improved No change No change No change No change
Verbrugge[25] NHIS 1958–1980	US population 65 years of age and over	Limitation in activity: any limitation major activity limitation	Trend unclear Trend unclear
	45–64 years 65+ years	Secondary activity limitation	Trend unclear May be a slight increase in major and any activity limitation after 1970

Table 4.1 (*cont.*)

Reference	Population	Disability measure	Findings
		Total restricted activity days	For both sexes, declines through 1970 then increases
		Total bed disability days	Steady
Palmore[23] NHIS 1961–1981	US population 65 years of age and over	Days of restricted activity	No change
	45–64 years 65+ years	Days of bed disability	Slight decrease
Crimmins[26] NHIS 1969, 1970, 1971, 1979, 1980, 1981	US population 65 years of age and over Age-specific	Limitation in major activity	Increased for males up to 74 years of age Increased for females up to 72 years of age
		Unable to perform major activity	Increased for males up to 74 years of age No change for females
		Restricted activity days	Increased for both sexes at nearly all ages
		Bed disability days	No change
Wilkins and Adams[28] Canada Health Health Survey 1978–79	Canadian population 65 years of age and over	Short-term disability: bed days	Unchanged for males Increased for females
		total days	Unchanged for males Increased for females
Canadian Sickness Survey 1950–51		Long-term disability percentage (males)	Unchanged to slight increase

Table 4.1 (*cont.*)

Reference	Population	Disability measure	Findings
Life expectancy 1951 and 1978		percentage (females)	Increased

and 1976 to detect improving quality of life concomitant with increasing life expectancy.[22] The increase in prevalence of long-term disability was greatest among those with severe limitation of activity (main activity impossible). Long-term disability was higher among men than women. Cases of moderate and slight limitation of activity were more frequent among women than men. For the latter two limitation of activity measures, there was a statistically significant decline in prevalence among the men.

Using data from the NHIS for the years 1961–1981, Palmore concludes that the United States has experienced a trend toward improved health among the aged.[23] Using the confounded measures of days of restricted activity and days of bed disability, he concludes that there has been no change in the days of restricted activity, and a corresponding decline in days of bed disability among persons 65 years of age and older from 1961 to 1981. Palmore attempts to separate out the age, period, and cohort effects from the cross-sectional NHIS data by computing a ratio of the relative health of persons 65 years of age and older compared with all persons surveyed. While he shows declines in the two ratios reported, his argument is unconvincing. Actual decline in the ratio indices reported by Palmore may reflect deterioration in the health indicators among persons 45–64 years of age or improvements in health indicators among the aged. A change in the numerator of the ratios is dismissed as an implausible explanation for the values computed despite evidence to the contrary. Colvez and Blanchet, utilizing the same NHIS data, found the greatest increases in disability measures among those in the age groups 45–64 years.[22] These findings would attenuate the ratios constructed by Palmore.

The National Survey of the Aged was a special survey of the US population of age 65 years and over for the years 1962 and 1975. Shanas employed comparable measures for degree of mobility, ambulation, and index of incapacity to search for disability change among the aged across these years.[24] No change was observed in degree of mobility, the prevalence of bedfast and homebound, or the prevalence ambulation across the 13-year interval. While the data are disaggregated by age, sex, and marital status, no concomitant evaluation of institutional status is provided.

Shanas has created a six-item index of incapacity for self-care. Respondents were asked whether they were able to: go outdoors, walk up and down stairs, walk around the house, bathe themselves, dress themselves and trim their own toenails. In the 13 year period between the surveys, the overall index of incapacity was essentially unchanged. Stair walking showed improvement in the 1975 sample compared with the 1962 sample. However, in both years, stair walking was the most difficult task to perform. The reamining five items showed no change across the time period.

Verbrugge plotted trends in NHIS data for the years 1965 to 1980 for several indices of disability.[25] Using the prevalence of limitation in activity, total restricted activity days, and total bed disability days, she identifies few distinguishable trends over these years. For limitation in activity, the prevalence of any limitation, major activity limitation, and secondary activity limitation are described by sex, but no trend is evident. For total restricted activity days, there is a decline in the averages to 1970 followed by an increase in average restricted days for both sexes. Total bed disability days, which is the more sensitive indicator of severity of disability, is relatively stable across these years.

Crimmins has improved on previous studies by assuring comparability of data over time and age-specific prevalences.[26] Using NHIS data from the years 1969, 1970, and 1971 and 1979, 1980, and 1981, she reports an increase in the prevalence of chronic disease (activity limitation) among the younger old people but no significant changes in chronic disease among the remaining older population. Crimmins uses a three-year-moving-average to compute the prevalence of activity limitation centred on the census years 1970 and 1980. Activity limitations were classified as either 'limited in activity' or 'unable to perform major activity'. If the limitation was of any kind, that is major activity or secondary activity, then the individual was classified as limited in activity. For males 1970 and 1980, there is a significant increase in prevalence of both 'limited in activity' and 'unable to perform major activity' for men aged 65 to 74. Thereafter, there is no detectable difference between either activity limitation at the advanced ages.

For women, a similar increase in prevalence was observed in limitations in activity up through 72 years of age. There were no statistically significant differences in limitations of activity thereafter. No differences in major activity limitation are seen between 1970 and 1980 for the women.

Similar analysis performed for restricted activity days and bed disability days show striking similarities in the 1970 and 1980 curves. Moreover, when differences are present between the two years the magnitude is generally small, in the range of 3 to 5 per cent.

Crimmins used self-reporting of how long the respondents had had an activity-limiting condition and their current ages to estimate ages of onset of these conditions. Between the years of 1970 and 1980, this proxy measure suggests the older males are reporting small decreases in the age of onset of limiting conditions. The youngest of the old, who had experienced the largest increases in the prevalence of limitation of activity, was the same group to experience the most dramatic declines in the age of onset of limiting condition.

Since this measure is sensitive to the onset of chronic limitation at any age prior to their present age, Crimmins looked at the age of onset of chronic disease within the previous 5 years. The evidence does not support an ongoing compression of morbidity. There appears to be no change in age of onset of limiting condition for either men or women in the three older age groups analysed. The data suggests increasing duration of time with chronic disease.

The only study reviewed that incorporates an evaluation of the institutionalized population is based on Canadian data. Wilkins and Adams detected no change in short-term impairment measures, but did identify an increase in long-term disability.[27, 28] These authors propose a comprehensive index of a population's health, which they call a 'health expectancy index'. This population-based statistic is a composite of mortality data, institutional data from long-term care facilities, and survey data on disability. The authors report that from birth the quality-adjusted life expectancy amounted to over 90 per cent of the total life expectancy. Based on a comparison of data from 1951 and 1978, the increase in life expectancy for each sex represented increased disability expectancy. For men, 70 per cent of the gain was in the form of increased disability expectancy, compared with 80 per cent for the women. These findings are consistent with those of Colvez and Blanchet,[29] who similarly conclude that the gains in life expectancy in Canada for both sexes have come in the form of increased disability years.

PROBLEMS WITH CURRENT RESEARCH AND FUTURE DIRECTIONS FOR RESEARCH

Throughout this discussion, we have attempted to relate the problems with current research to underlying difficulties in interpreting nuances of prevalence data. Many of the current studies fail to separate the effects of age, time period, and cohort. In terms of age effects, only the research by Crimmins and Shanas disaggregates the data into small age groups. Time period effects include changes in attitudes toward disability.[30] For example, regulations may make it easier to retire or claim disability benefits. There may be increased social acceptance of retirement associated with disability. Other than several Canadian studies, no research using the United States population has evaluated institutionalization concomitant with trends in disability.

Future studies of the United States population that use prevalence as a frequency measure must simultaneously consider the institutionalized population. Moreover changes in severity, or case mix, among the institutionalized must be considered, as well as changes in the overall threshold for institutionalization.

A number of unanswered questions remain about risk factors, which are central to Fries' argument. First, most of the current knowledge about prevention relates to chronic disease risk factors which directly impact on mortality, and not morbidity.[18] Thus, risk factor modification is more likely to impact the extension of life expectancy, rather than increase active life expectancy. Evans has raised questions about the malleability of risk factors for many of the conditions associated with morbidity.[31] For example, in the case of hypertension as a risk factor for cardiovascular disease, diastolic blood pressures are modifiable using existing treatment methods, but the success of treating elevated systolic pressures remains to be demonstrated.

The published research has not identified the extent of recovery from morbidity and how much morbidity is irreversible or permanent. The measures most frequently reported in the literature are relatively insensitive to changes from pre-existing disease states. Kovar has suggested that long-term disability is more likely to be irreversible, and that restricted activity days as a measure of disability would be better excluded from future discussions.[12] Future research may better be directed toward a consideration of the transitional probabilities between irreversible and reversible disability. Answering this type of question requires longitudinal studies of the population, following respondents through long observation periods.

Type of major activity is important when evaluating restriction of major activity. Comparability of wording of questions over time is essential, but it may mean using less than optimal questions originally.

Undoubtedly, no single data set will adequately answer every facet of the compression of morbidity argument outlined above. In the best of all worlds, the researcher needs incidence measures of disability, termination data (rates of recovery, case fatality rates, and duration of disability), and mortality rates over time to evaluate accurately whether compression of morbidity is occurring. At present, the concept remains an attractive but unsubstantiated theory.

Although research cannot confirm a decrease in morbidity, experienced clinicians have noted that the health status of elderly persons seems to have improved greatly in the last two decades. A 65-year-old person today is a much more vital person than a similarly aged individual 20 years ago. The apparent discrepancy between this clinical observation and the general expectation that improved survival may leave behind a wake of impaired elders may be reconciled by considering the possibility of a bipartite effect. In essence, the proportion of healthy, intact elders has increased, but at the same time so has the proportion of impaired persons.

This apparent paradox can be accounted for by a consistent improvement in health status. As a possible model to aid future research on this concept of bimodality, consider health conditions at two points in time, before and after some progress has been made in reducing mortality rates. It is at least conceptually possible to divide the population alive under the more favourable conditions into two groups—those who also would have been alive under the less favourable conditions and those who would have died but have been saved as a result of the progress in reducing mortality rates.[32]

Suppose the first group is healthier than before: for them, the benefit of health progress has been a reduction in morbidity. The second, resuscitated group may also be considered healthier than before: for them, the benefit is that they are alive. Many of the resuscitated may, however, be living in an impaired state of high morbidity. Hence the average level of morbidity may increase because of this influx of impaired lives, even though everyone's life status is better than before.

ACKNOWLEDGEMENT

The authors thank Dr Alan Lopez for his thoughtful review and comments on an earlier draft. The responsibility for the final text, however, remains with the authors.

References

1. Katz, K., Branch, L. G., Branson, M. H., Papsidero, J. A., Beck, J. C., and Greer, D. S. (1983). Active life expectancy. *New England Journal of Medicine*, November 17, **309**, 1218–24.
2. Gruenberg, E. M. (1977). The failure of success. *Milbank Memorial Fund Quarterly/Health and Society*, Summer, **55**, 3–24.
3. Kramer, M. (1980). The rising pandemic of mental disorders and associated chronic diseases and disabilities. *Acta Psychiatrica Scandinavica*, (Supplementum) 285, **62**, 382–97.

4. Fries, J. F. (1980). Aging, natural death, and the compression of morbidity. *New England Journal of Medicine*, **303**, 130–6.
5. Fries, J. F. and Crapo, L. M. (1981). *Vitality and aging.* W. H. Freeman and Company, San Francisco.
6. Fries, J. F. (1983). The compression of morbidity. *Milbank Memorial Fund Quarterly/Health and Society*, Summer, **61**, 397–419
7. Fries, J. F. (1987). An introduction to the compression of morbidity. *Gerontologica Perspecta*, **1**, 5–8.
8. Hayflick, L. (1976). The cell biology of human aging. *New England Journal of Medicine*, **295**, 1302–8.
9. Hayflick, L. (1980). The cell biology of human aging. *Scientific American*, **242**, 58–65.
10. Hayflick, L. (1965). The limited *in vitro* lifetime of human diploid strains. *Experimental Cell Research*, **37**, 614–36.
11. Brody, J. A., and Schneider, E. L. (1986). Diseases and disorders of aging: an hypothesis. *Journal of Chronic Diseases*, **39**, 871–6.
12. Kovar, M. G. (1987). Some comments on measuring morbidity. *Gerontologica Perspecta*, **1**, 49–54.
13. World Health Organization. (1980). *International classification of impairments, disabilities, and handicaps: a manual of classification relating to the consequences of disease.* World Health Organization, Geneva.
14. Kleinbaum, D. G., Kupper, L. L., and Morgenstern, H. (1982). *Epidemiologic research: principles and quantitative methods.* Van Nostrand Reinhold, New York.
15. Guralnik, J. M. and Schneider, E. L. (1987). The compression of morbidity: a dream which may come true someday! *Gerontologica Perspecta*, **1**, 8–14.
16. Manton, K. G. (1982). Changing concepts of morbidity and mortality in the elderly population. *Milbank Memorial Fund Quarterly*, **60**, 183–244.
17. Manton, K. G. (1986). Past and future life expectancy increases at later ages: their implications for the linkage of chronic morbidity, disability, and mortality. *Journal of Gerontology*, **41**, 672–81.
18. Manton, K. G. (1987). Response to 'an introduction to the compression of morbidity' and 'the compression of morbidity: a dream which may come true, someday!'. *Gerontologica Perspecta*, **1**, 23–30.
19. Myers, G. C. and Manton, K. G. (1984). Compression of mortality: myth or reality? *The Gerontologist*, **24**, 346–53.
20. Spenser, G. (1986). The first-ever examination of the characteristics of centenarians in the 1980 census. Unpublished paper. Annual Meeting of the Population Association of America, San Francisco.
21. Kovar, M. G. (1977). Elderly people: the population 65 years and over. *Health—United States—1976–1977*, DHEW Publication No. (HRA) 77–1232. US Department of Health, Education, and Welfare, Washington DC.
22. Colvez, A. and Blanchet, M. (1981). Disability trends in the United States population 1966–76: analysis of reported casues. *American Journal of Public Health*, **71**, 464–71.
23. Palmore, E. B. (1986). Trends in the health of the aged. *The Gerontologist*, **26**, 298–302.
24. Shanas, E. (1982). *National survey of the aged.* DHHS Publication No. (OHDS) 83–20425. US Department of Health and Human Services, Wash-

ington DC.

25. Verbrugge, L. M. (1984). Longer life but worsening health? trends in health and mortality of middle-aged and older persons. *Milbank Memorial Fund Quarterly/Health and Society*, **62**, 475–519.

26. Crimmins, E. M. (1987). Evidence on the compression of morbidity *Geronto-logica Perspecta*, **1**, 45–9.

27. Wilkins, R. and Adams, O. B. (1983). Health expectancy in Canada, late 1970's: demographic, regional, and social dimensions. *American Journal of Public Health*, **73**, 1073–980.

28. Wilkins, R. and Adams, O. B. (1987). Changes in the healthfulness of life of the elderly population: an empirical approach. *Revue Epidemologique et Santé Publique*, **35**, 225–35.

29. Colvez, A. and Blanchet, M. (1983). Potential gains in life expectancy free of disability: a tool for health planning. *International Journal of Epidemiology*, **12**, 224–9.

30. Chirikos, T. N. (1983). Accounting for the historical rise in work-disability prevalence. *Milbank Memorial Fund Quarterly/Health and Society*, **61**, 430–44.

31. Evans, J. G. (1984). Preventation of age-associated loss of autonomy: Epidemiological approaches. *Journal of Chronic Diseases*, **37**, 353–63.

32. Vaupel, J. W. and Yashin A. I. (1985). Heterogeneity's ruses: some surprising effects of selection on population dynamics. *The American Statistician*, 39, 176–85.

5

How are the elderly different?

J. GRIMLEY EVANS

One of the basic issues in planning for the consequences of demographic aging is whether the elderly should be regarded as a specific 'target' group or whether their needs should be catered for within the context of planning for the population as a whole. Both strategies have their proponents whose experience has been drawn exclusively from a limited number of economically developed countries. The theme of this essay will be to review the nature of human aging and its implications for the design and deployment of health services in aging populations. A general model of aging can establish the principles which health services for aging populations need to embody and can identify some of the impediments likely to be encountered. At an operational level, however, the widely different social and cultural contexts of economically developed and developing countries probably preclude there being a single appropriate response to what should be recognized as a range of unique situations.

THE NATURE OF HUMAN AGING

Aging in the sense of senescence comprises a loss of adaptability of an individual organism over time. All multicellular organisms display this phenomenon although many wild animals live in such dangerous environments that few individuals survive long enough for aging to become apparent. In less dangerous environments, loss of adaptability of an individual may not be readily apparent since it consists of a loss of functional reserve and a non-dangerous environment will rarely test individuals to their functional limits. None the less, aging of the individual members of populations will be reflected in risk of death computed as the age-specific mortality rate of the population. In humans, age-specific mortality rates fall from birth until the age of 12 or 13 years, after which they begin to rise again. After some initial perturbations due to deaths from accident and violence, particularly in men, mortality rates rise steadily as a function of age. In biological terms this can be seen as an initial phase of natural selection against individuals whose innate adaptability is insufficient to cope with the harsher variants of the environment or for whom parental protection is inadequate, followed somewhat before the age of puberty by the emergence of the effects of senescence.

Although the association of mortality rates with age has been conventionally regarded as exponential since Gompertz first examined the issue, and a great deal of gerontological theorizing has started from this assumption, it is not strictly true. Economos[1] among others has pointed out that mortality rates at ages above 80 years are lower than the exponential function would predict by a degree that is probably of biological as well as statistical significance. In the English population at ages over 104 years mortality rates in men seem to fall—a phenomenon that Barrett has suggested may reflect the emergence by survival of a biologically distinct subgroup of the population.[2, 3]

Differences between young and old

A starting point for the scientific appraisal of human aging is to compare young and old people, and the general public's view of aging is also derived explicitly or implicitly from comparison. Differences between young and old people can arise through processes other than aging, however, so the comparison can be deceptive. Table 5.1 outlines some of the sources of differences between young and old.

Differences not due to aging

Some differences have come about not because the old people have changed due to aging, but because they have always been different from the young with which they are being compared. *Selective survival* is one factor, although it is difficult to estimate how important this is in human populations. In order to identify specific characteristics undergoing selection by differential survival, it would be necessary to compare those members of an identified birth cohort who live into the ninth or tenth decade of age with those of the same cohort who die at younger ages. For obvious reasons such a research design is impractical and researchers have to fall back on comparisons of the very old with those from younger

Table 5.1 Differences between young and old

Aging	Non-aging
Primary	Selective survival
Intrinsic	Cohort effects
Extrinsic	Differential challenge
Secondary	
Individual adaptation	
Specific adaptation	

cohorts as yet unwinnowed by selective survival. This method requires the two assumptions that successive birth cohorts were equally equipped to face the selective pressures of adult life and also that those pressures remained the same over the time between the birth cohorts compared. The second assumption is usually less secure than the first. The method is essentially restricted to the study of genetic correlates of survival, and the more interesting and probably more powerful behaviourable and cultural variables remain unexamined.

Cohort effects refer to the differences between generations of people born at different times and therefore exposed, in developing societies, to different environmental factors, particularly early in life. Such cohort differences can be considerable and are important in changing societies. Schaie and Strother demonstrated that a major part of what appears to be age-associated change in psychological functioning in cross-sectional studies may be due to cultural differences between generations.[4] Although most obtrusive in the sphere of psychological function, which reflects educational standards and practices during childhood, cohort effects will contribute to cross-sectional estimates of age-associated variation in physical variables such as height, serum lipids, and obesity, as well as to risk of diseases such as lung cancer. The cross-sequential studies of aging Swedes in Göteborg suggests that cohort differences in bone density[5] and mental function,[6] even over periods as short as 5 years, may be comparable in magnitude to age-associated changes over the same period of years. Cohort differences should not be regarded as the inevitable effects of generations being passively moulded by their early environment; they will reflect differences between generations in lifestyle and behaviour at least as much as by changes in the physical environment.

The phenomenon of *differential challenge* is of great concern. If aging is to be defined in terms of reduced adaptability it can only be assessed by offering equal challenges to people at different ages. Social policy may lead to our offering more severe challenges to older people than to younger and then attributing the difference in response to the effects of aging. A classic example of this is the genesis of hypothermia among the elderly of Britain. Although hypothermia must be in part attributed to age-associated changes in an individual's ability to adapt to a cold environment,[7] it is precipitated by social policies that lead to old people being in worse and colder housing than is provided for the young.[8] Differential challenge is also a feature of health services where older patients may be the victims of negative discrimination.[9] An American study showed that doctors spend less time on consultation with older than with younger patients,[10] and the problem is sufficiently pervasive for there to be discussion of techniques of 'defensive' use of health services by which the elderly may overcome such discrimination.[11]

Such discrimination may be even more intense against the disabled and vulnerable old. A study in Tyneside, England, compared two hospitals in the survival of their patients aged 65 and over admitted with proximal femoral fractures. At one hospital there was a significantly higher fatality among mentally impaired patients, probably due to a lower provision of nursing than at the other hospital.[12,13] However, the majority of patients with mental impairment were admitted to the hospital with the poorer results. Because mentally impaired old people are expected to do badly after hip fracture, no one had noticed that because of inferior care they were dong worse than necessary. The poorer accommodation and facilities provided for geriatric departments compared with other medical departments in many parts of the United Kingdom is notorious and there is justifiable concern lest the increasing development of separate geriatric medical departments providing services that parallel those in general medical departments may lead to older people receiving inferior care, particularly in access to newer developments in therapy.

True aging

Secondary aging, a term designating those adaptations made to overcome the effects of aging, is most obvious in the realm of psychological functioning. Obsessional behaviour making an ordered environment substitute for memory, and increased absent-mindedness as we cope with reduced information-processing capacity by narrowed attention, are common and successful adaptations. It has recently been suggested that some features of the remodelling of long bones during aging may be an adaptive response to the diminishing strength of bones due to age-associated osteoporosis.[14] At a species level the female menopause seems to be an evolved adaptation to aging. In all mammalian species the chances of a successful outcome to pregnancy decline with age. In the unique context of the human species with a social structure centred round the family and with a cumulative culture mediated by speech, there will come a time in a woman's life when, in terms of the probability of her genes surviving into the next generation (the fundamental parameter of evolutionary success), it will be more profitable on average for her to give up increasingly unsuccessful attempts to produce children of her own, each containing 50 per cent of her genes, and to devote her biological resources instead to contributing to the survival and success of her grandchildren, even though each of these contains only 25 per cent of her genes. For the male, with so much less to lose biologically speaking in unsuccessful pregnancies, the best strategy for his genes is for him to stay sexually active as long as his life lasts. This interpretation of the biological origin of the menopause depends on the observation that it is an exclusively human phenomenon. The menopause may be defined as a genetically determined species characteristic of total cessation of reproductive capability occurring with low age variance at an age approximately halfway through the species maximum lifespan; otherwise it may be confused with the senescent changes in the reproductive system seen in all species and to which it was an adaptive response.

Although few clear-cut instances have so far been identified, we must expect that there will be both physiological and biochemical manifestations of secondary aging. The significance of the concept of secondary aging for health workers is to recognize that some age-associated changes may be adaptive and that attempts to 'correct' them may do more harm than good.

Once we have accurately delineated *primary aging*, it is here that the most important determinants of longevity and age-associated morbidity lie. Primary aging is due to the interaction of *extrinsic* (environmental) influences with *intrinsic* (genetic) factors. Extrinsically determined aging is recognized in variations in aging patterns exhibited by people living under different environments, or in the results of interventive trials in which age-associated patterns of morbidity or mortality are altered by environmental manipulation. Approached in this way, intrinsic aging is assumed to be contained within those age-associated changes which cannot be demonstrated as being modified by environmental influences. Such definition by exclusion or default is clearly unsatisfactory and there is interest in trying to specify the characteristics of intrinsic aging by which it might be recognizable directly; this can only be achieved within the context of evolutionary biology.

There is a long history of flawed or incomplete attempts at a comprehensive theory of intrinsic aging, but Kirkwood's analysis of the implications of selective pressure on different strategies for energy allocation by organisms,[15] coupled with modern perceptions of the strength of evolutionary selective pressure diffusing outwards from genetic to organismic level,[16] has produced an approach that seems likely to prove definitive. Kirkwood suggests that intrinsic aging comes about through failure to repair random environmentally induced damage to the organism leading to cumulative impairment of adaptability.[15] In principle, the organism could evolve means to detect and repair much of this damage and the achievement of some lineages, including our own hominid ancestors,[17] in lengthening their maximum lifespan is produced by this means. There is, however, an energy cost in repair, and an organism which develops a faultless system and no longer undergoes aging will, despite the evolutionary advantage of a longer potential reproductive life, be at a selective disadvantage compared with an otherwise similar organism that devotes less energy to repair in order to produce a higher reproduction rate. This disadvantage arises because the individual organism could not expect immortality even if aging were abolished since death would occur eventually from accident, predation, or warfare. The balance of benefit, therefore, between the length of reproductive life and the rate of reproduction is a dynamic one and will vary with the dangerousness of the environment since the higher the danger the greater is the selective pressure favouring high reproductive rates. There will also be pressure favouring greater complexity of organisms in their capacities to avoid the dangers of the environment, and this complexity will emerge only as lifespan becomes long enough for the necessary growth and development and for the survival benefits of complexity to emerge.

There are three lines of evidence to suggest that a fairly small number of genetic loci may have an important effect on the determination of maximum lifespan of a species. The segmental aging syndromes,[18] in which single gene effects produce a picture of accelerated aging in some of the body systems, probably indicate some of the relevant loci. The genetic distance, measured in terms of amino acid differences in homologous proteins[19] and DNA sequences,[20] between the chimpanzee and the much longer-lived human is so small that the number of loci involved must be small. Less directly, Cutler[17] has produced evidence from the estimated lifespan of our precursors that the length of life of the hominid line increased so rapidly over a small number of generations some 200 000 years ago that, unless mutation rates were much higher then than they are now, only a fairly small number of loci must have been involved.

Such evidence offers hope that biochemical interference in the action of certain genes might have important effects on the maximum lifespan and possibly on some of the manifestations of intrinsic aging that emerge as causes of disease and disability in old age. Kirkwood's theory, however, warns us that, despite this evidence that a relatively small number of genetic loci may have an important effect on intrinsic aging, its mechanisms are likely to be so numerous and complex that an attack on them does not offer immediate hope of modifying the human pattern of aging. Moreover, as Medawar[21] and Hamilton[22] have discussed, selection pressure on individual organisms declines with time from sexual maturation. There will therefore have been little selection pressure to foster the emergence of systems of repair for bodily defects which appear only late in life. These may include some of the important mechanisms of disability in old age arising through actual loss of unreplaced units, for example neurones or nephrons. The conclusion seems ineluctable that we cannot expect in the short term to increase the maximum lifespan of the species, which is genetically determined, nor to remove those aspects of disability in late life that reflect intrinsic constraints, but we may seek by modifying extrinsic aging to increase the proportion of the population who achieve, in an undisabled state, their genetic potential for longevity.

As noted above, extrinsic aging can be recognized in variation in aging patterns of people living in different circumstances, and can be evaluated in interventive trials. Short-term interventive experiments will detect only the early and reversible components of extrinsic aging, which largely comprise irreversible changes that can only be fully assessed in long-term preventive studies. A common alternative approach to identifying extrinsic aging is to compare the health or functional status of people in a population with different exposures to environmental factors postulated to be linked to age-associated changes. This is the classical 'risk factor' approach of analytical epidemiology. There are several reasons why this method may underestimate the importance of extrinsic effects on aging if only the elderly are studied.[23] Perhaps the most important is that relevant risk factors may lie in the past rather than the present. In a prospective study of stroke incidence in a Tyneside population aged 65 and over it was found that those subjects destined to suffer later stroke did not differ from controls in terms of weight and height at the time of entry to the study, but they had been significantly heavier for their height earlier in life.[24] Whether obesity in early life in this study should be regarded as the mechanism whereby environmental factors wrought their effects on the victims' arteries, or whether it was merely a marker for metabolic processes leading later to atherosclerosis, remains uncertain. Whatever the mechanism, the finding reminds us that aging is a lifelong process and needs to be studied as such.

Extrinsic aging, like intrinsic processes, can also be placed in a biological context. Several workers have suggested that part of the human aging process may come about because the human species evolved under different circumstances from those under which we now live. Thus genes may have been selected for that are maladaptive under modern circumstances. Neel[25] was among the first to explore this idea in postulating a 'thrifty gene' which enables its possessor to lay down excess calorie intake in the form of fat. This would enable him or her to survive subsequent periods of famine, cold, and exposure. Under the conditions of lifelong calorie excess enjoyed by the inhabitants of economically advanced nations, Neel postulated that the same gene might predispose to maturity onset diabetes and its associated diseases. Those populations that had undergone most selective pressure due to recurrent famine in the past would possess such genes in highest prevalence and this might lead to racial differences in susceptibility to coronary heart disease in economically advanced environments. A variant of such an evolutionary lag theory has recently been put forward by Hutton as a possible explanation for the age-associated disorder of osteoarthritis.[26] Hutton postulates that, since the adoption of bipedal gait by the precursors of *Homo sapiens* is comparatively recent in evolutionary terms, those joints which now bear the body weight have had a shorter time to become adapted to their role and so are relatively 'underdesigned' compared with those joints which have either retained their former function or now come under less stress than when gait was quadripedal. Given that selection pressure on maladaptive traits will be inversely proportional to the age from sexual maturity, this theory will explain both the distribution of joints most commonly affected by generalised osteoarthritis and also the age distribution of the condition.

Such 'maladaptive' evolution theories may seem to offer promise of reducing age-associated morbidity by a return to some primitive style of life closer to that under which the human species evolved. There is no empirical evidence to support such ideas. Economic development and the consequent changes in nutrition, housing, and health services has been consistently associated with improving mortality rates and there is no evidence that this is balanced by any disproportionate increase in age-associated morbidity. It must also be borne in mind that an essential feature of the circumstances under which early man evolved was a very high childhood mortality rate and the genetic benefits of selective pressure was to enable survival in childhood, not to reduce morbidity or mortality in later life. There is therefore a real danger that uncritical atavism might add to the burdens of extrinsic aging rather than lightening them.

Sex differences in aging

Biological considerations also apply to the sex differences in aging and longevity. In economically advanced nations the female outlives the male and analogies have been drawn with the greater longevity of the female in some other species in which the need of the female to nurture the eggs and perhaps the offspring has apparently led to her evolving greater resistance than the male to environmental challenge. This analogy is false, however, for in *Homo sapiens* the male is to a greater or lesser extent involved in the nurturing and protection of offspring. Moreover, from demographic and archaeological evidence it seems that the biological superiority of the human female as manifested in mortality is of recent origin historically.

At the time of the Neolithic revolution when human communities gave up the hunter–gatherer mode of subsistence and settled down to herd animals and grow crops, it became necessary to develop a warrior caste to defend territory and in times of famine to raid the lands and stores of neighbouring tribes. In such conditions human society inevitably becomes male dominant and the dedication of scarce resources to the maintenance of an effective army of young males a necessity of survival. Females become discriminated against particularly as regards nutrition, and thus under stronger selective pressure than the male to overcome the susceptibility to infections produced by chronic subnutrition. Presumably, given that the male and female share the same genes, the mechanism will lie in a metabolic switch diverting energy resources in the male to muscular strength and in the female to resistance to infections albeit at the price of generally smaller stature and feebler physical development than the male. When, under conditions of adequate nutrition, the two sexes come to compete on equal terms the female will emerge as biologically the more resistant to some forms of environmental challenge because of the greater selective pressure her female forebears underwent in the past. Clearly, grafted on to this biological difference, will be the consequences of environmental and behavioural differences between the sexes. In the United Kingdom, the ratio of male to female mortality was constant over the adult age span at about 1.2 in 1911 but subsequently developed two peaks of ratios higher than 2.0 at ages around 20 and 65, reflecting the consequences of lifestyle differences between the sexes during the twentieth century.[27] Whether these peaks of excess in male deaths will be eroded as women come to take on lifestyles closer to that of men remains to be seen.

There seems no reason to doubt that as economic advance takes place women will live longer than men, and, unless there is a change in the widespread tradition of men marrying women younger than themselves, a disproportionate increase in the numbers of elderly widows is the inevitable consequence. Few, if any, developed nations have produced systems of social and financial support appropriate to this challenge.

Aging and disease

The analytical approach to aging set out above is rooted in a fundamentally different conceptual ground from the traditional medical model of a distinction between 'aging' and 'disease'. There are several objections to this traditional model, of which the most telling is the variable or absent basis for defining what the two terms mean and the implications they carry. Proponents of the aging and disease model do not define aging but imply that it is whatever remains unexplained when all definable diseases have been diagnosed and/or that it is what happens to everybody, whereas diseases happen to only some people. In practice neither criterion is applied with any intellectual rigour or consistency.

In the earliest development of scientific medicine, disease was described (in pathological terms) rather than defined. The recognition of infectious diseases in the nineteenth century led to the hope that diseases might all eventually be definable in terms of a single necessary and sufficient cause. Before the end of the century it had become recognized, particularly from the epidemiology of tuberculosis, that even infectious diseases could not be defined by a single sufficient cause, since the susceptibility of the exposed person was also relevant. In this phase of the 'seed and ground' model of disease it still seemed possible to define diseases in terms of a single necessary cause. The chronic afflictions of economically advanced nations do not seem to fit this model. Conditions like coronary heart disease appear to be the final common pathways of a wide variety of possible antecedent causative chains, and to some extent medical science has come full circle in defining diseases in terms of their pathological descriptions rather than their aetiology. As any textbook of medicine will reveal, all these concepts of disease now coexist in different contexts appropriate to specific conditions, but none can be applied *a priori* to an entity of which the aetiology is unknown and the pathology non-specific—as is the case for many of the important forms of age-associated disability.

There have been attempts to distinguish aging and disease on epidemiological grounds. Kurtzke suggested that stroke was a manifestation of aging because, among other things, its mortality rates varied little in different environments and followed an exponential relationship to age, like the total mortality rates assumed without justification to reflect intrinsic aging.[28] In fact stroke incidence is now known to vary with time and from country to country, while the age-specific incidence of stroke follows a power-law and not an exponential relationship to age.[29] The power-law relationship may be a marker of a largely extrinsically caused condition. Age is a marker of length of time of exposure to environmental pathogens, and hence cumulative dose, and as Peto and colleagues[30,31] have demonstrated this appears to explain the monotonic relationship of cancer incidence to age. The incidence of most adult cancers follows a power-law relationship to age[32] and epidemiological evidence indicates that the great majoirty of such cancers are extrinsically caused.[33]

Disease is often defined operationally, and legitimately, as a condition that requires or is susceptible to specific treatment. It is also a designation that has implications for social labelling. A person with a disease is expected to adopt the privileges and obligations of the 'sick role' and to receive the sympathy and support of society. Aging by contrast is seen as the common lot, deserving no particular sympathy, and not the concern or responsibility of the medical profession. The difference in social attitudes towards someone who attempts to overcome or conceal the inroads of 'disease' compared with those towards someone who attempts to conceal or overcome the ravages of 'aging' makes the point clearly enough.

Rather than regarding the diagnosis of disease as the ultimate aim of care, those caring for older patients need to identify the patients' problems in functional terms. Typically these problems arise from discrepancies between what the patient is able to do and what the environment demands. In this approach care requires the specification of objectives, again in functional terms, and identification of the options for achieving them. Diseases thus may appear as the mechanisms of problems and impediments to care objectives; they do not automatically become objects of treatment in themselves. The 'aging' versus disease' model has been used by the medical profession to abrogate responsibility for caring for an arbitrarily defined category of human affliction and may delay or inhibit research. As Katzman implies it was only when 'senile dementia' ceased to be categorized as a manifestation of 'aging' and became 'Alzheimer's disease' that it attracted significant research effort and resources.[34] The disease/aging distinction is best remembered as an example of the way progress may be impeded by inappropriate models.

THE PATTERN OF AGING

As described earlier, the relationship of total mortality rates to age is continuous and approximately exponential. The same applies to a wide range of other correlates of age in later life. The prevalence of chronic disease and of dementia, mean length of hospital stay, general practitioner consultation rates, and use of a variety of domiciliary services in the United Kingdom show this phenomenon. Although the relationship is approximately exponential, the slope of the increase with age varies greatly. In Table 5.2, the slope of the gradient of a number of illustrative processes against age is indicated in the form of '10-year age factors', that is to say the proportional increase in the prevalence of a disability or use of a service for each 10 years of age from 65 onwards. Thus the prevalence of stroke increases 1.6 times from age 65 to 75 and then 1.6 times from 75 to 85. These figures are imprecise estimates based on averaging a range of published data and are specific to the United Kingdom over the last decade. They are therefore of no more than illustrative value but they do provoke some reflections on the relationship between aging and social responses to aging populations.

The epidemiology of aging is characterized by increasing incidence of many disabilities, but also by increasing fatality so that prevalence increases less steeply with age than does incidence. This is seen in the modest increase with age in the prevalence of stroke in Table 5.2. Dementia is a notable exception to this general rule in that fatality appears to diminish with age at onset, thus producing a large age factor for prevalence and making dementia the most challenging consequence of aging of a population.

A striking feature of the table is the difference in age factors between *prosthetic* and *therapeutic* services. Prosthetic services are those which simply compensate for a recipient's disability, whereas therapeutic ser-

Table 5.2 Ten-year age factors (see text) for selected disabilities, medical conditions and use of health and social services; United Kingdom, 1973–1983.

Activities of daily living:	
difficulty with household tasks	2.9
inability to do shopping	3.2
Specific medical conditions:	
stroke prevalence	1.6
dementia prevalence	4.4
proximal femoral fracture incidence	3.5
Prosthetic services	
home helps	4.0
meals-on-wheels	5.3
Therapeutic services:	
general practitioner consultations	1.2
chiropody	2.3
hospital admission	1.5

vices are aimed at removing the disability. Prosthetic services tend to be deployed by social workers and therapeutic services by medical and nursing personnel. The contrast in slopes raise questions of whether social workers may respond to the age rather than the assessed needs of their clients in deploying services, since this would also explain why the age factors for services such as home helps and meals-on-wheels are greater than those for the disabilities (difficulty with household tasks and inability to do shopping) for which they are prosthetic. The low age factor for the therapeutic service of general practitioner consultations suggests that primary medical care may fail to respond appropriately to the pattern of need among elderly people, a finding for which there is other evidence.

Provision of a prosthetic service to a disabled elderly person will confirm the level of disability and accelerate further decline in function. Ideally a prosthetic service should not be deployed until therapetuic possibilities have been competently explored. The administrative allocation of the two services to different professions working to different models of aging and care is therefore undesirable.

IMPLICATIONS FOR HEALTH CARE

Treatment

The analytical approach to human aging exemplified above leads to the identification of several ways in which the needs of older people have to be considered in the design and deployment of health services. For example some of the properties of illness in old age that need to be planned for in the design of acute medical services are as follows:

—— multiple pathology;

—— non-specific presentation of disease;

—— rapid deterioration if untreated;

—— high incidence of secondary complications of disease and treatment;

—— need for rehabilitation;

—— importance of environmental factors.

The best recognized of these is *multiple pathology*. Older people who develop acute illnesses typically do so against a background of pre-existing, often chronic, disability and disease that adds to the complexity of presentation and managment. More crucial factors are comprised in the concept of aging as loss of adaptability. Many of the diagnostic features of disease represent not so much the disease itself as the body's response to the disease. In many cases it is some aspect of the inflammatory response together with localization of the disease process by the body's defences that produce the characteristic clinical picture of disease that is recognized by the patient or the clinician. If the body's defences are impaired in the age-associated loss of adaptability, illnesses may have *non-specific presentation* that make them difficult to diagnose. Impaired defences will also lead to *rapid deterioration* in the patient's condition unless appropriate treatment is instituted, and to a *high incidence of secondary complications* both of the illness and as side-effects of treatment. Recovery from illness is likely to be delayed and older patients will often have a *need for rehabilitation* from services that would not be required by younger patients possessing greater functional reserve. Although the consequences of inadequate diagnosis and treatment of illness in older people will include unnecessarily high mortality rates, inadequacy of the rehabilitative dimension of health services will result primarily in increased disability and dependency in the elderly population, with the expected social and economic consequences.

The loss of physical adaptability in the older patient may be compounded by loss of psychological adaptability, so rendering him or her more at the mercy of the immediate environment in the determination of mood, self-image, perspective on the future, and hence personal commitment to recovery. This *importance of environmental factors* is further compounded by loss of social and economic adaptability so that the availability and range of rehabilitative and therapeutic environments are generally reduced for older compared with younger adults unless facilities for social as well as medical rehabilitation are made available.

Prevention

The nature of aging also has implications for preventive approaches to disease and disability in later life. As discussed earlier, we must assume that, while some of the afflictions of later life will relect intrinsic processes that are unlikely to prove modifiable in the near future, there is a much greater contribution from extrinsic processes than has been generally recognized. As already noted, epidemiological evidence suggests that 70 per cent or more of adult cancers are environmentally caused.[33] The overview of blood cholesterol and ischaemic heart disease by Peto and colleagues[35] confirms the long-claimed association between the two and indicates that efforts to reduce blood cholesterol may be expected to reduce the risk of heart disease for an individual and to do so within a small number of years. An acceleration of the age-associated decline in lung function by cigarette smoking is generally accepted, and beneficial effects of exercise in determining functional capacity[36] and bone density[37] in later life seem promising. Although the effects of some environmental exposures may be cumulative and irreversible, there is promising evidence that some preventive measures instituted in later life can be effective. Data from the follow-up of Harvard alumni[38] and from the Alameda County study[39] provide strong evidence that aspects of lifestyle under voluntary control have a significant effects on longevity and disease incidence, and the beneficial effects are seen in middle life and later.[40] Blood-pressure control appears to have contributed to the decline in stroke incidence in some countries.[41]

It would be overoptimistic to assume that the benefits of advances in knowledge such as these could become rapidly deployed within a population. People vary widely in their appraisal of the value of future benefits compared with present inconvenience both as individuals and as members of cultural subclasses. Much has been made in Britain, for example, of the differences between social classes in their perceptions of personal control over their own futures, and only recently have there been adequate explorations of the conceptual barriers to communicating the messages of preventive health education. Unless such cultural barriers can be overcome the effects of health education will be to widen the social class differentials in health as the intelligent and affluent classes appraise the evidence and adopt healthier lifestyle, while the lower classes remain the victims of their subculture. It seems that, for widely distributed benefits to be obtained in the short term from knowledge about preventive approaches to health, governments have to play a direct hand by manipulating incentives as well as disseminating knowledge. The reduction in related mortality produced by increasing the cost of alcohol and cigarettes is well known, although ignored by governments committed to sharing in the profits of the tobacco and alcohol industries.

THE ELDERLY IN SOCIETY

The status and role of the elderly in society are discussed extensively elsewhere in this volume. We have noted earlier the tendency for health services to discriminate against older people by offering them inferior care. This comes about partly because the contribution of aging to vulnerability is overestimated so that the consequences of inferior care are not recognized, and partly because of inadequate auditing of services, but more fundamentally from discriminatory attitudes towards older people that diminish concern for whether the services they receive are good or not. Studies have revealed that health care workers may make unjustified assumptions, for example that older patients are necessarily demented[9] and about the outcome of care, which is often regarded uncritically as being determined by age itself rather than by the variable correlates of age.

Discriminatory attitudes may arise from conventional approaches to establishing relative priorities in allocating health care resources. Usually these give weighting, directly or indirectly, to estimates of remaining years of life expectancy; this will automatically discriminate against older people. The ideological assumptions that underlie such paradigms for resource allocation have been insufficiently questioned since they are at variance with the overt values of the societies that adopt them. In essence there are three premises to which democratic societies are morally obliged to assent. Health services are provided for the benefit of the recipients not the convenience or profit of the providers; all citizens are equal in their rights to the resources of society and are not differentially valued according to biological characteristics for which they have no personal responsibility; the value of life can be judged only by the individual who possesses it and must not be equated to that individual's value to the State.[42] If these premises are accepted there can be no moral justification for discriminating against older people in the allocation of health care resources on the grounds of age alone. None the less in developed nations it appears that older people as a group are undervalued because they are perceived as economically unproductive, even though unproductivity may have been forced upon them by a compulsory retirement age. An important issue for the governments of the developing world is whether such undervaluing of older people is inseparable from economic advancement. Traditional patterns of support within families will be eroded by migration of young people to cities and by reduction in family size, as well as by changing mores. The claim made by some countries in evidence to the World Congress on Aging that their traditional modes of family care for their elderly will remain intact during economic development is no more that wishful thinking. Clearly, if national policy, whether of economic growth or population control, leads to withdrawal of traditional modes of support for the dependent in society, then democratic governments have a responsibility to substitute some alternative system of statutory care. The time necessary to devise and evaluate such a system, recruit and train the personnel, and deploy them effectively is probably measurable in decades rather than years.

CONCLUSION

Old people differ from younger adults in greater physical and psychological vulnerability. Too often this vulnerability is compounded by a more adverse environment and by social discrimination. There is reason to expect that these environmental and social factors are likely to accompany economic development. But is this inevitable? To what extent can nations learn from others' experience?—certainly no more than to the extent that the experience has been relevant. It is a widely held fallacy that today's developed countries were necessarily once in the same situation that developing countries are now in terms of their culturally determined patterns of caring for the old and dependent. Historical research establishes that there never has been a uniform pattern of social and family organization that transcends national and cultural frontiers. Nations and tribes have always been different. Historical research also warns us that even within a country customs may differ widely between localities. Whatever their planned future development, statutory services for the elderly should seek to implement principles derived from a study of the specific problems associated with population aging, but an operational level must initally blend and co-operate with existing informal practices. Imposition of models of care developed in other cultures may fail completely or lead to the premature or unnecessary destruction of traditional care. The emphasis in some recent WHO-supported research of identifying the normal social information networks of different societies as channels for extended health and self-care information is commendable.

Perhaps the most valuable lesson for nations to learn from others is how to avoid repeating some mistakes, and how to recognize and anticipate the side-effects of some approaches to care of aging populations. None of the economically advanced nations took the opportunity of planning ahead for their aging populations, partly because they lacked the necessary political will and partly because during the crucial years they were preoccupied in other matters such as warfare. They were therefore forced into applying inappropriate models of care and pressing services that were originally devised for other purposes into the care of the elderly. It is probable that not one of the developed countries would reproduce its present system of health and social care for its aging population if it had the opportunity to start again from scratch. This presents an exciting challenge to the developing nations, but even for them time is running out.

References

1. Economos, A. C. (1982). Rate of aging, rate of dying and the mechanism of mortality. *Archives of Gerontology and Geriatris*, **1**, 3–27.
2. Barrett, J. C. (1985). The mortality of centenarians. *Archives of Gerontology and Geriatrics*, **4**, 211–8.
3. Barrett, J. C. (1986). The mortality of centenarians: a correction. *Archives of Gerontology and Geriatrics*, **5**, 81.
4. Schaie, K. W. and Strother, C. R. (1968). A cross-sequential study of age changes in cognitive behavior. *Psychological Bulletin,* **70**, 671–8.
5. Svanborg, A. (1983). The physiology of ageing in man: diagnostic and therapeutic aspects. In *Advanced Geriatric Medicine 3* (ed. Caird, F. I. and J. G. Evans), pp. 175–82. Pitman, London.
6. Berg, S. (1980). Psychological functioning in 70- and 75-year old people. A study in an industrialized city. *Acta Psychiatrica Scandinavica*, Suppl. **288**, 1–47.
7. Fox, R. H., Woodward, P. M., Exton-Smith, A. N., Green, M. F., Donnison, D. V., and Wilks, M. G. (1973). Body temperatures in the elderly: a national study of physiological, social and environmental conditions. *British Medical Journal*, **1**, 200–6.
8. Collins, K. J., Dore, C., Exton-Smith, A. N., Fox, R. H., MacDonald, I. C., and Woodward, P. M. (1977). Accidental hypothermia and impaired temperature homeostasis in the elderly. *British Medical Journal*, **1**, 353–6.
9. Wetle, T. (1987). Age as a risk factor for inadequate treatment. *Journal of the American Medical Association*, **258**, 516.
10. Keeler, E. H., Solomon, D. H., Beck, J. C., Mendenhall, R. C., and Kane, R. L. (1982). Effect of patient age on duration of medical encounters with physicians. *Medical Care*, **20**, 1101–8.
11. Kane, R. A. and Kane, R. L. (1986). Self-care and health-care: inseparable but equal for the wellbeing of the old. In *Self-care and health in old age* (ed. Dean, K., T. Hickey, and B. E. Holstein), pp. 251–83. Croom Helm, London.
12. Evans, J. G., Wandless, I., and Prudham, D. (1979). A prospective study of fractured proximal femur: factors predisposing to survival. *Age and Ageing*, **8**, 246–50.
13. Evans, J. G., Prudham, D., and Wandless, I. (1980). A prospective study of fractured proximal femur: hospital differences *Public Health (London)*, **94**, 149–54.
14. Hayes, W. C. and Ruff, C. B. (1986). Biomechanical compensation mechanisms for age-related changes in cortical bone. In *Current concepts of bone fragility* (ed. Uhtoff, H. K), pp. 371–7. Springer-Verlag, Berlin.
15. Kirkwood, T. B. L. (1981). Repair and its evolution: survival versus repro-

duction. In *Physiological ecology: an evolutionary approach to resource use*, (ed. Townsend, C. R. and P. Callow), pp. 165–89. Blackwell Scientific, Oxford.

16. Dawkins, R. (1982). *The extended phenotype*. Oxford University Press, Oxford.
17. Cutler, R. G. (1975). Evolution of human longevity and the genetic complexity governing aging rate. *Proceedings of the National Academy of Science, USA*, **72**, 4664–8.
18. Martin, G. M. (1978). Genetic syndromes in man with potential relevance to the pathobiology of aging. In *Genetic effects on aging*, (ed. Bergsma, D., D. E. Harrison, and N. W. Paul), pp. 5–39. AR Liss, New York.
19. King, M. C. and Wilson, A. C. (1975). Evolution at two levels in humans and chimpanzees. *Science*, **188**, 107–16.
20. Ruvolo, M. and Pilbeam, D. (1986). Hominid evolution: molecular and palaeontological patterns. In *Major topics in primate and human evolution* (ed. Wood, B., L. Martin, and P. Andrews), pp. 157–60. Cambridge University Press, Cambridge.
21. Medawar, P. (1952). *An unsolved problem in biology*. Lewis, London.
22. Hamilton, W. D. (1966). The moulding of senescence by natural selection. *Journal of Theoretical Biology*, **12**, 12–45.
23. Evans, J. G. (1984). Prevention of age-associated loss of autonomy: epidemiological approaches. *Journal of Chronic Diseases*, **37**, 353–63.
24. Evans, J. G. (1983). Hypertension and stroke in an elderly population. *Acta Medica Scandinavica*, Suppl. **676**, 22–32.
25. Neel, J. V. (1962). Diabetes mellitus: a 'thrifty' genotype rendered detrimental by 'progress'? *American Journal of Human Genetics*, **14**, 353–62.
26. Hutton, C. W. (1987). Generalised osteoarthritis: an evolutionary problem? *Lancet*, **1**, 1463–5.
27. Evans, J. G. (1981). The biology of human ageing. In *Recent advances in medicine 18* (ed. Dawson, A. M. N. Compston and G. M. Besser), pp. 17–37. Churchill Livingstone, Edinburgh.
28. Kurtzke, J. F. (1969). *The epidemiology of cerebrovascular disease*. Springer-Verlag, Berlin.
29. Evans, J. G. and Caird, F. I. (1982). Epidemiology of neurological disorders in old age. In *Neurological disorders in the elderly* (ed. Caird, F. I.), pp. 1–16 John Wright and Sons, Bristol.
30. Peto, R., Roe, F. J. L., Levy, I., and Clack, J. (1975). Cancer and ageing in mice and men. British Journal of Cancer, **32**, 411–26.
31. Peto, R., Parish, S. E., and Gray, R. G. (1986). There is no such thing as aging and cancer is not related to it. In *Age-related factors in carcinogenesis* (ed. Likhachev, A. *et al.*), pp. 43–53. International Agency for Research on Cancer, Lyons.
32. Doll, R. (1970). The age distribution of cancer: implications for models of carcinogenesis. *Journal of the Royal Statistical Society (A)*, **134**, 133–55.
33. Doll, R. and Peto, R. (1981). *The causes of cancer*. Oxford University Press, Oxford.
34. Katzman, N. (1988). Discussion. In *Research and the ageing population*, Ciba Symposium No. 228, p. 47. Wiley, Chichester.
35. Peto, R. *et al.* (1988). In press.
36. Sherwood, D. E. and Selder, D. S. (1979). Cardiorespiratory health, reaction

time and ageing. *Medical Science of Sport*, **11**, 68–9.

37. Pocock, N. A., Elsman, J. A., Yeates, M. G. *et al.* (1986). Physical fitness is a major determinant of femoral neck and lumbar spine bone mineral density. *Journal of Clinical Investigation*, **78**, 618–21.

38. Paffenbarger, R. S., Hyde, R. T., Wing, A. L., and Hsieh, C. (1986). Physical activity, all-cause mortality and longevity of college alumni. *New England Journal of Medicine*, **314**, 605–13.

39. Wingard, D. L., Berkman, L. F., and Brand, R. J. (1982). A multivariate analysis of health-related practices. *American Journal of Epidemiology*, **116**, 765–75.

40. Schaie, K. W. and Strother, C. R. (1968). A cross-sequential study of age changes in cognitive behavior. *Psychological Bulletin,* **70**, 671–8.

40. Breslow, L. and Enstrom, J. E. (1980). Persistence of health habits and their relationship to mortality. *Preventive Medicine*, **9**, 469–83.

41. Garraway, W. M. and Whisnant, J. P. (1987). The changing incidence of hypertension and the declining incidence of stroke. *Journal of the American Medical Association*, **258**, 214–17.

42. Evans, J. G. (1988). Age and equality. *Annals of the New York Academy of Sciences*, **530**, 118–24.

6

Assessment of health and functional status: an international comparison

GERDA G. FILLENBAUM

The World Health Organization (WHO) defines health as a state of complete physical, mental, and social well-being. Accordingly it is clear that assessment of health should not be limited to an evaluation of physical and mental state, and the consequences of these as manifested in the performance of activities of daily living, but should also take into account social and economic conditions, and the general environmental situation.

While such complete assessments obviously represent a substantial undertaking, evaluations designed to examine several areas of functioning are being successfully carried out, and more are planned. References 1-17 give only a partial listing of studies.

Our focus here is twofold: to compare selected cross-nationally used multidimensional assessments designed for population level evaluation of the elderly, and to consider some of the basic characteristics which the measures and the samples to which they are applied must possess if the resulting information is to be meaningful and valuable. Linking both matters is our concern with whether we now have the start of a truly international data base which will provide information on overall personal functioning, rather than, as is presently the case, surveys or estimates providing information on specific but unintegrated aspects of well-being. The data we seek demand measures which are valid and reliable, equivalence of content across assessments, and information from representative samples.

SELECTED CROSS-NATIONAL MULTIDIMENSIONAL EVALUATIONS: SOME CONSIDERATIONS

The main multidimensional evaluations to be considered are those used in the WHO 11-country study,[12] referred to here as WHO Eurpoe, since all sites but one were in Europe, the four-country study carried out under WHO auspices in the Western Pacific (WHO Pacific[2]), the 13-country Pan American Health Organization-sponsored study in South America and the Carribean (PAHO[3]), the OARS Multidimensional Functional

Assessment Questionnaire (OARS[18]), and FACE (Fast Assessment of Community Elderly[19]), an internationally relevant rapid screen to identify those elderly urgently in need of care, which is currently being developed under WHO auspices.

WHO Europe

WHO Europe[12] is a sociomedical survey carried out in 1979 at 16 sites in 10 European countries (Belgium, Finland, France, Germany (FDR), Greece, Italy, Poland, Romania, the USSR, and Yugoslavia) and in Kuwait. The investigators decided to use an age- and sex-stratified sampling system to obtain 100 men and 100 women in six consecutive 5-year age groups starting with age 60 and ending with age 89.

In selecting subjects the assumption was typically made that census data, electoral lists, and population registers were complete, and provided accurate information on date of birth, sex, name, and address. No preliminary household surveys were carried out to identify accurately the presence of persons of the desired age range. Reflecting differential prevalence in the population aged 60 and over, different sampling ratios were used to attain the desired numbers for each 5-year age group.

With some exceptions, the number of respondents in each age group is large enough to permit comparison across age groups. However, since the proportional representation of each age group is not given (it may be forthcoming in future publications) and the characteristics of non-respondents has not yet been adequately presented, the extent to which current data accurately represent the status of the elderly in the sampled areas cannot be determined. These data must therefore be used with great caution. While cross-age comparison within each country may be legitimate, cross-national comparison remains hazardous. Such considerations notwithstanding, the study does show that multidimensional evaluation of the elderly is feasible.

WHO Pacific

The WHO Pacific study[2] obtained information on persons aged 60 and over in four countries: Fiji, Malaysia, the Philippines, and the Republic of Korea. Recognizing the desirability of using random sampling but noting the extraordinary costs of this approach, a multistage sampling approach was used. While sampling details varied from country to country, generally a restricted but most typical geographic area was purposively selected. Within that a major administrative district was selected at random. There then followed consecutive random sampling of successively smaller administrative units, ending with minor units within which all persons aged 60 and over became potential study members. A sample size of 800 was aimed for in each country. The demographic characteristics of the sample obtained was weighted to reflect the known distribution in the sample area. The non-response rate, where reported, was low.

Item reliability and validity were examined. Reliability was assessed by determining the extent to which subjects, presented after a brief interval with the same items, gave the same responses as they had initially. Validity was examined by comparing the subjective responses to certain items, for example visual capacity, with the results of objective testing, and by determining whether certain theoretically expected relationships among selected items held.

The results indicate that reliance can be placed on the findings and that, with appropriate weighting, they represent the status of the populations represented.

WHO PAHO

WHO PAHO[3] uses a common core of questions and site-specific additions. Data are being gathering in 13 countries: Argentina, Barbados, Brazil, Chile, Colombia, Costa Rica, Cuba, El Salvador, Guyana, Honduras, Jamaica, Trinidad and Tobago, and Venezuela. This study is in various stages of completion. Data have been gathered for most countries and are now being cleaned prior to extensive analysis, but one country is still in the planning stage, while the final report has been completed for another. Sampling procedures have not yet been publicly reported but they vary from country to country.

OARS Multidimensional Functional Assessment Questionnaire

OARS[18] is a standardized questionnaire whose reliability and validity has been established for a North American population. It was among the first questionnaires to be developed with the specific aim of obtaining a global view of personal functioning. It permits assessment of functional status in each of five areas: activities of daily living, mental health, physical health, social resources, and economic resources. For each area the resulting information can be summarized, and across all five areas a profile of functional status can be obtained. In addition to gathering information on functional state, information is obtained on use of and need for each of 24 generically defined services, a mutually exclusive but broadly encompassing set. Linked to functional status, service use information indicates which services are needed, and permits assessment of service impact.

FACE (Fast Assessment of Community Elderly)

Under the auspices of the European office of the World Health Organization, FACE[19] is being developed as an internationally applicable screen to identify rapidly those elderly persons in urgent need of attention. Pretesting in five different languages (French, Hebrew, Romanian, Russian, and Spanish) is in progress; translation into Arabic is planned.[20] This screen takes a multidimensional functional view. It is intended to be of particular help to countries which do not currently maintain a sophisticated information base on their older residents. Designed to be useful at the individual level, data can be aggregated to yield population statistics.

Purpose and problems

The measures used in the first three studies mentioned above were designed for population-based assessment. OARS and FACE were intended to be clinically applicable at the individual level with data aggregatable to provide population statistics. While all are intended to provide a multidimensional evaluation, none can be used independently of a professional to indicate what services should be provided to a specific individual. The data they provide, however, is appropriate for analyses which will help to indicate the type and amount of service needed by the populations they assess.

Of these measures, reported information on validity (whether the assessment measures what it says it measures) and reliability (consistency of response under essentially the same conditions, and consistency of interpretation of the responses obtained) is available only for OARS and for some aspects of WHO Pacific. The items for WHO Europe, PAHO, and FACE were taken largely from standardized assessments. Establishment of the validity and reliability of the PAHO and FACE measures is in progress. WHO Europe has focused on careful training of interviewers to ensure uniform administration; further analysis of WHO Europe data may provide information on validity.

Cross-national studies have their own agenda of problems, among them being the cross-site relevance of items and assuring the equivalence of meaning of items across different languages and different cultures. Items reflecting common practice at a particular time in one country may not apply to another. For instance, while WHO Pacific includes the same housing categories and medical services as WHO Europe, it also necessarily enquires about types of housing and medical services extant in its region alone. WHO Europe, WHO Pacific, and FACE have used standard back-translation procedures. That is, they have translated their questionnaires from English into the desired foreign languages and back to English again and compared the two English versions. Some of the results, however, suggest that problems in meaning equivalence still exist. For instance, 27 per cent of the men aged 60 to 64 years in Leuven indicated that they had difficulty feeding themselves, as compared with roughly 3 per cent averaged over the other WHO Europe sites and less than 1 per cent in the US. This suggests that the intended meaning of the item—whether food can be transferred from plate or cup to mouth—is not the perceived meaning, and that perhaps here the perceived meaning of 'Can you feed yourself?' reflects the broader view of meeting the family's basic welfare.

In the case of self-feeding, sound baselines exist against which the response can be compared. Such baselines do not exist for all items. Consequently care must be taken in comparing cross-national differences, since they may reflect differences in the perceived meaning of the questions asked rather than in the status of those assessed. It should also be noted that even when it is clear that the questions asked are identical, differences may be obtained because of different response tendencies and expectations, and also differences in familiarity with surveys.

AREAS OF FUNCTIONAL ASSESSMENT

In assessing the condition of the elderly, there is general agreement that information is needed in seven areas, each of which is itself multi-dimensional: (1) activities of daily living, (2) mental health, (3) physical health, (4) social resources, (5) economic resources, (6) environmental matters, and (7) strain on the caregiver. These areas and their usual constituent topics will be briefly summarized (fuller reports are available elsewhere[21]) and their representation in the five reviewed assessments described. Specific details are given in Table 6.1.

Activities of daily living

Many of the problems from which the elderly suffer tend to be chronic rather than acute. Under such conditions, adequacy of treatment cannot be measured in terms of cure. Rather, there must be concern to amelio-rate the health conditions present, and to facilitate independence. While reflecting level of both mental and physical health functioning, assessment of activities of daily living (ADL) provides important information on ability to live independently. ADL-based information supplements in-formation on health status. It does not replace it.

ADL activities are most logically grouped into three types:[22] mobility, instrumental ADL, and physical ADL.

Mobility refers to the ability to get around: to go from here to there. It may encompass activities covering very short distances (e.g. moving from bed to chair) to long-distance travel. Instrumental ADL is concerned with domestic tasks (shopping, cooking, cleaning) and activities required to be

Table 6.1 Basic content of five international assessments

	WHO Europe	WHO Pacific	PAHO	OARS	FACE
Demographic:					
Country	+		+		+
Sex	+	+	+	+	+
Age	+	+	+	+	+
Race		+		+	+
Date of birth (month, day)	+	+	+	+	+
Year of birth	+	+	+	+	+
Address	+	+	+	+	+
Education	+	+	+	+	+
Religion		+			+
Marital status	+	+	+	+	+
Area of residence			+		
Literacy	+		+		+
Activities of daily living:					
Instrumental ADL					
use of telephone		+		+	
shop		+		+	+
prepare meals		+(W)	+	+	+
housework:					
—light	+			+	+
—heavy	+			+	
take medicine		+	+	+	+
personal finances		+	+	+	+

	1	2	3	4	5
Mobility					
travel		+	+	+	+
move outdoors/go out	+		+	+	+
move indoors			+		+
stairs	+				+
walk/traverse (m)	50			300	400
drive car					+
strength/stamina					
carry 5 kg for 100 m					–
Physical ADL					
feed self	+	+	+	+	+
dress	+	+	+	+	+
groom		+	+	+	
walk	+	+	+	+	+
in/out of bed	+	+	+	+	+
bath/shower	+	+	+	+	+
continence	+	+	+	+	+
use toilet	+			+	+
cut toenails					+
bite/chew hard food	+		+	+	+
Mental health:					
Cognitive status		+			
SPMSQ	+				
four items					+
abbreviated MMSE				+	
interviewer's name				+	
right ear, left hand				+K	
Personality change					

Table 6.1 (*cont.*)

	WHO Europe	WHO Pacific	PAHO	OARS	FACE
Memory, coping					
forgetfulness	+	+K			+
handling problems		+KI		+KI	
Symptoms: psychotic					
auditory hallucinations		+			
visual hallucinations		+			
subject of plots		+		+	
receives special messages		+			
Symptoms: other mental					
no. of items	17	5K		15	
Self-assessment, quality					
no. of items	12		2	5	
behaviour in interview	I	I		I	I
Physical health:					
Illnesses and conditions, symptoms					
illness, conditions	+	+	+	+	+
symptoms	+	+	+		+
impact on daily life	+	+K	+	+K	
Medications					
number or presence	+	+	+	+	
Level of activity	+			+	
Disability days	+	+		+	
Self-assessed health	+	+ K	+	+K	+
Communication					+
Health habits					
smoking	+	+			
drinking	+	+		+	

Social:					
Contact with others	-	+	+	+I	+
Help from family, friends	+	+KI	+	+KI	+
Social participation	+	+	+	+	+
Household composition	+	+	+	+	
Religious participation	+		+		+
Use of free time			+		
Economic:					
Income					
source, amount	+	+	+	+	
adequacy	+	+KI	+	+KI	
Home ownership	+	+	+	+	
Occupation					
past	+	+	+		
present	+	+	+		
Housing:					
No. of rooms	+I	+I		+I	
Facilities present	+I	+I			+
Elevation (storey)	—	+I			—
Type		+			—
Adequacy		+			+
Safety	+	+			
Service access	+	+	+		
Service use:					
Transportation			+	+	+
Social/recreational			+	+	
Employment				+	
Sheltered employment				+	
Educational (employment)				+	

Table 6.1 (*cont.*)

	WHO Europe	WHO Pacific	PAHO	OARS	FACE
Remedial training				+	+
Mental health	+			+	+
Psychotropic drugs	+			+	+
Personal care			+	+	
Nursing care	+			+	
Medical services	+	+	+	+	
Supportive devices, prostheses	+	+	+	+	
Physical therapy	+			+	
Continuous supervision				+	
Checking				+	
Relocation and placement				+	
Homemaker-household	+			+	
Meal preparation	+			+	
Administrative, legal, and protective				+	
Systematic multidimensional evaluation				+	

	WHO Europe	WHO Pacific	PAHO	OARS	FACE
Financial assistance	+	+		+	
Food, groceries		+		+	
Housing	+	+		+	
Co-ordination, information, and referral			+	+	
Open-ended item on service use			+		
Summary scores:					
Activities of daily living		+	+	+	
Mental health		+		+	
Physical health		+		+	
Social		+		+	
Economic		+		+	
Danger flags					+

WHO Europe = 11-country European study;[12] WHO Pacific = 4-country Western Pacific Study;[2] PAHO = 13-country collaborative Pan American Health Organization study;[3] OARS = OARS Multidimensional Functional Assessment Questionnaire;[28] FACE = Fast Assessment of Community Elderly.[19]
+ = item present.
K = information from knowledgeable other.
I = interviewer assessment.
W = women only.
SPMSQ = Short Portable Mental Status Questionnaire.[30]
MMSE = Mini-Mental State Examination.[29]
Some inclusions are open to interpretation.

a functioning member of society (e.g. handling personal finances). Physical ADL is concerned with basic self-care (e.g. bathing, eating, dressing, grooming). Of the three aspects of ADL, mobility is the least developed.

In well-standardized measures of ADL the activities considered are typically hierarchically ordered. For physical ADL the best established ordering is that of Katz and his colleagues (e.g. ref. 23). From most to least difficult (percentage of community resident US elderly aged 65+ experiencing the difficulty given in parentheses[24,25] the items are: bathing (9.8 per cent), dressing (6.2 per cent), using the toilet (4.3 per cent), transfer, continence, and eating (1.8 per cent). For instrumental ADL the ordering is: housework (23.8 per cent), shopping (11.3 per cent), preparing meals (7.1 per cent), and handling personal finances (5.1 per cent).

Table 6.1 shows that, with the exception of mobility (which is barely represented in OARS), the ADL information gathered is highly similar across the three surveys and two measures. Such similarity allows for cross-national comparison of findings. A comparison of data from six of the WHO Europe sites with OARS-based North American data[26] indicates that with some exceptions (probably due to translation difficulties) the same hierarchical ordering of physical ADL items holds across all settings and for both sexes. Marked decline in performance comes around age 75 to 79. However, where instrumental activities are concerned, decline starts roughly 5 years earlier, and the order of item difficulty varies as a function of sex at five of the six European sites. Only in the US and in Tampere, Finland are gender-based differences absent. This suggests strongly that physical ADL items reflect very basic functioning, while instrumental items are culturally influenced. Mobility was not examined in this comparison. Other data indicate that problems with mobility are among the first to appear and may vary as a function of race and sex.[27]

Mental health

Assessment of mental health of the elderly is typically concerned with some combination of the following four overlapping areas: adequacy of cognitive functioning, the presence of symptomatology indicative of psychiatric disorder or the establishment of a psychiatric diagnosis, personal assessment of emotional well-being, and indicators of the quality of mental health functioning.

All the assessments considered here, with the possible exception of the WHO PAHO study, include a measure of cognitive status. WHO Europe and FACE both include only a minimum set of the most sensitive items (i.e. age, date of birth, address) typically included in cognitive screens.[28]

However, the WHO Pacific study includes an abbreviated form of the Mini-Mental State Examination,[29] while OARS includes the 10-item Short Portable Mental Status Questionnaire.[30] Since level of education and cultural factors markedly influence performance on these cognitive measures, cross-site conclusions must be drawn with great caution.[2] In no case is sound cross-national validation reported.

Three of the five comparison assessments (WHO Europe, WHO Pacific, OARS) obtain information on psychiatric symptomatology. None specifically seeks psychiatric diagnosis although, with the availability of the Composite International Diagnostic Interview,[31] uniform cross-national psychiatric diagnosis now appears feasible.

Table 6.2 gives information on the percentage reporting mental health symptoms at six of the WHO Europe sites and in the WHO Pacific study. (Note that the symptoms enquired about and the time frame used were not identical in the two assessments.)

Within each country there is a tendency for reported symptomatology to increase with age. Thus the major groups likely to have problems can be identified. However, the percentage reporting the presence of mental health symptoms varies considerably from country to country. The reason for this is unclear. It may reflect problems of translation, cultural factors, true differences, or some combination of these and other factors. Because of this, these findings should not be used for cross-national comparison, (e.g. to indicate that those in one country are 'healthier' than those in another).

The third-mentioned indicator of mental health is personal assessment of emotional well-being. Three assessments gather varying amounts of information on this aspect (WHO Europe, PAHO, and OARS).

Finally, two assessments (WHO Pacific and OARS) provide information on quality of mental health functioning. In both cases information relies on reports from the interviewer and from an informant familiar with the subject regarding the subject's ability to handle problems. All except the PAHO study capitalize on the presence of the interviewer to provide additional information on directly observed behaviour.

Physical health

In order to assess current functional capacity attributable to physical health condition, some combination of the following topics is generally considered: self-assessment of health; presence of physical symptomatology; diagnosed illnesses and conditions, medications and use of medical services; level of activity; and measures of incapacity (e.g. bed days, disability days).

All the assessments under review include a self-appraisal of health.

Table 6.2 Percentage reporting mental health symptoms at selected sites in the WHO Europe and the WHO Pacific study, by sex and age category

	Men						Women					
	60–64	65–69	70–74	75–79	80–84	85–89	60–64	65–69	70–74	75–79	80–84	85–89
WHO Europe:[a]												
Leuven	48	52	64	64	50	52	76	65	76	67	69	70
Berlin (West)	52	49	47	56	63	62	69	71	66	73	70	77
Tampere	62	67	60	64	71	71	62	60	66	69	79	83
Florence	46	54	56	43	58	62	81	71	77	73	74	79
Kiev	55	55	61	64	52	67	72	81	83	79	85	87
Belgrade	45	54	54	54	57	60	61	67	59	68	74	68
WHO Pacific:[b]												
Fiji	67	68	70	81		76	66	80	70	85	86	
Rep. of Korea	44	54	50	56		58	57	54	62	66	70	
Malaysia	52	54	50	54		66	55	63	64	69	68	
Philippines	23	29	37	55		71	38	39	55	50	49	

[a] Percentage with marked occurrence of any of 17 psychosomatic signs or symptoms in previous 2 weeks (from Table 23, ref. 12).
[b] Highest percentage reporting any one of five current mental health symptoms (from Table 30, ref. 2).

Table 6.3 Percentage reporting that they feel healthy, by sex and age group. Selected sites from WHO Europe study and WHO Pacific study.

	Men						Women					
	60–64	65–69	70–74	75–79	80–84	85–89	60–64	65–69	70–74	75–79	80–84	85–89
WHO Europe:[a]												
Leuven	79	81	78	77	81	84	74	81	65	79	83	83
Berlin (West)	53	56	54	45	44	43	52	50	36	34	33	34
Tampere	30	21	32	41	30	35	34	25	35	29	23	39
Florence	87	76	69	82	83	80	63	62	68	66	61	64
Kiev	28	25	18	19	21	12	17	16	10	11	8	6
Belgrade	65	58	58	48	55	48	55	50	43	43	38	41
WHO Pacific:[b]												
Fiji	56	58	52	48		41	66	56	62	78	56	56
Rep. of Korea	59	54	52	48		54	46	46	48	34	50	50
Malaysia	79	78	76	68		55	72	72	68	78	54	54
Philippines	86	78	89	83		76	87	88	81	88	72	72

[a] Abstracted from Table 19.[12]
[b] Calculated from Figure 5.[2]

Selected data presented in Table 6.3 indicate that self-assessed health based on apparently identical questions differs markedly from country to country. However, since in the WHO Pacific countries the expected relationship was found between self-assessed health and ADL performance, and in most countries reports of good health are inversely related to age, some reliance can be placed on these data. Further investigation is needed in order to determine the cause of the substantial cross-national differences found. In particular, differences in translation, administration, and scoring need to be checked.

It is generally more appropriate to enquire about physical symptomatology than about diagnosis, since diagnosis implies access to skilled medical services, accurate identification of the disorder, and receipt and recall of that information. Regardless of whether symptoms or diagnosis are sought, it is advisable to determine the extent to which health problems interfere with daily life (i.e. to determine whether they have a functional impact).

All the assessments under review gather information on diagnosis and (except for OARS) on symptoms, and also ask about their impact on daily life. Enquiry is generally open ended, allowing freedom to report or describe any problems—and so demanding considerable coding skills. All the current assessments also gather information on medications used (where relevant enquiring about both Western and traditional types), and also ask about use of medical services, frequently in great detail. If coding is accurate cross-national comparison should be feasible.

In contrast to direct enquiry into specific health problems, only two assessments obtain information on physical activity level (WHO Europe and OARS) and three ask about disability days (WHO Europe, WHO Pacific, and OARS). This suggests that it will be possible to develop measures in which levels of poor health can be graded, but where levels of good physical health cannot be distinguished.

Social resources

The main focus in assessing the social resources of the elderly is typically on two issues: the extent and adequacy of contacts with family and friends, and the extent of availability of help in time of need.

All the assessments under review obtain information on the extent of contacts with others. All also seek full information on household composition. In addition some enquire about specific aspects of social participation, including religious observance, and also ask about the use of free time.

Information on the extent to which help is available from family and friends is included in all assessments except the WHO Europe survey.

Economic resources

At a minimum, concern focuses on determining whether income is adequate. Defining 'adequate' is not easy, however, for standards may vary considerably from place to place and country to country. Possibly Townsend's[32] definition of an adequate income as that level which permits unashamed participation in society is the most reasonable.

Enquiry may range from the very general (e.g. a rough estimate of total income), to detailed investigation of precise sources and amounts. The detail with which information is obtained should reflect the purposes for which that information is intended. If only a rough estimate of income adequacy is needed, it may be sufficient to know whether income is above or below a particular standard, such as the poverty level. However, if concern is that the elderly obtain all economic rights to which they are entitled, very detailed enquiry is necessary. In addition to asking about financial status, it is quite common to seek a subjective assessment of income adequacy, although the value of doing so is questionable.

To round out the picture of economic condition and provide a fuller view of socio-economic status information may be sought on assets, particularly home ownership, and on occupational history (main lifetime job, work history, and whether currently employed).

With the exception of FACE, which is interested only in whether income is above or below the poverty level, all the assessments considered here obtain information on source and amount of income (in varying levels of detail), self-assessed adequacy of income, home ownership, and present occupational status. Information on main lifetime occupation is obtained by WHO Europe, WHO Pacific, and OARS. Thus here also direct cross-national comparison seems quite feasible.

Environmental matters

The condition of the dwelling, its social milieu, and location with respect to needed services all influence personal independence. Each of the assessments surveyed gathers some information in this area. All enquire about housing. All but OARS seek information on the adequacy of the residence as a safe place to live and identify the facilities present. There is particular emphasis on such matters as overcrowding, fresh water (and whether or not it is piped in), temperature control, and the availability of toilet, bathing, and cooking facilities. Only two assessments (WHO Europe and FACE) are concerned with access to basic services (transportation, financial institutions, shops, post office, medical care), while only WHO Pacific asks about the safety of the milieu.

Strain on the caregiver

A larger number of severely disabled elderly live outside institutions than in them. Very often continued community residence is only feasible because of care given by the family—care which can place a severe strain. If such strain is not recognized and alleviated continued care may not be available for the older disabled person, and institutionalization may be unavoidable. FACE is the only assessment which recognizes that attention must be paid to the caregiver of an impaired person, but, as a screen, FACE tries only to identify which caregivers should have a full evaluation.

Information on services

While information on functional status is important, indicating the extent to which independent living is feasible and identifying areas where help is needed, without knowing what services are currently being received and the adequacy of those services any planning to facilitate continued independence, health, and well-being is hindered. To maximize the value of the multidimensional functional status data gathered, related information on service use and its adequacy is critical.

OARS, which was specifically designed to assess the impact of services on functional state, developed an extensive list of 24 generically defined services: a mutually exclusive, broadly encompassing set. For each service, information is sought on whether the service is currently being used, who provides it (whether family, friends, or agency), and whether it is needed. The other assessments were not specifically service oriented. Nevertheless, WHO PAHO enquires about six services and makes provision for more, while WHO Europe, WHO Pacific, and FACE ask about 10, five, and three basic services respectively. Information on the specific services included is given in Table 6.1. All ask about medically related services, with further enquiry focusing on personal care, housing, financial assistance, and social/recreational services. Thus they enquire about those services most salient to an older population.

Aggregating information

Multidimensional assessment of the type used here involves substantial amounts of detailed information. To increase reliability and to maximize usability the information should be aggregated. Within each area of enquiry, various approaches to aggregation are possible: summation of similar information (e.g. counting reported symptoms, noting number of medications taken), ordering information hierarchically as is done with ADL scales, and identifying the psychometric structure of area items in order to obtain unidimensional measures. With the latter it is possible to determine for which precise dimension a problem exists or a service has an effect. This may be particularly important in such areas as mental health and social resources, which are designed to measure a diversity of issues. Finally, although many areas are multidimensional, there may nevertheless be interest in obtaining an area summary score. This is done, for instance, in OARS. Using specific guidelines, subjects receive a single rating on a six-point scale (1 = excellent functioning; 6 = totally impaired) for each of the five areas included in that assessment. Plotted across the five areas these ratings provide a profile of functioning. The five area ratings can also be summed, resulting in values which can range from 5 to 30. In the US, scores above the midpoint of 17.5 indicate that institutionalization is appropriate, while scores below the midpoint suggest that continued community residence is feasible.

The final section of Table 6.1 indicates the availability of total area summaries for each of the assessments reviewed here. Area summaries are most extensively available for OARS and WHO Pacific (which was closely modelled on OARS) and are being developed for aspects of the PAHO data. FACE uses a dichotomy to identify elderly in urgent and emergent need of attention, but it could provide a broader range of ratings. While WHO Europe includes no area summaries, their development would seem to be feasible for all areas except mental health (which is barely covered), and could in each case range from excellent to totally deficient functioning.

COMPARATIVE OVERVIEW

Each of the assessments reviewed has unique characteristics designed to make it particularly relevant for the populations it was intended to assess. But there is also substantial agreement among them. All seek extensive information in the areas of ADL, physical health, social resources, and economic resources. Mental health is not adequately represented in all measures, but epidemiological determination of psychiatric diagnosis is only now becoming viable, while cultural and educational factors raise particular difficulties in assessing cognitive status. Housing-related issues, but not necessarily other environmental characteristics, are well covered in most of these assessments; however, concern for the condition of the caregiver is typically lacking. All seek some information regarding service use, typically focusing on the health and personal maintenance services of greatest import to the impaired and disabled elderly. Within each of the areas examined, there is overlap in the specific topics included; indeed, identical questions are sometimes asked.

Such basic comparability suggests that it should be possible to develop summary ratings for each area which are equivalent across assessments, and hence to develop functional profiles. Based on a larger number of items, they could be expected to be more reliable than the information provided by individual questions and so might reduce some of the variation currently found among countries. Further, profiles also provide the multidimensional view which these assessments seek, but which they do not obtain when they scrutinize their information item by item.

Considerable information is available world-wide on the health, economic, social, and environmental conditions of populations (although admittedly, some is of dubious value). Such information, however, is rarely available within a multidimensional framework. Rather, we have discrete pieces of information; we know what proportion of a particular population is able to carry out particular activities, the average length of stay in a hospital, how many live alone, and the number in poverty. We do not know whether those who have problems in one area have problems in other areas also. As a result we lack crucial information about populations. The validity and reliability of most of the assessments examined here remain to be established or confirmed (when used in settings other than that in which they were developed). Nevertheless, these multidimensional assessments, each of which has been used in different cultures, countries, and continents, show that multidimensional assessment is feasible, and suggest that there is sufficient similarity in the current assessments that, with further analysis and evaluation and given appropriately selected samples, valuable cross-national/cross-continental comparisons can be made, an international data base developed, and important findings gleaned in one area applied to another.

References

1. Alvarez Gutierrez, R. A. and Brown, M. J. (1983). Encuesta de las necesidades de los ancianos en Mexico. *Salud Publica de Mexico*, **25**, 21–75.
2. Andrews, G., Esterman, A. J., Braunack-Mayer, A. J., and Rungie, C. M. (1986). *Aging in the western Pacific*. Who Regional Office for the Western Pacific, Manila.
3. Pan American Health Organization (1985). *General plan of action for establishment of policies and programs for the elderly population in the Americas*. PAHO, Washington DC.
4. Chaney, E. M. (1984). *Women of the world, WID-1: Latin America and the Caribbean*. US Department of Commerce, Washington DC.
5. Newman, J. S. (1984). *Women of the world. WID-2: Sub-Saharan Africa*. US Department of Commerce, Washington DC.
6. Chamie, M. (1985). *Women of the world. WID-3: Near East and North Africa*. US Department of Commerce, Washington DC.

7. Shah, N. M. (1985). *Women of the world. WID-4: Asia and the Pacific.* US Department of Commerce, Washington DC.
8. United Nations (1987). *Development of statistics for monitoring the implementation of the World Program of Action concerning disabled persons, 1983–1992.* Report prepared by the Statistical Office, Department of International Economic and Social Affairs of the United Nations Secretariat (CSDHA/DDP/GME/4). Paper prepared for Global meeting of experts to review the implementation of the World Program of Action concerning disabled persons at the mid-point of the United Nations Decade of Disabled Persons. August 17–22, Stockholm, Sweden.
9. Gerontology, Culture and Development (1987). A global dialogue, 2, no. 1 International Association of Gerontology, New York.
10. Gurland, B. J., Copeland, J., Kuriansky, J. *et al.* (1983). *The mind and mood of aging: mental health problems of the community elderly in New York and London.* Haworth Press, New York.
11. Hawaii, State of (1983). *Statewide needs assessment of individuals age 60 and over.* State of Hawaii, Executive Office on Aging, Office of the Governor, Honolulu, HI.
12. Heikkinen, E., Waters, W. E., and Brzezinski, Z. J. (1983). *The elderly in eleven countries: a sociomedical survey.* Public Health in Europe, No. 21. WHO, Copenhagen.
13. ORS in collaboration with INSERM unit 164 (1986). *Conditions de vie et état de santé des personnes âgées en Ile-de-France.* Unit 164 INSERM, 44 Chemin de Ronde, 78110 Vesinet, France.
14. Palmore, E. (ed.) (1980). *International handbook an aging: contemporary developments and research.* Greenwood Press, Westport, CT.
15. Ramos, L. (1987). Growing old in Sao Paulo, Brazil: assessment of the health status and family support of the elderly living in the community in different socio-economic strata. Ph.D. thesis, University of London.
16. United Nations (1986). *Development of statistics of disabled persons: case studies.* ST/ESA/STAT/SER.Y/2 New York.
17. National Indian Council on Aging (1981). *American Indian elderly: a national profile.* National Indian Council on Aging, Albuquerque, NM.
18. Fillenbaum, G. G. (1988). *Multidimensional functional assessment of older adults: the Duke Older Americans Resources and Services Procedures.* Lawrence Erlbaum Associates Hillsdale, NJ.
19. WIIO Regional Office for Europe (1987). *Consultation on review of ADL measures in care of the elderly.* Meeting no. 2. ICP/HEE 215(S) 7985E.
20. Davies, M. (1987). Personal communication.
21. Fillenbaum, G. G. (1984). *The wellbeing of the elderly: approaches to multidimensional assessment.* Offset publication No. 84, WHO, Geneva.
22. Katz, S. (1983). Assessing self-maintenance: activities of daily living, mobility, and instrumental activities of daily living. Journal of the American Geriatrics Society, **31**, 721–7.
23. Katz, S. and Akpom, C. A. (1976). A measure of primary sociobiological functions. *International Journal of Health Services*, **6**, 493–507.
24. Dawson, D. and Hendershot, G. (1987). Aging in the eighties: functional limitations of individuals age 65 years and over. *NCHS Advancedata*, No. 133.

25. Fillenbaum, G. G. (1985). Screening the elderly: a brief instrumental ADL measure. *Journal of the American Geriatrics Society*, **33**, 698–706.
26. Fillenbaum, G. G. (1986). Development of a brief, internationally usable screening instrument. In *Aging: the universal human experience. Highlights of the 1985 International Congress of Gerontology*. (ed. Maddox, G. L. and E. W. Busse). Springer, New York pp 328–34.
27. Fillenbaum, G. G., Hughes, D. C., Blazer, D. G., and George, L. K. (1986). *Race and functional status*. MS. Center for the Study of Aging and Human Development, Duke University.
28. Fillenbaum, G. G. (1980). A comparison of two brief tests of organic brain impairment: the Mental Status Questionnaire and the Short Portable Mental Status Questionnaire. *Journal of the American Geriatrics Society*, **28**, 381–84.
29. Folstein, M. F., Folstein, S. E., and McHugh, P. R. (1975). Mini-mental state. A practical method for grading the cognitive state of patients for the clinician. *Journal of Psychiatric Research,* **12**, 189–98.
30. Pfeiffer, E. (1975). A Short Portable Mental Status Questionnaire for the assessment of organic brain deficit in elderly patients. *Journal of the American Geriatrics Society*, **10**, 433–41.
31. Robins, L. N., Wing, J., and Helzer, J. (1985). *The Composite International Diagnostic Interview (CIDI)*. Geneva, WHO.
32. Townsend, P. (1979). *Poverty in the United Kingdom: a survey of household resources and standards of living*. Penguin Books, Harmondsworth, England.

7

Aging, quantitative health status assessment and the effectiveness of medical care

ROBERT B. WALLACE and JAMES E. ROHRER

In industrialized nations, the elderly consume a substantial proportion of the available health services. Yet, to the extent that various individual treatments and programmatic innovations and interventions are quantitatively evaluated, most studies are conducted on young and middle-aged adults. Evaluation of health system performance and clinical therapy requires measurement of health status. Recent advances in health status measurement of the elderly have allowed higher quality health care intervention studies, though limitations remain. Here we briefly review these methods and limitations, consider their implications for assessing health status and care needs of the community-based elderly, and examine their application to evaluating the effectiveness of selected elderly medical care programmes.

ASSESSING HEALTH STATUS IN THE ELDERLY

Longevity and mortality

Longevity (survivorship) and mortality rates have been applied as indicators of biological aging phenomena, demographic predictors of future population size, and outcome measures of disease and health care interventions. Yet such applications must be carefully considered. Population longevity may not accurately reflect human biological aging and lifespan. Similarly, prediction of future population trends, critical for determining the medical and social burden, is subject to great uncertainty as the prediction interval increases.[1] For example, the recent increase in actuarial survivorship of older Americans was unexpected and has not occurred in all Western countries.[2] Particular attention must be paid to cohort analyses of mortality, as the survivorship of each successive birth cohort may not coincide with actuarial calculations derived from current data.

Death serves as the end point for many types of health care studies. It is easily measurable and accurate information is widely available. While the use of medical services is on average increased in the year before death,[3] there is substantial variation in that use and thus the fact of death *per se* does not predict very well the prior resource consumption for individuals, though it certainly has value in the aggregate. As a corollary, very little research has been done on the natural history of health status decline prior to death, which would be extremely useful in evaluating elderly health services.

Inferring prior health status or receipt of care by cause of death is also problematic, as there are substantial errors in designating such causes;[4] concordance with autopsy findings and clinical records is on balance modest. This dilemma is compounded in the elderly by the presence of multiple, interactive clinical conditions and less homeostatic capacity, making the concept of 'underlying cause' of death relatively less useful than in younger age groups. However, ancillary conditions and clinical information on the death record may be of value when used cautiously, and offer added insight into rates of comorbid events present at death and their impact on death rates from specific underlying causes.[5]

Morbidity

This refers to the signs, symptoms, syndromes, and described diseases that form the basic language of medical care. Signs, symptoms, and their regularly recurring clusters (syndromes) are probably underutilized as population phenomena in characterizing the health of the elderly, though surveys documenting their distributions and correlates are appearing.[6] They subsume by definition much of the discomfort and explain some of the dysfunction older persons experience, and are key predictors of health services use.[7] Major problems in application include their often subjective nature and unstandardized vocabulary, though advances in medical nomenclature are continuing. One example is a systematic approach to the taxonomy of pain.[8]

Using named diseases and conditions in studying the health of the elderly is clearly valuable. They form the basis of clinical thought and separate patients into groups with common prognosis and resource use, though individual variation here is great. This is highlighted by the controversy over the use of 'diagnosis-related groups' as a basis for paying American hospitals for care of the elderly.[9] While the basic concept of morbidity is not in question, the use of disease names to characterize the health of populations or medical care efficacy has several limitations. Among the important conceptual problems is that morbidity is a labelling process occurring in the clinical setting; morbidity rates are extremely sensitive to participation in formal medical care and the intensity of such care. Thus, variation in access to and receipt of care, and the possibly decreased intensity of care given to the oldest old, may bias population assessment of the elderly's health status using this technique. Also, since the language of morbidity is evolving and highly technical, and cognitive decline due to illness or aging may be present, elderly patients may not always be able to recall fully the diagnostic labels given them. This is a central issue in the interpretation of health surveys in the clinical or community setting based solely on self-report.

The problem of valid morbidity designation is not fully solved by medical record scrutiny since, like patient reporting, such records may have concurrent and historical inaccuracies. The varied course and gradual onset of many chronic conditions impede easy summary of their natural histories and time course. Also, the problems of conceptualizing and analysing multiple simultaneous diseases are great, and better methods are needed. Finally, and perhaps most critically, with some exceptions (e.g. diabetic coma, spastic paraparesis) the lexicon of morbidity reveals little of individual functional status or disease impact in the elderly.

Functional status

The gerontological and geriatric literature contains substantial work concerning the characterization of health by measuring individual function, and only selected major issues are considered here. Measures of function, like morbidity, predict physiological parameters,[10] utilization of health resources, and long-term health outcomes. As with other elements of health status, evaluating functional status measures requires consideration of their proposed application. Functional status is multidimensional and often divided into physical, mental, and social components, though these are highly interrelated. Ware suggested that role functioning and general well-being should also be included in any definition of health.[11] The World Health Organization characterizes the progressive functional consequences of disease in terms of impairment, disability, and handicap.[12] Functional status measures, either alone or with other health status indices, have been applied to complex constructs such as the quality of life and wellness. Even community levels of life satisfaction and happiness have been measured and evaluated.[13] Functional status may be reported, observed, or objectively tested, and thus measurement issues often dominate their consideration. Like morbidity, these measures generally concentrate on the dysfunctional end of the function spectrum to reflect the sickest individuals; the highly functional end of the spectrum is less well studied and discriminated. Functional status measures may assess and summarize overall health status or be constructed for specific diseases, demographic groups, or clinical situations.

The rationale for functional status measures and indices is clear. For both research and practical applications they summarize at both the organism and population levels the net impact of incompletely understood or characterized pathobiological processes and morbid conditions. They can be used to assess and determine individual and programmatic health care needs, match personal care needs to available resources, and measure individual and programmatic outcomes after health care interventions.[14] They can be used at the clinic or bedside to characterize more fully the patient status and guide the therapeutic process.[15] Finally, they can assist health professionals in learning to conceptualize and assess individual health status for clinical practice or quantitative study.[16] There are many useful reviews of function status measures and methods (e.g. see refs. 17, 18, 19).

However, functional status indices (FSIs) have various constraints, problems, and defects that may limit their use. Each implies a particular conceptualization of health and social utility, which may vary depending on goals and values. This and the difficulties in defining health may impede their development.[20] While FSIs characterize the physical, social, and emotional impact of disease, they do not contain some information residing in named conditions, such as prognosis. For example, inability to rise from a low chair has different implications when due to degenerative arthritis rather than septic arthritis or stroke. Thus, combining FSIs with disease nomenclature yields information not contained in either alone. In the same vein, the methodological evolution toward more global, combined indices and measures allows easier summarization and analysis, but with a loss of application and relevance to specific personal or public health problems. Furthermore, combining multiple measures into indices implies utility weighting that is not always overtly considered or justified.[21]

A major impediment to assessing functional status concerns the measurement process. Measures may be insensitive to changes in health status[21] or inadequately evaluated for such sensitivity; in one summary evaluation only 10 of 145 geriatric health status tests, rating forms, checklists, and questionnaires had such information.[22] As noted above, there is less developmental work at the healthy end of the function spectrum and thus less ability to measure change there. Even when describing major dysfunction, such as dependency in the Activities of Daily Living (ADL),[23] FSIs may not sufficiently characterize the breadth or adequacy of the remaining function. Measurement error is a particular problem in all assessments, and reliability issues are important in clinical and even in physiological measures.[24] In the frequent situation where self-report is the sole means of data collection, respondents may be unwilling or unable to provide accurate information, not only in emotionally sensitive areas but also in hypothetical, untested situations (e.g. can you walk half a mile?). Thus, functional status measures and indices must also be considered in terms of actual versus potential functional capacity. The elderly person's environment may not demand or encourage maximal function or behaviour, which would only be revealed by formal testing. FSIs may inadequately consider the time required to complete a given function or task—an important psychomotor dimension of biological aging. In population surveys, respondents also tend to offer socially desirable responses to various items, the normatively 'correct' response,[25] and this may vary by ethnic group and social status.[26] Single measurements may misclassify individuals and be unresponsive to health care interventions because they do not capture the natural fluctuation in functional status.

Perhaps the biggest problem for functional status measures is validation. This is a particular issue for many psycho-behavioural constructs, but may occur in other areas. In some cases, self-reported function has not been validated by actual functional testing. In many cases, no 'gold standard' for validation exists.[27] Since the various dimensions of functional status are correlated with one another,[28] regardless of the causal mechanism, there is added concern for validity. For example, if mental or cognitive function is impaired, self-report of other functional dimensions may be suspect. Clinical depression is associated with frequent reporting of somatic complaints, which may complicate assessment of physical illness. Our group has shown that objectively measured memory function is related to response reliability and amount of missing data in a large survey of the elderly.[29] None of this disputes the current utility of functional status measures, but it highlights the urgent need for additional research, particularly with respect to assessing medical interventions.

In order to assess better the functional capacity in contrast to current performance, formal functional and physiological testing seems desirable. This is a promising area that is difficult to summarize easily, and it too has limitations. Aside from general measurement issues, such testing may be time consuming, expensive, and a physical burden to frail persons. Basic physiological measures or abstract cognitive test scores may not be easily related to complex personal and social function. Further, testability in many areas requires sufficient motivation, comprehension, and stamina. In some instances, normative test standards for the elderly may not fully exist, particulary in the face of intercurrent illnesses, disability, and impairments. Physiological measures of function, as all others, should be sensitive to secular change as well as health care interventions.

AGING, FUNCTIONAL STATUS, AND DEVELOPING COUNTRIES

While in many less developed countries (LDCs) life expectancy often does not exceed 50 years and the proportion of elderly is low, they will sustain substantial growth in the next few decades, perhaps at a rate of

3–4 per cent per year. To the extent that LDCs progressively urbanize and industrialize, this will tend to dissolve the traditional family and social structure that supported older persons, as it has done world-wide. These trends will increase elderly dependency in a setting of meagre health care and social resources, little geriatric expertise, and frequently a low national priority for the elderly.

In LDCs, as a first step systematic, population-based surveys are needed which critically characterize morbidity and functional status, and such surveys are being performed. However, function status measures for LDCs may require special developmental efforts. Data may be inadequate to define normative levels of function and personal values concerning function loss. The distribution of illnesses leading to or sustaining dysfunction in tropical countries may be somewhat different from that in temperate climates, necessitating special approaches and taxonomy. Standardized interpretation of items across diverse cultures will require major validation efforts. Evaluating health services should emphasize self and family care and folk-healing practices as well as formally structured programmes.

THE HEALTH OF THE COMMUNITY-BASED ELDERLY

Periodic quantitative determination of the health status of elderly populations in any country is required for accurately assessing health care needs and the outcomes of health care programmes. This in turn requires population surveys using the health status measures noted above. In the United States of America, longevity of the elderly has recently been increasing,[30] but the trend in morbidity and functional status is less certain. Fries[31] made a series of predictions on the health status of older Americans in the next few years. He noted that with increasing preventive measures in the population, such as dietary modification and less cigarette smoking, the onset of many chronic illnesses would be postponed to older ages. Thus, morbidity and dysfunction rates, at least in the seventh and eighth decades, would decline and there would be a 'compression' of morbidity toward the last years of an increasing lifespan. Further, encouragement to maintain physical activity and other environmental modification among the elderly might also lead to a compression or retardation of senescence, the fundamental aging process, or at least an improvement in mean age-specific functional levels in the older population, as functional decrements due to disuse are slowed.

However, these optimistic predictions have been contested by others.[32] With increasing survivorship would come increasing numbers and proportions of elderly persons, where the incidence of many chronic illnesses is most common. Thus, the net medical care burden could still increase. Also, recent analyses of serial population surveys conducted by the US National Center for Health Statistics have suggested that disability levels and illnesses prevalence rates in the elderly have remained unchanged or have actually increased.[33, 34] While these surveys do not include the institutionalized population of the United States, a preliminary analysis combining both population and long-term care facility surveys showed that recent increases in chronic disease morbidity rates and related declines in function levels may be even more pronounced.[35]

However, most of the information in these national surveys is obtained from self-report, and all of the potential limitations of these data noted earlier pertain here and limit interpretation of these trends. Further, these periodic surveys may suffer from subtle secular changes in data collection methods as well as temporal variation in sampling errors, differential response bias, and a variety of non-sampling errors,[36] suggesting further caution. Particularly for the oldest old, the changing character and distribution of persons admitted to long-term care facilities, as noted above, may alter apparent secular health trends. Yet, if these trends ultimately prove correct, they raise important issues for primary and secondary prevention of disease as well as major research questions for demography, epidemiology, and human population biology. These secular trends in health status of the elderly, if real, also have major implications for the health and health care of future elderly cohorts.

THE EFFECTIVENESS OF HEALTH CARE FOR THE ELDERLY

Given the improving but still limited methods for characterizing the health status in the elderly, the possibly increasing medical care burden, and the limited availability of health care resources, it has become extremely important to assess the effectiveness of care for that age group. Clearly the best approach is to conduct appropriate randomized clinical trials. Older persons, and particularly the 'oldest old', may be systematically excluded from clinical research and trials, making it difficult to extend findings to this age group. However, for several reasons, such trials, with or without elderly subjects, are uncommon and one frequently resorts to observational evaluation methods. There follows a brief review of trials and studies of selected therapies and medical services for the elderly, to explore the extent to which modern health status measures have been applied to care effectiveness questions. One basic if indirect approach to the effectiveness question is to contrast effectiveness in the elderly with that of other age groups. Throughout the discussion an effort will be made to distinguish among the various ways health services have been shown to be effective: their impact on physical, mental and social health, quality of life, and on the health of family members.

Acute Medical and Surgical Services

Intensive care

Diagnosis, severity of illness, and age are the major determinants of both the use of and the outcomes of intensive care.[37] Patients most likely to have unfavourable outcomes are those with cardiac arrest, chronic respiratory or hepatic disease, or multisystem organ failure. Patients under 30 years of age have increased survival even after controlling for illness severity. This causes considerable policy concern since patients over 65 constitute a high percentage of intensive care unit (ICU) cases, and unnecessary use of ICUs is a waste of scarce health system resources. It may also have iatrogenic effects: nosocomial infection, overtreatment, unnecessary pain, stress, limitations on visitors, reduced autonomy, and a potentially crippling drain on family resources.

However, closer examination reveals some legitimacy to the treatment of elderly patients in ICUs. Since they are at greater risk of heart failure, the elderly may benefit more from ICU care for illnesses of moderate severity than younger patients. In a study of 2-year survival of general medical and surgical ICU patients, age was found to be the least important of the variables predicting death,[38] which included coma, cardiopulmonary resuscitation, renal failure, infection, shock, white blood count, and the number of intravascular lines. When cardiac surgery patients were eliminated from the sample, only cardiac arrest, age, renal failure, and shock were significant variables. When Parno et al.[38] examined the relationship between age and regaining ability to perform activities of daily living, no significant improvement ($P < 0.10$) occurred in patients younger than 40 years, but patients over 40 had significantly better function after hospitalization than before. Of patients 41–65 years of age, more than 71.4 per cent improved ($P < 0.05$); 84.6 per cent of patients over 65 improved ($P < 0.01$).

In a study of admissions to a medical intensive and coronary care unit, Campion et al.[39] found that patients over 75 years were less likely to survive than younger patients. However, 1-year survivial for those over 75 years was still 56 per cent (as compared with 67 per cent for patients of 65–74 years and 78 per cent for those aged 55–64). In this study older patients did not regain their pre-admission activity levels when returned to their pre-admission living situation. However, they did not incur greater hospital charges than their younger counterparts, even though they were more likely to receive major life-support interventions such as mechanical ventilation.

A reasonable conclusion to draw from the evidence available is that age alone is not a sufficient criterion for excluding patients from ICUs, because poor prognosis is the result of a variety of factors. Elderly injury patients with a young physiological age generally can be expected to benefit from intensive care. On the other hand, net benefits may be negative when the patient is terminal.

Hip replacement

This is an example of a medical procedure which clearly benefits elderly patients. Hip replacements are more successful for patients 50 to 60 than for patients under 30.[37] The failure rate after 5 years and operative mortality are low, and there are few early complications. The procedure improves mobility and reduces pain, and functional improvement is demonstrable.

Dialysis

Kidney dialysis serves as the classic example of a medical technology which may be withheld from the elderly on the grounds that benefits will not justify the cost. The 10-year survival rate for dialysis patients is less than 20 per cent.[37] Dialysis patients under 50 years of age experience a 10 per cent annual death rate; in those over 50 years it is 20 per cent. Patients with complicating diseases, a more common situation among the elderly (e.g. diabetes), have poorer prognoses. Great Britain has reported higher survival rates than the above, which is attributed to the exclusion from therapy of older patients and those with complicating conditions. For those who survive the quality of life varies, as is evidenced by the increased risk of suicide.[37]

This suggests that the elderly sustain relatively less benefit than younger dialysis patients, though the quality of life of survivors requires further characterization. Better results for patients between the ages of 44 and 72 have been reported recently and some critics of Great Britain's National Health Service argue that dialysis has more merit than other services which enjoy greater availability, such as intensive treatment of metastatic cancer.[37]

Coronary artery bypass surgery (CABS)

CABS is another medical technology which critics argue has been over-utilized. Once again, however, it appears that the available evidence does not support refusal of treatment solely on the basis of age. In a study of survival of patients over 65 years, Rahimtoola *et al.*[40] found 5-year and 10-year survival rates of 81 and 65 per cent respectively. Operative mortality was low (3 per cent) and did not increase with age. They concluded that the outcomes in elderly patients were similar to those seen in a young patient group and that the surgery should be 'offered to the older members of our society for the usual indications'. Again, more work is needed on functional status after the procedure.

Services and organizational innovations targeted at the elderly

Stroke rehabilitation units

Special stroke units are intended to reduce medical complications in stroke patients, optimize adaptation to neurological deficits, and reduce the need for long-term hospitalization. A prospective, controlled trial of a Swedish stroke unit confirmed that these objectives can be met.[41] While patients treated in the stroke unit had mortality rates similar to controls treated on general medical wards, the former were less likely to be rehospitalized in the year after admission and more likely to be independent in walking, personal hygiene, and dressing.

In a similar study in Great Britain, Stevens *et al.*[42] found that patients treated in a stroke unit received more rehabilitation therapy and better discharge planning. They had higher survival rates and were more likely to return to the community. The only difference between the two groups was the initial level of consciousness. A smaller percentage of the treatment group subjects were drowsy or comatose and more of them were graded in Rankin scale IV and V. However, this difference may be critical to the findings. Johnston and Keister[43] evaluated the effects of early rehabilitation on stroke patients and found that early admission was related to better outcomes. However, this effect disappeared when functional status on admission, prior improvement in acute care, and level of consciousness shortly after the stroke were controlled. They concluded that the timing and intensity of rehabilitation must be matched to the capacity and needs of patients in order to maximize benefits.

Other investigators have been even less supportive of rehabilitation services for stroke patients. In an Edinburgh study, Garraway *et al.*[44] reported that patients treated in a stroke unit received more health and social services after discharge than did controls but during follow-up did not experience better functional outcomes. In a synthesis of studies on stroke rehabilitation, Lind[45] noted that true experimental studies were less likely to find that rehabilitation is effective and concluded that functional gains experienced by stroke patients are primarily due to spontaneous recovery. However, rehabilitation may reduce dependence in activities of daily living for patients with moderate levels of impairment.

A reasonable conclusion to draw from this selection of studies is that special rehabilitation services for stroke patients have not yet demonstrated a general, substantial improvement in functional outcomes, and should be targeted to patients most likely to benefit from them. While older patients may have more frequent and severe strokes, age is not an important criterion for determining whether a patient will benefit from rehabilitation therapy. As with other therapies, severity of illness, prognosis, and the effectiveness of the therapy should be considered directly, and not inferred from the age of the patient. (See also Chapter 12).

Geriatric assessment units (GAU)

GAUs are designed to assess patient needs fully and implement a comprehensive plan of care, including rehabilitation services when appropriate. GAUs are now an established part of the health care system of several countries. Most of the reports on the effectiveness of GAUs have been positive; apparently comprehensive assessment and rehabilitation lead to improved patient outcomes.[46] Most studies used impact on functional status as a measure of programme effectiveness. However, others also report favourable effects on placement location, diagnostic accuracy, and drug prescribing. Thus, almost all of the evidence to date attests to the GAU's effectiveness. However, as Rubenstein *et al.*[46] note, most of the studies were observational and more experimental data are required before a final judgement can be made. (See also Chapter 25).

Home care

Perhaps 20–40 per cent of the institutionalized elderly in the United States could be cared for at home if home care services were available.[47] The assumption underlying this observation is that home care is better than institutional care. This assumption was tested by Mitchell in a Veterans Administration setting.[48] Mitchell compared the outcomes of home care patients with those of patients in hospital-based and community nursing homes. She hypothesized that worse outcomes would occur in institutionalized patients, as measured by the FSI of Fanshel and Bush.[49] Home care patients indeed suffered from slightly but significantly less physical disability after 3 months than did community nursing home or hospital-based nursing home patients. However, this was not true of patients with poor prognoses.

In general, it has been difficult to show that home care results in less physical disability than does nursing home care. Perhaps this is why Hughes *et al.*[47] compared home care patients to those not receiving either specialized home or nursing home care. They showed that, while self-rated mental health outcomes may have been better in the treatment group, self-reported ability to function independently in activities of daily living was worse.

Zimmer *et al.*[50] also compared home care patients with other patients not in nursing homes. Using the Sickness Impact Profile to measure health status, they found that home care patients did not have better outcomes. However, for patients who had been in the programme for at least 6 months, satisfaction with care was higher. Caregivers at home also showed higher satisfaction throughout the study period, and findings such as these led Haug[51] to argue that the benefits from home care were almost entirely psychological. However, easing the stress felt by patient and family constitutes a mental health benefit.

While there are isolated exceptions, home care has not generally been shown to be superior to institutional care overall. This may partly be a result of failing to conceptualize and measure the full range of potential benefits.

Case management

Case management systems are based on the premise that in order to take advantage of the benefits of noninstitutional services, clients must be matched to the services which offer the greatest benefit for their particular needs. Such programs are varied and pose complex problems in coordination.

One such programme was the Triage experiment in co-ordinated care for the elderly.[52] Triage operated with wide discretion to match the elderly with the services they required. Services provided ranged from medical devices, transportation, and friendly visits to home health care, outpatient care, and nursing home or hospital placement. Triage was thus a comprehensive and almost heroic effort to meet the needs of the elderly in Connecticut. It was not surprising that programme evaluations found costs to be higher for Triage clients than for potential clients randomized into usual community care. Triage clients had better mental function, but there was no effect on physical and social functioning. Thus, little was purchased for the additional cost.

Another case management system was evaluated in Georgia.[53] Once again, potential clients were randomly assigned to the usual community care or a treatment programme referred to as Alternative Health Services (AHS). AHS clients were offered either alternative living arrangements, adult day care, or home-delivered services. The programme evaluation revealed that AHS clients had higher survival rates and used fewer nursing home days.

The On Lok project, a consolidated model of long-term care implemented in the Chinatown/North Beach area of San Francisco, was found by Yordi and Waldeman[54] to have no effect no functional impairment in four categories: cognition, upper/lower extremities, continence, or ADLs. Home-making skills of study clients declined more than did those of the controls.

It is perhaps unfair to conclude that research evidence does not support the advantages of case management programmes. There are many ways to organize these programmes, and innovative approaches might be devised that improve health outcomes. Furthermore, newly emerging studies may be more encouraging. Nevertheless, at this point case management programmes have not yet shown substantial benefit for the elderly patient, even when many functional status measures are considered.

CONCLUSION

The determination of health status in the elderly is complex and, while improving, is still limited. It begins with the difficult problem of defining health, or at least determining its most important elements and dimensions. This determination requires considerable creativity and is clearly laden with cultural and ethical values. It requires contributions from many disciplines as well as from consumers of health services.

Once operational definitions of health are produced, their measurement becomes the critical issue in both the community and clinical setting and, as reviewed above, substantial measurement problems remain. Health measures must be easy to acquire, reproducible over long periods, and sensitive to important changes in health status and to medical therapies and programmes. New and sophisticated health status measures have been suggested and, while all have precautions and potential limitations, many have unfortunately not been fully applied. Once the criteria for appropriate health status measures are satisfied, they can then be used to assess population health status and health care effectiveness, and more critically contribute to the policy decisions which must be made in all health care systems. Based on our selected review of various health programmes for the elderly, the advent of critical, multidimensional health status measures may offer an unanticipated benefit: they may free us from dependence on chronological age as a prime indicator of the need for or utility of our health care activities.

ACKNOWLEDGEMENT

Supported in part by contract NO1 AG 2106 for the US National Institute on Aging.

References

1. Vaupel, J. W. and Gowan, A. E. (1986). Passage to Methuselah: some demographic consequences of continued progress against mortality. *American Journal of Public Health*, **76**, 430–33.

2. Demeny, P. (1984). A perspective on long term population growth. *Population Development Review*, **10**, 103–26.
3. National Center for Health Statistics (1984). *Use and costs of Medicare services in the last years of life, United States, 1983*. DHHS Publication No. (PHS) 84–1232. Public Health Service, Government Printing Office. Washington DC.
4. Gittelsohn, A. and Senning, J. (1979). Studies on the reliability of vital and health records: I. Comparison of cause of death and hospital record diagnoses. *American Journal of Public Health*, **69**, 680–8.
5. Manton, K. (1982). Changing concepts of morbidity and mortality in the elderly population. *Milbank Memorial Fund Quarterly*, **60**, 183–244.
6. Cornoni-Huntley, J., Brock, D. B., Ostfeld, A. M., Taylor, J. O., and Wallace, R. B. (ed.) Established populations for epidemiologic study of the elderly. *Resource Data Book*. US DHHS, NIH Publication No. 86–2443. National Institute on Aging.
7. Aday, L. and Anderson, R. (1981). Equity of access to medical care; a conceptual and empirical overview. *Medical Care*, **19**, (Suppl), 4–27.
8. Melzack, R. (1975). The McGill pain questionnaire: major properties and scoring methods. Pain, **1**, 277–99.
9. Jencks, S. F. and Dobson, A. (1987). Refining case-mix adjustments. The research evidence. *New England Journal of Medicine*, **317**, 679–86.
10. Kaplan, S. H. (1987). Patient reports of health status as predictors of physiologic health measures in chronic disease. *Journal of Chronic Diseases*, **40** (Suppl. 1), 27S–35S.
11. Ware, J. E. (1987). Standards for validating health measures: Definition and content. *Journal of Chronic Diseases*, **40**, 473–80.
12. World Health Organization (1980). *Classification of Impairments, Disabilities and Handicaps. A manual of classification relating to the consequences of disease*. WHO, Geneva.
13. Najman, J. and Levine, S. (1981). Evaluating the impact of medical care and technologies on the quality of life. *Social Science and Education*, **151**, 107–15.
14. Falcone, A. R. (1983). Comprehensive functional assessment as an administrative tool. *Journal of the American Geriatrics Society*, **31**, 642–50.
15. Palmer, R. H. (1987). Commentary: assessment of function in routine clinical practice. *Journal of Chronic Diseases*, **40** (Suppl. 1), 65S–69S.
16. Besdine, R. W. (1983). The educational utility of comprehensive functional assessment in the elderly. *Journal of the American Geriatrics Society*, **31**, 651–6.
17. Katz, S. (ed.) (1987). The Portugal Conference: measuring quality of life and functional status in clinical and epidemiologic research. *Journal of Chronic Diseases*, **40**, 459–650.
18. Lohr, K. N., Ware Jr, J. R. (ed.) (1987). Proceedings of the Advances in Health Assessment Conference. *Journal of Chronic Diseases*, **40** (Suppl. 1), 1S–191S.
19. Kane, R. A. and Kane, R. L. (1981). *Assessing the Elderly. A practical Guide to Measurement*. Lexington Books, Lexington, MA.
20. Goldsmith, S. B. The status of health status indicators. *Health Service Reports*, **87**, 213–18.
21. Jette, A. M. (1980). Health status indicators: their utility in chronic-disease

evaluation research. *Journal of Chronic Diseases*, **33**, 567–79.

22. Israel, L., Kozarevic, D., and Sartorius, N. (1984). *Source book of geriatric assessment, Vol. 1, Evaluations in gerontology*. S. Karger, New York.

23. Katz, S. *et al.* (1963). Studies of illness in the aged: the index of ADL: a standardized measure of biological and psychosocial function. *Journal of the American Medical Association*, **185**, 914–18.

24. Koran, L. M. (1975). The reliability of clinical methods, data and judgments. *New England Journal of Medicine*, **293**, 642–702.

25. Ross, C. E. and Mirowsky, J. (1983). The worst place and the best face. *Social Forces*, **62**, 529–36.

26. Ross, C. E. and Mirowsky, J. (1984). Socially-desirable responses and acquiescence in a cross-cultural survey of mental health. *Journal of Health and Social Behaviour*, **25**, 189–97.

27. Spitzer, W. O. (1987). State of science 1986: quality of life and functional status as target variables for research. *Journal of Chronic Diseases*, **40**, 465–71.

28. Wolinsky, F. D., Coe, R. M., Miller, D. K., and Prendergast, J. M. (1984). Measurement of the global and functional dimensions of health status in the elderly. *Journal of Gerontology*, **39**, 88–92.

29. Colsher, P. and Wallace, R. B. (1987). *Relationship of memory function and affect to response reliability in a survey of the elderly*. Presented at the annual meeting of the Society for Epidemiologic Research, Amherst, MA, 17 June.

30. Rice, D. P. and Feldman, J. J. (1983). Living longer in the United States: demographic changes and health needs of the elderly. *Milbank Memorial Fund Quarterly*, **61**, 362–91.

31. Fries, J. F. (1983). The compression of morbidity. *Milbank Memorial Fund Quarterly*, **61**, 397–419.

32. Schneider, E. L. and Brody, J. A. (1983). Aging, natural death, and compression of morbidity: another view. *New England Journal of Medicine 1983*, **309**, 854–6.

33. Verbrugge, L. (1984). Longer life but worsening health? Trends in health and mortality of middle-aged and older persons. *Milbank Memorial Fund Quarterly*, **62**, 475–519.

34. Colvez, A. and Blanchet, M. (1981). Disability trends in the United States population 1966–76: Analysis of reported cases. *American Journal of Public Health*, **71**, 464–71.

35. Tracy, K. B. (1987). *Personal care dependency in the older population: 1962–1984*. Presented at the annual meeting of the American Public Health Association, New Orleans, LA, 19 Oct.

36. Wilson, R. W. and Drury, T. F. (1984). Interpreting trends in illness and disability; Health statistics and health status. *Annual Review of Public Health*, **5**, 83–106.

37. Jennett, B. (1986). *High technology medicine: benefits and burdens*. Oxford University Press London.

38. Parno, J. R., Teres, D., Lemeshow, S. *et al.* (1984). Two-year outcome of adult intensive care patients. *Medical Care*, **22**, 167–76.

39. Campion, E. W., Mulley, A. G., Goldstein, R. L. *et al.* (1981). Medical intensive care for the elderly; study of current use, costs, and outcomes. *Journal of the American Medical Association*, **246**, 2052–6.

40. Rahimtoola, S. H., Grunkemeier, G. L., and Starr, A. (1986). Ten year survival after coronary artery bypass sugery for angina in patients aged 65 years and older. *Circulation*, **74**, 509–17.

41. Strand, T., Asplund, K., Eriksson, S. *et al.* (1985). A non-intensive stroke unit reduces functional disability and the need for long-term hospitalization. *Stroke*, **16**(1), 29–34.

42. Stevens, R. S., Ambler, N. R., and Warren, M. D. (1984). A randomized controlled trial of a stroke rehabilitation ward. *Age and Ageing*, **13**, 65–75.

43. Johnston, M. V. and Keister, M. (1984). Early rehabilitation for stroke patients: a new look. *Archives of Physical Medicine and Rehabilitation*, **65**, 437–41.

44. Garraway, W. M., Walton, M. S., Akhtar, A. J., and Prescott, R. J. (1981). The use of health and social services in the management of stroke in the community: results from a controlled trial. *Age and Ageing*, **10**, 95–104.

45. Lind, K. (1982). A synthesis of studies on stroke rehabilitation. *Journal of Chronic Diseases*, **35**, 133–149.

46. Rubenstein, L. Z., Rhee, L., and Kane, R. L. (1982). The role of geriatric assessment units in caring for the elderly: an analytic review. *Journal of Gerontology*, **37**, 513–21.

47. Hughes, S. L., Cordray, D. S., and Spiker, V. A. (1984). Evaluation of a long-term home care program. *Medical Care*, **22**, 460–75.

48. Mitchell, J. V. (1978). Patient outcomes in alternative long-term care settings. *Medical Care*, **16**, 439–52.

49. Fanshel, S. and Bush, J. W. A health status index and its application to health service outcomes. *Operations Research*, **18**, 1021–66.

50. Zimmer, J. G., Groth-Junker, A., and McCusker, J. (1985). A randomized controlled study of home health care teams. *American Journal of Public Health*, **75**, 134–41.

51. Haug, M. R. (1985). Home care for the ill elderly–who benefits? *American Journal of Public Health*, **75**, 127–8.

52. Hicks, B., Raisz, H., Segal, J., and Doherty, N. (1981). The triage experiment in coordinated care for the elderly. *American Journal of Public Health*, **71**, 991–1003.

53. Skellie, F. A., Mobley, G. M., and Coan, R. E. (1982). Cost-effectiveness of community-based long-term care: current findings from Georgia's alternative health services project. *American Journal of Public Health*, **72**, 353–8.

54. Yordi, C. L. and Waldeman, J. (1985). A consolidated model of long-term care: service utilization and cost impacts. *Gerontologist*, **25**, 389–97.

8

Social factors affecting the health of the elderly

M. S. GORE

The awareness that social factors affect the health of individuals has probably always been there. Every medical practitioner is generally aware that his poorer patients cannot afford the medicines he prescribes for them, that workers who work in coal mines or stone quarries tend to develop certain types of diseases special to their type of work, that the health of people living in slums and generally poor environments suffers because of unclean and insanitary conditions in which they live, and that epidemics often leave the poorer segments of a city or town more devastated than others. What is probably new is our awareness that not only physical and economic but even psychological and social factors affect the well-being of persons.

The term 'social' is used here in a comprehensive sense to include economic, social, and psychological factors. We will not address the specifically biological and biomedical aspects of the health of the elderly.

At the outset we must recognize that hard facts about the morbidity patterns among the elderly and their variation in relation to socio-economic factors are not easy to come by. This is particularly true in respect of developing countries. Vital statistics are more readily available and they will be used. These will be supplemented by data drawn from some sample studies, results of which are available in published form. At the national level, data from sample studies in India will be utilized because they are more readily available to the author.

ECONOMIC CONDITIONS

Income and health

At the level of inter-country or inter-regional comparison it is known that countries or regions with developed economies have higher life expectancy at birth than countries with lower levels of economic development. One would assume that longer life expectancy is also generally indicative of better health over a longer span of the extended life. At the intra-national level we rarely get data which would help examine the proposition that individuals with higher income levels have generally better levels of health. Yet, among non-biological factors the most important single factor that might affect the health of the elderly is the economic condition of the elderly individuals. Based on the proceedings of a meeting on socio-economic determinants and consequences of mortality in Mexico City, June 1979, Jacob B. Siegel points out that mortality rates are related to income levels independent of the national levels of economic development. One would expect morbidity to be so related as well, though data on establishing such a relationship are not available.[1] Siegel also suggests, on the basis of a study by M. Nag in India and H. Behm in Latin America, that lack of education is an important factor in explaining high mortality,[2] though it is always difficult to distinguish between the relative influence of education and economic status.

The level of income must influence a person's ability to meet his needs for nutritious diet, adequate housing, access to medical facilities, the availability of leisure, and chances of his withdrawal from the labour force.

Need for continued income

Data on the distribution of the elderly by income or economic status are not easily available but one indirect index is the proportion of the elderly who are still economically active and are engaged in manual occupations. The United Nations document *The world aging situation* observes, on the basis of an ILO report on problems of employment and occupation for older workers (A/CONF-113/15), that 'approximately 70% of the older workers in the developing countries are active in the sectors of agriculture, fishing, hunting and forestry, while the remaining 30% are employed in offices, businesses, service jobs, manual occupations, liberal professions or hold technical or administration posts'.[3] From the kind of occupations in which the majority of the elderly are engaged, it should be clear that most of them are in the labour market because they cannot afford to withdraw from it. They may be less productive in their work, but continuity in employment is probably necessary for their physical sustenance.

This situation is different from the developed world where the nature of the organized, urban economy generally tends to push the elderly out of the employment market and where policies are now in vogue to extend the age up to which a person can continue to be active beyond 60. The situation is different in two ways. The developed countries have a proportionately high dependency ratio of the aged to the working population. The withdrawal of the elderly from employment means an increase in the number and proportion of the population that has to be supported by the smaller economically active group. Besides, the developed countries also tend to have a variety of economic support systems—social security, social assistance, and welfare—which, while they provide for the care of the aged, also become a burden on the economy when the population as a whole begins to age in a demographic sense. In the developing countries where the percentage of the elderly in the total population is small, the total number of individuals involved is still large and these countries are characterized by a near absence of adequate systems of economic support for the aged. The poor, self-employed elderly who continue in the employment market do so at the cost of their health.

Continued involvement of the elderly in the work role may, however, have other positive social and psychological consequences for the individual within his family. Rural elderly individuals continue in the employment market in the developing world in response more to poverty than to their desire or ability to remain productively engaged. These rural elderly may also suffer from a poorer diet, poorer access to medical services, and continued physical exertion. Based on a study conducted in four areas in and around Delhi, Dr R. S. Srivastava observes 'The population of the *unhealthy* is the highest in the rural areas. Rural areas are greater victims of economic and family problems but almost immune from *disease*. It is the other way about with the rich urban people'.[4] Dr Srivastava distinguishes between 'poor health' and 'disease'. He seems to suggest that infirmity and physical disability—as distinguished from disease—are the main causes of what he considers poor health. He attributes the high incidence of physical disability to the lack of medical specialists (in the rural areas).

Access to health services

Data on the relative health status of the urban and rural elderly population are available for India as given in the National Sample Survey in its 28th round (1973), and summarized by H. B. Chanana and P. P. Talwar of the National Institute of Health and Family Welfare in their unpublished paper submitted to the XI World Congress of Sociology. According to this survey, summarized in Table 8.1, 28.8 per cent of the rural elderly and 25.8 per cent of urban elderly had experienced temporary ailments lasting on an average for a period of 9 days. As shown in Table 8.2, about 7.4 per cent of the rural elderly and 7.9 per cent of the urban elderly suffered from some type of chronic complaint. The prevalence rate of ailments and chronic disabilities among males is generally higher than among females.

Not only is the prevalence of temporary ailments higher in the rural areas; health services are less easily available than in the urban areas. In

Table 8.1 Prevalent rate of temporary ailments among the elderly by place of residence and sex: All-India

Place of residence	Male	Female	Both
Rural	31.32	25.96	28.78
Urban	26.05	25.06	25.57

Data taken from an unpublished paper by H. B. Chanana and P. P. Talwar of the National Institute of Health and Family Welfare, entitled Implications of demographic goals in 2000 AD for aging population of India, submitted to XI World Congress of Sociology, New Delhi, 1986.

the LDCs about two-thirds of all elderly people live in rural areas. In 1980, the rural-dwelling elders of the less developed regions were 145.24 million out of a total of 375.76 million of the world's elderly (i.e. 38 percent).[5]

In the urban areas the poorest segment of the population is unable to benefit fully from the free services offered by the general hospitals run by the municipality or the government.[6] The time involved in commuting and in waiting to be seen by a doctor and collecting the medicines dispensed means the loss of about half a day's daily wage or income. In India those who are self-employed as hawkers and vendors or employed in the unorganized small workshop sector have no wage or earning protection during periods of illness. Workers in the organized sector, however, are protected and they have also the option of going to a private doctor who is compensated directly by the Employees State Insurance Programme.

Thus residence (rural or urban), type of employment, and level of income all tend to establish a hierarchy in the access of individuals to available health services in developing countries. Based on the NSS tenth round data, P. C. Mahalanobis pointed out in 1958 that the proportional expenditure on medicines and medical services continued to increase with an increase in the expenditure class and observed that 'medical care

Table 8.2 Prevalence rate of chronic disease among the elderly by place of residence and sex All-India

Place of residence	Male	Female	Both
Rural	9.25	5.34	7.40
Urban	9.45	6.39	7.89

Data taken from the same paper as mentioned above. Original source mentioned—but not checked by present author—*National Sample Survey*—28th Round, 1973.

would seem to be the highest luxury of India which only the richer people could afford'.[7]

Nutritional status

Studies of diets by the National Sample Survey have also shown that, as the level of total expenditure rises, the level of the total intake of calories, protein, and fat also rises. Table 8.3 displays data adopted from a survey of 8626 villages covering a population of 72 270 households.[8]

The data in the table relate to *persons of all ages* and do not help to identify the consumption levels of the elderly population. But one assumes that the relationship between expenditure level and nutritional status given in the table holds true for the elderly. If we regard an intake of less than 2000 kilocalories (8400 kJ) per day as unsatisfactory for a rural sample, then 43 per cent of the households are in this category and we would expect approximately the same proportion of the elderly to be in that group.

The United Nations' *Periodical on aging*[9] reported that 7 out of 19 governments from the developed regions had a policy on nutrition for the poor and underprivileged elderly in their countries. In the developing regions, only 8 out of 47 claimed to have such a policy.

Table 8.3 Nutritional Components of daily diet as related to level of expenditure. All Ages

Range of monthly average per capita expenditure in rupees	Percentage estimate of number of persons covered	Per capita per diem intake of		
		Energy (kcal)	Protein (Grams)	Fat (Grams)
I 10.38 to 22.41	17.90	776	21.8 to 44.9	5.6 to 12.2
II 25.91 to 30.86	25.67	1747 to 1944	49.7 to 54.5	13.6 to 16.4
III 38.14 to 63.20	47.19	2210 to 2929	61.1 to 80.8	21.8 to 36.4
IV 85.26 to 342.81	9.24	3439 to 6991	93.6 to 177.8	50.1 to 138.9
All classes 43.91	100.00	2266	62.7	24.5

Data derived and abridged from. Government of India, (1982). *National Sample Survey Organization*. Sarvekshana, January–April. p. 5–5.

Housing

Housing is another area where income differentials make for a considerable difference in the quality of construction of the dwelling and the environment in which households and, therefore, the elderly live. This is particularly the case in the urban areas. In the metropolitan cities of the developing regions of the world over 60 to 70 per cent of all households live in single room tenements and shanty towns. The water supply, sanitation, and drainage facilities in these areas are notoriously bad. Noise, air pollution, and overcrowding are common. Even in the rural areas people live in similar conditions so far as inadequate and unprotected water supply, insanitary conditions, and absence of drainage are concerned.

The housing and environment conditions of the elderly in the developed countries are definitely better in comparison with those in the developing countries. Yet, the UN document *The world aging situation* observes that the level of comfort in dwellings inhabited by the elderly tends to be below the average for the general population.[10] In the United Kingdom, the English Home Conditions Survey (1976) found that, among households headed by persons aged 65 and over, 37 per cent were in need of rehabilitation and 44 per cent lacked amenities. Generally, the elderly live in older housing in several countries. The older houses often do not have a bath and, in the rural areas, may also lack the amenities of hot water and central heating.

The elderly who live in cities in the developing countries face special problems. Life in the city demands a greater degree of physical mobility. This is made difficult for the elderly not only because of their own disabilities, but also because of the absence of supportive facilities. The elderly cannot expect to get on and off crowded buses, trams, or suburban trains without running the risk of accidents. In the developing countries, residential buildings and often public buildings, railway stations, and airports are not provided with elevators. To have to climb up or down two to three flights of steps poses a barrier to mobility. All these factors increase dependence on others, reduce mobility, and affect the quality of life of the elderly persons. Physical and social communication gets increasingly limited to the household and to members of the immediate family. Limited space and social mores that separate age groups as well as the two sexes make the elderly feel stifled and isolated.

A study of the elderly done in Bombay in the 1960s showed that 189 out of a sample of 600 middle class individuals who had recently retired from service experienced physical difficulties in walking, climbing stairs, boarding trains or buses, etc.[11]

The *Periodical on aging*[12] reports that 3 out of 17 of the responding governments in the developed countries indicated that housing of the elderly in their countries was unsatisfactory. In the developing countries, 13 out of 44 indicated the housing conditions to be unsatisfactory and an additional 19 governments expressed no view! One assumes that these latter did not consider the housing of the elderly to be satisfactory in their countries. This is not surprising because most households in the developing world, whether in the rural or urban area, live in substandard structures which are often not adequate to provide security or protection against the elements.

Housing and environment are still physical aspects of the context in which human beings live, though these aspects are also influenced by economic considerations of what the occupants can afford and what they consider desirable or adequate. More specifically social are the living arrangements, the household composition, and the network of relationships between those who occupy the houses.

LIVING ARRANGEMENTS

Household composition

At a very general level it can be said that in both the developing and developed countries the overwhelming majority of the elderly live in families; however, an appreciable proportion of elderly males and females live in single person households in the developed world. A small but growing percentage of the very elderly live in institutions because they need special care. The UN document *The world aging situation* reports that between 1 and 10 per cent of the elderly live in institutions in different countries of the developed world.[13] Since women generally live longer than men in the developed countries, the percentage of women living singly or in institutions of special care is also consistently larger than men.

One important implication of this situation is that if elderly individuals living alone have to meet their health and other needs adequately, there is a need for a whole set of domiciliary and community services to be created by the community. Many of these services are public supported, though sometimes, as in England, they may be operated by voluntary agencies. Home-maker services, visiting nurses, meals-on-wheels, and community welfare centres for the elderly are all efforts to meet the physical, social, and health needs of elderly individuals living on their own.

Despite these services, the risk of accidents and of acute health conditions going unnoticed is necessarily higher in the case of those who live alone. Even within institutions, because of the degree of individuation fostered as a value, many elderly individuals prefer to maintain their privacy by occupying single rooms. This requires establishing a system of periodic personal checks and alarm devices to ensure that no emergency goes unattended in respect of a very elderly person living by herself.

In the developing countries the elderly generally live within the family context, usually with their children or other relatives. In the rural areas there are situations where the elderly may be left on their own because the children have migrated to the city. This phenomenon is noticed particularly in the villages of Konkan—the coastal strip immediately south of Bombay. Here village after village have at times only aged males and females left behind while the young males and their spouses have moved to Bombay in search of livelihood. The economy of these villages depends on money order remittances from the younger members living in Bombay. But usually neighbourhood and village community contacts facilitate their living by themselves. Also, life in the villages is less physically demanding on the elderly than life in the cities.

A study of 600 retired persons, consisting of former gazetted and non-gazetted officers of the government and of school teachers, by Desai and Naik[14] and another study by Kirpal Singh Soodan[15] covering 390 households in the city of Lucknow are used here to give an idea of the living arrangements of the elderly in urban India. The chronological definition for the elderly used by Desai and Naik was the age of 58+; while Soodan used 55+.

Table 8.4 Percentage distribution of the elderly by type of household

	Desai & Naik	Soodan
Living alone	3.01	7.18
With spouse	8.3	10.52
Living with unmarried son/members	61.0 ⎫	73.34
Living with married sons/daughters	30.0 ⎭	
Living with married daughter	Category not used	4.61
Living with other relative	—	4.35
Total (*N*)	100 (600)	100 (390)

Data drawn from two studies—one in Bombay and the other in Lucknow. The two authors do not follow exactly the same categories for deciding households. Desai and Naik only speak of unmarried and married 'members'; Soodan uses the word 'children'. Desai and Naik have no data on female elders; Soodan has. Bibliographic details given at the end of the paper.

Table 8.4 gives the living arrangements of the two urban samples. The Bombay sample was limited to the middle class of retirees; the Lucknow study covered a cross-section of city population and included 70 per cent from the low-income group in its sample. The modal living arrangement for the elderly in both studies is to live with their children—married or unmarried. The percentage of those living alone is 3.01 in Bombay and 7.18 in Lucknow. Those living with the spouse are 8.3 and 10.52 respectively. In the Lucknow sample, 18 respondents live with their married daughters—an uncommon arrangement in India.

Familial relationship

Life within the family also poses many problems. These are problems of social relationship arising out of changing values, limited space, and the state of economic dependence of the elderly. These social problems may affect physical health but more commonly they express themselves in strained relations, mental tensions, ennui, and a loss of interest in life. The intensity of these problems varies from household to household, but generally we would expect them to be greater in urban households than in rural ones and greater in situations of economic dependence of the elderly than those where they have resources to meet their needs; there is also likely to be a sex difference in the type of problems the elderly face. We will discuss some of these briefly.

Although the traditional family values of respect for the elders and acceptance of responsibility for them still persist in developing countries, the changing social and economic context is raising new problems. In the traditional land-owning family in the village, the elderly male had a sustained feeling of being a sharer in the property of the family and, therefore, of economic self-sufficiency. In the urban economy the elder individual often loses his economic role and status altogether on his ceasing to be active in the economy. To the extent that he has savings—as in the middle class—he may still retain a sense of worth. But the sudden withdrawal from the daily activity of his occupation poses social problems. If he has no savings and is really dependent upon his son or other relatives the adjustment is more difficult, because he may have to ask for money to meet even his small day-to day-needs. If the son is economically well off the financial problem is minimized, but then the problem of differing lifestyles between a father of humble origin and a son who has achieved urban sophistication and, more particularly, the daughter-in-law who does not have the same emotional tie with the old man may become an irritant.

The elderly woman has an advantage in that she experiences no sudden discontinuity in her familial role or her daily activities, but she is likely to have more problems than her husband in making adjustments at home. The male can keep out of minor frictions at home by keeping to himself or spending part of his time out of the house. The woman may find that her desire to continue to perform her usual housewife role interferes or clashes with the preferred lifestyles of her daughter-in-law. She does not have the option of withdrawal from household responsibilities because that can also give rise to misunderstandings. In the Western countries this has at times led to an elderly widow living in the house of her daughter rather than her daughter-in-law. The American syndicated comic strip Hubert by Dick Wingert (King Features Syndicate, Inc.), would have no relevance or appeal except in a cultural context where a man not uncommonly has to cope with his wife's mother as a permanent member of his household.

On the whole, however, life within the family still helps the vast majority of the elderly to cope with their livelihood as well as 'care' needs, to the extent that the family resources will permit. The adjustment of the elderly to the state of dependence on their children is somewhat facilitated in India by the value that as age advances an individual must gradually withdraw from the concerns of daily life and engage himself in religious, spiritual pursuits or assume a role of community responsibility.

As already mentioned, data on social aspects of the life of the elderly are not available on a national level, nor are data available on conditions of mental stress and tensions. For these, we have to depend on small sample studies conducted by individual scholars. The studies reported upon below were done in India.

Perception of who is the head of the household

Dasai and Naik give a breakdown of the respondent's perception of who is the head of the household in which he lives (Table 8.5). Comparable data are not available for the Soodan study.

This view about who is the head of the household was generally corroborated by the younger generation as well. The fact that 93 per cent of the retirees consider themselves to be head of their households suggests three possibilities:

(1) the house they occupy is owned or was rented by the retiree;

(2) the middle class retiree is still economically not a total dependent;

(3) irrespective of the above factors, the tradition that the eldest male is considered the head of household still prevails in most households.

This self-perception as being the head of the household may be psychologically satisfactory, especially if it is supported by a measure of economic self-reliance.

Table 8.5 Responses of the elderly retirees about who is the head of the household

Head of the household	Percentage
Self	93.1
Spouse	0.4
Siblings	1.4
Sons	3.6
Others	1.5
Total	100.0 (*N* = 600)

Data from the Bombay study by K. G. Desai and R. D. Naik.

On this point, Naik[16] gives further information in a separate paper based on the same data. The retirees reported different modes of maintaining their families, as shown in Table 8.6. Approximately 48 per cent of the retirees seemed to maintain the households on their own income or savings.

Thus, it would seem that in the middle class households represented by the retiree, the elderly individuals self-perception of being the head of the household is largely supported by a high degree of financial independence. Naik gives further data to say that in 44 per cent (of 68 cases) where children contribute to family maintenance, their contribution is less than half of the total household expenses; in the other 56 per cent of the cases the contribution is larger than half the total expenditure.

This pattern of autonomy and dependence is not characteristic of the lower-income household, as argued by Soodan.[17] Based on a comparison of data from different studies he argues: 'maintenance of income in old age is one of the major unsolved problems of the aged in India'. He says on the basis of his own study in Lucknow that 50 per cent of the aged had no income of their own, about 30 per cent had an income of less than Rs. 100/- per month, and that a majority of the aged live in households where the average household size is five and the total monthly income is less than Rs. 200/- per month. He points out that even the Delhi study by S. N. Ranade had shown that more than half of the elderly interviewed had no income of their own.[18]

Desai and Naik give data on the types of financial liabilities their retirees had still to meet. About 68 per cent of the sample had still to meet their liabilities for the education of their children, marriages of their daughters, or had to repay the money they had borrowed from the bank for home construction and other such purposes.

Table 8.6 Distribution of retirees by different modes of family maintenance

Modes	Percentage	
Own income	33.7 ⎫	Indicate maximum
By withdrawing from saving	14.2 ⎬	autonomy
Through assistance from children	26.5 ⎫	
Through assistance from other relative	4.5 ⎬	Partial dependence
Through assistance and own income	5.3 ⎭	
By joint pooling of all income	15.8	Traditional pattern
Total	100.0	

Table from R. D. Naik (1981). An analysis of a change in family economy, *Indian Journal of Social Work* (January). Order of data presentation is slightly altered.

ADJUSTING TO THE NEW STATUS

Apart from economic self-reliance, living with adult children and other relatives raises other questions of adjustment. Desai and Naik say that while 56 per cent of the elderly in their sample experienced no difficulty in getting along with the younger generation, 44 per cent admitted to such problems and, of these, 17 per cent had not been able to cope with the problem. When asked whether they would like to live independently, about 66 per cent of the total sample preferred not to live on their own, but 20 per cent said they would like to live by themselves if it were possible. In the Indian context this latter percentage is significantly high.

Desai and Naik asked certain important questions about relationship of the elderly with other members of the family before and after retirement. While the general trend is that the position of the retiree head is largely the same as before, there are some changes. Whereas 81 per cent of the respondents said that they made all the major decisions in the family while they were still economically active, this dropped to 69 per cent after retirement.

Fifty-four per cent of the respondents indicated that members of the family always or often agreed with them in the decisions they made. Of the rest, 33 per cent said they agreed 'sometimes'; about 10 per cent gave no answer to the question.

Sixty-eight per cent said they experienced no change in the behaviour of others toward them after retirement, but the rest thought either their sons, spouse, or some others had changed in their attitude to them.

In all three cases the change which would adversely affect the ego of the retiree is limited, but again in the Indian context the fact that 20 to 30 per cent of the elderly feel that they have experienced such a change is indicative of potential strain in relationship.

When it was directly asked of the elderly respondents whether they agreed with the view that it is difficult to get on with the younger generation, only 52 per cent said they experienced no such difficulty; of the rest, some said that it was difficult (15.5 per cent) and others that while it was difficult one could adjust to it (27 per cent) or gave no reply.

In a review of studies of the elderly entitled *Social situation of the aged*, authored jointly by Desai and Rekha Bhalla,[19] a study of the rural elderly is cited which suggests that the elderly do not enjoy a uniformly high status and that their status varies with age, physical health, material condition, and interpersonal relationships. The older and more physically helpless a person is, the less economically independent, or the less capable of adjusting to new roles, the lower is the likelihood of his enjoying high status. In fact, they say that only a minority of men continued to enjoy prestige, authority, and security beyond the age of 60. Unlike the study by Desai and Naik, a study of village elders in village Burail in Punjab by J. Singh[20] showed that 66 per cent of the elderly were not regarded as heads of the family and were rarely consulted by family members. Based on a comparison of the results of three village studies, Desai and Bhalla conclude that the aged occupy a precarious position in rural households, unless their economic status and education enables them to assume village leadership roles.

Desai and Bhalla refer to still another study of the rural elderly, that of Gurusheran Kaur,[21] in which the author found that 50 per cent of her sample lived alone and not with any relative; half this number were widows and had their sons living in the same village!

The picture that emerges from these studies of the elderly is very different from the stereotype of the family support role of the extended family. As suggested earlier, while reviewing the study by Desai and Naik, the status of the elderly in the family seems to greatly depend upon the individual's economic status. A majority of the elderly do not enjoy any effective authority in the family though they may be 'formal' heads of households. Most dissatisfactions arise over minor matters. The elderly individual gives the impression of resenting his changed role and his loss of status because he may have grown up at a time when in retrospect the elderly seemed to be respected.

NEED TO BE USEFUL

The loss of familial status, increasing economic dependence, and, sometimes, one's inability to meet familial obligations such as educating the younger sons, the inability to pay a sufficient dowry for the marriage of a daughter, or decreasing physical abilities—all these give rise to tensions and aggravate problems of interpersonal relationships as well as physical health. If the elderly have to migrate to the city to live with their children they lose the companionship of their friends from 'home' and have to live in cramped space and get used to the problems of living in urban neighbourhoods.

Data from all the studies show that the elderly seek to reduce their sense of uselessness as well as lonesomeness by trying to take some responsibility for household chores, by developing religious interest, or by gathering in small groups in public parks.

A study done by Saraswati Mishra[22] showed that the elderly who participate in activities of voluntary associations or who can keep themselves living in some meaningful activity tend to be better adjusted than those who remain inactive. The study also showed that the more the conflicts at home, the lower is the adjustment to one's old age.

Many of the physical problems associated with age such as aches and pains, vascular problems, and even metabolic disorders are sensitive to psychological conditions and can become aggravated by familial worries. The ability to withstand tension is lower and so is the ability to recover from illness. Unhappy social relationships may intensify health problems and unhealthy, dependent elders who require care can be a source of irritation to others. The elders may tend to keep their health worries to themselves in order not to appear to be a nuisance.

MARITAL STATUS AND HEALTH

Jacob S. Siegel in the paper referred to above mentions marital status as an important social factor that seems to be related to mortality.[23] In the developed countries it has been noticed that married men and women have lower death rates and divorced men and women have higher death rates. The situation in the developing countries is not known. But Siegel argues that 'health is related to marital status both as "determinant" and "consequence"; one's marital status may influence one's health'.

If this is true then women who live longer than men are more likely to be widowed and, therefore, more exposed to health problems than men, partly as a result of their more advanced age and partly as a result of their marital status as widows. In India there is the additional factor that an elderly widowed woman enjoys less status than one whose husband is still alive.

In the context of changing values it might be helpful for those individuals who would like to live on their own or only with their spouses to be enabled to do so by creating an infrastructure of community services. But the developing countries lack the resources to support such services. As it happens the old-age dependency ratios are currently low, but in the next few decades the situation may begin to alter; if this shift in population structure occurs without an appreciable expansion and growth of the economies of these countries, we may find increased longevity will be a situation to be dreaded rather than looked forward to by the elders.

In the meanwhile, the ability of the elderly to continue to remain in the employment market has the value of reducing their burden on the family and also keeping their mind off their individual and familial problems. This ability of the elderly to remain in the employment market, however marginally, depends upon a person's state of health. This factor is critical in the area of manual work in agriculture or handicraft in rural areas, as it also is in the unorganized sector in the urban area. On the other hand, the elderly person's sense of health is itself dependent on his being meaningfully occupied.

In the organized market, as well as the white collar market, an individual's ability to continue in the labour market is severely limited by clear-cut rules governing superannuation. One would expect that this factor would adversely affect their health, though the fact of their having belonged to the 'salaried' class is more likely to ensure a greater degree of economic independence compared with that of the manual worker. In the sample of retired persons studied by Desai and Naik it was noticed that, while a small number of the respondents had complained of health problems prior to their retirement, a much larger number became aware of their ailment and impairment only after their retirement. Some of this increase would be considered natural since aging involves a progression of degenerative diseases, but the fact of being without any occupation must itself contribute to the awareness of this degenerative condition.

OVERVIEW

The data presented in the paper are too meagre to permit the drawing of any conclusions. But some general observations may be permissible.

While there are no data showing direct relationship between income level and health of elderly individuals, one would assume that the nutritional and clinical care needs of the elderly are better met with adequate income than without it. If so, the poor countries and the poorer segments of the elderly population within each country would experience greater problems of health and well-being.

While income is an important determinant of access of elderly individuals to health services in less developed countries, rural urban residence is another important factor that would influence such access to services. In India, we would also expect a male–female differential to exist in access to services.

In poorer countries and in less developed economies there are no state support systems for maintaining the incomes of the elderly. But in these countries, it is also possible for the elder individuals to continue in employment beyond the normal age of 'superannuation' in the agrarian sector of the economy and the unorganized sector of the urban economy. This need not ensure adequacy of earning.

In the less developed countries, the family system is still the major system of support for the elderly. Support of parents and respect for them are culturally prescribed. While there is a general conformity to this norm, the familial status of an elderly person seems to be related to the degree of financial autonomy he enjoys.

In predominantly agrarian societies, the elderly male continues to be the formal head of the household. The actual authority he enjoys may, however, be small.

The social adjustment to old age may be less difficult in the case of a woman than in the case of a man because the latter experiences a sudden change in his social–occupational role on retirement. For the same reason, a working woman may experience greater difficulties in adjusting to 'old' age and loss of work role than a woman who is a housewife.

While elderly individuals are generally looked after within the family in most developing societies, the phenomenon of migration of young people to cities may occasionally leave the elders on their own in the village home without the younger generation to provide care.

The elderly have to cope with their sense of uselessness and lonesomeness. This problem is somewhat reduced in the case of the elderly who live within the family in comparison with those who may live in institutions. Studies in India show that the elderly, even while living in the family, seek to increase their involvement by taking some responsibility for household chores, by developing religious interest, and by participating in small groups of other elderly persons.

Living with one's grown-up son occurs naturally in the village where the house the family occupies is inherited from father to son. But in the city, the elderly father or mother living with the son may often involve a decision on the part of the elder as well as the son to do so. This situation emphasizes the dependent status of the elderly.

Also, life in the household of one's son may raise problems of relationships.

All these problems—of change of social role, of loss or decrease of income, of loss of status, of potential conflict of authority—have the potential for raising anxiety levels and affecting the health of the elderly individuals.

In the developed countries where the elderly live either on their own or in institutions the sense of being without a meaningful social role and the sense of isolation is likely to be accentuated. The problems of financial support and access to health services, on the other hand, are greatly minimized by a network of publicly financed services; however, there is probably a discernible difference between the quality of life of the well-to-do and economically self-sufficient elderly and those that are wholly dependent on social security or social assistance.

References

1. Siegel, J. S. (1982). *Demographic aspects of the health of the elderly to the year 2000 and beyond, WHO/AGE/82.3*, Geneva.
2. Siegel, J. S. *ibid.*, pp. 45–47.
3. United Nations, (1985). *The world aging situation: strategies and policies*. Department of International and Social Affair, ST/ESA/150–1985, p. 88. United Nations, New York.
4. Srivastava, R. S. (1986). The aged and society, background paper No. 10, in *Care of the elderly* (ed.) P. C. Bhatla, a Round Table Discussion, 6–8 December. International Conference on Health Policy, I.M.A. House Indra Prastha Marga, New Delhi.
5. United Nations, *op. cit.*, Table 9, p. 32.
6. Yesudian, A. (1981). Differential utilisation of health services in a metropoli tan city. *Indian Journal of Social Work*, **XLI**, 381–92.
7. Mahalanobis, P. C. (1961). Anniversary address of the President: *science and national planning*, National Institute of Sciences of India, *Sankhya*, **20**, 69–206. (This reference has been taken from a quotation from the *Report on Mortality*, National Sample Survey of India).
8. Government of India, NSS. (1982). *Sarvekshan*, January–April, 5.
9. United Nations (1985). *Periodical on aging*, Vol. 2, No. I, Table No. 7. Department of International Economic and Social Affairs.
10. United Nations, *The world aging situation, op. cit*, p. 246.
11. Desai, K. G. and Naik, R. D. (196x). *Problems of retired people in Greater Bombay*, 45. Tata Institute of Social Science, Bombay.
12. United Nations, (1985). *Periodical on aging*, Vol. 2, No. 1, Department of International Economic and Social Affairs.
13. United Nations, *The world aging situation, op. cit*, Table 48, p. 247.
14. Desai, K. G. and Naik, R. D. *op. cit*, p. 25.
15. Soodan, K. S. (1975). *Aging in India*, Minerva Calcutta: Associates (Publication) Pvt. Ltd, p. 50–1.
16. Naik, R. D. (1981). An analysis of a change in family economy. *Indian*

Journal of Social Work, **XLI**, 335–41.
17. Soodan, K. S. (1982). Problems of the aged—field study and implications. In *Aging in India* (ed. Desai, K. G.), pp. 143–58. Institute of Social Sciences, Bombay.
18. Ranade, S. N. (1974). *A study of the aged in Delhi*. Delhi School of Social Work (Mimeographed), Delhi.
19. Desai, K. G. and Bhalla, R. (1978). *Social situation of the aged* (mimeographed), February. Tata Institute of Social Sciences, Bombay.
20. Singh, J. (1962). *Problems of old men in Burail*, quoted in Desai, K. G. and R. Bhalla, *op. cit*, p. 36 (no bibliographic reference given).
21. Kaur, G. *The problem of aged women in Batala*. A field work monograph, Sociology Department, Punjab Univesity as quoted in Desai, K. G. and R. Bhalla, *op. cit.* p. 47.
22. Mishra, S. (1976). *Social adjustment in old age*. Unpublished Dissertation, Department of Sociology, Punjab University, as quoted in Desai, K. G. and R. Bhalla, *op. cit.*, p. 44.
23. Siegel, J. S. *op. cit.*, p. 40.

Part II

Progress in specific areas

9

Introduction

J. GRIMLEY EVANS

Aging as manifested in the loss of adaptability of an individual with time is the result of the accumulation and interaction of many impairments, both functional and anatomical. Some of these impairments have been traditionally designated as 'diseases' and have therefore been long under the scrutiny of the medical sciences. Others, dismissed as 'normal aging' or whose functional importance was underestimated, have only recently received scientific attention.

A central dilemma in medical research is whether priorities should be determined by the likelihood of success or the importance of the subject. Both those who fund and those who work in research are tempted to follow those paths where progress seems certain even if that progress in social tems is unimportant or even undesirable. Funding of research is irrational in other ways. Charitable funding is easily raised for emotive diseases even if these make minimal contributions to the total sum of human suffering. Where funding is from governmental sources there may be a hidden political agenda. Research will be done in those areas that placate noisy lobbies or offer the appearance rather than necessarily the substance of concern for the public good. In some nations we now see medical research priority being directed towards those areas that give promise of commercial profitability. Only by chance, it seems, will the needs of the poor and weak of the world be met.

The traditional exclusion of elderly subjects from trials of new treatments and the failure to direct attention to afflictions commonest in old age have long been a mute indictment of a lack of epidemiological awareness and social responsibility among medical scientists and their sponsors. There are signs of change—in some countries due to elderly people forming effective political lobbies, in others to advocacy by social idealists. It is only a beginning, but more research is now being done on aging and age-associated impairments, and the more enlightened clinical investigators are including older patients in their treatment trials. In this section reviewers set out some of the first fruits of this new awareness of human aging.

10

Progress in the biology of aging

CALEB E. FINCH

INTRODUCTION AND BRIEF HISTORICAL PERSPECTIVE

This paper describes some major trends and major gaps in knowledge in biogerontology. In its focus on humans and animals, it cannot be comprehensive. Three areas are growing spectacularly: physiology–pathology, biochemistry–cell biology, and molecular genetics. A major theoretical theme in biogerontology has concerned the possible accumulation of random damage in the genetic apparatus, as hypothesized from various mechanisms by Harmon,[1] Szilard,[2] Medvedev,[3] Orgel,[4] Burnet,[5] and others. However, many types of recent evidence do not support random genomic damage as a prominent cause of age-related dysfunction at either the cell or organ level, though the age-related increase of cancer may involve cumulative effects from mutations over the lifespan. Consequences of limited cell proliferation are another major theme in all three areas, drawing from the finite replication of diploid human fibroblasts *in vitro*.[6] While many mammalian cells show clonal senescence through a finite number of cell cycles *in vitro* and *in vivo*, the role of this phenomenon in age changes *in vivo* is not generally established. The impaired proliferation of cultured human lymphocytes[7] could be a related phenomenon, and there may also be indirect consequences from limited clonal proliferation during development (e.g. through the inability to replace damaged neurones in the adult brain). Physiological–pathological changes are being analysed from the molecular level upwards. A remarkable diversity of age changes can be manipulated through diet, hormones, and drugs. These laboratory and clinical manipulations provide powerful tests of hypotheses about the many different types of cell and molecular mechanisms in aging. Suffice it to say that few biologists expect a comprehensive theory of biological aging and that most recognize a multiplicity of mechanisms.

It is useful to distinguish age changes according to whether they are *universal* and occur in all individuals of a species or *adventitious* and reflect varying environmental influences. Ovarian oocyte depletion at midlife is clearly universal in mammals because of programmed but hormonally dependent cell loss.[8] In contrast, the generality of neurone loss during aging remains controversial; it is also difficult to establish because of the prevalence of cerebrovascular disease in the elderly and because neurone shrinkage may be confused with neurone loss. Although specific neurones are likely to be lost in humans (e.g. pyramidal neurones in the hippocampus and cerebral cortex[9]), no brain region has been established as *always* losing neurones during the average lifespan of humans and laboratory rodents. Certainly, neurones and postmitotic cells in heart and other organs are at risk of irreparable damage throughout the lifespan, and many age-related losses appear to be due to accidental or haphazard damage. Vascular disease, cancer, and many other age-related changes also vary so widely between individuals that environmental factors are widely suspected. Evaluating the relative contributions of universal and adventitious causes to aging and their interactions is a major issue in nearly all areas of biogerontology. For example, the maximum lifespan of highly inbred C57BL/6J male mice has increased 40 per cent from 29 months in the early 1960s at the Jackson Laboratory[10] to 42 months by 1970 in the author's colony,[11] presumably because of reduced respiratory disease; by hearsay, this trend continues in some rodent genotypes. We must therefore question whether even present conditions are suboptimal, and whether current data are confounded by age-related diseases, especially of the kidney,[12, 13] that will be further reduced in the future. These issues also support the major revision of the previously widely held view that functions must decline linearly with age.[14] Recent studies show that there is considerable variation between individuals in the age at which a particular function starts to decline, if it does so at all (e.g. intelligence[15] or kidney function[16]). Many functional impairments in older age groups probably reflect specific diseases, rather than an elusive universal aging process.

LIFESPAN AND DISEASE

A major question concerns the role of diseases in limiting the lifespan of humans and other mammals. Because older individuals in all species so far examined show one or more major degenerative diseases, most researchers concede the importance of specific age-related diseases in determining the maximum lifespan. The postmortem data on the diseases present at death in very old humans and rodents, although embarrassingly limited, give no support for the mythical 'natural death' in the absence of definable pathological conditions. Most mammals in older age groups have at least one major degenerative change.[17, 18, 19] Strong support for the linkage of lifespan to disease *per se* comes from increasingly sophisticated studies of rodents on different diets, in which changing the diet can effect an increase in the average and maximum lifespan of 10–25 per cent, together with a delayed incidence of age-related diseases.[13] Diet restriction is so far the only manipulation that reduces the Gompertz (exponential) mortality rate in mammals.[20] A major puzzle is that the age-related diseases of laboratory rodents and humans can vary widely between populations, yet the exponential (Gompertz) mortality rate co-efficients and maximum lifespans are not all that different between populations.[21]

A related issue concerns the search for biomarkers of aging (i.e. indices of molecules, cells, or organ functions that might be predictors of the individual lifespan[22]). So far, no markers have been found that are distinctively better than chronological age in predicting residual lifespan in humans or in laboratory rodents, even highly inbred strains.[23] Blood-pressure and lipids, however, are useful in identifying risk for premature mortality. Major efforts continue.

GENETICS OF LONGEVITY

Strong genetic determinants for short lifespans are well recognized in the progeroid syndromes of humans[24] and in laboratory rodents strains which develop early onset diseases[23,25]. The *B10.F* mouse strain, for example, is susceptible to a vertically transmitted virus that causes leukaemia and greying of hair and death about 12 months before the usual mouse lifespan of 30 months.[25] Other related mice have longer lifespans that are being identified with different alleles in the main histocompatibility complex on chromosome 17.[26] These inbred strains differ in the age of onset and types of diseases[27] and in their patterns of female reproductive senescence.[27A] Another short-lived variant is the *senescence-accelerated mouse*, which develops hair loss, hunched back, and amyloid deposits in many tissues. An amino acid difference was recently found in the amyloid protein by comparison with several strains with longer lifespans but without amyloid deposits.[28] Most agree that genes predisposing to progeroid syndromes and other early onset diseases should be considered as a special category.[24] They do not accelerate most aspects of biological aging and their relation to genes that enhance lifespans beyond the average is not clear. The rare genotypes, hypobeta- and hyperalpha-lipoproteinaemias, appear to add 5–10 years to the human lifespan by protecting against vascular disease.[29] Other such genotypes may be found.

The first example of a mutation that increases lifespan beyond the wild type (exciting news!) comes from *Caenorhabditis*, a nematode with a 3-week lifespan. A recessive mutant, *Age-1*, increased lifespan 50 per cent by reducing the Gompertz mortality rate.[30] The relatively small genome and short lifespan favours isolation of such genes. Although few expect that maximum lifespan in mammals is determined by a single gene locus, biogerontology is proving to be a subject of many surprises.

ALZHEIMER'S DISEASE AND OTHER AGE-RELATED NEUROLOGICAL CONDITIONS

Alzheimer's disease is attracting great attention because of its increase as a result of the greater human survival to advanced age in many countries throughout the world. There is no evidence that the age-related risk has changed, or that it is a new condition. The major symptom of Alzheimer's disease is loss of recent memory, which is associated with selective degeneration of large neurones in the frontal lobes and hippocampus. Degenerating regions are characterized by neurones containing aggregates of cytoskeletal proteins (neurofibrillary tangles), degenerating terminals (neuritic plaques), and amyloid deposits. Yet, not all large neurones are damaged, and some brain regions seem quite protected. Several neurotransmitter systems are diminished, particularly certain cholinergic, noradrenergic, and glutaminergic pathways. Major efforts are being made to develop a treatment through precursor therapy.

Genes which predispose to Alzheimer's disease may be located soon. Chromosome 21 gets particular attention because trisomy 21 (Down's syndrome) increases the incidence of neurofibrillary tangles, neuritic plaques, and amyloid by middle age. Moreover, a strong genetic marker on chromosome 21 was found in one family with multigeneration Alzheimer's disease by analysis of restriction-fragment length polymorphisms.[31] The mapping of an amyloid gene in a nearby region of chromosome 21 may be fortuitous, since no segregants have been found with this locus so far. These findings must be considered preliminary. Isolation of an Alzheimer gene could lead to fundamental mechanisms by studying the controls on its expression after transfection into cultured cells or into mice. Other genes may influence the age of onset; these are suspected for Huntington's chorea[32] and are shown for the latency of infections with the scrapie agent in mice.[33] The scrapie 'prion' is a non-conventional 'slow virus', apparently without RNA or DNA,[34] which causes a global neurodegenerative disease with amyloid-like deposits and is sometimes considered as a model for Alzheimer's disease.[35]

AGE-RELATED CHANGES IN NEURONES

Changes seen by the average lifespan may begin much earlier, as shown by the decrease of receptors for the neurotransmitters dopamine and serotonin, in which the loss of the D2 and S2 receptor types can be detected before midlife in humans and rodents by analysis of postmortem tissues or by position emission tomography (PET) scanning.[36, 37] Many other types of receptors do not change.[36] Loss of D2 and S2 receptors is among the few brain age changes which occur in short- and long-lived mammals; it exceeds loss of the corresponding presynaptic transmitter pools. The cause of these receptor decreases is not clear, and could be due to loss of neurones, or loss of neural processes without neurone loss. The consequence of receptor loss may be slowed neural processing, in view of the slowing reaction times caused by partial pharmacological blockade of these receptors,[38] which models the age-related receptor loss. As is being realized for so many biochemical markers, diet restriction slows the age-related loss of D2 receptors.[39] Diet restriction of rodents also increases the lifespan, retards the onset of cancers and kidney diseases, among others (e.g. ref. 13), and decreases the exponential mortality rate.[20] The effect of diet restrictions on age changes in the primate brain is being studied at the National Institute on Aging in Baltimore.

Steroids are another factor in age changes of neurones in rodents. A large literature documents hypothalamic–pituitary age changes in female rodents which are slowed by ovariectomy or accelerated in the young by chronic exposure to oestradiol.[40, 41, 42] Hippocampal neurone aging can also be slowed by adrenalectomy or accelerated by stress.[43, 44] A variety of age changes in rodent neuroendocrine functions are hypothesized to be caused by cumulative effects from hormones acting on the same brain centres that control them.[41, 44] These add to the examples of manipulation of aging through physiological variables. Their mechanisms and the generalizability to humans and other species are unknown.

ACTIVITIES OF THE CELL NUCLEUS AND THE GENOME

The cell nucleus is the seat of control in most organs throughout the body. Through dynamic regulation of gene activity by hormones, diet, and other physiological factors, humans and other organisms adapt to their environment and combat infectious disease. How aging influences the cell nucleus is thus of major significance, as reflected in the emphasis of the mutation and error theories of aging.[1–4]

RNA and protein synthesis

A controversy concerns the possible effect of age on the metabolism of RNA and proteins. Although the literature is generally consistent that total organ RNA and protein synthesis in liver and muscle decreases progressively after maturity across the lifespan of rodents,[45, 46] there are many technical uncertainties. For example, it is difficult to make appropriate corrections for age changes in precursor pool kinetics in studies with radiolabelled precursors. Moreover, not all studies find major decrements in the brain[47] or other cells. Any slowing in synthesis and turnover must be in close balance because the organ content of messenger RNA,[48, 49] protein, or most enzymes[50] does not change notably; this close balance implies continuing, precise regulation of gene activities throughout the lifespan.

Individual genes vary widely in their activities across the lifespan. Two regularly show increased activities: albumin production, with variably increased mRNA,[51, 52] increases in aging rats as a compensation for the albumin lost in urine from the endemic kidney disease of old rats; the hypersecretion of gonadotrophins[8, 53] by the pituitary increases in aging mice and humans, a consequence of the loss of ovarian steroids as ovarian follicles become depleted (in this case, studies of RNA and protein synthesis remain to be done). Recently, an 'anti-proliferative' mRNA was found to be increased in fibroblasts that had lost the ability to divide during clonal senescence.[54] It would be remarkable if altered activities of a few genes proved to be primarily responsible for clonal senescence: the manipulation of such gene activities might be an approach for many types of interventions and therapies to counteract senescence. On the other hand, other genes show decreased activity. For example, transcription of alpha$_{2u}$-globulin and its mRNA decreases strikingly in old male rodents.[55, 56] Another case is the lymphokine IL-2, whose induction after mitogenic stimulation of lymphocytes is much reduced in aging rodents and humans.[57, 58] The smaller stimulation of IL-2 and its mRNA parallel the smaller mitotic response of these cells. The underlying cause may be a shrinkage in the responding subpopulation of T lymphocytes, rather than a defect in the mitotically responsive cells to make Il-2.[59] Parenthetically, the reader might consider that the dramatic decrease in some cellular immune responses and decrease of thymus hormones as widely observed during aging[57] do not cause defects as gross as those in AIDS. The immune system must have tremendous reserves that suffice for present lifespan at least. On another front, the recent demonstration that intact and clonable RNA can be obtained postmortem from the brains of normal elderly or Alzheimer's patients[60] will enable a host of interesting questions about our own species. The emergent data suggest that relatively few genes show major changes in Alzheimer's disease.[61, 62]

There are many examples of possible effects of age on the physiological systems which influence gene regulation. In livers of old rats, the gene for tyrosine aminotransferase shows unimpaired transcriptional responses to corticosteroids.[52] However, the activation of this gene during stress is slower, presumably because of changes in neuroendocrine regulation of the liver.[63] Altered physiological regulation is also implied in slowing of bulk protein synthesis in old rats which is blunted by diet restriction,[49, 64, 65] and which also increases transcription of alpha$_{2u}$-globulin and other genes.[56, 66] Another major group of changes in gene function is implied in cells that are influenced by ovarian steroids, particularly the oestrogen-sensitive cells in the reproductive tract which tend to atrophy after menopause unless there is replacement of oestrogens. Clinical inter-ventions into the adverse aspects of the menopause are becoming more effective, including reduction in bone loss in osteoporosis in at least some women.[8] These exciting findings bridge the gap between aging changes in physiology and in gene regulation. Moreover, many other changes in gene and cell functions could be due to regulatory changes at the physiological level, rather than some intrinsic or random aging mechanism.

Altered proteins and slowed cell metabolism

The mutational and error hypotheses of aging lead to a search for altera-tions in enzymes. There are many examples in senescing cells and organ-isms of altered enzymes which have no activity but retain immunological cross-reactivity by which they are detected.[67, 68] In some cases, the cross-reactivity is negligible between the native and altered forms.[68] These altered forms have the same polypeptide chains as the 'young' forms, and in some cases can be transformed into active enzymes.[69] They appear to be degradation intermediates,[70] which are also detectible in young cells but in much smaller amounts.[71] The level of altered enzymes can be manipulated. For example, hepatectomy transiently purges the remaining cells of several altered forms in old rats; during the subsequent 9 days as the liver regenerates, the usual complement of inactive enzymes reappears.[72, 73] The accumulation of altered forms is attributed to slower protein turnover.[74, 75, 76] Altered enzymes also accumulate in cells with no protein synthesis, such as in the lens of the eye[77, 78] and circulating erythrocytes.[79, 80, 81] It is possible to speculate that the neurofibrillary tangles accumulated in aging and Alzheimer's disease may also be a consequence of altered protein degradation. The presence of ubiquitin in the tangles[82] suggests impaired degradative mechanisms that may be shared by other cells, but with different consequences.

Glycosylation is another cause of altered molecules. Drawing from their observations that diabetics have increased amounts of glycosylated haemoglobins (Hb A_{1c}), Cerami and colleagues[83] have strong evidence to implicate glycosylation of collagen and lens crystallins as a source of molecular damage during aging. The non-enzymatic glycosylation of amine groups in proteins can lead to cross-linking of adjacent chains, which may, for example, favour the trapping of plasma proteins during arteriosclerosis. The brown fluorescence in membranes and cataracts which is common during aging appears to arise in this way. The inten-sification of arteriosclerosis, cataracts, and other common aging condi-tions by diabetes may thus represent a greater cumulative impact of endogenous sugars. Diet restriction might oppose their effects, and results of such studies are forthcoming.

Spontaneous gene reactivation

Some repressed genes may spontaneously re-activate during the lifespan. X-linked genes in mammals are useful for studying this question, since one X chromosome is genetically repressed (Lyonization) in somatic cells. This phenomenon probably differs fundamentally from the increased activities of some genes through physiological signals as described above. Autosomal genes influencing coat colour, introduced to the X chromosome by translocation, showed increased expression at later ages.[84, 85] Their closeness to the inactive X heterochromatin is thought to have prevented their expression initially. However, select patches of fur in some mice became progressively darker between 3 and 12 months, indicating changes in melanocyte enzyme functions in which the translocated genes became derepressed. Moreover, the adjacent translocated autosomal coat colour genes were re-activated in a temporal sequence that was inverse to their distance from the inactivating X heterochromatin. Similarly, the X-linked gene for ornithine carbamoyl transferase, which can be histochemically discriminated, shows a progressive, apparently random increase in activation in mice, increasing 50-fold between 2 and 17 months.[86] Although it is possible that mutations could contribute to these phenomena, the most likely explanation is a spontaneous change in chromatin structure permitting transcription. These changes may be related to other phenomena; according to one study,[87] women show a progressive age-related decrease in the number of Barr bodies, the heterochromatinized X chromosome, and murine leukaemia viruses show sporadic age-related increased expression which does not penetrate in all carriers.[88, 89, 90] Erosion of the mechanisms of selective gene regulation, a non-programmed sporadic event as conceptualized by Getz[90] and seen in the above examples, could be important at many levels of function. It need not involve primary damage to DNA itself.

Does damage accumulate in DNA?

Attempts to document the extent of damage to DNA according to the intrinsic mutagenesis hypothesis[5] (see above) continue to give a mixed picture. No phenomenon of physiological aging has been related to DNA damage. The survivors of acute radiation exposure from the atomic bomb have not shown a different pattern of aging,[91] although an increased level of somatic mutations persist in erythroid cells.[92] A very sensitive assay for errors in the fidelity of DNA polymerase failed to show alterations in polymerases isolated from cerebral cortex neurones[93] or livers[94] of old rodents. No age change was seen in the frequency of resistance to thioguanine by primary clones from kidney or muscle of mice.[95] The increase in chromosomal abnormalities in cells of old mice[96] could originate in chromosomal or spindle proteins, as well as in DNA.

The first definitive demonstration of age-associated changes in DNA was recently reported. Modified DNA bases occur increasingly in tissues of aging rats, reaching 1–10 modifications per cell nucleus.[97] Their structure is unknown, but chromatographically they resemble heterocyclic adducts of carcinogens formed *in vivo* with DNA.[98] Such changes, even at low levels, could be mutagenic steps in the age-related increase of cancer.

The methylation of cytosine in DNA attracts interest in aging research because of general correlations between the extent of DNA demethylation and transcription. DNA methyl groups are decreased during aging in several specific sequences in livers of rodents and birds, and during clonal senescence of fibroblasts.[99, 100] No functional consequences are proved, but the trend is consistent with increased gene expression (see above).

SYNOPSIS: PROSPECTS FOR INTERVENTION

The manipulations of age-related changes described above suggest a major new approach to identifying fundamental mechanisms in aging that will surely lead to potential interventions applicable to humans. A great reduction in age-related bone disorders may be possible in the next decade, for example, through diet and hormones. The effects of diet in reducing the incidence of cancer and kidney disease in rodents may also yield approaches for humans. There also are hints from rodents that some aspects of brain aging can be extensively manipulated by diet and hormones. It is thus conceivable that the expression of genetic determinants for Alzheimer's disease may be modified to reduce its impact or even prevent its onset. It is now possible that a large number of age changes are not due to intrinsic processes of aging in molecules and cells, but rather represent specifiable extrinsic influences.[101] Although biological aging is clearly very complex, particularly in long-lived species like humans, major advances can be expected as specific phenomena are tackled one by one.

References

1. Harmon, D. (1957). Prolongation of the normal life span by radiation protection chemicals. *Journal of Gerontology*, **11**, 298–300.
2. Szilard, L. (1959). On the nature of the aging process. *Proceedings of the National Academy of Sciences, USA*, **45**, 30–45.
3. Medvedev, Zh. A. (1961). *Protein biosynthesis*. Oliver and Boyd, London.
4. Orgel, L. E. (1963). The maintanence of the accuracy of protein synthesis and its relevance to ageing. *Proceedings of the National Academy of Sciences USA*, **49**, 517–21.
5. Burnet, F. M. (1974). *Intrinsic mutagenesis: a genetic approach to aging*. Wiley, New York.

6. Hayflick, L. (1965). The limited in vitro lifespan of human diploid cell strains. *Experimental Cell Research*, **37**, 614–36.
7. Hefton, J. M., Darlington, G. J., Casazza, B. A., and Weksler, M. E. (1980). Immunologic studies of aging. V. Impaired proliferation of PHA responsive human lymphocytes in culture. *Journal of Immunology*, **125**, 1007–10.
8. Finch, C. E. and Gosden, R. G. (1986). Animal models for the human menopause. In *Aging reproduction and the climacteric* (eds Mastroianni, L. and C. A. Paulsen), pp. 3–34. Plenum Press, New York.
9. Coleman, P. D. and Flood, D. G. (1987). Neuron numbers and dendritic extent in normal aging and Alzheimer's disease. *Neurobiology of Aging* **8**, 521–45.
10. Russell, E. S. (1966). Lifespan and ageing patterns. In *Biology of the laboratory mouse* (ed. Green E. L.), pp. 511–19. McGraw Hill, New York.
11. Finch, C. E. (1971). Comparative biology of senescence: Evolutionary and developmental considerations. In *Animal models for biomedical research IV*, pp. 47–67. National Academy of Science, Washington DC.
12. Coleman, G. L., Barthold, S. W., Osbaldiston, G. W., Foster, S. J., and Jonas, A. M. (1977). Pathological changes during aging in barrier-reared Fischer 344 male rats. *Journal of Gerontology*, **32**, 258–78.
13. Iwasaki, K., Gleiser, C. A., Masoro, E. J., McMahan, C. A., Seo, E. J., and Yu, B. P. (1988). The influence of dietary protein source on longevity and age-related disease processes of Fischer 344 rats. *Journal of Gerontology*, **43**, B5–12.
14. Shock, N. W. (1961). Physiological aspects of aging in man. *Annual Review of Physiology*, **23**, 97–122.
15. Schaie, K. W., and Labouvie-Vief, G. (1974). Generational versus ontogenic components of change in adult cognitive behaviour: a fourteen-year cross sequential study. *Developmental Psychology*, **10**, 305–20.
16. Lindeman, R. D., Tobin, J., and Shock, N. W. (1985). Longitudinal studies on the rate of decline in renal function with age. *Journal of the American Geriatrics Society*, **33**, 278–85.
17. Simms, H. S. and Berg, B. N. (1957). Longevity and the onset of lesions in male rats. *Journal of Gerontology*, **12**, 244–52.
18. Howell, T. H. (1963). Multiple pathology in nonagenarians. *Geriatrics*, **18**, 899–902.
19. Zeman, F. D. (1962). Pathologic anatomy of old age. *Archives of Pathology*, **73**, 48–65.
20. Sacher, G. A. (1977). Life table modification and life prolongation. In *Handbook of the biology of aging*, (1st ed) (ed. Finch, C. E. and L. Hayflick, pp. 582–638 Van Nostrand, New York.
21. Jones, H. B. (1956). A special consideration of the aging process, disease, and life expectancy. *Advances in Biology, Medicine and Physics*, **4**, 281–337.
22. Reff, M. E. and Schneider, E. L. (ed.) (1982). *Biological markers of aging*. NIH Publication No. 82–2221 Bethesda MD.
23. Harrison, D. E., Ingram, D. K., and Archer, J. R. (1989). The ability of tests of 13 physiological, behavioural, and growth parameters to predict subsequent longevities in 6 mouse genotypes. *Mechanisms of Aging De-*

velopment, (in press).
24. Martin, G. M. (1982). Syndromes of accelerated aging. *National Cancer Institute Monographs,* **60**, 241–7.
25. Morse, H. C., Yetter, R. A., Stimpfling, J. H., Pitts, O. M., Frederickson, T. N., and Hartley, J. W. (1984). Greying with age in mice: relation to expression of murine leukemia viruses. *Cell,* **41**, 439–48.
26. Smith, G. S. and Walford, R. L. (1977). Influence of the main histocompatibility complex on ageing in mice. *Nature,* **270**, 727–9.
27. Meredith, P. and Walford, R. L. (1977). Effect of age on response to T and B cell mitogens in mice congenic at the H-2 locus. *Immunogenetics,* **5**, 109–28.
27A. Lerner, S. P. Anderson, C. P., and Finch, C. E. (1988). Genotypic influences on female reproductive senescence in mice. *Biology of Reproduction* **38**, 1035–44.
28. Kunisada, T., Higuchi, K., Aota, S., Takeda, T., and Yamahishi, H. (1986). Molecular cloning and nucleotide sequence of cDNA for murine senile amyloid protein: nucleotide substitutions found in ap[olipoprotein A-II cDNA of senescence accelerated mouse (SAM). *Nucleic Acids Research,* **14**, 5729–40.
29. Glueck, C. J., Garside, P. S., Fallat, R. W., Sielski, J., and Steiner P. M. (1977). Longevity syndromes: familial hypobeta and familial hyperalpha lipoprotenemia. *Journal of Laboratory and Clinical Medicine,* **88**, 941–57.
30. Johnson, T. (1987). Aging can be genetically dissected into component processes using long-lived lines of *Caenorhabditis elegans. Proceedings of the National Academy of Sciences, USA,* **84**, 3777–81.
31. St George-Hyslop, P. H., Tanzi, R. E. *et al.* (1987). The genetic defect causing familial Alzheimer's disease maps on chromosome 21. *Science,* **235**, 885–90.
32. Farrer, L. A., Connealy, P. M., and Yu, P. I. (1984). The natural history of Huntington's disease: possible role of 'aging' genes. *American Journal of Medical Genetics,* **18**, 115–23.
33. Carlson, G. A., Kingsbury, D. T., Goodman, P. A. *et al.* (1986). Linkage of prion and scrapie and incubation time genes. *Cell,* **46**, 503–11.
34. Prusiner, S. B. (1982). Novel proteinaceous infectious particles cause scrapie. *Science,* **216**, 136–44.
35. Gibbs, C. J. Jr, and Gajdusek, D. C. (1972). Amyotrophic lateral sclerosis, Parkinson's disease, and the amyotrophic lateral sclerosisparkinsonism-dementia complex on Guam: a review and summary of attempts to demonstrate infection as the aetiology. *Journal of Clinical Pathology,* **25** Suppl. 6, 132–40.
36. Morgan, D. G., May, P. C., and Finch, C. E. (1987). Dopamine and serotonin systems in human and rodent brain: effects of age and degenerative disease. *Journal of the American Geriatrics Society,* **35**, 334–45.
37. Wong, D. F., Wagner *et al.* (1984). Effects of age on dopamine and serotonin receptors measured by positron tomography in the living human brain. *Science,* **226**, 1393–6.
38. Amalric, M. and Koob, G. F. (1987). Depletion of dopamine in the caudate nucleus but not nucleus accumbens impairs reaction-time performance in rats. *Journal of Neuroscience,* **7**, 2129–34.

39. Levin, P., Janda, J. K., Joseph, J. A., Ingram, D. K., and Roth, G. S. (1981). Dietary restriction retards the age-associated loss of rat striatai dopaminergic receptors. *Science*, **214**, 561–2.

40. Schipper, H., Brawer, J. R., Nelson, J. F., Felicio, L. S., and Finch, C. E. (1981). Role of the gonads in the histologic aging of the hypothalamic arcuate nucleus. *Journal of Gerontology*, **24**, 784–94.

41. Finch, C. E., Felicio, L. S., Mobbs, C. V., and Nelson, J. F. (1984). Ovarian and steroidal influences on neuroendocrine aging processes in female rodents. *Endocrine Review*, **5**, 467–97.

42. Telford, N., Mobbs, C. V., Sinha, Y. N., and Finch, C. E. (1986). The increase of anterior pituitary dopamine in aging C57BL/6J female mice is caused by ovarian steroids, not intrinsic pituitary aging. *Neuroendocrinology*, **43**, 135–42.

43. Landfield, P. W., Waymire, J. C., and Lynch, G. (1978). Hippocampal aging and adrenocorticoids. Quantitative correlations. *Science*, **202**, 1098–102.

44. Sapolsky, R. M., Krey, L. C. and McEwen, B. S. (1986). The neuroendocrinology of stress and aging: the glucocorticoid cascade hypothesis. *Endocrine Review*, **7**, 284–301.

45. Rothstein, M. (1982). *Biochemical approaches to aging*. New York, Academic Press.

46. Richardson, A., Roberts, M. S., and Rutherford, M. S. (1985). Aging and gene expression. *Review of Biological Research of Aging*, **2**, 395–419.

47. Cosgrove, J. W. and Rapaport, S. (1987). Absence of age differences in protein synthesis by rat brain, measured with an initiating cell-free system. *Neurobiology of Aging*, **8**, 27–34.

48. Colman, P. D., Kaplan, B. B., Osterburg, H. H., and Finch, C. E. (1980). Brain poly(A)RNA during aging: Stability of yield and sequence complexity in two rat strains. *Journal of Neurochemistry*, **34**, 335–45.

49. Birchenall-Sparks, M. C., Roberts, M. S., Staecker, J., Hardwick, J. P., and Richardson, A. (1985). Effect of dietary restriction on liver protein synthesis in rats. *Journal of Nutrition*, **115**, 944–50.

50. Finch, C. E. (1972). Enzyme activities, gene function and ageing in mammals (review). *Experimental Gerontology*, **7**, 53–67.

51. Horbach, G. J. M. J., Princen, H. M. G., Van Der Kroef, M., Van Bezooijen, C. F. A., and Yap, S. H. (1984). Changes in the sequence content of albumin mRNA and its translational activity in the rat liver with age. *Biochimica et Biophysica Acta*, **783**, 60–6.

52. Wellinger, R. and Guigoz, Y. (1986). The effect of age on the induction of tyrosine aminotransferase and tryptophan oxygenase genes by physiological stress. *Mechanisms of Ageing Development*, **34**, 203–17.

53. Gee, D. M., Flurkey, K., and Finch, C. E. (1983). Aging and the regulation of luteinizing hormone in C5BL/6J mice: Impaired elevations after ovariectomy and spontaneous elevations at advanced ages. *Biology of Reproduction*, **28**, 598–607.

54. Lumpkin, C. K., McClung, J. K., Pereira-Smith, O. M., and Smith, J. R. (1987). Existence of high abundance antiproliferative mRNA's in senescent human diploid fibroblasts. *Science*, **232**, 393–5.

55. Roy, A. K., Nath, T. S., Motwani, N. M., and Chatterjee, B. (1983).

Age-dependent regulation of the polymorphic forms of a2u-globulin. *Journal of Biological Chemistry*, **258**, 10123–7.

56. Richardson, A., Butler, J. A., Rutherford, M. S. *et al.* (1987). Effect of age and dietary restriction on the expression of alpha$_{2u}$-globulin. *Journal of Biological Chemistry*, **262**, 12821–5.

57. Weksler, M. (1985). Changes in the immune response with age. In *Handbook of the biology of aging* (2nd edn) (ed. Finch, C. E. and Schneider), pp. 414–32. Van Nostrand, New York.

58. Wu, W., Pahlavani, M., Cheung, H. T., and Richardson, A. (1986). The effect of aging on the expression of interleukin-2 messenger ribonucleic acid. *Cellular Immunology*, **100**, 224–31.

59. Holbrook, N. and Adler, W. (1987). *Gerontologist*, **27**, 132.

60. Johnson, S. A., Morgan, D. G., and Finch, C. E. (1986). Extensive postmortem stability of RNA from rat and human brain. *Journal of Neuroscience Research*, **16**, 267–80.

61. May, P. C. and Finch, C. E. (1988). RNA changes as marker for neuronal atrophy and hyperactivity during Alzheimer's and other age-related brain diseases. In, *Molecular Biology of Alzheimer's Disease*. CE Finch and P Davies (eds.), pp. 43–7. Cold Spring Harbor Laboratories, Cold Spring Harbor NY.

62. Johnson. S. A., Pasinetti, G. M., May, P. C., Ponte, P. A., Cordell, B., and Finch, C. E. (1988). Selective reduction of mRNA for the B-amyloid precursor protein that lacks a Kuntiz-type protease inhibitor motif in cortex from AD. *Experimental Neurology*, 102: 264–268.

63. Finch, C. E., Huberman, H. S. and Mirsky, A. E. (1969). Regulation of tyrosine aminotransferase by endogenous factors in the mouse. *Journal of General Physiology*, **54**, 675–89.

64. Ricketts, W. G., Birchenall-Sparks, M. C., Hardwick, J. P. and Richardson, A. (1985). Effect of age and dietary restriction on protein synthesis by isolated kidney cells, *Journal of Cellular Physiology*, **125**, 492–8.

65. Ward, W. F. (1988). Enhancement by food restriction of liver protein synthesis in the aging Fischer 344 rat. *Journal of Gerontology,* **43**, B50–3.

66. Richardson, A., Semsei, I., Rutherford, M. S., and Butler, J. A. (1987b). Effect of dietary restriction on the expression of specific genes. *Federation Proceedings*.

67. Rothstein, M. (1982). *Biochemical approaches to aging*. Academic Press, New York.

68. Dovrat, A., Scharf, J., Eisenbach, L., and Gershon, D. (1986). G6PD molecules devoid of catalytic activity are present in the nucleus of the rat lens. *Experimental Eye Research*, **42**, 489–96.

69. Sharma, H. K. and Rothstein, M. (1978). Age-related changes in the properties of enolase from Turbatrix aceti. *Biochemistry*, **17**, 2869–78.

70. Reznick, A. Z., Dovrat, A., Rosenfelder, L., Shpund, S., and Gershon, D. (1985) Defective enzyme molecules in cells of aging animals are partially denatured, totally inactive normal degradation intermediates. In *Modification of proteins during aging* (ed. Adelman, R. C.) pp. 926–82. Liss, New York.

71. Reznick, A. Z., Rosenfelder, L., Shpund, S., and Gershon, D. (1985). Identification of intracellular degradation intermediates of aldolase B by

antiserum to the denatured enzyme. *Proceedings of the National Academy of Sciences, USA*, **82**, 6114–18.

72. Schapira, H. C., Weber, A., Guillouzo, C., and Dreyfus, J. C. (1978). Search for alterations of three enzymes with a different turnover rate in the liver of senescent rats. In *Liver and aging* (ed. Kitani, K.) pp. 47–54. Elsevier.

73. Hiremath, L. S. and Rothstein, M. (1982). Regenerating liver in aged rats produces unaltered phosphoglycerate kinase. *Journal of Gerontology*, **37**, 680–3.

74. Lavie, L., Reznick, A. Z., and Gershon, D. (1982). Decreased protein and puromycinyl-peptide degradation in livers of senescent mice. *Biochemical Journal*, **202**, 47–51.

75. Reiss, U., Reznick, A. Z., and Gershon, D. (1979). Characterization and possible effects of age-associated alterations in enzymes and proteins. *Aging Vol. 8: Physiology and cell biology of aging*, pp. 1–26.

76. Reiss, U. and Rothstein, M. (1975). Age-related changes in isocitrate lyase in the free-living nematode *Turbatrix aceti*. *Journal of Biological Chemistry*, **250**, 826–30.

77. Dovrat, A., Scharf, J., and Gershon, D. (1984). Glyceraldehyde 3-phosphate dehydrogenase activity in rat and human lens and the fate of enzyme molecules in the aging lens. *Mechanisms of Aging Development*, **28**, 187–91.

78. Gracy, R. W., Yuksel, K. U., Chapman, M. L. *et al.* (1985). Impaired degradation may account for the accumulation of 'abnormal' proteins in aging cells. In *Modifications of proteins during aging* (ed. Adelman, R. C.), pp. 1–18. Liss, New York.

79. Low, P. S., Waugh, S. M., Zinke, K., and Drenckhahn, D. (1985). The role of hemoglobin denaturation and band 3 clustering in red blood cell aging. *Science*, **227**, 531–3.

80. Mennecier, F. and Dreyfus, J. C. (1974). *Biochimica et Biophysica Acta*, **364**, 320–6.

81. Oliver, C. N., Ahn, B., Moerman, E. J., Goldstein, S., and Stadtman, E. R. (1987). Age-related changes in oxidized proteins. *Journal of Biological Chemistry*, **262**, 5488–91.

82. Mori, H., Kondo, J., and Ihara, Y. (1987). Ubiquitin is a component of paired helical filaments in Al; zheimer's disease. *Science*, **235**, 1641–4.

83. Cerami, A., Vlassara, H., and Brownlee, M. (1987). Glucose and aging. *Scientific American*, **256**, 90–6.

84. Cattenach, B. M., Pollard, C. F., and Perez, J. N. (1969). Controlling elements in the mouse X-chromosome. *Zeitschrift für Vererbungslere*, **96**, 313–23.

85. Cattenach, B. M. (1974). Position effect variegation in the mouse. *Genetics Research*, **23**, 291–306.

86. Wareham, K. A., Lyon, M. F., Glenister, P. H., and Williams, E. D. (1987). Age-related reactivation of an X-linked gene. *Nature*, **327**, 725–7.

87. Voitenko, V. P. (1980). Aging, diseases, and X-chromatin. *Zeitschrift Gerontologie*, **13**, 18–23.

88. Florine, D. L., Ono, T., Cutler, R. G., and Getz, M. J. (1980). Regulation of endogenous murine-leukemia virus-related nuclear and cytoplasmic RNA

complexity in C57BL/6J mice of increasing age. *Cancer Research*, **40**, 519–23.

89. Peters, R. L., Hartley, J. W., Spahn, G. J., Rabstein, L. S., Whitmire, C. E., Turner, H. C., and Huebner, R. J. (1972). Prevalence of the group-specific (gs) antigen and infectious virus expressions of the murine C-type RNA viruses during the lifespan of BALB/cCr mice. *International Journal of Cancer*, **10**, 283–9.

90. Getz, M. J. (1985). Molecular mechanisms for age-related virus expression. In *Handbook of the biology of aging*, (2nd edition) (ed. Finch, C. E. and E. L. Schneider) pp. 255–72. Van Nostrand, New York.

91. Hollingsworth, J. W., Hashizume, A., and Jablon, S. (1965). Correlations between tests of aging in Hiroshima subjects—an attempt to define 'physiologic age'. *Yale Journal of Biology and Medicine*, **38**, 11–26.

92. Langlois, R. G., Bigbee, W. L., Kyoizumi, S., Nakamura, N., Bean, M. A., Akiyama, M., and Jensen, R. H. (1987). Evidence for increased somatic cell mutations at the glycophorin a locus in atomic bomb survivors. *Science*, **236**, 445–8.

93. Rao, K. S., Martin, G. M., and Loeb, L. A. (1985). Fidelity of DNA polymerase-B in neurons from young and very aged mice. *Journal of Neurochemistry*, **45**, 1273–8.

94. Silber, J. R., Fry, M., Martin, G. M., and Loeb, L. A. (1985). Fidelity of DNA polymerases isolated from regenerating liver chromatin of aging Mus musculus. *Journal of Biological Chemistry*, **260**, 1304–10.

95. Horn, P. L., Turker, M. S., Ogburn, C. E., Disteche, C. M., and Martin, G. M. (1984). A cloning assay for 6-thioguanine resistance provides evidence against certain somatic mutational theories of aging. *Journal of Cellular Physiology*, **121**, 309–15.

96. Martin, G. M., Smith, A. C., Ketterer, D. J., Ogburn, C. E., and Disteche, D. J. (1985). Increased chromosomal abnormalities in the first metaphase of cells isolated from kidneys of aged mice. *Israel Journal Medical Science*, **21**, 296–301.

97. Randerath, K., Reddy, M.V., and Disher, R. M. (1986). Age- and tissue-related DNA modifications in untreated rats: detection by ^{32}P-postlabelling assay and possible significance for spontaneous tumor induction and ageing. *Carcinogenesis*, **7**, 1615–17.

98. Reddy, M. V. and Randerath, K. Nuclease P_1-mediated-enhancement of sensitivity of ^{32}P-postlabelling test for structurally diverse DNA adducts. *Carcinogenesis*, **7**, 1343–51.

99. Mays-Hoopes, L. L. (1985). Macromolecular methylation during aging. *Advances in Biological Research in Aging*, **2**, 361–94.

100. Mays-Hoopes, L., Chao, W., Butcher, H. C., and Huang, R. C. C. (1986). Decreased methylation of the major mouse long interspersed repeated DNA during aging and in myeloma cells. *Developmental Genetics*, **7**, 65–73.

101. Finch, C. E. (1987). Neural and endocrine determinents of senescence: investigation of causality and reversibility of laboratory and clinical interventions. In *Modern biological theories of aging* (ed. Warner, H. *et al.*), pp. 261–306. Raven Press, New York.

11

Osteoporosis

INTRODUCTION
J. GRIMLEY EVANS

Osteoporosis, conceptualized as a condition characterized by a low amount of histologically normal bone tissue per volume of anatomical bone, is a multifactorial disorder. This implies that it may be the final common pathway of a wide variety of aetiological and pathogenic causal chains. The relative importance of these different pathways may well vary between populations and between groups within a population, and such heterogeneity may underlie some of the contradictory results of epidemiological and interventive studies in osteoporosis. For example, dietary calcium intake is less likely to emerge as an important risk factor for osteoporosis in a population with a uniformly high dietary intake than in one with a lower and more variable intake. In a population with uniformly low levels of physical activity the importance of activity as a determinant will be underestimated and oestrogen deficiency may seem to account for more of the variance between the osteoporotic and the normal than in a population with wider variation in physical activity levels.

A second common cause of confusion lies in the relationship between osteoporosis, as defined above, and fractures. There is no doubt that the incidence of proximal femoral fractures (PFF) varies with time and place. There has been a doubling of incidence in the UK since the 1950s,[1] an increase that is probably still going on in women if not in men.[2] Is this increase necessarily due to a rise in the prevalence of osteoporosis and is this in turn due to some factor that may afflict other developed or developing nations? A number of studies have pointed out that the relationship between PFF and osteoporosis is apparently less close than is commonly thought[3] and is reduced in the very old.[4] The great majority of fractures of the proximal femur occur as a consequence of a fall, and the prevalence of falls increases with age above 65 years.[5] It is not surprising therefore that the incidence of PFF also increases with age above 65. The incidence of distal forearm fracture does not show an increase over the same age range;[6] this indicates that with increasing age people are not only more likely to fall they are also less likely to get their arm out in time to break their fall (and their forearm)—therefore, perhaps, they are more likely to fall on their hip and fracture their femur.[7] Although at young ages, where falls are infrequent and protective responses intact, osteoporosis will emerge as the main difference between those members of a populations who fracture their hips and those who do not, in old age where osteoporosis is universal the variance between those who break their hips and those who do not will be accounted more by liability to falls and the state of the protective responses.[8] The overall incidence of PFF in the population may still be determined largely by the average population severity of osteoporosis, but osteoporosis will not reliably identify those members liable to PFF.

In its contribution to fracture incidence, osteoporosis is the main form of bone weakness that can be identified in elderly groups but is not necessarily the only one. Osteomalacia occurs in some populations,[9] though it may be getting rarer, and there may be other forms of bone weakness in old age, including dystrophic changes characterized by abnormal crystalline forms of bone mineral or perhaps defective matrix. It may also be important that osteoporosis comes about through an imbalance between the continuous remodelling activities of bone-resorbing osteoclasts and bone-producing osteoblasts. The biological function of this continuous turnover of bone is presumably to remove the microfractures ('fatigue fractures') that would inevitably accumulate in and weaken bone that was not being regularly replaced by new tissue.[10] Conceivably, therefore, bone weakness in an elderly person might arise through a reduction in the turnover rate of bone, with increase in the accumulation of fatigue fractures, independently of any reduction in the amount of bone to produce osteoporosis as normally defined. The presence of this, or other unidentified forms of bone weakness, in a population may confound the results of studies that focus only on osteoporosis.

Some of the current approaches to treatment employ processes that are probably unrelated in the great majority of patients to the underlying causes of osteoporosis. More is becoming known about the intricate linking of the activities of the osteoclasts and osteoblasts through local tissue factors and their modulation by influences, for example hormonal and physical stress, from outside the bone tissue.[11] There is evidence that, since bone reconstitution after osteoclast activity requires the presence of enough trabecular structure to form a template, osteoporosis may be to some extent a self-accelerating and essentially irreversible process. If this is true, the search for a cure for established osteoporosis may be vain. There is perhaps some hope in the hints that physical exercise may be able to increase bone mass,[12,13] while other treatments merely retard rate of loss. The scope for prevention, however, seems large, but the scale of the trials necessary to evaluate preventive programmes is daunting. The British National Osteoporosis Society has recently issued a consensus statement[14] recommending improved levels of physical activity and dietary calcium intake throughout life but especially during childhood and adolescence, and also the availability of carefully supervised hormone therapy to all menopausal women who desire it and who are free of medical contraindications. In drawing up this statement the Society worked from the two premises that the first requirement is to do no harm but the second is that it may not be wise to wait until the results of adequate trials are available. The Society also enjoins the public to co-operate in such trials.

Although adequately supervised oestrogen therapy in carefully selected cases carries only minimal risk, it would be desirable to restrict it to that minority of women who are liable to suffer the problems of osteoporosis if untreated. This may require the measurement of bone mass and its rate of decline, but present methods for doing this require expensive equipment and are accurate only in skilled hands. Newer techniques involving ultrasound attenuation[15] are promising but not yet reliable. The suggestion by Christiansen *et al.*[16] that a combination of anthropometric measurement with a few simple laboratory tests can identify the majority of women with rapid bone loss is of great interest, but it needs to be replicated in large numbers.

SCOPE FOR THE PREVENTION AND TREATMENT OF OSTEOPOROSIS

B. E. CHRISTOPHER NORDIN

BACKGROUND

'Osteoporosis' implies a low quantity of bone without any obvious abnormality in its quality. As a definition, osteoporosis can be said to be present in a bone or skeleton in which the amount of bony tissue per unit volume of anatomical bone falls below the lower normal limit in young adults of the same sex.[1,2] In simple terms, therefore, it represents a reduction in bone 'density' bearing in mind that it is the density of the whole (anatomical) bone rather than the density of the bony tissue itself which is implied.

Whole bone density falls with age in all human races so far studied; the same is probably true of other higher vertebrates. In women the process starts, or at least greatly accelerates, at the menopause, and in men it probably starts at about the age of 50–55, though this is less well documented. Because young women have a lower bone density than young men, because of the menopausal effect, and because women live longer than men, the social and medical complications of osteoporosis are far more significant in women than in men and this review will therefore concentrate largely on the former.

Table 11.1 Mean age ($\pm$ SE), forearm mineral density (FMD), forearm mineral content (FMC) and cross-sectional area of ulna and radius in 557 normal post-menopausal women divided into those who had fractured or never fractured in adult life

Variable	Fracture ($n = 135$)	Non-fracture ($n = 422$)	t	P
Age	58.5 $\pm$ 0.29	60.1 $\pm$ 0.52	2.8	<0.01
FMD (mg/cm^3)	359 $\pm$ 5.6	394 $\pm$ 3.5	5.0	<0.001
FMC (mg/cm)	973 $\pm$ 15.8	1031 $\pm$ 9.2	3.1	<0.001
Area (mm^2)	274 $\pm$ 3.6	264 $\pm$ 1.8	2.6	<0.01

Note that the difference in FMD between the two groups is more significant than the difference in FMC because the bone area is significantly greater in the fracture than non-fracture subjects.

There is a wide dispersion of bone mass in young adult women (normal range 30 per cent above and below the mean)[3] and this 'peak bone mass' is correctly regarded as playing a major role in the subsequent liability to osteoporosis. However, some of the variation in this peak bone mass is due to variation in bone size between individuals; when this is allowed for, the range of peak bone density is reduced to 22 per cent above and below the mean.[3] Since osteoporosis is defined in terms of density, and since fracture risk is more closely related to bone density than to bone mass (Table 11.1), it is peak bone density that is more truly relevant to osteoporosis in later life.

The loss of bone, which starts for practical purposes at the menopause, is rapid at first but slows down with time. The rapid component can be attributed to the menopause and the slower component to aging[4,5] (Fig. 11.1). This reflects the fact that the rate of bone loss is an inverse function of initial bone density.[4] it follows that those with the highest peak bone density lose bone most rapidly, at least in the early stages, and that those with the lowest peak bone density lose bone more slowly. Independently of the effect of initial density, there is a tendency for the rate of bone loss to diminish with time elapsed since menopause.[4] By definition, subjects at the bottom of the normal range must fall into the osteoporotic bone range very shortly after the menopause, whereas those with the highest initial densities may never fall below the normal lower limit even if they live into their 80s or 90s (Fig. 11.1). Those starting in the middle of the normal range cross the lower limit about 10 years after menopause (age about 60), at which point 50 per cent of women are suffering from osteoporosis by definition.

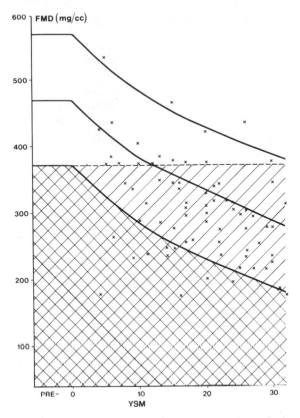

Fig. 11.1 Fall in forearm mineral density with time elapsed since menopause as calculated from data on 77 premenopausal and 557 normal postmenopausal women. The interrupted line represents the young normal lower limit. The single shading represents simple osteoporosis, and the double shading accelerated osteoporosis. The crosses represent postmenopausal women who have had vertebral and peripheral fractures.

The determinants of peak bone density are uncertain. Since there is little if any change in bone density from the early twenties until the menopause, the peak value must be established by the time growth ceases and is determined therefore in childhood and adolescence. It follows that there are likely to be genetic factors in peak bone density, a probable nutritional component during adolescence when calcium requirement is very high,[6] and possibly an effect of age at puberty—late puberty being associated with lower peak bone density.[7] (Late puberty may limit the time available for the normal adolescent rise in bone density[8,9] (Table 11.2).)

The peak bone density is the main determinant of subsequent bone

Table 11.2 Probable determinants of peak bone density in young women and of rates of bone loss after the menopause

Variable	Probable determinants
Peak bone density	Genetic factors Nutrition in adolescence (?) Age at puberty
Rate of bone loss	Initial bone density Years since menopause Plasma oestrogen Body mass index Calcium intake and absorption (?) Obligatory calcium loss Alcohol intake Tobacco consumption Caffeine intake (?)

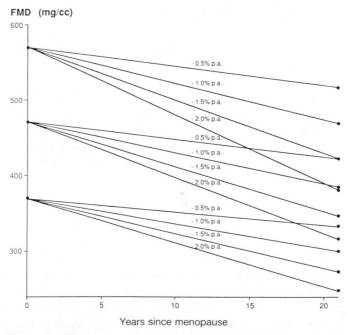

Fig. 11.2 The importance of peak bone density: the lines represent four different rates of bone loss after the menopause starting from the top, middle, and bottom of the normal range.

density for at least 10 years after the menopause because the premenopausal range of densities (±22 per cent) is large relative to the subsequent rate of loss (1–2 per cent per annum) (Fig. 11.2). After 10 to 15 years postmenopause, peak bone density plays a progressively diminishing role because of inter-individual variation in the rate of bone loss. Because of this variation, the bone density of some individuals—particularly those who start with low values—comes to fall below the lower limit of the *age-corrected* normal range; this condition has been called 'accelerated osteoporosis'.[1,2]

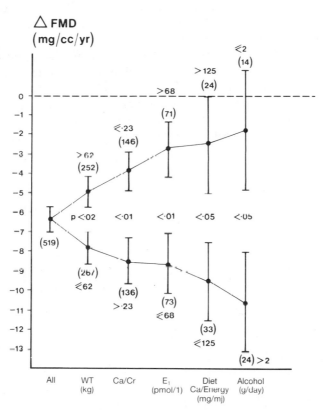

Fig. 11.3 Mean rate of change in forearm mineral density in 519 normal postmenopausal women (extreme left). The upper line represents those with high body mass index, low urine calcium, high serum E_1, high dietary calcium, and low alcohol intake. The lower line represents those with low body mass index, high urine calcium, low serum E_1, low dietary calcium, and high alcohol intake. The residual numbers after each subdivision are shown in parenthesis. Each subdivision was made at the median value of the independent variable and these criteria are shown at the top and bottom.

In normal women, the principal factors responsible for these inter-individual differences in the rates of bone loss—at least in peripheral (cortical) bone—are body mass index (BMI) (the higher the weight the slower is the loss), serum oestrogen (the higher the level the slower is the loss), alcohol (the higher the intake the faster is the loss), obligatory calcium excretion in the urine (the higher the output the faster is the loss), and dietary calcium intake (the higher the intake the slower is the loss,[4] though this has been questioned[10, 11] (Fig. 11.3; Table 11.2). These factors are probably operative on trabecular bone as well, but an additional important risk factor in spinal osteoporosis appears to be malabsorption of calcium,[12] which some workers attribute to a deficiency of $1,25 (OH)_2D$[13] but others more to gastrointestinal 'resistance' to the action of this vitamin D metabolite.[14]

The fall in bone density after the menopause is associated with a significant rise in fracture risk,[15–17] which is a continuous inverse function of bone density (Fig. 11.4) probably throughout life; there is no clearly defined threshold above which fractures do not occur and below which they do occur. However, if the fracture risk at the middle of the young adult range of bone density is defined as 1, then at one standard deviation

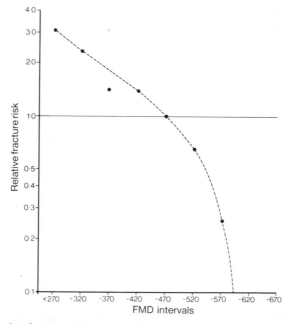

Fig. 11.4 Relative fracture risk as a function of forearm mineral density calculated from a study of 557 normal postmenopausal women of whom 135 had suffered fractures at some time in their adult life.

(SD) below the mean it is about 1.5, at two SD below the mean it is about 2, and at three SD below the mean (i.e in the osteoporotic range) it is about 3.[15] The cumulative rate of fracture in women is at least 30 per cent by the age of 80.[15]

BIOCHEMICAL EVENTS AT THE MENOPAUSE

The menopause is associated with a significant rise in plasma calcium concentration and an associated rise in obligatory calcium loss which raises the mean calcium requirement from about 550 mg to at least 700 mg per day.[6] The suggested calcium allowance for young adults is 800 mg per day and for postmenopausal women 1000 mg per day[6] but some would regard the latter as less than optimal.[18] There is an associated rise in urinary hydroxyproline (representing increased bone resorption) and in plasma alkaline phosphatase (representing a compensatory but inadequate increase in bone formation).[4] It has been suggested that the increase in plasma calcium (and consequent increase in urinary calcium) is the result of increased sensitivity of the bone to parathyroid hormone (PTH) in the absence of oestrogens[19, 20] but also that the changes are the result of a raised parathyroid gland set-point[21] which serves to maintain the plasma calcium (and therefore the urinary calcium) at a higher level in post- than in premenopausal women. Whichever is the correct explanation, and there may be some truth in both, the essential controversy centres on whether the increased obligatory loss of calcium is the *cause* or the *result* of osteoporosis. If it represents a genuine increase in calcium requirement, then calcium supplementation should play a role in prevention. If it is simply the result of the disease, then any therapy would have to be directed at the processes within the bone itself. In this connection, it should be noted that calcium deficiency causes osteoporosis in experimental animals[22] and that the loss of bone produced by oophorectomy in rats is much more significant when the animals are on a low-calcium than on a high-calcium intake.[23]

Reversibility of menopausal biochemical changes

There is general agreement that the biochemical abnormalities which appear at the menopause are reversible with oestrogen therapy; this is certainly true of the elevated plasma and urinary calcium, plasma alkaline phosphatase, and urinary hydroxyproline.[24, 25] Much less work has been done on the effect of calcium on these variables. Calcium supplements would not be expected to lower plasma or urinary calcium but possibly rather to lower urinary hydroxyproline (and ultimately plasma alkaline

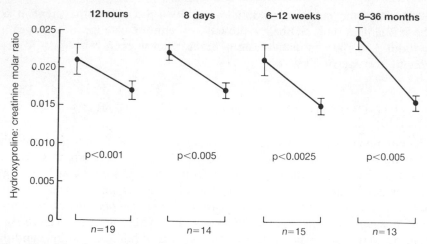

Fig. 11.5 Morning fasting urinary hydroxyproline before and at various time intervals after the regular administration of 1 gram effervescent calcium at 9 p.m. to osteoporotic women with normal calcium absorption. (Separate studies but some patients appear in more than one group.)

phosphatase), particularly if the high bone turnover was a response to loss of calcium in the urine operating through the parathyroid glands, since it is clear that calcium administration lowers serum PTH level in both normal and osteoporotic subjects.[26–28] In one study on 14 normal post-menopausal women,[29] calcium carbonate supplements had no effect on urinary hydroxyproline or plasma alkaline phosphatase, but in another study from the same group[30] there was a consistent rise in bone gla-protein (BGP) (which reflects bone turnover) when calcium supplements were stopped. In another study[27] urinary hydroxyproline fell after calcium administration in 10 normal subjects. In three other studies[31–33] the administration of 1 gram of effervescent calcium supplement each night had an immediate and sustained effect on the fasting urinary hydroxyproline of osteoporotic women with normal calcium absorption (Fig. 11.5) and a slower but equally sustained effect on plasma alkaline phosphatase, though neither to the extent produced by oestrogen. There is therefore a strong presumption that oral calcium inhibits bone turnover as oestrogen does, but not in the same way and not perhaps so effectively.

PREVENTION AND TREATMENT OF OSTEOPOROSIS

Introduction

Various agents have been used in attempts at prevention and treatment of osteoporosis. Preventive trials are generally directed at normal women close to the menopause but sometimes involve older subjects. They are designed to establish whether bone loss can be prevented or even reversed in a population that is normally losing bone at a significant rate.

Treatment trials are somewhat different. In clinical practice, the diagnosis of osteoporosis is generally made in subjects presenting with one or more crush fractures of the spine. This dates from the time when quantitative bone densitometry was not available but is still widely used as an entry criterion and can be justified by the fact that women with vertebral crush fractures (on average) have significantly less cortical and trabecular bone than do age-matched controls.[34–6] It follows that most studies on the treatment of osteoporosis have been confined to the treatment of women with vertebral compression. The treatments used can be broadly classified into those which are designed to prevent further loss of bone and those which are designed to increase bone density. Unfortunately, there are very few randomized controlled trials of treatment in spinal osteoporosis because the condition is widely recognized to be a progressive disorder in which vertebral compression is an irreversible event that increases pain and disability. In this situation, clinicians are reluctant to offer placebo to such patients and feel under pressure to prescribe treatment which they have reason to believe may be at least partially effective.

Hormones

There is general agreement that oestrogen administration delays or prevents bone loss in postmenopausal women, particularly when administered within a few years of the menopause when the bone loss is normally most rapid[373–41] There is also considerable evidence from case control studies[42, 43] and at least one prospective study[44] that oestrogen therapy reduces fracture rate.

It must be remembered, however, that oestrogens inhibit not only bone resorption but also bone formation because of the coupling of resorption and formation. Oestrogen treatment cannot therefore be expected to produce more than a marginal gain in bone—such as has been reported in subjects within about 3 and 6 years of the menopause.[45]

Moreover, the oestrogen effect on bone is dose dependent. The beneficial effects recorded have been obtained at doses of 0.625 mg daily of conjugated oestrogens or the equivalent in other preparations. At lower oestrogen doses (0.3 mg conjugated oestrogens or 10 mcg ethinyl oestradiol) bone loss continues at a rate not significantly different from that in untreated controls.[46–49]

Oestrogen therapy has been widely used on a largely empirical basis in postmenopausal osteoporosis, as originally recommended by Albright and colleagues[50] probably for the wrong reasons. The treatment reduces

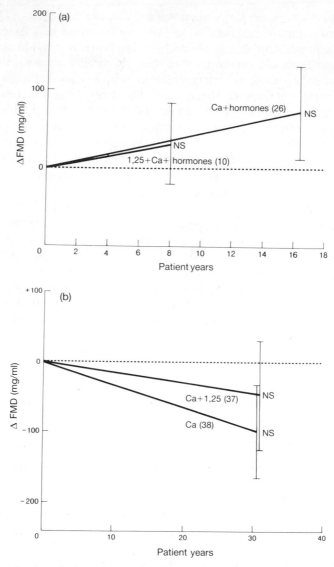

Fig. 11.6 (a) Cumulative change in forearm mineral density in osteoporotic women given oestrogen or progestogen in addition to calcium or calcium plus calcitriol. (b) Cumulative change in FMD in osteoporotic women with normal calcium absorption given calcium supplements (lower line) and in osteoporotic subjects with calcium malabsorption given both calcitriol and calcium (upper line). (c) Cumulative change in FMD in osteoporotic women given anabolic steroid treatment at the doses indicated for an average of 7 months. (Note this figure includes all treated cases irrespective of what other treatment was given at the same time.)

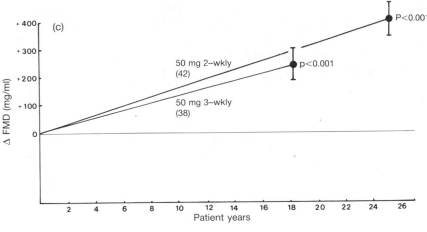

Fig. 11.6 (*cont.*)

urinary calcium in osteoporotic women[51, 52] and has also been reported to increase calcium absorption by some workers,[51] but not by others.[52] However, since the average age of women presenting with crush fractures is approximately 65 years, the uterine bleeding associated with oestrogen therapy may be unacceptable to the patient and oestrogens may confer a risk of cardiovascular complications in subjects with established atheroma. Moreover, since the most consistent effect of oestrogen therapy is that it lowers obligatory calcium loss *if the latter is high*, it is of doubtful value if the obligatory calcium is normal. If hormone therapy is to be used in such cases, it is probably preferable to use one of the progestogens, which has a similar effect on obligatory calcium loss without the dangers or side-effects of oestrogen[53, 54] and may even stimulate bone formation.[55, 56] There is therefore only a limited place for oestrogen treatment in established spinal osteoporosis and this mainly in younger patients in whom there may be other indications for such therapy. However, having said this, there may be a small but significant gain of bone in hormone-treated osteoporotic women compared with the small but non-significant loss seen in those on other forms of antiresorptive treatment[57] (Fig. 11.6).

Calcium supplementation

There has been much less work on the effects of calcium supplements than those of oestrogens on postmenopausal bone loss and the results with calcium are somewhat more controversial. In two early studies[38, 39] based on metacarpal morphometry and forearm densitometry (mainly cortical bone), calcium-supplemented subjects lost bone at a rate inter-mediate between those of untreated controls and of oestrogen-treated patients. In both studies, the rate of bone loss was not significantly different from zero in the calcium-treated subjects, but neither was it significantly different from the rate of loss in the controls. In another study in 14 postmenopausal women,[29] there was no significant loss of bone from the proximal forearm or whole skeleton in calcium-treated subjects but there was significant loss in the controls; the difference was significant in the proximal forearm. In another study on 24 70-year-old women, there was no loss of bone from the forearm during 12 months of calcium therapy.[58] (The metacarpal measurements in the paper are not valid because they do not allow for expansion of the bone.) In a 3-year study of the effect of exercise and/or calcium supplements in 80-year-old women,[59] forearm mineral content declined significantly in the controls, increased in the activity and calcium groups at a rate significantly differ-ent from the controls, and fell at a non-significant rate in the combined treatment group. In a 4-year study,[60] bone mineral content was measured in the forearm and humerus in 34 calcium-supplemented postmenopausal women and 33 controls. The authors reported a significant correlation between total calcium intake and bone loss in the humerus, but not in the radius. In another study on 70-year-old women[61] there was a just-significant increase in phalangeal bone after 6 months of calcium supple-mentation in 20 subjects, but there were no controls. In another study of just-postmenopausal women,[46] there was no significant loss of bone from the radius in 35 women given calcium supplements for 2 years, but the treated subjects were not significantly different from the controls who lost bone at a significant rate. (The cortical thickness measurements in this paper are again not valid for the reasons stated above.) In the most recently reported study,[62] there was a non-significant gain of forearm bone in 133 calcium-supplemented subjects and a significant loss in 72 controls over a period of 9 months. The difference between the treated and control subjects was significant (Table 11.3).

All the above studies are based on peripheral (cortical) bone or whole body calcium. In two recent studies[29, 46] trabecular bone loss from the spine in the immediate postmenopausal period was not prevented by calcium in 14 and 36 women respectively, but in one of these studies[46] calcium supplementation prevented spinal bone loss when given with a small dose of oestrogen, which given alone did not have any effect.

There have been no controlled trials of calcium therapy alone in clinical osteoporosis but in two uncontrolled studies it has been reported to reduce the vertebral fracture recurrence rate.[63, 64] Since malabsorption is a common feature of spinal osteoporosis[12, 13] and since oral calcium does not reduce hydroxyproline in such malabsorbing subjects,[65] calcium treat-

Table 11.3 Effects of dietary manipulation on forearm mineral content (FMC) in normal postmenopausal women observed for 9 months[4,62]

Regimen	n	Percentage change in FMC (annual rate)
Ca supplementation	133	+0.19 ± 0.23
Controls	71	−0.70 ± 0.33[a]
P		<0.05
Protein and/or salt restriction	84	−0.37 ± 0.34
Controls	60	−0.96 ± 0.38[a]
P		NS

[a] Significance of difference from zero: $P < 0.05$.

ment in this condition should probably be confined to subjects with normal calcium absorption or combined with a suitable vitamin D metabolite to correct calcium malabsorption (see below). In two uncontrolled clinical studies[57,64] there was no significant loss of bone in osteoporotic women with normal calcium absorption who were treated with calcium supplements (Fig. 11.6). In another study[66] there was significant bone loss in untreated postmenopausal women, no significant loss in osteoporotic women on calcium, and a significant gain with other forms of treatment. In an unpublished study in which calcium-supplemented patients were treated as controls for fluoride and calcium combination therapy, there was a very significant gain of cortical bone in the calcium-treated controls.[67]

The overall conclusion from these reports must be that calcium supplementation almost certainly reduces the rate of bone loss in postmenopausal women, at least in cortical bone, which comprises 80 per cent of the skeleton and the density of which is related to fracture risk.[15,17] Whether it can prevent the rapid loss of trabecular bone from the spine which immediately follows the menopause is at present much more doubtful but it must be remembered that in the sociomedical sense spinal osteoporosis (though important) is much less significant than peripheral fractures. Moreover, the apparent effect of calcium on vertebral fracture recurrence in osteoporotic patients[63,64] suggests that it may also play some role in the prevention of bone loss from the spine.

Vitamin D metabolites

At one time, heroic doses of vitamin D were used to overcome malabsorption of calcium in osteoporosis. This treatment is not effective either in correcting the calcium malabsorption[68] or in preventing further bone loss—in fact it may do more harm than good.[64]

The potent vitamin D metabolites, 1αOHD and 1,25 $(OH)_2D$, are increasingly used in the management of osteoporosis particularly, but not only, where malabsorption of calcium is present. There is no doubt about the positive effect of these metabolites on calcium absorption in osteoporotic women[65, 69] nor that they lower urinary hydroxyproline (indicating inhibition of bone resorption) particularly when combined with a calcium supplement.[65] They do involve a significant risk of hyper-calcaemia (particularly when combined with calcium) but this can be probably avoided if the dose if 1,25 $(OH)_2D$ is limited to 0.25 μg daily or the dose of 1αOHD to 0.5 μg daily. The effect of vitamin D analogues combined with calcium in subjects with malabsorption is similar to the effect of calcium alone in those with normal absorption—there is a small but non-significant loss of bone (Fig. 11.6). A possible reduction in vertebral fracture recurrence rate has been recorded in one small control-led trial.[70]

Calcitonin

It has been suggested that calcitonin deficiency may be a cause of osteoporosis, although the plasma calcitonin levels seems to be normal in this condition.[71, 72] Calcitonin is a powerful inhibitor of bone resorption; it is very effective in Paget's disease and has also been advocated for the treatment of osteoporosis. However, there have been very few controlled trials. In the most widely quoted study, synthetic salmon calcitonin in a daily dosage of 100 units was given for 24 months to 24 osteoporotic patients and the effect on total body calcium was compared with 21 controls.[73] At the end of 18 months, the total body calcium had increased by 2 per cent in the treated subjects; this was a significantly change compared with the fall of about 2 per cent in the controls ($P < 0.01$), but in the final 6 months of the trial there was a decline in total body calcium in the treated patients and an increase in total body calcium in the controls, with the result that the difference between the two was only just significant ($P < 0.05$) by the end of this period. In another study[74] total body calcium also rose in the first 18 months by nearly 3 per cent but once again declined in the next 6 months; there were no controls. In a much larger multicentre study,[75] relief of back pain and other subjective im-provement was reported to be better in the treated cases than in the controls but no objective measurements were made. However, a very significant inhibition of bone resorption by calcitonin has been reported in immobilization following paraplegia[76] when bone resorption is very high; it is possible that calcitonin therapy will find its greatest use in osteoporo-tic conditions of high, or very high bone turnover.

Diphosphonates

Since the diphosphonates are powerful inhibitors of bone resorption, and are used for this reason in the treatment of Paget's disease, attempts have been made to use them in the treatment of osteoporosis. In balance studies, a favourable effect has been reported in 12 osteoporotic patients with improvement in calcium absorption.[77] In a double-blind controlled study[78] osteoporotic patients were treated intermittently with 1200 to 1600 mg of chlodronate daily and their total body calcium was compared with that of controls. After 18 months, there was a 6 per cent increase in total body calcium in nine treated subjects, and a non-significant reduction in total body calcium in nine controls. The difference between the two groups was significant. In an unpublished study, favourable results were reported with the use of another diphosphonate (APD) in osteoporosis.[79] In the study referred to above[76] diphosphonate therapy was also found to inhibit bone loss after paraplegia. It must be remembered, however, that some diphosphonates produce 'osteomalacic'—type bone similar to that produced by sodium fluoride therapy and their long-term safety is therefore uncertain; this stricture may not apply to the new diphosphonate APD.

Thiazides

Thiazide diuretics have also been tested in the prevention of postmenopausal bone loss because they tend to reduce urinary calcium. In the only prospective study, there was an initial delay in bone loss lasting a few months, after which the treated subjects lost bone at the same rate as the controls.[41] On the other hand, there is one report that postmenopausal women taking thiazides have a slightly higher mean bone density than do controls.[80] There are no reports of the use of thiazides in the treatment of osteoporosis.

Protein, salt, and caffeine

In so far as urinary calcium excretion is a positive function of protein[81] and sodium[82] intake, it might be anticipated that protein and/or salt restriction would tend to inhibit postmenopausal bone loss. The only prospective study of the effect of protein and/or salt restriction on bone loss in postmenopausal women yielded results which were suggestive but not conclusive[4, 62] (Table 11.3). However, it has been suggested that the ability of some Third World populations to maintain skeletal integrity on lower calcium intakes than appear to be necessary in the Western world may be due to their lower dietary protein and salt, and therefore lower obligatory urinary calcium. It has also been reported[83] that calcium balance is adversely affected by caffeine, which increases urine calcium, but there has been no prospective trial of the effect of caffeine restriction on the rate of bone loss.

Exercise

Several attempts have been made to demonstrate the preventive value of exercise. In one study[84] on 27 women, vertebral density rose by about 3 per cent in 2 years in subjects undergoing 'physical training' but fell by about 2 per cent in the controls ($P < 0.01$). In another study,[85] total body calcium increased by about 3 per cent in 1 year in the exercise group and fell by nearly the same amount in the controls ($P < 0.001$). In another study,[86] there was a significant loss of bone in controls and 'walkers' but no significant loss in 'dancers' over a 6 month period. The favourable effect on bone density in 80-year-old women has already been mentioned.[61] The conclusion seems to be that fairly severe exercise can delay or prevent bone loss in postmenopausal women. Whether this effect is due to stimulation of bone formation or to inhibition of resorption is not clear—exercise may do both.

THERAPY DESIGNED TO PROMOTE BONE FORMATION

Anabolic steroids

In accordance with Albright's concept[50] that osteoporosis was due to impaired bone formation and should be treated with agents which promoted protein synthesis, a number of compounds appeared on the market in the 1960s which were essentially weak androgens and have come to be known as anabolic steroids. Their usefulness in osteoporosis was not tested by modern densitometric or histological techniques and with the progressive realization that high bone resorption was the main cause of osteoporosis they gradually fell into disrepute. More recently, it has come to be appreciated that control of bone resorption is not by itself an adequate treatment for osteoporosis, particularly since it leads to a secondary suppression of bone formation and cannot be expected to produce an actual gain of bone.[87] There has therefore been a resurgence of interest in these compounds, two of which have now been tested with modern densitometric techniques, both with positive results.

The first agent to be tried was stanozolol, an oral agent which was given in a dose of 2 mg three times a day for 3 out of every 4 weeks.[88] Twenty-one patients and 17 controls completed a study in which all subjects were maintained on a calcium intake of not less than 100 mg for a total period of 29 months. The total body calcium of stanozolol-treated subjects rose by just over 4 per cent; it was unchanged in the controls. The difference was significant ($P < 0.03$). Three new compression fractures occurred in the control group and none in the treated group.

The other anabolic agent which has been tested with modern techniques is 19-nortestosterone (nandrolone decanoate). In the first study, 11 osteoporotic patients were given 50 mg nandrolone decanoate by injection every 3 weeks for 2 years and their progress was followed by FMD.[89] Bone mineral content rose by almost 5 per cent in the treated group (mainly in the first year) but did not change in 'control' groups receiving 1αOHD or calcium infusions.

In an uncontrolled study in which nandrolone decanoate in a dose of 50 mg every 2–3 weeks was added to current anti-resorptive treatment, there was a very significant gain of bone in 80 patients[57] (Fig. 11.6c). In 52 of these patients, bone changes were recorded before or after the treatment as well as during therapy.[90] There was significant gain in forearm mineral content during nandrolone decanoate therapy and a non-significant loss of bone in the same subjects before or after this treatment. The difference between the rates of change on and off treatment was highly significant ($P < 0.001$) and the average gain of bone on treatment corresponded to an annual rate of over 5 per cent. Any other treatments being given at the same time were continued throughout the study.

These studies appear to show that osteoporotic patients can gain bone on anabolic steroid treatment, though how long this gain can continue is unknown.

Sodium fluoride

The high bone density which is a feature of patients with fluorosis has served as the basis for the extensive use of sodium fluoride in the treatment of osteoporosis extending back to the 1960s—despite the fact that fluorotic bone is known to be liable to fracture. There is a significant incidence of side-effects on the usual daily dose of about 50 mg sodium fluoride[91] and blood level monitoring is recommended. Iliac crest biopsies have demonstrated an increase in trabecular bone density in about half the subjects so treated[92] but the new bone formed is abnormal and coated with osteoid, as if osteomalacic. A very significant reduction in fracture recurrence rate has been reported in an uncontrolled study[65] but the most convincing report to date of a significant increase in vertebral (but not cortical) bone has not yet been published.[69]

Interpretation of the response to fluoride has been complicated by the fact that this treatment is usually combined with large doses of calcium and/or vitamin D,[93] designed to prevent 'osteomalacia', however, whether this 'osteomalacia' can in fact be prevented in such a way is itself a controversial subject. Moreover, the advocates of fluoride treatment claim only an effect on trabecular bone; it is unlikely therefore to prevent peripheral, including hip, fractures.

There is only one published trial of the preventive action of sodium fluoride on bone loss in normal women.[41] In this study, the bone loss in treated postmenopausal women was no less than in a placebo-treated control group. It has been reported that there is less osteoporosis in areas where water fluoride is high than where it is low,[94] but this report predated the modern techniques of bone densitometry. A recent report from Finland showed no difference in the incidence of hip fractures between regions of high and low water fluoride.[95]

Parathyroid hormone

The stimulatory effect of PTH on bone formation (as well as resorption) has been used as the basis for cyclical treatment with PTH injections as part of the so-called ADFR regime. The object of ADFR (activation, depression, formation, and repetition) is to activate bone formation by activating bone resorption, then to depress resorption in the hope that the high formation rate will be sustained, and then to repeat the cycle. This highly theoretical approach to treatment has not yet been in use long enough to demonstrate its efficacy but a recent report offered persuasive evidence of increased vertebral density in a group of osteoporotic patients treated in this way.[96] In other variants of this approach, inorganic phosphate has been given continuously to stimulate bone resorption (and so formation) and calcitonin intermittently to depress the resorption;[97] in yet another variant fluoride therapy has been given on a cyclical basis.[98] None of these treatments can yet be said to have reached the stage of practical application or widespread use.

CONCLUSIONS

Present evidence suggests that bone density in young adult life is determined during childhood and adolescence by genetic, hormonal, and nutritional factors. Once established in the early twenties it does not change significantly in most women until the menopause. There follows a relatively rapid loss of bone immediately after the menopause; this continues at a diminishing rate for about 20 years. It is associated with a sharp rise in the incidence of fractures of all kinds, the individual fracture risk being an inverse function of bone density. Because there is a wide range of peak bone density in young adults, this value is a major determinant of bone density and therefore of fracture risk for at least 10 to 15 years after the menopause. Although the overall pattern is similar in men, the fracture prevalence is much lower because they have a higher peak bone density, no acute menopausal bone loss, and die younger than women.

There is little doubt that postmenopausal bone loss is wholly or partly preventable, definitely with medium- or high-dose hormone therapy, probably with calcium therapy, and very probably with a combination of low-dose hormone therapy and calcium. However, the main determinant of postmenopausal bone density, and therefore of fracture risk, for many years after the menopause is the initial bone density at menopause. For all practical purposes, preventive therapy need not be directed at women whose initial bone density is high because they are unlikely to develop significant osteoporosis unless they live a very long time or suffer from significant risk factors to accelerate their bone loss—some of which (low body weight, significant alcohol intake) can easily be identified. It should be directed instead at those whose initial density is low. The only way in which those with low initial bone density can be identified is by some form of mass screening densitometry, of which the only practical type is forearm densitometry. The introduction of such densitometry on a wide scale is being delayed for several reasons. First, some workers believe that spinal densitometry is more appropriate, despite the fact that the cost of its use for screening purposes would be prohibitive and the information obtained similar to that from the forearm;[99] second not everyone is convinced of the relationship between bone density and fracture risk; third, the effectiveness of preventive measures is still not generally recognized; fourth, perhaps, there is the fear that large-scale screening densitometry may yield inappropriate profits to the owners of densitometers.[100] Also the medical insurance agencies and government bodies are alarmed at the possible costs incurred by screening despite the probable long-term saving. These issues will need to be resolved in the near future.

As far as the treatment of established osteoporosis is concerned, the condition is poorly managed by all but a few specialist clinicians, largely out of ignorance of specific therapy. Many patients with established bone disease are still not receiving the anti-resorptive agents which are now available to prevent deterioration, and only a very small proportion are receiving therapy calculated to promote bone formation and increase bone mass, as appears to be possible with certain at least of the anabolic steroids and perhaps with sodium fluoride.

ACKNOWLEDGEMENT

Prepared for the Expert Committee on Health of the Elderly, Geneva, November 1987.

References

Introduction

1. Boyce, W. J. and Vessey, M. P. (1985). Rising incidence of fracture of the proximal femur. *Lancet*, **1**, 150–2.
2. Evans, J. G. (1985). Incidence of proximal femoral fracture. *Lancet*, **1**, 925–6.
3. Aitken, J. M. (1984). Relevance of osteoporosis in women with fracture of the femoral neck. *British Medical Journal 1984*, **288**, 597–601.
4. Cooper, C., Barker, D. J. P., Morris, J., and Briggs, R. S. J. (1987). Osteoporosis, falls, and age in fracure of the proximal femur. *British Medical Journal*, **295**, 13–15.
5. Prudham, D. and Evans, J. G. (1981). Factors associated with falls in the elderly: a community study. *Age and Ageing*. **10**, 141–6.
6. Miller, S. W. M. and Evans, J. G. (1985). Fractures of the distal forearm in Newcastle: an epidemiological survey. *Age and Ageing*, **14**, 155–8.
7. Evans, J. G. (1982). Epidemiology of proximal femoral fracture. In *Recent advances in geriatric medicine 2* (ed. Isaacs, B.) pp. 201–14. Churchill Livingstone, Edinburgh.
8. Boyce, W. J. (1987). Osteoporosis, falls, and age in fracture of the proximal femur. *British Medical Journal*, **295**, 444–5.
9. Aaron, J. E., Gallagher, J. C., Anderson, J., Stasiak, L., Longton, E. B., Nordin, B. E. C., and Nicholson, M. (1974). Frequency of osteomalacia and osteoporosis in fractures of the proximal femur. *Lancet*, **1**, 229–33.
10. Burr, B., Martin, R. B., Schaffler, M. B., Radin, E. L. (1985). Bone modelling in response to in vivo fatigue microdamage. *Journal of Biochemistry*, **18**, 189–200.
11. Raisz, L. G. (1988). Local and systemic factors in the pathogenesis of osteoporosis. *New England Journal of Medicine*, **318**, 818–28.
12. Krolner, B., Toft, B., Nielsen, S. P., and Tondevold, E. (1983). Physical exercise as prophylaxis against involutional vertebral bone loss: a controlled trial. *Clinical Science*, **64**, 541–6.
13. Chow, R., Harrison, J. E., and Notarius, C. (1987). Effect of two randomised exercise programmes on bone mass of healthy postmenopausal women. *British Medical Journal*, **295**, 1441–4.
14. National Osteoporosis Society (1987). *Consensus statement*. National Osteoporosis Society, Bath.
15. Rubin, C. T., Pratt, G. W., Porter, A. L., Lanyon, L. E., and Poss, R. (1987). The use of ultrasound in vivo to determine acute change in the mechanical properties of bone following intense physical activity. *Journal of Biomechanics*, **20**, 723–7.

16. Christiansen, C., Riis, B. J., and Rodbro, P. (1987). Prediction of rapid bone loss in post-menopausal women. *Lancet*, **1**, 1105–8.

Prevention and treatment

1. Nordin, B. E. C., Crilly, R. G., and Smith, D. A. (1984). Osteoporosis. In *Metabolic bone and stone disease* (ed. Nordin, B. E. C.), pp. 1–70. Churchill Livingstone, Edinburgh.
2. Bancroft, J., Burger, H. G., Devi, P. K. *et al.* (1981). *Research on the menopause*. Report of a WHO Scientific Group. World Health Organization Technical Report Series 670, Geneva.
3. Nordin, B. E. C., Chatterton, B. E., Steurer, T. A., and Walker C. J. (1986). Forearm bone mineral content does not fall with age in premenopausal women. *Clinical Orthopaedics and Related Research*, **211**, 252–6.
4. Nordin, B. E. C. and Polley, K. J. (1987). Metabolic consequences of the menopause. A cross-sectional, longitudinal and intervention study on 557 normal postmenopausal women. *Calcified Tissue International*, **41**, Suppl., (in press).
5. Johnston, C. C. Jr, Norton, J. A. Jr, Khairi, R. A., and Longcope, C. (1979). Age-related bone loss: In *Osteoporosis* II (ed. Barzel, U.S.) pp. 91–100. Grune & Stratton, New York.
6. Nordin, B. E. C. (1986). Calcium. *Commonwealth Department of Health Journal of Food and Nutrition*, **42**, 67–82.
7. Johnell, O. and Nilsson, B. E. (1984). Life-style and bone mineral mass in perimenopausal women. *Calcified Tissue International*, **36**, 354–6.
8. Garn, S. M. (1970). *The earlier gain and later loss of cortical bone*. Charles C. Thomas, Springfield, Illinois.
9. Riis, B. J., Krabbe, S., Christiansen, C., Catherwood, B. D., and Deftos, L. J. (1985). Bone turnover in male puberty: a longitudinal study. *Calcified Tissue International*, **37**, 213–17.
10. Nilas, L., Christiansen, C., and Rodbro, P. (1984). Calcium supplementation and postmenopausal bone loss. *British Medical Journal*, **289**, 1103–6.
11. Riggs, B. L., Wahner, H. W., Melton III, L. J., O'Fallon, W. M., Judd, H. L., and Richelson, L. S. (1986). In women dietary calcium intake and rates of bone loss from midradius and lumbar spine are not related. *Journal of Bone Mineral Research*, (Suppl.) **1**, Abstr. 167.
12. Nordin, B. E. C., Robertson, A., Seamark, R. F. *et al.* (1985). The relation between calcium absorption, serum dehydroepiandrosterone, and vertebral mineral density in postmenopausal women. *Journal of Clinical Endocrinology and Metabolism*, **60**, 651–7.
13. Gallagher, J. C., Riggs, B. L., Eisman, J., Hamstra, A., Arnaud, S. B., and DeLuca, H. F. (1979). Intestinal calcium absorption and serum vitamin D metabolites in normal subjects and osteoporotic patients. *Journal of Clinical Investigation*, **64**, 729–36.
14. Morris, H. A., O'Loughlin, P. D., Need, A. G., Horowitz, M., Hartley, T. F., and Nordin, B. E. C. (1987). Gastrointestinal resistance to 1,25 $(OH)_2D_3$ as a risk factor for osteoporosis in postmenopausal women. In *Calcium regulation and bone metabolism* (ed. Cohn, D. V., T. J. Martin, and P. J. Meunier), p. 616–25. Elsevier, Amsterdam.

15. Nordin, B. E. C., Chatterton, B. E., Walker, C. J., and Wishart, J. (1987). The relation of forearm mineral density to peripheral fractures in postmenopausal women. *Medical Journal of Australia*, **146**, 300–4.

16. Wasnich, R. D., Ross, P. D., Heilbrun, L. K., and Vogel, J. M. (1985). Prediction of postmenopausal fracture risk with use of bone mineral measurements. *American Journal of Obstetrics and Gynecology*, **153**, 745–51.

17. Jensen, G. F., Christiansen, C., Boesen, J., Hegedus, V., and Transbol, I. (1983). Relationship between bone mineral content and frequency of postmenopausal fractures. *Acta Medica Scandinavica*, **213**, 61–3.

18. Heaney, R. P., Recker, R. R., and Saville, P. D. (1977). Calcium blance and calcium requirements in middle-aged women. *American Journal of Clinical Nutrition*, **30**, 1603–11.

19. Jasani, C., Nordin, B. E. C., Smith, D. A., and Swanson, I. (1965). Spinal osteoporosis and the menopause. *Proceedings of the Royal Society of Medicine*, **58**, 441–4.

20. Heaney, R. P. (1965). A unified concept of osteoporosis. *American Journal of Medicine*, **39**, 877–80.

21. Francis, R. M., Peacock, M., Taylor, G. A., Kahn, A. J., and Teitelbaum, S. L. (1985). How do oestrogens modulate bone resorption? In *Vitamin D, chemical, biochemical and clinical update* (ed. Norman, A. W., K. Schaefer, H.-G Grigoleit, and D. V. Herrath) pp. 479–82. Walter de Gruyter, Berlin.

22. Nordin, B. E. C. (1960). Osteomalacia, osteoporosis and calcium deficiency. *Clinical Orthopaedics*, **17**, 235–58.

23. Hodgkinson, A., Aaron, J. E., Horsman, A., McLachlan, M. S. F., and Nordin, B. E. C. (1978). Effect of oophorectomy and calcium deprivation on bone mass in the rat. *Clinical Science and Molecular Medicine*, **54**, 439–46.

24. Nordin, B. E. C. and Peacock, M. (1983). Calcium and bone metabolism. In *Progress in clinical medicine* (ed. Horler, A. R. and J. B. Foster), pp. 287–315. Churchill Livingstone, Edinburgh.

25. Christiansen, C., Rodbro, P., and Tjellesen, L. (1984). Serum alkaline phosphatase during hormone treatment in early postmenopausal women. *Acta Medica Scandinavica*, **216**, 11–17.

26. Goddard, M., Young, G., and Marcus, R. (1986). Short-term effects of calcium carbonate, lactate, and gluconate on the calcium-parathyroid axis in normal elderly men and women. *American Journal of Clinical Nutrition*, **44**, 653–8.

27. Reid, I. R., Schooler, B. A., Hannan, S. F., and Ibbertson, H. K. (1986). The acute biochemical effects of four proprietary calcium preparations. *Australian and New Zealand Journal of Medicine*, **16**, 193–7.

28. Horowitz, M., Morris, H. A., Hartley, T. F. *et al.* (1987). The effect of an oral calcium load on plasma ionized calcium and parathyroid hormone concentrations in osteoporotic postmenopausal women. *Calcified Tissue International*, **40**, 133–6.

29. Riis, B., Thomsen, K., and Christiansen, C. (1987). Does calcium supplementation prevent postmenopausal bone loss? *New England Journal of Medicine*, **316**, 173–7.

30. Podenphant, J., Christiansen, C., Catherwood, B. D., and Deftos, L. J. (1985). Serum bone Gla protein and other biochemical estimates of bone

turnover in early postmenopausal women during prophylactic treatment for osteoporosis. *Acta Medica Scandinavica*, **218**, 329–33.

31. Horowitz, M., Need, A. G., Philcox, J. C., and Nordin, B. E. C. (1984). Effect of calcium supplementation on urinary hydroxyproline in osteoporotic postmenopausal women. *American Journal of Clinical Nutrition*, **39**, 857–9.

32. Horowitz, M., Need, A. G., Philcox, J. C., and Nordin, B. E. C. (1985). The effect of calcium supplements on plasma alkaline phosphatase and urinary hydroxyproline in postmenopausal women. *Hormone Metabolic Research*, **17**, 311–12.

33. Need, A. G., Horowitz, M., Philcox, J. C. and Nordin, B. E. C. (1987). Biochemical effects of a calcium supplement in osteoporotic postmenopausal women with normal absorption and malabsorption of calcium. *Mineral Electrolyte Metabolism*, **13**, 112–16.

34. Cohn, S. H., Aloia, J. F., Vaswani, A. N., Yuen, K., Yasmura, S., and Ellis, K. J. (1986). Women at risk for developing osteoporosis: determination by total body neutron activation analysis and photon absorptiometry. *Calcified Tissue International*, **38**, 9–15.

35. Seeman, E., Wahner, W., Offord, K. P., Kumar, R., Johnson, W. J., and Riggs, B. L. (1982). Differential effects of endocrine dysfunction on the axial and the appendicular skeleton. *Journal of Clinical Investigation*, **69**, 1302–9.

36. Johnston, C. C., Norton, J., Khairi, M. R. A. *et al.* (1985). Heterogeneity of fracture syndromes in postmenopausal women. *Journal of Clinical Endocrinology and Metabolism*, **61**, 551–6.

37. Lindsay, R., Aitken, J. M., Anderson, J. B., Hart, D. M., MacDonald, E. B., and Clarke, A. C. (1976). Long-term prevention of post-menopausal osteoporosis by oestrogen. *Lancet*, **i**, 1038–41.

38. Recker, R. R., Saville, P. D., and Heaney, R. P. (1977). Effect of estrogens and calcium carbonate on bone loss in postmenopausal women. *Annals of Internal Medicine*, **87**, 649–55.

39. Horsman, A., Gallagher, J. C., Simpson, M., and Nordin, B. E. C. (1977). Prospective trial of oestrogen and calcium in postmenopausal women. *British Medical Journal*, **2**, 789–92.

40. Nachtigall, L. E., Nachtigall, R. H., Nachtigall, R. D., and Beckman, M. (1979). Estrogen replacement therapy I: a 10-year prospective study in the relationship of osteoporosis. *Obstetrics and Gynecology*, **53**, 277–81.

41. Christiansen, C., Christiansen, M. S., McNair, P., Hagen, C., Stocklund, E., and Transbol, I. (1980). Prevention of early postmenopausal bone loss: controlled 2-year study in 315 normal females. *European Journal of Clinical Investigation*, **10**, 273–9.

42. Hutchinson, T. A., Polansky, S. M., and Feinstein, A. R. (1979). Postmenopausal oestrogens protect against fractures of distal hip and radius. *Lancet*, **ii**, 705–9.

43. Paganini-Hill, A., Ross, R. K., Gerkins, V. R., Henderson, B. E., Arthur, M., and Mack, T. M. (1981). Menopausal estrogen therapy and hip fractures. *Annals of Internal Medicine*, **95**, 28–31.

44. Ettinger, B., Genant, H. K., and Cann, C. E. (1985). Long-term estrogen replacement therapy prevents bone loss and fractures. *Annals of Internal Medicine*, **102**, 319–24.

45. Abdalla, H., Hart, D. M., and Lindsay, R. (1984). Differential bone loss and effects of long-term estrogen therapy according to time of introduction of therapy after oophorectomy. In *Osteoporosis* (ed. Christiansen, C., Arnaud, C. D., B. E. C. Nordin, A. M. Parfitt, W. A. Peck, and B. L. Riggs) Proceedings of Copenhagen International Symposium on Osteoporosis, pp. 621–3. Glostrup Hospital, Denmark.

46. Ettinger, B., Genant, H. K., and Cann, C. E. (1987). Postmenopausal bone loss is prevented by treatment with low-dosage estrogen with calcium. *Annals of Internal Medicine*, **106**, 40–5.

47. Horsman, A., Jones, M., Francis, R., and Nordin, B. E. C. (1983). The effect of estrogen dose on postmenopausal bone loss. *New England Journal of Medicine*, **309**, 1405–7.

48. Christiansen, C., Christensen, M. S., Larsen, N.-E., and Transbol, I. B. (1982). Pathophysiological mechanisms of estrogen effect on bone metabolism. Dose-response relationships in early postmenopausal women. *Journal of Clinical Endocrinology and Metabolism*, **55**, 1124–30.

49. Lindsay, R., Hart, D. M., and Clark, D. M. (1984). The minimum effective dose of estrogen for prevention of postmenopausal bone loss. *Obstetrics and Gynecology*, **63**, 759–63.

50. Albright, F. and Reifenstein, E. (1948). *The parathyroid glands and metabolic bone disease*. Williams and Wilkins, Baltimore.

51. Gallagher, J. C., Riggs, B. L., DeLuca, H. F. (1980). Effect of estrogen on calcium absorption and serum vitamin D metabolites in postmenopausal osteoporosis. *Clinical Endocrinology and Metabolism*, **51**, 1359–64.

52. Crilly, R. G., Horsman, A., Peacock, M., and Nordin, B. E. C. (1981). The vitamin D metabolites in the pathogenesis and management of osteoporosis. *Current Medical Research and Opinion*, **7**, 337–47.

53. Abdalla, H. I., Hart, D. M., Lindsay, R., Leggate, I., and Hooke, A. (1985). Prevention of bone mineral loss in postmenopausal women by norethisterone. *Obstetrics and Gynecology*, **66**, 789–92.

54. Gallagher, J. C. and Nordin, B. E. C. (1975). Effects of oestrogen and progestogen therapy on calcium metabolism in post-menopausal women. In *Estrogens in the post-menopause* (ed. van Keep, P. A. and C. Lauritzen, Frontiers of Hormone Research, Vol. 3, pp. 150–76. Karger, Basel.

55. Christiansen, C., Nilas, L., Riis, B. J., Rodbro, P., and Deftos, L. (1985). Uncoupling of bone formation and resorption by combined oestrogen and progestagen therapy in postmenopausal osteoporosis. *Lancet*, **ii**, 800–1.

56. Lindsay, R., Hart, D. M., Purdie, D., Ferguson, M. M., Clark, A. S., and Kraszewski, A. (1978). Comparative effects of oestrogen and a progestogen on bone loss in postmenopausal women. *Clinical Science*, **54**, 193–5.

57. Need, A. G., Chatterton, B. E., Walker, C. J., Steurer, T. A., Horowitz, M., and Nordin, B. E. C. Comparison of calcium, calcitriol, ovarian hormones and nandrolone in the treatment of osteoporosis. *Maturitas*, **8**, 275–80.

58. Jensen, G. F., Christiansen, C., and Transbol, I. (1982). Treatment of post menopausal osteoporosis. A controlled therapeutic trial comparing oestrogen/gestagen 1,25-dihydroxy-vitamin D_3 and calcium. *Clinical Endocrinology*, **16**, 515–24.

59. Smith, E. L., Reddan, W., and Smith, P. E. (1981). Physical activity and

calcium modalities for bone mineral increase in aged women. *Medical Science of Sports Exercise*, **13**, 60–4.

60. Freudenheim, J. L., Johnson, N. E., Smith, E. L. (1986). Relationships between usual nutrient intake and bone-mineral content of women 35–65 years of age: longitudinal and cross-sectional analysis. *American Journal of Clinical Nutrition*, **44**, 863–76.

61. Lee, C. J., Lawler, G. S., and Johnson, G. H. (1981). Effects of supplementation of the diets with calcium and calcium-rich foods on bone density of elderly females with osteoporosis. *American Journal of Clinical Nutrition*, **34**, 819–23.

62. Nordin, B. E. C., Polley, K. J., Need, A. G., Morris, H. A., and Marshall D. (1987). The problem of calcium requirement. *American Journal of Clinical Nutrition*, **45**, 1295–304.

63. Riggs, B. L., Seeman, E., Hodgson, S. F., Taves, D. R., and O'Fallon, W. M. (1982). Effect of the fluoride/calcium regimen on vertebral fracture occurring in postmenopausal osteoporosis. *New England Journal of Medicine*, **306**, 446–50.

64. Nordin, B. E. C., Horsman, A., Crill, A. G., Marshall, D. H., and Simpson, M. (1980). Treatment of spinal osteoporosis in postmenopausal women. *British Medical Journal*, **280**, 451–4.

65. Need, A. G., Horowitz, M., Philcox, J. C., and Nordin, B. E. C. (1985). 1,25-dihydroxycalciferol and calcium therapy in osteoporosis with calcium malabsorption. *Mineral and Electrolyte Metabolism*, **11**, 35–40.

66. Aloia, J. F., Ross, P., Vaswani, A., Zanzi, I., and Cohn, S. H. (1982). Rate of bone loss in postmenopausal and osteoporotic women. *American Journal of Physiology (Endocrinology and Metabolism 5)*, **242**, E82–E86.

67. Riggs, B. L. (1987). Data presented to the Fourth International Conference on Bone, Sydney, March.

68. Francis, R. M., Peacock, M., Taylor, G. A., Storer, J. H., and Nordin, B. E. C. (1984). Calcium malabsorption in elderly women with vertebral fractures: evidence for resistance to the action of vitamin D metabolites on the bowel. *Clinical Science*, **66**, 103–7.

69. Gallagher, J. C., Jerbak, C. M., Jee W. S. S., Johnson, K. A., DeLuca, H. F., and Riggs, B. L. (1982). 1,25-dihydroxyvitamin D_3: short- and long-term effects on bone and calcium metabolism in patients with postmenopausal osteoporosis. *Proceedings of the National Academy of Sciences, USA*, **70**, 3325–9.

70. Gallagher, J. C. (1983). The use of calcitriol (1,25 dihydroxyvitamin D) in osteoporosis. In *Clinical disorders in bone and mineral metabolism* (ed. Frame, B. and J. T. Potts Jr), pp. 364–7. Excerpta Medica, Amsterdam.

71. Chesnut, C. H. III, Baylink, D. J., Sisom, K., Nelp, W. J., and Roos, B. A. (1980). Basal plasma immunoreactive calcitonin in postmenopausal osteoporosis. *Metabolism*, **29**, 559–62.

72. Tiegs, R. D., Body, J. J., Wahner, H. W., Barta, J., Riggs, B. L., and Heath, H. III (1985). Calcitonin secretion in postmenopausal osteoporosis. *New England Journal of Medicine*, **312**, 1097–100.

73. Gruber, H. E., Ivey, J. L., Baylink, D. J. *et al.* (1984). Long-term calcitonin therapy in postmenopausal osteoporosis. *Metabolism*, **33**, 295–303.

74. Aloia, J. F., Vaswani, A., Kapoor, A., Yeh, J. K., Cohn, S. H. (1985).

Treatment of osteoporosis with calcitonin, with and without growth hormone. *Metabolism*, **34**, 124–9.

75. Mazzuoli, G. F., Passeri, M., Gennari, C. *et al.* (1986). Effects of salmon calcitonin in postmenopausal osteoporosis: a controlled double-blind clinical study. *Calcified Tissue International*, **38**, 3–8.

76. Minaire, P., Meunier, P., Edouard, C. *et al.* (1982). Acute osteoporosis in paraplegic patients: pathophysiology and effects of treatment with calcitonin or dichlorodimethylene diphosphonate. In *Osteoporosis*(ed. Menczel, J., G. C. Robin, M. Makin, and R. Steinberg), pp. 421–8. Wiley, New York.

77. Heaney, R. P. and Saville, P. D. (1976). Etidronate disodium in postmenopausal osteoporosis. *Clinical Pharmacology and Therapeutics*, **20**, 593–604.

78. Chesnut, C. H. III (1984). Synthetic salmon calcitonin, diphosphonates, and anabolic steroids in the treatment of postmenopausal osteoporosis. In *Osteoporosis* (ed. Christiansen, C., C. B. Arnaud, B. E. C. Nordin, A. M. Parfitt, W. A. Peck, and B. L. Riggs) pp. 549–55, Munksgaard, Copenhagen.

79. Sorensen, H. (1987). Data presented to the Consensus on Osteoporosis Conference, Washington, February.

80. Wasnich, R. D., Benfante, R. J., Yano, K., Heilbrun, L., and Vogel, J. M. (1983). Thiazide effect on the mineral content of bone. *New England Journal of Medicine*, **309**, 344–7.

81. Linkswiler, H. M., Zemel, M. B., Hegsted, M., and Schuette, S. (1981). Protein-induced hypercalciuria. *Federation Proceedings*, **40**, 2429–33.

82. Goulding, A. (1983). Effects of varying dietary salt intake on the fasting urinary excretion of sodium, calcium and hydroxyproline in young women. *New Zealand Medical Journal 1983*, **96**, 853–4.

83. Heaney, R. P. and Recker, R. R. (1982). Effects of nitrogen, phosphorus, and caffeine on calcium balance in women. *Journal of Laboratory and Clinical Medicine*, **99**, 46–55.

84. Krolner, B., Toft, B., Pors-Nielsen, S., and Tondevold, E. (1983). Physical exercise as prophylaxis against involutional vertebral bone loss: a controlled trial. *Clinical Science*, **64**, 541–6.

85. Aloia, J. F., Cohn, S. H., Ostuni, J. A., Cane, R., and Ellis, K. (1978). Prevention of involutional bone loss by exercise. *Annals of Internal Medicine*, **89** (3), 356–8.

86. White, M. K., Martin, R. B., Yeater, R. A., Butcher, R. L., and Radin, E. L. (1984). The effects of exercise on the bones of postmenopausal women. *International Orthopaedics*, **7**, 209–14.

87. Riggs, B. L. and Melton, J. III (1986). Involutional osteoporosis. *New England Journal of Medicine*, **314**, 1676–85.

88. Chesnut, C. H. III, Ivey, J. L., Gruber, H. E., Matthews, M., Nelp, W. B., Sisom, K., and Baylink, D. J. (1983). Stanozolol in postmenopausal osteoporosis: therapeutic efficacy and possible mechanisms of action. *Metabolism*, **32**, 571–80.

89. Dequeker, J. and Geusens, P. (1985). Anabolic steroids and osteoporosis. *Acta Endocrinologica*, Suppl. **271**, 45–51.

90. Need, A. G., Horowitz, M., Morris, H. A., Walker, C. J., and Nordin, B. E. C. (1987). Effects of nandrolone therapy on forearm bone mineral content in osteoporosis. *Clinical Orthopaedics and Related Research*, **225**, 273–8.

91. Riggs, B. L., Hodgson, S. F., Hoffman, D. L., Kelly, P. J., Johnson, K. A., and Taves, D. (1980). Treatment of primary osteoporosis with fluoride and calcium. *Journal of the American Medical Association*, **243**, 446–9.
92. Meunier, P. J., Galus, K., Briancon, D., Edouard, X., and Charhon, S. A. Treatment of idiopathic osteoporosis with sodium fluoride. In *Clinical disorders of bone and mineral metabolism*. (ed. Frame, B. and J. T. Potts Jr), pp. 360–3. Excerpta Medica, Amsterdam.
93. Jowsey, J., Riggs, B. L., Kelly, P. J., and Hoffman, D. L. (1972). Effect of combined therapy with sodium fluoride, vitamin D and calcium in osteoporosis. *American Journal of Medicine*, **53**, 43–9.
94. Bernstein, D. S., Sadowsky, N., Hegsted, D. M., Guri, C. D., and Stare, F. J. (1966). The prevalence of osteoporosis in high-and low-fluoride areas in North Dakota. *Journal of the American Medical Association*, **198**, 499–504.
95. Arnala, I., Alhava, E. M., Kivivuori, R., and Kauranen, P. (1986). Hip fracture incidence not affected by fluoridation. Osteofluorosis studied in Finland. *Acta Orthopaedica Scandinavica*, **57**, 344–8.
96. Slovic, D. M., Daly, M. A., Doppelt, S. H., Potts Jr, J. T., Rosenthal, D. I., and Neer, R. M. (1987). Increases in vertebral bone density of post-menopausal osteoporosis after alternating treatment with hPTH-(1–34) fragment + 1,25-$(OH_2)D_3$: an interim report. In *Calcium regulation and bone metabolism* (ed. Cohn, D. V., T. J. Martin, and P. S. Meunier) pp. 119–22. Elsevier, Amsterdam.
97. Rasmussen, H., Bordier, P., Marie, P. *et al.* (1980). Effect of combined therapy with phosphate and calcitonin on bone volume in osteoporosis. *Metabolic Bone Disorders and Related Research*, **2**, 107–11.
98. Delmas, P. D., Casez, J. P., Boivin, G. Y. *et al.* (1984). Cyclic fluoride therapy for postmenopausal osteoporosis. In *Osteoporosis* (ed. Christiansen, C., C. D., Arnaud, B. E. C. Nordin, A. M. Parfitt, W. A. Peck, and B. L. Riggs) pp. 581–5, Munksgaard, Copenhagen.
99. Ott, S. M., Kilcoyne, R. F., and Chesnut, C. H. III (1987). Ability of four different techniques of measuring bone mass to diagnose vertebral fractures in postmenopausal women. *Journal of Bone and Mineral Research*, **2**, 201–10.
100. Ott, S. M. (1986). Should women get screening bone mass measurements? *Annals of Internal Medicine*, **104**, 874–6.

12
Stroke

INTRODUCTION

J. GRIMLEY EVANS

Stroke is one of the most dreaded of afflications of old age and one that puts heavy strains on both statutory and informal caregivers. The incidence of stroke increases as a power-law function of age,[1] in which respect it resembles most adult cancers.[2] The fatality of stroke, however, also increases with age so that the rise in prevalence with age is less steep than the incidence figures might lead one to expect. Other things remaining equal, the aging of populations will have less effect on the numbers of stroke victims in the community than it will on the numbers of those suffering from some other impairments, particularly dementia—for which prevalence rises more steeply with age. For example, projections for the period 1981 to 2001 for England and Wales[3] suggest that, although the number of people afflicted by moderate to severe dementia will increase by 20 per cent the increase in numbers of stroke victims in the community will increase by only 3 per cent. The number of acute hospital admissions for stroke, reflecting incidence rather than prevalence, will increase by 12 per cent. These projections were made on the assumption of no change taking place in the incidence of stroke or in the deployment or efficacy of treatment. This section examines these assumptions and the following section goes on to review current good practice in the treatment of acute stroke.

The major source of information on the frequency of stroke is mortality data. Variations in mortality rates of stroke over time and between countries offer hope that the disease may have environmental determinants that could be modified as a means of primary prevention. As Ostfeld[4] and others have commented, the interpretation of mortality data for stroke is complicated by greater diagnostic uncertainties than attend the study of some other disorders such as ischaemic heart disease.

Stroke has a heterogeneous pathology. To the traditional three pathogenic processes of thrombosis, haemorrhage, and embolism we must now add a fourth, the haemodynamic stroke, which may make a greater contribution than has generally been recognized.[5] Even within the pathological category of infarctive stroke a variety of causal mechanisms may be responsible.[6] Haemorrhagic strokes may also be the product of a wide variety of pathological mechanisms and precursors including blood dyscrasias, mycotic aneurysms, and amyloid angiopathy.[7] These considerations do not invalidate the epidemiological approach if the majority of strokes share common aetiological factors.

Hatano[8] has shown that stroke can be diagnosed accurately enough for epidemiological purposes if care is taken over standardization of definitions and procedures. It is the quality of routine mortality data that is more commonly called into question. At a clinical level, only 70 per cent of strokes produce hemiplegia[9] and neurological deficits of sensory or cognitive type are easily missed, particularly in confused or demented patients. The differential diagnosis of stroke in a clinical context is wide; some patients presenting with a stroke syndrome may subsequently prove to have disorders ranging from hypoglycaemia to subdural haematoma[10] or intracerebral tumour. The question is whether these conditions occur and remain undiagnosed sufficiently commonly to distort mortality data to a serious extent.

Kagan *et al.*[11] examined autopsy data from restricted areas in Czechoslovakia, Japan, and Sweden as a means of validating mortality rates for those three countries. Autopsy-verified rates of cerebrovascular disease mortality in the study areas were similar in rank to death-certificate-based mortality rates in the three countries as a whole. The authors note that, although overall mortality rates for stroke as a group of disorders has been generally validated by their study, accuracy of clinical attribution to different pathological categories of stroke was less satisfactory. Clinicians tended to overdiagnose haemorrhagic and underdiagnose infarctive strokes.

Florey *et al.*[12] compared death certificate diagnosis of stroke with the results of autopsy and with clinical records. Overall, there was an agreement between autopsy and clinical records of 79 per cent, and between autopsy and certification of death of 65 per cent. This study also revealed a tendency to clinical overdiagnosis of haemorrhagic strokes.

De Fairc[13] studied the accuracy of cause-of-death certification among subjects enrolled in a Swedish national study of twins by collating death certificates with information from other forms of medical documentation. For cerebrovascular disease the sensitivity of death certificates was 96 per cent cause of death was supported from other sources in 97 per cent and autopsy evidence was available in 53 per cent. In Sweden, therefore, mortality data seem surprisingly accurate for stroke, although the subjects in this study were young, ranging in age at death from approximately 48 to 72 years.

Corwin *et al.*[14] have reviewed the accuracy of death certification of stroke among the participants in the Framingham study. Of 280 subjects who died and who had been known to have suffered a stroke according to study criteria, 113 (40 per cent) had no mention of this diagnosis on their death certificate. The proportion of such strokes mentioned on the death certificates diminished with the age at death of the subject and with increasing time between the stroke episode and death. These findings presumably reflect the certifiers' statutory concern with the immediate cause of death rather than with accurately listing multiple pathology or past medical history. There was a false positive rate of 21 per cent in the Framingham mortality data in that, for 46 for the 216 deaths certified as being due to stroke, no evidence supporting this diagnosis could be found in a study of the medical records or from interview with attending doctors and the families of the decedents. With regard to subtypes of stroke there was over-reporting of cerebral haemorrhage and under-reporting of cerebral embolism.

These studies, reviewed as representative of work spanning two decades, suggest that mortality data for stroke are more accurate than many have feared, but are likely to be unreliable in distinguishing between the different pathological types of stroke. There is evidence that, over recent decades, doctors in the Western countries have tended to reduce their frequency of diagnosing cerebral haemorrhage in favour of thromboembolic stroke[15] and this is probably the explanation for the secular increase in the proportion of infarctive strokes at the expense of haemorrhagic strokes since the 1950s that Yates[16] and others have noted.

Mortality rates from stroke have been falling in the USA since 1900.[17-19] This decline is strikingly different from the trends shown by coronary heart disease mortality over the same period, which showed a rise from the 1920s until the late 1960s followed by a fall in the 1970s.[20] The decline in stroke mortality in the USA has accelerated in recent years. Ostfeld[21] calculates the decline between 1975 and 1977 as 4 per cent per annum compared with 1.5 per cent per annum between 1951 and 1974, and 1 per cent per annum between 1900 and 1950.

In England and Wales, also, mortality rates for stroke have been falling during this century.[21] Among men aged 45 to 84, rates have been falling since the early 1950s. At ages 25 to 44, rates were constant until the late 1960s and since then have been falling. At ages 85 and above, rates were constant or still rising until the early 1970s; since then they have been falling in the same proportion as at younger ages. The picture is essentially similar in females except that there is more suggestion of declining rates prior to 1950 in the middle-aged group (45 to 64). At ages under 45 there is little evidence of the decline seen in men except in the most recent years. For the age group 85 and above (and to a smaller extent the 75- to 84-year age group) the rise in incidence rates from the 1940s to the 1970s may partly reflect an increasing precision of diagnosis among older people, evidence for which has been found in other contexts.[22] This may have obscured a decline in mortality which was able to emerge from this certification artefact only in the last decade. The striking feature of the graphs is that, except among the very old, the decline was almost simultaneous in onset and proportionately similar in all age groups. This is difficult to reconcile with any kind of cohort effect or indeed with preventive treatment of hypertension which might be expected to have a larger effect at younger age groups since it is only very recently that high blood-pressure at older ages has begun to be generally treated in the UK. It is also incompatible with the hypothesis that cerebrovascular disease fell as a consequence of the rise in coronary heart disease which began to kill in their middle age those subjects with vascular disease who would previously have suffered from strokes at older ages.[23]

There is no evidence in Britain of the recent acceleration in decline of mortality rates which Whisnant[19] attributes in the American data to increasingly effective detection and treatment of hypertension which has undoubtedly occurred in the USA.[24] Reid and Evans[25] examined mortality data from England and Wales and found that death rates from hypertension and nephritis combined declined steadily from the 1920s into the Second World War. This would have been compatible with a decline in nephritis as a cause of hypertension. Paffenbarger *et al.*[26] had also suggested that there may have been a decline during this century in the prevalence of some infective cause of renal disease and hypertension. Alternatively, it is likely that before the role of hypertension in causing vascular and renal damage was sufficiently understood, deaths due to uncontrolled hypertensive disease would have been attributed to nephritis.

It seems then, that the decline in mortality from hypertension, both in England and Wales and in the USA,[24] started before effective hypotensive therapy could have been deployed widely in the community and suggests that some environmental cause of hypertension may have become less active between 1920 and 1960. This might in turn explain the fall in stroke mortality. Joossens[27] has suggested that a secular decline in dietary sodium has reduced the prevalence of hypertension.[28] However, as Borhani[24] has pointed out, there is no direct evidence from community surveys for a secular decline in the prevalence of higher levels of blood-pressure before the advent of effective therapy. Indeed, Whisnant,[19] citing data from a blood-pressure survey in the 1930s in a comparison with more recent data, suggests that, if anything, the prevalence of the higher levels of pressure may have been lower in the earlier data. Problems in observer variation in measurement of blood-pressure are too well known, however, for much weight to be attached to comparisons between data collected in surveys 20 or 30 years apart. There is more reliable evidence of a decline in prevalence of high blood-pressure in

United States population samples over the period that hypotensive therapy has been effectively deployed in the community.[19]

Dobson[29] has reported on mortality rates from cerebrovascular disease in Australia which fell from 1950 onwards in all age groups above 35 years. Bonita and Beaglehole[30] have demonstrated a decline in mortality from cerebrovascular disease in New Zealand, which is greater in men than in women, and which accelerated in the late 1970s—possibly due to more effective community control of hypertension.

Not all studies have found a decline in mortality rates from cerebrovascular disease. Data collected by the World Health Organization apparently show no evidence of a secular decline in stroke mortality in some countries of Eastern Europe—Bulgaria, Czechoslovakia, Rumania, Hungary, and Poland.[31] Nor is the secular trend observed throughout the Western world. Krueger *et al.*[32] for example, found no secular trend in overall mortality rates from cerebrovascular disease in Memphis, Tennessee for the years 1920 to 1960, although they did note, (as had Yates[16] in British data), a rise in deaths attributed to cerebral thrombosis which was balanced by a fall in those attributed to cerebral haemorrhage. Acheson[33] recorded an increase in mortality rates from cerebrovascular disease in the Republic of Ireland from 1926 to 1956. Anderson and MacKay[34] found no evidence of a decline in mortality rates from stroke in Ontario over the years 1901 to 1961, but their method of investigation, based on a sample of death certificates drawn from one year in ten, would not have been sensitive to a decline after the Second World War.

Partly because of the inconsistencies of these reports, the decline in mortality rates from stroke has been often assumed to reflect nothing more than changes in death certification practice with perhaps a particular contribution from an increasing tendency to attribute sudden deaths to coronary heart disease rather than apoplexy. Alternatively, a decline in mortality might reflect improved treatment and a fall in case fatality rather than a decline in frequency of the disease. Garraway *et al.*[35] have documented improvements in survival following stroke in the Rochester population from 1945–1959 to 1975–1979. Thirty-day survival in cerebral infarction changed little, from 76 to 84 per cent, over the 30 years, but survival in intracerebral haemorrhage increased from zero to 42 per cent and in subarachnoid haemorrhage from 43 to 63 per cent. Three-day survival also improved in cerebral haemorhage from 38 to 63 per cent but showed little change in cerebral infarction (92 to 95 per cent) or subarachnoid haemorrhage (64 to 70 per cent). These changes presumably reflect, to at least some degree, improvements in management but there may also have been changes in diagnostic criteria. At earlier stages in the period reviewed, fatality may have been an implicit criterion for the diagnosis of cerebral haemorrhage. None the less, taken with the Framingham finding that the longer a patient survives following a stroke the less likely is stroke to appear on his or her death certificate,[14] a prolongation of average survival due to improved care would have reduced the proportion of strokes appearing as cause of death.

However, evidence has now accumulated confirming that, at least in some areas, the incidence and not just the mortality or certification of stroke has been declining. Incidence data from the Community Data Bank of Rochester have confirmed a decline in incidence rates for cerebral haemorrhage and cerebral thrombosis since the 1950s in all age groups.[36, 37] The incidence of subarachnoid haemorrhage, which forms a larger component of the total stroke incidence at younger ages than at older, has not changed over this time. There is also a report of declining incidence rates of stroke in the Japanese community of Hisayama,[38] and evidence that incidence rates in Japan in 1975–1979 were lower than in 1960–1969.[39]

Garraway and Whisnant[40] have analysed the data from the Rochester population to compare the decline in stroke incidence with evidence on the detection and control of hypertension. The data showed no evidence for an overall lowering of the blood-pressure distributions, although the prevalence of hypertensive levels (160/95 or greater) diminished over the decades from the 1950s to the 1970s. The pattern of control of hypertension and that of the decline in stroke show some concordance in that hypertension in women appeared to be controlled better and earlier than in men and this was mirrored in the pattern of decline of stroke. In conclusion, therefore, the evidence suggests that the incidence of stroke has been falling in several economically advanced nations since the 1950s. Part of this fall in incidence is probably due to public health programmes leading to the detection and control of hypertension but it seems likely that some other factors were already operating, perhaps through reducing the prevalence or the pathological consequences of extreme degrees of hypertension. Reduced case fatality due to improved treatment probably contributed to the decline in mortality in the 1950s. However, it is not clear why, despite these consistent trends in some countries, stroke mortality rates appear to be stable or increasing in others.

The first of the next two chapter subparts is an exposition of current optimal care for the patient with acute stroke. The second reviews the case for detection and treatment of high blood pressure as a means of reducing stroke incidence. Although studies from North America show that hypertension is a risk factor for cardiovascular disease at ages above 70, as at lower ages, studies from other countries raise the possibility that this might not be true for all populations of elderly people. Because the extrinsic determinants of aging will vary from country to country we must expect that the old of different countries will differ more than the young, at least until cultures have converged through economic and social development. The Bergen study[41] showed that the relationship between blood-pressure and stroke mortality apparent at young adult ages disappeared the elderly. A study from Finland[42] found that the relationship between mortality and blood-pressure in a population sample of people aged 85 and over was actually inverse—higher levels of blood-pressure being associated with lower mortality. A study in a population sample aged 65 and over in northern England found no relationship between blood-pressure and stroke incidence in women, and the relationship in men was too slight to justify a screening programme aimed at reducing stroke incidence.[43] These findings are a warning that among the elderly, more perhaps than among the young, it is necessary to be sure that research findings in one population are applicable to another.

CARE OF THE PATIENT WITH ACUTE STROKE
TAKENORI YAMAGUCHI AND TERUO OMAE

This section reviews recent trends in the treatment of cerebral infarction and parenchymatous intracerebral haemorrhage. Intracranial haemorrhage due to rupture of an aneurysm or leakage from arteriovenous malformations, for which definitive surgical treatment may be required, will not be considered.

Traditionally, the management of acute cerebrovascular disease aims firstly at saving the patient's life, secondly at minimizing neurological disability, and thirdly at preventing further attacks. In the initial stages, the emphasis is on general medical care, including the maintenance of fluid and electrolyte balance, respiratory and cardiac care, and the prevention and management of medical complications. Many measures for specific treatment of the brain lesion have been proposed but few are well established in adequately conducted clinical trials. Surgical treatment, for example the evacuation of haematomata, has only a limited role.

EMERGENCY TREATMENT

Emergency treatment in acute cerebrovascular disease is not essentially different from that in other disorders associated with an acute deterioration in consciousness. The maintenance of a good airway by positioning and suction of the mouth and pharynx, if necessary, is essential. Insertion of a cuffed endotracheal tube, and aspiration of the stomach through a nasogastric tube, may be required if the patient is in danger of inhaling vomitus. Arterial gas estimation may be appropriate. Venous access should be established and fluid given to maintain a blood pressure sufficient to ensure adequate cerebral perfusion. An indwelling catheter will facilitate maintenance of fluid balance in the unconscious or uncooperative patient. Nursing care must be scrupulous and 1-hour or 2-hour turning will be essential to prevent pressure sores, particularly in the older patient. For the first 24 hours intravenous fluids are usually sufficient but feeding, if necessary through a nasogastric tube, should be started as soon as feasible.

MANAGEMENT OF SPECIFIC COMPLICATIONS

Convulsions

Convulsions are not uncommon immediately following the onset of stroke, particularly in cerebral haemorrhage and embolic infarction. As the convulsion may itself exacerbate brain ischaemia and produce anoxia by interfering with respiration, treatment should be started promptly. Phenytoin in a dose of 500–1000 mg by intravenous infusion over 20 minutes is the treatment of choice. In addition to a higher therapeutic index than other anticonvulsants, phenytoin has little effect on the electroencephalogram or the level of consciousness. Diazepam, 5–10 mg by slow intravenous injection, has recently gained popularity in the treatment of convulsive disorders, although its anticonvulsant action is short lived and it may depress respiration and the level of consciousness.

High blood-pressure

High blood-pressure is common after the onset of stroke, particularly if haemorrhagic. Its management is controversial and depends to some extent on the type of cerebrovascular disease.

Cerebral infarction

Rapid lowering of high blood-pressure should be avoided in the first 2 weeks following ischaemic stroke, unless pressures are extremely high (systolic pressure 250 mmHg (33 hpa) or more, diastolic pressure 120 mmHg (16 hpa) or more). Reasons for this approach are as follows:

1. In the acute stage of cerebrovascular disease, particularly in ischaemic stroke, autoregulation of cerebral blood flow around the ischaemic focus is almost always impaired or abolished and flow becomes dependent on perfusion pressure.[1] Many stroke victims have had longstanding high blood-pressure. The lower limit of systemic blood-

pressure at which cerebral autoregulation ceases and cerebral blood flow falls with blood-pressure is higher in patients with long-standing hypertension.[2] In such patients a small lowering of blood-pressure to within the 'normal range' may provoke a disproportionate fall in cerebral blood flow.

2. High blood-pressure seen in the first few days after the onset of a stroke may be due to a temporary increase in catecholamine release and often falls gradually without treatment.

Parenchymatous intracerebral haemorrhage

The treatment of hypertension in the acute phase of intracerebral haemorrhage is controversial. Severe hypertension soon after the haemorrhage may prolong the period of active bleeding, promote recurrence, and also accelerate the development of brain oedema. On the other hand there is some evidence that acute lowering of blood-pressure may have an unfavourable effect on the cerebral microcirculation[3] and attempts to halt the bleeding by lowering the systemic blood-pressure have not been successful.

Our current policy is that extreme hypertension, a systolic pressure of 250 mmHg (33 hPa) or more, should be reduced to a level below 200 mmHg (27 hPa), but a precipitate decline in pressure should be avoided.

Subarachnoid haemorrhage

High blood-pressure in the acute stage of subarachnoid haemorrhage should be lowered to normal levels, if possible, to prevent re-rupture of a saccular aneurysm. It is reported that autoregulation in this type of stroke is less impaired than in other forms.[4]

SPECIFIC TREATMENT

Brain oedema

Patients with massive brain infarction or with lacunar infarction may have brain oedema. If signs of oedema on CT scanning (shift of midline structures, compression of the ventricular system, and disappearance of cortical sulci) are present, anti-oedema agents are given to prevent brain herniation and to reduce functional disturbance. Ten per cent glycerol in fructose-added solution is commonly used, in doses of 10 to 15 ml per kg. Rapid infusion of 10 per cent glycerol in solution without fructose has been reported to cause haemoglobinuria. Glycerol may also be given orally or by means of a nasogastric tube in a 20 per cent solution.

In clinical trials, 10 per cent glycerol infusions have been reported to be safe and more effective than physiological saline,[5] adrenocorticosteroids,[6] and mannitol.[7] The usefulness of adrenocorticosteroids in reducing brain oedema in cerebrovascular disease appears to have been disproved in repeated trials over the last decade.[8]

Anticoagulants

In theory these might be expected to be useful in preventing completed stroke in patients with transient ischaemic attacks (TIA), or reversible ischaemic neurological disability (RIND). Anticoagulant medication might also be expected to be effective in halting progression of stroke-in-evolution.

TIA and RIND
Anticoagulants were widely used for the prevention of stroke following TIA or RIND during the last two decades, but the place of these agents has recently been taken by platelet anti-aggregants. The efficacy of anti-coagulants in preventing stroke after TIA or RIND has not been fully established as there have been no well-controlled double-blind clinical trials of adequate size.[9] Anticoagulation for a limited time is empirically recommended for patients with TIA in whom a thrombus is radiologically visible in a major artery, and/or failure to respond to platelet anti-aggregants.[9, 10]

Stroke-in-evolution (progressing stroke)
The concept of stroke-in-evolution seems to be widely recognized, and it seems reasonable to consider anticoagulant therapy if ischaemic neurological impairment is worsening. However, the number of clinical studies of anticoagulant therapy in this situation is surprisingly small. Moreover, although a few randomized studies have shown a trend towards benefit, the number of patients involved was too small to justify anticoagulation as standard therapy.

Cardiogenic cerebral embolism
Recent development of neuroradiological techniques and imaging devices allows more accurate diagnosis of cerebral embolism. If intracardiac thrombi are found by two-dimensional echocardiography, anticoagulant therapy is appropriate for prevention of recurrent systemic embolization.[11, 12] Studies on rheumatic heart disease[13, 14] and myocardial infarction[15] led to the conclusion that patients on anticoagulants have fewer embolic events than those without therapy, although the number of patients included in these studies was, again, not large enough to provide convincing evidence.

Anticoagulants are also recommended for patients with cardiac disorders, such as atrial fibrillation, prosthetic heart valves, cardiomyopathy, and valvular lesions, if the patient has shown evidence of embolization and has not responded to aspirin.[9]

The optimal time after an episode of cerebral embolism to institute anticoagulants has not been established. There is a risk of converting an ischaemic infarct into a hemorrhagic one in the acute phase of embolic stroke,[16] a transition that is not infrequent.[17] On the other hand, recurrent embolization is apt to occur within 2 weeks (up to 20 per cent,[18, 19] so that anticoagulation is desirable as soon as compatible with reasonable safety.

The Cerebral Embolism Study Group reported that the risk of recurrent embolization appeared to be lower than the risk of haemorrhagic transformation of ischaemic infarct following early anticoagulation with heparin (starting at an average of 32 hours after the epidsode, continuing for 14 days), if the infarct was not haemorrhagic on CT performed at 48 hours, and if the patient was not hypertensive.[17] Larger infarcts and advanced age appeared to increase the risk of haemorrhagic transformation and an unfavourable outcome.

Platelet anti-aggregants

Since microembolism is widely accepted as the major pathogenetic mechanism of TIA, studies have focused on drugs which alter platelet function and prevent thrombus formation in the arterial system. Aspirin, sulphinpyrazone, and dipyridamole are known to have such properties.

Most of the clinical trials of platelet anti-aggregants have been conducted on patients with specific types of TIA using modern methods and biostatistics. To date, there have been two trials in which a reasonably large number of patients were entered and followed up for considerable length of time which revealed a 50 per cent reduction in stroke occurrence and stroke death.[20, 21] Results of other smaller trials have been variable, but the accumulated data suggest the usefulness of aspirin for prevention of ischaemic stroke from TIA and recurrence of stroke.[22, 23]

Other platelet anti-aggregants—sulphinpyrazone, dipyridamole, and suloctidil—have not been shown consistently to reduce recurrences in patients with TIA and stroke. Ticlopidine, a new platelet anti-aggregant, is now being evaluated in TIA and stroke patients in the USA. A preliminary short-term double-blind trial of ticlopidine (200 mg/d) or aspirin (330 mg/d) conducted in Japan showed that cumulative occurrence rates for TIA, stroke, and myocardial infarction were nearly equal in the two groups.[4] The results of a large randomized study are awaited.

The optimal dosage of aspirin has been the matter of controversy.

Aspirin reduces both the production of thromboxane—the thrombogenic and vasoconstricting substance released from platelets—and that of prostacyclin—the antithrombotic and vasodilating substance produced by the endothelial cell—through inhibition of cyclo-oxygenase. In theory, a smaller dosage will interfere with prostacyclin production less than thromboxane release, so that a smaller dose would be expected to be more effective than a large dose in preventing thrombogenesis.

Studies which have demonstrated the efficacy of aspirin, however, have used a dosage of 1.0 to 1.3 g/d rather than a smaller dosage.[20, 21] Although an antithrombotic effect in the plastic tubing of haemodialysis circuits has been shown with a daily dosage of 165 mg,[25] a smaller dosage cannot be recommended for stroke-threatened patients, until it is proved to be beneficial by an acceptable controlled clinical trial.

Fibrinolytic agents

Fibrinolytic (thrombolytic) therapy might be expected to be helpful in restoring blood flow by thrombolysis in patients with acute cerebral infarction. One randomized trial in patients with acute cerebral infarction using intravenous streptokinase, however, failed to prove its efficacy because of the risk of converting an ischaemic infarction into a haemorrhagic lesion.[26] Another uncontrolled study using a large amount of urokinase (UK: 1 400 000 3 300 000 U) in 31 patients with hyperacute stroke, produced four cases of fatal intracerebral haemorrhage within 24 hours.[27] Thus, these drugs are considered, in the United States, to be without any benefit and to have to potential hazard of haemorrhagic transformation of ischaemic infarcts. It is, however, thought that massive hemorrhagic infarction occurs only in cerebral embolism. A randomized controlled trial with a double-blind design, using small doses of urokinase (60 000 U) against placebo has demonstrated some beneficial effect on a general improvement index in patients with non-embolic cerebral infarction.[28]

A new thrombolytic agent, tissue-type plasminogen activator (t-PA), has been shown to induce thrombolysis without any systemic fibrinogenolysis, and is considered to be less hazardous and more effective than urokinase for treatment of thrombotic disorders.[29] A randomized controlled trial of this agent in patients with non-embolic cerebral infarction is awaited.

Haemodilution therapy

Normovolaemic or hypervolaemic haemodilution therapy has been suggested to improve the ischaemic microcirculation.[30] One technique for haemodilution involves phlebotomy and simultaneous infusion of 10 per cent dextran-40-saline (250 ml of venesection and 150 to 200 ml infusion of dextran-40 followed by 300 to 350 ml infusion of the latter, over the succeeding 2 to 4 hours.[31]) If the patient's haemoglobin is above 12 g/dl on the next day, further venesection (250 to 400 ml accompanied by 500 ml infusion of dextran solution) is performed to maintain the haemoglobin below 12 g/dl.

A preliminary study demonstrated significant improvement of the neurological scores over the first 10 days in the haemodiluted patients as compared to the controls, although the number of the study subjects was small.[31]

Vasodilators

Conventional vasodilators such as papaverine hydrochloride, cyclandelate, hexobendine, etc. are not used in the acute phase of ischaemic stroke (within 2 weeks after onset) for the following reasons:

1. Cerebral blood flow (CBF) in the ischaemic brain is not increased by inhalation of carbon dioxide, which is known to be the most potent vasodilator.[32] Regional CBF may decrease in the ischaemic focus owing to intracerebral steal.[33] Intra-arterial injection of papaverine has a similar effect on the ischaemic microcirculation.[34]

2. Vasodilators reduce systemic blood-pressure, which may have a detrimental effect on ischaemic brain where autoregulation of CBF is totally or partially impaired.[1]

Although calcium-entry blockers are potent vasodilators, some investigators suggest they may have potential in suppressing expansion of focal ischaemia by blocking Ca^{2+} influx into anoxic cells.[35, 36] Therapeutic benefits from these drugs in patients with acute cerebral ischaemia have not yet been demonstrated.

Pharmacological brain protection

Potential for recovery lies in the area surrounding the acute lesion where nerve cell damage is thought to be reversible, ('penumbra'). Several agents such as barbiturates, naloxone, and phenytoin have been assessed for protective effects in focal cerebral ischaemia.

Despite encouraging results of barbiturate therapy in experimental animal models of stroke,[37, 38] effects in human cerebral infarction are uncertain, partly because of difficulty in evaluating effectiveness. Even if positive results are obtained, barbiturate therapy seems to be not univer-

sally applicable for stroke patients, because of depression of consciousness and respiration, which complicates the management.

Naloxone, a morphine antagonist, was shown to have a beneficial effect
in reversing focal cerebral ischaemia in post-operative patients with ruptured aneurysms. The clinical and experimental results, however, have
not yet shown uniform and predictable benefit.[39, 40]

Conflicting reports on the value of these agents in acute ischaemia
emphasize the need for prospective randomized controlled trials; the use
of these agents as immediate therapy for stroke is not recommended at
present.

Surgical treatment

Extracranial–intracranial bypass surgery

Extracranial–intracranial (EC-IC) bypass surgery was introduced in
1969;[41] it has been widely applied to patients with stenosis or occlusion of
the internal carotid or middle cerebral arteries in an effort to improve
blood flow to potentially ischaemic brain or to prevent stroke recurrence.

Although early uncontrolled clinical studies appeared encouraging, a
well-controlled, prospective study failed to prove favourable effects of
EC-IC bypass in 1377 randomly assigned patients with known ischaemic
cerebrovascular diseases.[42] Surgery did not reduce the frequency of TIAs,
major strokes, or death below that observed in patients receiving
appropriate medical therapy. Analyses of subgroups of patients, including
those with carotid occlusion or stenosis of the intracranial carotid or
middle cerebral arteries, also failed to show evidence of benefit in outcome after follow up lasting as long as 5 years.

Carotid endarterectomy

There have been only two randomized trials published in which the effect
of carotid endarterectomy was assessed in patients with TIAs.[43, 44]
Although a favourable outcome was reported by the Cooperative Study
Group in the United States in 1970,[43] careful analyses of the data provided no evidence in favour of surgical treatment when the surgical
fatality and morbidity were added to the probability for stroke occurrence
in follow-up.[45]

Another trial in the United Kingdom was abandoned early because of
high fatality and morbidity at the time of, and within the first 30 days
after, the carotid endarterectomy.[44]

Despite the lack of convincing evidence favouring carotid endarterectomy, this procedure has been performed with increasing frequency in
the hope of preventing TIAs and strokes related to extracranial carotid
occlusive disease. A great variation in the surgical fatality and morbidity

of this procedure is seen in the published reports,[46-9] and the results of endarterectomy appears to depend largely on patient selection and the surgeon's skill. The Committee on Health Care Issues of the American Neurological Association has published the opinion that carotid endarterectomy may be of value if the surgical complication rate is very low, but that the overall results of this procedure in the United States are unfavourable.[45] The Committee estimated that a combined surgical fatality and stroke morbidity of 4 per cent and a stroke rate of 2 per cent per year following the first 30 days after the surgery, would balance the negative effect of the surgical treatment after a little more than one year, yielding a 33 per cent reduction in stroke occurrence at the end of 5 years. If the surgical fatality/stroke morbidity is less than 1 per cent, a 50 per cent reduction in stroke could be expected.

Intracerebral hemorrhage

There is no specific medical treatment for intracerebral haemorrhage (ICH) except for infusion of an anti-oedema agent. Management of patients with ICH must be determined by the location and size of haematoma, age, blood-pressure, and presence or absence of various complications. Whether or not high blood-pressure in the acute stage of ICH should be actively treated was discussed earlier.

Management for brain oedema

Intravenous infusion of hyperosmolar agents, such as mannitol or glycerol, is the treatment of choice. Dosage and technique in ICH are essentially the same as in cerebral infarction (see above). As it has a more rapid oedema-reducing effect than glycerol, mannitol is recommended for patients with impending brain herniation due to ICH. Mannitol given in a concentration of 20 per cent produces such a remarkable diuresis that dehydration and electrolyte imbalance should carefully be watched for.

Surgical treatment

Two surgical techniques are applied for ICH: the transcortical or trans-Sylvian approach with craniotomy and needle aspiration of the haematoma. Although it seems plausible that damage to the surrounding brain tissue due to ICH can be reduced by evacuation, solid indications for surgical treatment of ICH have not yet been established. There is a lack of well-controlled clinical studies comparing the efficacy of medical and surgical treatments.

Provisional guidelines for surgical treatment are as follows:

1. Cerebellar haemorrhage occasionally causes a life-threatening syndrome which can be reversed by prompt surgical removal of a haematoma. The general recommendation is that haematomas greater than 3

cm in diameter should be operated on if the patient is seen within the first week. Patients with hematomas smaller than 3 cm should be treated medically unless unpredictable deterioration occurs, in which case surgical intervention is indicated.[50]

2. Most lobar haematomata can be treated conservatively. If the patient shows progressive deterioration, however, surgical evacuation is indicated.

3. Whether surgery can improve the functional outcome of putaminal haemorrhage is controversial. Surgical treatment can sometimes be life saving, but does not always improve functional outcome.[50]

4. There is no evidence that surgery for patients with thalamic and pontine haemorrhage is beneficial. Emergency ventricular drainage is at times needed, however, to treat obstructing hydrocephalus.

5. Needle aspiration of haematomas has been re-introduced since the advent of CT and new instrumental devices.[52] This technique is attractive because decompression and relief of increased intracranical pressure can be accomplished less invasively. It may be indicated for elderly or high-risk patients if it proves in adequately controlled trials to be superior to conventional evacuation or medical management.

In conclusion, the treatment of the acute stage of cerebrovascular accidents has advanced considerably in recent years, which may have contributed at least in part to a the reduction in mortality from cerebrovascular accidents. Many problems, however, still remain unsolved in reducing the recurrence rate of cerebrovascular accidents.

STROKE PREVENTION AND THE POPULATION CONTROL OF HYPERTENSION

C. J. BULPITT

INTRODUCTION

This section discusses the different types of stroke, their risk factors, the contribution of hypertension to the incidence of stroke, the decline in stroke rates over the years, and the possible causes for this reduction. How strokes may be prevented in the population is also considered and the problems, costs, and benefits of such an activity is discussed.

THE DIFFERENT TYPES OF STROKE

The World Health Organization definition of a stroke is: 'rapidly developing clinical signs of focal and at times global loss of cerebral function

(applied to patients in deep coma and to those with subarachnoid haemorrhage), and with symptoms lasting more than 24 hours or leading to
death with no apparent cause other than that of vascular origin'.[1]

Stroke-related conditions will be defined as having a similar aetiology
but not resulting in a sudden cerebrovascular accident. These include
transient ischaemic attacks (TIAs) and multi-infarct dementia. TIAs have
been defined as acute loss of focal cerebral or ocular function, with
symptoms lasting less than 24 hours, which after adequate investigation is
presumed to be due to emboli or thrombotic vascular disease.[2]

Table 12.1 provides a simplified but possibly practical classification of
cerebrovascular accidents and stroke-related diseases. Cerebral infarction
is considered first as the Oxfordshire Community Stroke project reported
that 85 per cent strokes occurring in this community in 1981–1982 were
infarcts. Only 9 per cent were due to intracerebral haemorrhage and 6 per
cent to subarachnoid haemorrhage.

A study at the Stroke Unit of the Austin Hospital in 1977–1979[3] found
that 59 per cent of their stroke patients had a *cortical* infarction (1.1 in
this classification). The Oxfordshire project reported that this condition
accounts for 75 per cent of their strokes. Infarction can lead to lacunae
in the internal capsule (*capsular* infarction: 1.2); also, when multiple, it

Table 12.1 Proposed classification of strokes and stroke related conditions. The
percentage figures are discussed in the text.

A. *STROKES*:
1. **Cerebral infarction** (85%)
    1.1   cortical infarction (75%)
           1.11 ipsilateral carotid occlusion (14%)
           1.12 non-stenotic atheromatous carotid lesion (44%)
           1.13 atrial fibrillation (10%)
    1.2   capsular (lacunar) infarction (10%)
2. **Intracerebral Haemorrhage** (9%)
    2.1 cerebrum (7%)
    2.2 brainstem (1%)
    2.3 cerebellum (1%)
3. **Subarachnoid haemorrhage** (6%)

B. *STROKE-RELATED CONDITIONS*:
1. **Transient ischaemic attacks (TIAs)**
    1.1 single attack
    1.2 repeated attacks
           1.21 embolic
           1.22 external compression of an artery
           1.23 failure of autoregulation
2. **Multi-infarct dementia**

---

leads to dementia and to TIAs. In Oxford in 1981–1982, cerebral haemorrhage was responsible for 9 per cent of strokes, but other studies suggest that it may be responsible for up to a third of major strokes; it is in the cerebrum in 82 per cent of cases, in the brainstem in 11 per cent, and in the cerebellum in 7 per cent[4]. Subarachnoid haemorrhage constitutes a slightly rare stroke occurrence (6 per cent in Oxford).

A further study at Austin Hospital[3, 5] found that 18 per cent of cortical infarcts were associated with an occlusion of the ipsilateral carotid artery, 59 per cent with a non-stenotic atheromatous carotid lesion, and 22 per cent with atrial fibrillation. The patients with atrial fibrillation presumably had embolism from thrombus in the heart. As the lumen of the carotid artery has to be reduced by 90 per cent to reduce cerebral blood flow significantly under normal conditions, it is probable that embolism from atheromatous lesions in the carotid is responsible for a large number of cases of cerebral infarction. On the other hand, variations in the circle of Willis may be present in over half of stroke patients and hypertension may also ensure that infarction occurs due to an impaired blood supply without embolization[6]. The Australian (Austin Hospital) study confirmed the results of the Harvard Co-operative Stroke Registry study,[7] namely that the arterial lesions occur mainly in the carotid arteries rather than in the smaller cerebral arteries. This is somewhat surprising. Although atheroma does not usually affect vessels less than 2 mm in diameter, in hypertension atheroma can be found in arteries penetrating the internal capsules, basal ganglia, and pons,[8, 9] and even the central retinal artery.[10, 11]

The occlusion of small arteries may lead to capsular or lacunar infarctions (listed as 1.2 in Table 12.1). These lacunae, or small trabeculated cavities,[6] when multiple are 0.5 to 1.5 mm in diameter and situated far from the cortex. When single they appear to have arisen from an infarction and may be up to 1 cm in diameter.[12] It has been suggested that infarction, haemorrhage or arterial pulsation may be responsible for multiple lacunae. They are part of the picture of 'small vessel disease'[13]. Atheromatous changes may be associated with aneurysm formation (for example the Charcot–Bouchard aneurysm).[14, 15] These aneurysms may be expected to lead to haemorrhage and are associated with dilation of the perivascular spaces, the 'état lacunaire' of Marie.[16] However, lacunes may also arise from infarction or exaggerated pulsation of the arteries.[6]

Cerebral haemorrhage arises mainly in the cerebrum.[4] The lenticulostriate artery supplies the basal ganglia and is often known as the 'artery of cerebral haemorrhage'. Less frequently the brainstem is involved (11 per cent of cerebral haemorrhages) and the cerebellum (7 per cent).

The prevalence of multi-infarct dementia is unknown but should be considered when dementia is associated with focal neurological signs and symptoms.[17] The condition is often associated with lacunar infarcts.

TIAs last, by definition, for less than 24 hours and usually from 2 to 15 minutes. It has been suggested that a third of patients with TIAs will develop a cerebral infarct within 5 years.[18]

Table 12.1 follows the suggestion of Graham *et al.* and divides TIAs into single and repeated episodes. A single episode may possibly be due to a small infarct or haemorrhage but repeated attacks are usually due to emboli, external compression of an artery (e.g. the vertebral artery in the presence of cervical spondylosis), and systemic hypertension and failure of autoregulation. With a reduction in arterial pressure, cerebral blood flow is kept constant by vasodilation and the mechanism operates effectively down to a mean arterial presure of 50 mmHg (6.7 hPa) in normal subjects.[19] In patients with a compromised circulation or at mean pressures less than 50 mmHg (6.7 hPa), blood flow may fall and TIAs or cerebral infarction may occur.

Subarachnoid haemorrhage arises from rupture of a saccular aneurysm on one of the arteries at the base of the brain. These are now thought to be most commonly due to atheroma and less often to congenital defects.[20, 21] Stress on the arterial wall due to turbulent flow rather than laminar flow in the neighbourhood of bifurcations and/or atheroma may certainly lead to aneurysmal dilation and eventual rupture. On the other hand, these aneurysms occur in association with polycystic disease of the kidneys in the absence of hypertension and in the connective tissue disorder known as Ehlers–Danlos syndrome, suggesting an abnormality of mesoderm.[6]

RISK FACTORS FOR STROKE

The risk factors for stroke to be considered are:

1. hypertension;

2. age;

3. atrial fibrillation and other cardiac causes;

4. diabetes mellitus;

5. high haematocrit;

6. high serum cholesterol;

7. cigarette smoking;

8. male sex;

9. high alcohol consumption.

Hypertension

We shall consider which types of stroke are statistically associated with an elevation of arterial blood pressure, and what proportion of any type of stroke is in fact caused by hypertension. Cole and Yates[22] examined the brains of hypertensive patients at autopsy. They found cerebral haemorrhage and capsular infarcts virtually only in hypertensive patients and not in controls known to be normotensive during life. However, they did find cortical infarctions in normotensive patients. Nevertheless, atheromatous stenosis of the larger cerebral vessels is more frequent and more severe in hypertensive patients.[23, 24] Moreover, atrial fibrillation is more common in hypertension than in normotension and a proportion of cortical infarcts may be expected to be causally associated with hypertension. The same argument applies to TIAs. As multi-infarct dementia is associated with capsular infarcts, hypertension must also be expected to play a part in this condition.

TIAs due to a small haemorrhage may be expected to be associated with hypertension, emboli from carotid atheroma are presumably more common in hypertension, and failure of auto-regulation occurs not merely below a mean arterial pressure of 50 mmHg (6.7 hPa) (as above) but below approximately 90 mmHg (12 hPa) in the presence of hypertension.[19]

Whether or not subarachnoid haemorrhage is associated with hypertension is disputed:[6] McCormick and Schmalsteig[25] examined both the prevalence of hypertension in patients dying with a ruptured or unruptured saccular aneurysm and its prevalence in an age- and sex-matched control autopsy series. No difference was discovered. However, as aneurysms are associated with both coarctation of the aorta and polycystic kidneys, and as both these conditions may lead to hypertension, some association between aneurysm and hypertension is to be expected although it may be weak.

In conclusion, nearly all cerebral haemorrhage and capsular infarction may result from hypertension. A proportion of patients with cortical infarction, multi-infarct dementia, and TIAs will have these conditions in association with hypertension. A small proportion of subarachnoid haemorrhage events may be associated with hypertension.

We are left with a few facts and many questions. We shall start with the facts:

1. Stroke mortality is declining.[26, 27, 28]

2. The case fatality rate for stroke has declined.[29]

3. The incidence of stroke (fatal and non-fatal) has declined.[33]

4. The treatment of hypertension has increased.

5. The treatment of hypertension reduces stroke mortality by about 40 per cent (data from the large trials). Thus, most studies agree that stroke mortality is declining by 1–2 per cent per annum, although maybe more in women than men.[27] This is due, at least in part, to the treatment of hypertension.

The questions include:

1. To what extent is the treatment of hypertension responsible for the fall in stroke mortality?
2. Does lowering blood-pressure reduce the incidence of cortical infarction?
3. Is the population's blood-pressure falling without treatment and what effect does this have on stroke incidence?

These questions are interrelated. Although stroke mortality was falling before the introduction of antihypertensive drugs, the decline accelerated with their introduction and cerebral haemorrhage has been greatly reduced. Spence[30] briefly reported some data given in Table 12.2. Following the introduction of a hospital CT scanner and a community-based programme that bought 92 per cent of 'hypertensives' under treatment (84 per cent were 'controlled'), he determined the number of stroke patients admitted to the corresponding district hospital. The reduction of hypertension-related strokes fell by 90 per cent with no change in the number treated with a cortical infarction. Spence therefore concluded that the treatment of hypertension does not reduce the incidence of cortical thrombosis. Nevertheless half of such events occur in the relatively few persons with hypertension.[31] Acheson and Fairbairn determined the stroke incidence in Oxfordshire in 1966.[32] This study did not have the benefit of CT scanning and presumably lacunar infarctions were included in the column headed 'cortical infarction' (Table 12.2). The area was also surveyed 16 years later by the Oxfordshire Community Stroke Project.[2] Despite the difference in methods it appears probable that stroke incidence declined over the 16 years and that this was mainly due to a reduction in cerebral haemorrhage (Table 12.2). On the other hand, Garraway and his colleagues in Rochester, Minnesota reported a reduction in both cerebral haemorrhage and cerebral infarction[33] in a community with an overall autopsy rate of 58 per cent (Table 12.2). As with the controversy as to whether or not treatment of hypertension reduces deaths from myocardial infarction,[34] it is probable that treatment will prove to have a beneficial effect on cortical infarction. It must be remembered, however, that blood-pressure may be declining irrespective of drug treatment. A reduction in the incidence of nephritis is one possibility, as is a reduction in salt intake following the introduction of refrigeration as a preservative method.[35]

Table 12.2 Four studies of stroke incidence and mortality[a]

	Cerebral haemorrhage + lacunar infarction	Cortical infarction	Other stroke	Total strokes	Percentage reduction
Stroke patients/year:					
Victoria Hospital (1977)	250	175	75	500	—
(1984)	25	175	50	250	50
Incidence/1000/year:					
Oxford (1966) Men 55+	10.6[b]	15.8	7.2	33.6	
Women 55+	11.9	13.1	6.5	31.5	
Oxford (1982) Men 55+	4.6	18.1	4.6	27.0	20
Women 55+	4.1	16.1	4.1	24.0	24
	(17%)[d]	(67%)	(17%)		
Incidence/100 000/year:					
Rochester (1947)	18[b]	140[c]	29	186	
(1972)	10	92	18	120	35[e]

[a] Spence *reporting* from the Victoria Hospital. Canada,[30] Acheson *et al.* from Oxford, UK in 1966,[32] the Oxfordshire Community Stroke Project in 1982,[2] and Garraway from Rochester, Minnesota.[33] The Canadian Study[30] was of stroke patients in a hospital; the other studies were of stroke incidence (in Rochester for all ages).
[b] These figures may have excluded lacunar infarcts.
[c] These figures may have included lacunar infarcts.
[d] Percentage of total strokes in both men and women in 1982. The percentages differ from Table 12.1 as they include strokes with site unknown.
[e] A 45% reduction if age adjusted.

The trials of antihypertensive medication reveal a reduction in stroke mortality in hypertensives averaging over 40 per cent. It is quite possible that hypertensive subjects suffer a high proportion of cerebral haemorrhage or lacunar infarcts and, if these represent 40 per cent of strokes in such patients, then prevention of these would account for the 40 per cent reduction in stroke mortality. In the general population in 1982, the proportion of strokes due to haemorrhage or lacunar infarction was less than 20 per cent (Table 12.1), which possibly reflects widespread antihypertensive treatment. Suppose all hypertensives in the population were identified and actually treated; Table 12.3 gives the possible benefits of such a programme. The table assumes all cerebral haemorrhage and lacunar infarct deaths are prevented, and that 0, 25, and 50 per cent of other strokes respectively are prevented in hypertensive patients. Prior to treatment, hypertensives are assumed to constitute 10 per cent of the population, and to have 100 per cent of deaths from cerebral haemorrhage and lacunar infarction and 50 per cent deaths from other types of stroke.[31]

Table 12.3 Possible improvement in stroke mortality over and above the Oxford situation in 1982. Treatment is expected to prevent all cerebral haemorrhage and lacunar infarction deaths and 0%, 25%, and 50% of other stroke deaths. Assume 100 deaths in 1982

| | Numbers of deaths | | |
	Cerebral haemorrhage and lacunar infarction (1)	Cortical thrombosis & subarachnoid haemorrhage (2)	Percentage reduction
Oxford (1982)			
normotensives	0	41	
hypertensives	19	40	
(Assume all hypertensives treated with prevention of (1))			
No effect on (2)	0	81	19
25% reduction in (2)			
normotensives	0	41	
hypertensives	0	30	29
50% reduction in (2)			
normotensives	0	41	
hypertensives	0	20	39

If stroke death rates decline by a further amount and in excess of 19 per cent it may be assumed that the incidence of cortical thrombosis is being reduced by antihypertensive treatment. A fall of this degree has not yet been observed. Moreover, risk factors for stroke other than hypertension may be declining and we shall briefly consider these in the following sections.

Age and male sex

Neither age nor being a male are reversible risk factors, nevertheless it is important to stress the dramatic increase in stroke incidence with increasing age and the fact that men of a given age experience more strokes than woman of the same age. The Royal College of Physicians' report[36] stressed that the incidence of stroke does not exceed 1 per 1000 per year until after the age of 55 years. The incidence at ages 55–64 is 3.5 per 1000 per year, at ages 65–74 it is 9, at ages 75–84 it is 20, and over the age of 85 years it is 40 per 1000 per year. The early fatality is about 50 per cent and the resulting prevalence of stroke survivors is 1 per cent at ages 55–64, 4 per cent at ages 65–74 and 8 per cent over the age of 75 years[36] Moreover, these patients account for about a quarter of the most disabled in a community.[37] These facts will be further considered in the section below on the cost-benefit of treating hypertension.

There are more elderly women than men and consequently more women with strokes than men. At any given age, however, a man is more likely to have a stroke than a women. The male excess in incidence of about 10 per cent (Table 12.2) is, however, much less than the male excess for other vascular diseases such as ischaemic heart disease.

Smoking and alcohol consumption

The evidence that smoking and a heavy consumption of alcohol may both be risk factors for stroke is supported to some extent by a recent study of 104 patients thought to have suffered an intracranial haemorrhage and 368 a cerebral infarction. Control subjects were obtained from a screening programme of factory workers. Despite the limitations of this case-control study a relative risk from smoking of 2.0 was reported in men but a normal risk (1.0) in women.[38] Male smokers may be 'health careless' in respects other than smoking, such as failing to take antihypertensive medication. Although the authors adjusted for alcohol intake and 'antihypertensive status', a confounding variable may well have produced a spurious association in men.

A high alcohol intake is associated with an increase in blood-pressure[39, 40] and in the above study a high intake of $\geqslant$ 400 g alcohol/week was associated with a relative risk greater than 2.0. However, a low intake of 10–90 g/week was associated with a low relative risk of 0.7.[41]

High serum cholesterol, high blood sugar and high haematocrit

Although there are data implicating high cholesterol, high blood sugar (or the presence of diabetes mellitus), and high blood haematocrit levels in the aetiology of stroke, these factors may be of declining importance in the elderly who suffer the most strokes, and these factors may be difficult to rectify. These possible risk factors will not be discussed further.

Atrial fibrillation and other cardiac causes

There is no doubt that a proportion of strokes arise as emboli from cardiac causes. No therapeutic trials of sufficient size have been mounted to assess the place of pharmacological treatment in the prevention of stroke from this cause. The benefits, or otherwise, of such treatment in, say, atrial fibrillation, remains unknown.

In conclusion, the only risk factor that appears worthy of dealing with to prevent stroke is hypertension. We shall now discuss the community control of hypertension and the cost-benefits of such an activity.

COMMUNITY CONTROL OF HYPERTENSION

The community control of hypertension requires four stages: the definition of hypertension and the age group of interest, the identification of the hypertensive subjects, the provision of antihypertensive care and ensuring that the care continues, and determining that the patient persists in taking his or her treatment.

Defining the objectives

As previously discussed, the elderly suffer from strokes and any definition of hypertension should include this age group. The definition of hypertension must be pragmatic, for example a level of blood-pressure above which treatment may be expected to do more good than harm. Applying this principle in a recent review for the elderly, I suggested that the definition should be 'a sustained diastolic pressure. (phase V Korotkoff sound) equal to or greater than 90 mmHg (12 kPa) in the standing position acompanied by a sustained systolic pressure equal to or greater than 160 mmHg (21 hPa)'. The word 'sustained' implies that this pressure must be maintained after, say, three measurements over a 6-week period[42] The age range could be any age under that of 80, as evidence for benefit from treatment exists for subjects up to this age. Taking the blood-pressure in the standing position is necessary in the elderly to exclude those incapacitated by a fall of blood-pressure on standing.

Identification of 'hypertensives'

In most societies with a reasonable level of medical care it is possible to identify the primary care physician who has a continuing remit for an individual's medical care. The vast majority of middle-aged and elderly patients attend these physicians over a 5-year period. There are therefore, broadly speaking, two methods of identifying hypertensive patients: 'case finding' and 'population screening'.

Case finding

Case finding may be very efficient *provided* that primary care physicians are motivated to check the blood-pressure of their patients who may come to see them for a variety of different reasons.

When the medical care system provides remuneration that increases when a hypertensive patient is diagnosed and treated, this financial income will often act as a sufficient incentive. However, this may lead to overdiagnosis and overtreatment.[43] The temptation may be great to treat for reward without determining whether the level of hypertension is sustained. The push to treat is aided and abetted by the Pharmaceutical Industry whose sales of antihypertensive drugs rose from 610 million US dollars world-wide in 1970 to 2800 million dollars in 1982.[43] Although the adverse effects of treatment and the effects of labelling an individual patient as hypertensive are real, nevertheless the problem of overtreatment is greatly overshadowed by the problem of undertreatment. In the 1970s the rule of halves was said to apply: half the hypertensives were aware of the diagnosis, half of these were on drug treatment and half of these (12.5 per cent of the total) had acceptable blood-pressure control. This rule is possibly now the three-quarters rule—34 per cent of US hypertensives having adequate treatment in 1976–1980.[43]

When the medical care system does not provide remuneration for the extra work involved in finding, treating, and following hypertensive patients, how can the primary care physicians be encouraged? In one study in London it was apparent that the primary care physicians were very well motivated but had difficulty in assessing their success rate. The vast majority of the population were registered with primary care physicians who knew who their patients were. What they did not know, was how many were hypertensives unknown to them. Their age–sex registers were therefore copied by a research team[44] and the general practitioners notified them of every hypertensive patient they found and treated. Every year the practitioners were informed in confidence of the proportion of their patients over the age of 40 who were being treated and the average proportion for their colleagues. The research team also contacted the patients annually to determine whether or not they continued with the follow-up and drug treatment. The doctors were encouraged by their annual audits to look for hypertensive patients. Their registration rates soared, especially in women, and there was evidence that stroke mortality declined.[45] The authors concluded that the cost of saving or postponing one stroke death in this study was £1400 at 1981 prices, though this figure does not take in account the time spent by the practitioners, nurses, senior researchers, and receptionists (and therefore their salaries).

Screening the population

The alternative to case finding is screening the whole population, say every 5 years. The yield from such an activity is unlikely to be worthwhile under the age of 40, the prevalence of hypertension being so low. Similarly, screening need not be repeated at shorter intervals than 5 years when the subject's blood-pressure is well within the normal range.[46] Nevertheless screening requires clerical effort in contacting the patients, special screening clinics, and the provision of antihypertensive treatment and follow-up. Alderman and Stanback have argued 'systematic worksite based treatment, relying heavily on nurses for the provision of care; produces a better blood pressure reduction at lower cost'.[47] Screening at the worksite, however, has obvious benefit for those at work but will not help the rest of the community, especially the elderly. It is unlikely, in most industrialized countries, that the additional cost of screening over those of case finding can be justified.

COSTS AND BENEFITS FROM TREATING HYPERTENSION

Table 12.4 gives the direct cost of the North Karelia Project hypertension program from 1972 to 1977 for a population of 175 000.[48] At 1975 prices this works out at 7 dollars per head of population per year.

Table 12.5 gives the direct and indirect costs of a stroke in the United States in 1976.[49] At 1976 prices this works out at 34 dollars per person in that year. If 40 per cent of these strokes were prevented, if this reduction

Table 12.4 Direct costs (at 1975 prices) of the North Karelia Project hypertension programme during the period 1972–1977[48]

	US dollars (× 1000)	Percentage of total costs
Case finding	170	3
Initial examination	168	3
Annual follow-up	415	7
Intermediate follow-up	1167	20
Drug treatment	3498	59
Visits to hypertension dispensary by borderline patients and normotensives	109	2
Hypertension register	83	1
Training of health personnel	206	3
Education, planning, & management	146	2
Total	5962	100

Table 12.5 US costs of stroke (1976) at 6% discount rate (Adelman[49])

Direct Costs	Millions ($)
Direct:	
In-patient (acute)	1376
Nursing care facilities	1029
Physicians	127
Non-physician services	699
Appliances	29
	3260
Indirect:	
Morbidity—earnings loss	
Out of hospital can't work	98
Out of hospital can't keep house	160
In hospital can't work, etc.	180
	438
Mortality costs	
Present value of future earnings	3666
Total	7364

were the only benefit from treating hypertension, and if indirect costs of such treatment are excluded, then the cost savings could be $14 - 7 - 7$ dollars/person/year. This calculation, however, relies heavily on many assumptions: the 40 per cent reduction in strokes, the treatment costs in Finland for hypertension, the treatment costs in the United States for stroke. It does not consider, for instance, whether the treatment costs for hypertension would be much higher in the USA. Alderman and Stanback calculate the cost of treating a hypertensive patient in the USA to be between 200 and 300 dollars per year.[47] If 3 per cent of the *total* population were treated this would amount to 6–9 dollars/person/year. Similarly Hartunian *et al.*[50] have calculated the 1975 USA costs to be 6456 million dollars, which is close to the 7364 million dollars of Adelman's study.[49]

The costs of treatment in the North Karelia Project were mainly those of drug treatment (59 per cent) and follow-up (27 per cent). The costs of stroke were mainly those of premature death (50 per cent), whereas loss of earnings due to morbidity accounted for only 6 per cent. Acute in-patient care accounted for 19 per cent of costs and chronic long-term care for 14 per cent. Such calculations will, however, depend on the age of the population. In the UK, the older population will increase direct costs and reduce mortality costs through lower potential future earnings.

Table 12.6 gives the calculations of Hartunian and colleagues[50] broken

Table 12.6 Estimated costs for four major diseases (USA, 1975—Hartunian *et al.*[50])

	Costs (millions US$)		
	Direct	Indirect	Total
Strokes			
haemorrhage	239	1470	1709
infarction	2015	2602	4617
TIA	114	16	130
all strokes	2368	4088	6456
All cancers	6411	16 737	23 148
Coronary heart disease	2491	11 225	13 716
Motor vehicle injuries	4773	9662	14 435

down into direct costs such as hospitalization costs and indirect costs such as loss of productivity. The Table considers not only strokes, including cerebral haemorrhage, infarction, and TIAs, but also cancers, coronary heart disease, and motor vehicle injuries. As expected, the ratio of indirect to direct costs is least for strokes as they occur in the oldest members of the population. Coronary heart disease and cancers are responsible for 22 per cent and 21 per cent of loss of life expectancy respectively, compared with 11 per cent for stroke.[51]

Another form of analysis, differing from the cost–benefit approach discussed above, is that of cost-effectiveness analysis.[52] In this analysis the sum of the direct and indirect costs is divided by a measure of outcome to give, for example, a cost per mmHg of blood-pressure reduction per hypertensive patient per year. This varies between 8 and 29 dollars per mmHg in certain studies.[53] Similarly, the cost of each year of life may be calculated; Table 12.7 gives the years of life lost when a person has an untreated diastolic blood-pressure of 115 mmHg (15¼ hPa).[54] The calculations are given for both men and women at ages 25, 45, 65, and 75. Note that high blood-pressure would not appear to be a risk indicator at the age of 75. This has been confirmed in the very elderly (average 88 years) in a study in Finland.[55] Few would disagree with one of these authors' conclusions. 'A moderately high blood pressure would seem to indicate an adequately functioning cardiovascular system' and the hypertensive subjects had a longer survival especially in comparison with these who had the lowest pressures.

Nevertheless this does not indicate whether lowering blood-pressure in these advantaged elderly subjects would be to their further advantage or detriment. It is not desirable for an elderly hypertensive patient to suffer

Table 12.7 Number of years lost due to elevated DBP of 115 mmHg (Waaler et al.[54])

Age	Men	Women
25	10.0	13.7
45	4.7	7.9
65	0.7	3.0
75	0	0.1

a stroke. Only randomized controlled trials of treatment can address this issue. In the meantime, cost–effectiveness in terms of years of survival has to be calculated from observational data as in Table 12.7.

A cost–utility analysis is employed when the divisor is not fall in pressure or increased years of survival, but years of survival adjusted for its quality (quality-adjusted life years or QALYs) Table 12.8 gives such a calculation for men and women aged 20 and 60. The surprisingly high cost of one QALY in men aged 60 may be due to calculations being based on observational data and not on experimental data from randomized trials of treatment. Such trials show not only a benefit in terms of prolonging survival and preventing stroke[56-8] but also that the proportional benefit of treatment in preventing stroke is the same in the elderly as in younger subjects. However, as the older patients have more strokes, the absolute benefits per annum are greater in the elderly. For example, less than 100 patients in the European Working Party on hypertension in the Elderly[57] have to be treated for a year to prevent one stroke compared with over 800 middle-aged patients in the Medical Research Council trial.[59]

Leaving aside the issue of age, Maynard has calculated that the lifelong treatment of hypertension in the UK in 1983–1984 costs £1700 to provide one QALY.[60] This compares favourably with heart transplantation (£5000) and hospital haemodialysis (£14 000), but not with aortic valve replacement (£900) or hip replacement (£850) where the emphasis must

Table 12.8 Net cost of 1 QALY (quality-adjusted life-year) from lifelong treatment of hypertension, (Weinstein and Stason[62]) ·

Age (years)	Costs ($)	
	Men	Women
20	3300	8500
60	16 300	5000

be on quality of life rather than increased survival. These cost–utility analyses depend heavily on the measurement of quality of life—a difficult procedure especially after a stroke.[61] Nevertheless, from the cost-benefit point of view the treatment of hypertension is well worthwhile, especially in young and in elderly women,[62] and almost certainly in elderly men.

Reference

Introduction

1. Evans, J. G. and Caird, F. I. (1982). Epidemiology of neurological disorders in old age. In *Neurological disorders in the elderly* (ed. Caird, F. I.), pp. 1–16. Bristol. Wright.
2. Doll, R. (1971). The age distribution of cancer: implications for theories of pathogenesis. *Journal of the Royal Statistical Society A*, **134**, 135–55.
3. Evans, J. G. (1983). Towards 2001—population changes: implications for care. The health services. *Journal of the Royal Society of Health*, **103**, 220–1.
4. Ostfeld, A. M. (1980). A review of stroke epidemiology. *Epidemiologic Reviews*, **2**, 136–52.
5. Mitchinson, J. J. (1980). The hypotensive stroke. *Lancet*, **1**, 244–6.
6. Critchley, E. M. R. (1984). Non-atheromatous causes of cerebral infarction. *Postgraduate Medical Journal*, **60**, 386–90.
7. Jellinger, K. (1977). Cerebral haemorrhage in cerebrovascular amyloid angiopathy. In *Cerebral vascular disease* (ed. Meyer J. S., H., Lechner and M. Reivich), pp. 170–3, Excerpta Medica, Amsterdam.
8. Hatano, S. (1976a). Variability of the diagnosis of stroke by clinical judgement and by a scoring method. *Bulletin of the World Health Organization*, **54**, 533–40.
9. Hatano, S. (1976b). Experience from a multicenter stroke register—a preliminary report. *Bulletin of the World Health Organization*, **54**, 541–53.
10. Caplan, L., Hier, D., Goodwin J. and Ferguson, L. (1980). Subdural hematoma mimicking other stroke syndromes. *Transaction of the American Neurological Association*, **105**, 167–9.
11. Kagan, A., Katsuki, S., Sternby, N., and Vanacek, R. (1967). Reliability of death certificate data on vascular lesions affecting the central nervous system. *Bulletin of the World Health Organization*, **37**, 477–81.
12. Florey, C. du V., Senter, M. G., and Acheson, R. M. (1969). A study of the validity of stroke in mortality data. II: Comparison by computer of autopsy and clinical records with death certificates. *American Journal of Epidemiology*, **89**, 15–24.
13. De Faire, U., Faiberg, L., Lorich, U., and Lundman, T. (1976). A validation of cause-of-death certification in 1156 deaths. *Acta Medica Scandinavica*, **200**, 723–8.
14. Corwin, L. I., Wolf, P. A., Kannel, W. B., and McNamara, P. M. (1982). Accuracy of death certification of stroke: the Framingham study. *Stroke*, **13**, 818–21.
15. von Arbin, M., Britton, M., De Faire, U., Helmers, C., Miam, K., and Murray, V. (1981). Accuracy of bedside diagnosis in stroke. *Stroke*, **12**, 288–93.

16. Yates, P. O. (1964). A change in the pattern of cerebrovascular disease. *Lancet*, **1**, 65–9.

17. Acheson, R. M. (1966). *Cerebrovascular disease epidemiology*. Public Health Monograph No. 76, US Department of Health Education and Welfare, Washington DC.

18. Stallones, R. A. (1979). Epidemiology of stroke in relation to the cardiovascular disease complex. *Advances in Neurology*, **25**, 117–26.

19. Whisnant, J. P. (1984). The decline of stroke. *Stroke*, **15**, 160–8.

20. Stallones, R. A. (1980). The rise and fall of ischaemic heart disease. *Scientific American*, **243** (5), 43–9.

21. Evans, J. G. (1986). The decline of stroke. In *Stroke: epidemiological, therapeutic and socioeconomic aspects* (ed. Rose, F. C.), pp. 33–8 Royal Society of Medicine, London.

22. Evans, J. G. (1971). Trends in mortality from ulcerative colitis in England and Wales. *Gut*, **12**, 119–22.

23. Yablonski, M., Behar, A., Ungar, H., Resch, J., and Alter, M. (1968). Cerebral atherosclerosis among Israeli Jews of European and Afro-Asian origin. *Neurology*, **18**, 550–8.

24. Borhani, N. (1979). Mortality trends in hypertension, United States, 1950–1976. In *Proceedings of the conference on the decline in coronary heart disease mortality* (ed. Havlik, X. and M. Feinleib), NIH Publication No. 79–1610, pp. 218–33. US Department of Health, Education and Welfare, Washington DC.

25. Reid, D. D. and Evans, J. G. (1970). New drugs and changing mortality from non-infectious disease. *British Medical Bulletin*, **26**, 191–6.

26. Paffenbarger R. S., Milling P. H., Poe N. D., and Krueger, D. E. (1966). Trends in death rates from hypertensive disease in Memphis, Tennessee 1920–1960. *Journal of Chronic Diseases*, **19**, 847–56.

27. Joossens, J. V. (1973). Salt and hypertension, water hardness and cardiovascular disease. *Triangle*, **12**, 9–16.

28. Joossens, J. V., Kesteloot, H, and Amery, A. (1979). Salt intake and mortality from stroke. *New England Journal of Medicine*, **300**, 1396.

29. Dobson A. J. (1981). Age-specific trends in mortality from ischaemic heart disease and cerebrovascular disease in Australia. *American Journal of Epidemiology*, **113**, 404–12.

30. Bonita, R. and Beaglehole, R. (1982). Trends in cerebrovascular disease mortality in New Zealand. *New Zealand Medical Journal*, **95**, 411–14.

31. Editorial (1983). Why has stroke mortality declined? *Lancet*, **1**, 1195–6.

32. Krueger, D. E., Williams, J. L., and Paffenbarger, R. G. (1967). Trends in death rates from cardiovascular disease in Memphis, Tennessee 1920–1960. *Journal of Chronic Diseases*, **20**, 129–37.

33. Acheson, R. M. (1960). Mortality from cerebrovascular accidents and hypertension in the Republic of Ireland. *British Journal of Preventive and Social Medicine*, **14**, 139–47.

34. Anderson, T. W. and MacKay, J. S. (1968). A critical reappraisal of the epidemiology of cerebrovascular disease. *Lancet*, **1**, 1137–41.

35. Garraway, W. M., Whisnant, J. P., and Drury, I. (1983). The changing pattern of survival following stroke. *Stroke*, **14**, 699–703.

36. Matsumoto, N., Whisnant, J. P., Kurland, L. T., and Okazaki, H. (1973). Natural history of stroke in Rochester, Minnesota, 1955 through 1969: an

extension of a previous study, 1945 through 1954. *Stroke*, **4**, 20–9.

38. Ueda, K., Omae, T., Hirota, Y., Takeshita, M., Katsuki, S., Tanaka, K., and Enjoji, M. (1981). Decreasing trend in incidence and mortality from stroke in Hisayama residents, Japan. *Stroke*, **12**, 154–60.

39. Komachi, Y., Tanaka, H., Shimamoto, T., Hanoa, K., Ioa, M., Isomura, K., Kojima, S., Matsuzaki, T., Ozawa, H., Takahashi, H., and Tsunetoshi, Y. (1984). A collaborative study of stroke incidence in Japan: 1975–79. *Stroke*, **15**, 28–36.

40. Garraway, W. M. and Whisnant, J. P. (1987). The changing pattern of hypertension and the declining incidence of stroke. *Journal of the American Medical Association*, **258**, 214–17.

41. Holme, I., Waaler, H. T. (1976). Five-year mortality in the City of Bergen, Norway according to age, sex and blood pressure. *Acta Medica Scandinavica*, **200**, 229–39.

42. Mattila, K., Haavisto, M., Rajala, S. and Heikinheimo, R. (1988). Blood pressure and five year survival in the very old. *British Medical Journal*, **296**, 887–9.

43. Evans, J. G. (1987). Blood pressure and stroke in an elderly English population. *Journal of Epidemiology and Community Health*, **41**, 275–82.

Acute stroke

1. Agnoli, A., Fieschi, C., Bozzao, L. *et al.* (1968). Autoregulation of cerebral blood flow. Studies during drug-induced hypertension in normal subjects and in patients with cerebral vascular diseases. *Circulation*, **38**, 800–12.

2. Strandgaard, S., Olesen, J., Skinhøj, E. *et al.* (1973). Autoregulation of brain circulation in severe arterial hypertension. *British Medical Journal*, **1**, 507–10.

3. Kawakami, H., Kutsuzawa, T., Uemura, K. *et al.* (1974). Regional cerebral blood flow in patients with hypertensive intracerebral hemorrhage. *Stroke*, **5**, 207–12.

4. Heilbrun, M. P., Olesen, J., and Lassen, N. A. (1972). Regional cerebral blood flow studies in subarachnoid hemorrhage. *Journal of Neurosurgery*, **37**, 36–44.

5. Bayer, A. J., Pathy, M. S. J., and Newcombe, R. (1987). Double-blind randomized trial of intravenous glycerol in acute stroke. *Lancet*, **1**, 405–8.

6. Gilsanz, V., Rebollar, J. L., Buencuerpo, J. *et al.* (1975). Controlled trial of glycerol versus dexamethasome in the treatment of cerebral oedema in acute cerebral infarction. *Lancet*, **1**, 1049–56.

7. Ishii, S., Tsubokawa, T., Tsuru, M. *et al.* (1977). Clinical effect of glycerol (CG-A30) on increased intracranial pressure—Double-blind controlled trial of glycerol versus mannitol (in japanese). *Shin-Yaku to Rinsho*, **26**, 1791.

8. Norris, J. W. (1976). Steroid therapy in acute cerebral infarction. *Archives of Neurology*, **33**, 69–71.

9. Barnett, H. J. M. (1986). Antithrombotic therapy in cerebral vascular disease; Antispasmodics and fibrinolysins. In *Stroke: pathophysiology, diagnosis and management* (ed. Barnett, H. J. M. *et al.*) pp. 989–99. Churchill Livingstone, New York).

10. Gates, P. C., Buchan, A. M., and Barnett, M. J. M. (1985). Luminal thrombus in cerebral circulation. *Stroke*, **16**, 140.

11. Keating, E. C., Gross, S. A., Schlamowitz, R. A. *et al.* (1983). Mural thrombi in myocardial infarctions. *American Journal of Medicine*, **74**, 989–95.
12. Weinreich, D. J., Burke, J. F., and Pauletto, F. J. (1984). Left ventricular mural thrombi complicating acute myocardial infarction. *Annals of Internal Medicine*, **100**, 789–94.
13. Szekely, P. (1964). Systemic embolism and anticoagulant prophylaxis in rheumatic heart disease. *British Medical Journal*, **1**, 1209–13.
14. Adams, G. F., Merrett, J. D., Hutchinson, W. M. *et al.* (1974). Cerebral embolism and mitral stenosis; survival with and without anticoagulants. *Journal of Neurology, Neurosurgery and Psychiatry*, **37**, 378–83.
15. Veterans Administration Hospital Investigators (1973). Anticoagulants in acute myocardial infarction. Results of a cooperative clinical trial. *Journal of the American Medical Association*, **225**, 724–9.
16. Yamaguchi, T., Minematsu, K., Choki, J. *et al.* (1984). Clinical and neuroradiological analysis of thrombotic and embolic cerebral infarction. *Japanese Circulation Journal*, **48**, 50–8.
17. Cerebral Embolism Study Group (1984). Immediate anticoagulation of embolic stroke; brain hemorrhage and management options. *Stroke*, **15**, 779–89.
18. Yamaguchi, T., Minematsu, K., Choki, J. *et al.* (1986). Recurrent cerebral embolism and factors rerated to early recurrence,—Analysis of 186 cases. In *Central nervous system control of the heart*, (ed. Strober, T. *et al.*) p. 237, Martinus Nijhof Publishing, Boston.
19. Cerebral Embolism Task Force (1986). Cardiogenic cerebral embolism. *Archives of Neurology*, **43**, 71–84.
20. Bousser, M. G., Eschwege, E., Haguenau, M. *et al.* (1983). 'AICLA' controlled trial of aspirin and dipyridamole in the secondary prevention of athero-thrombotic cerebral ischemia. *Stroke*, **14**, 5–14.
21. Canadian Cooperative Study Group (1978). A randomized trial of aspirin and sulfinpyrazone in threatened stroke. *New England Journal Medicine*, **299** 53–9.
22. Reuther, R. and Dorndorf, W. (1978). Aspirin in patients with cerebral ischemia and normal angiograms or nonsurgical lesions. Results of a double blind trial. In *Acetylsalicylic acid in cerebral ischemia and coronary heart disease* (ed. Breddin, K. *et al.*) p. 97. FK Schattauer Verlag, Stuttgart.
23. Fields, W. S., Lemak, N. A., Frankowski, R. F. *et el.* (1977). Controlled trial of aspirin in cerebral eschemia. *Stroke*, **8**, 301–15.
24. Murakami, M., Toyokura, Y., Omae, T. *et ul.* (1983). Effect of ticlopidine and aspirin on transient ischemic attacks; Multi-center double-blind controlled trial in Japan (in Japanese). *Igaku no Ayumi*, **127**, 950.
25. Harter, H. R., Burch, J. W., Majerus, P. W. *et al.* (1978). Prevention of thrombosis in patients on hemodialysis by low dose aspirin. *New England Journal of Medicine*, **301**, 577–9.
26. Meyer, J. S., Gilroy, J., Barnhart, M. E. *et al.* (1965). Therapeutic thrombolysis in cerebral thromboembolism. Randomized evaluation of intravenous streptokinase. In *Cerebral vascular diseases*, (ed. Millikan C. H. *et al*) p. 200 Grune & Stratton, New York.
27. Hanaway, J., Track, R., Fletcher, A. P. *et al.* (1976). Intracranial bleeding associated with urokinase therapy for acute ischemic hemispheric infarction. *Stroke*, **7**, 143–6.

28. Ohtomo, E., Araki, G., Ito, E. *et al.* (1985). Clinical efficacy of urokinase in the treatment of cerebral thrombosis-Multicenter double blind study in comparison with placebo. (in Japanese with English abstract). *Clinical Evaluation*, **13**, 711.

29. Zivin, J. A., Fisher, M., DeGirolami, U. *et al.* (1985). Tissue plaminogen activator reduces neurological damage after cerebral embolism. *Science*, **230**, 1289–92.

30. Wood, J. H. and Kee, D. B. (1985). Hemorheology of the cerebral circulation in stroke. *Stroke*, **16**, 765–72.

31. Strand, Y., Asplund, K., Eriksson, S. *et al.* (1984). A randomized trial of hemodilution therapy in acute ischemic stroke. *Stroke*, **15**, 980–9.

32. Yamaguchi, T., Regli, F., and Waltz, A. G. (1971). Effect of $PaCO_2$ on hyperemia and ischemia in experimental cerebral infarction. *Stroke*, **2**, 139–47.

33. Høedt-Rasmussen, K., Shinhøj, E., Paulson, O. B. *et al.* (1967). Cerebral blood flow in acute apoplexy. The 'luxury perfusion syndrome' of brain tissue. *Archives of Neurology*, **17**, 271–81.

34. Olesen, J. and Paulson, O. B. (1971). The effect of intraarterial papaverine on the regional cerebral blood flow in patients with stroke or intracranial tumor. *Stroke*, **2**, 148–59.

35. Kazda, S., Hoffmeister, F., Garthoff, B. *et al.* (1979). Prevention for the postischemic impaired reperfusion of the brain by nimodipine (BAY e 9736). *Acta Neurologica Scandinavica*, **60** (Suppl. 72), 302–5.

36. Newberg, L. A., Steen, P. A., Milde, J. H. *et al.* (1958). Effect of nimodipine on cerebral blood flow and neurologic function following complete global ischemia in dogs and primates. In *Nimodipine—pharmacological and clinical properties*, (ed. Betz, E. *et al.*) p. 99 FK Schattauer, Stuttgart.

37. Hoff, J. T., Smith, A. L., Hankinson, H. L. *et al.* (1975). Barbiturate protection from cerebral infarction in primates. *Stroke*, **6**, 28–33

38. Black, K. L., Weidler, D. J., Jallad, N. S. *et al.* (1978). Delayed pentobarbital therapy of acute focal cerebral ischemia. *Stroke*, **9**, 245–9.

39. Holaday, J. W. and D' Amato, R. J. (1982). Naloxon or TRH fails to improve neurological deficits in gerbil models of stroke. *Life Sciences*, **31**, 385–92.

40. Jabaily, J. and Davis, J. N. (1984). Naloxon administration to patients with acute stroke. *Stroke*, **15**, 36–9.

41. Yasargil, M. G. (1969). *Microsurgery applied to neurosurgery*. p. 105 Georg-Thieme, Stuttgart.

42. The EC/IC Bypass Study Group (1985). Failure of extracranial–intracranial arterial bypass to reduce the risk of ischemic stroke. Results of an international randomized trial. *New England Journal of Medicine*, **313**, 1191–200.

43. Fields, W. S., Maslenikov, V., Meyer, J. S. *et al.* (1970). Joint study of extracranial arterial occlusion. V. Progress report of prognosis following surgery or nonsurgical treatment for transient cerebral ischemic attacks and cervical carotid arterial lesions. *Journal of the American Medical Association*, **211**, 1993–2003.

44. Shaw, D. A., Venables, G. S., Cartlidge, N. E. F. *et al.* (1984). Carotid endarterectomy in patients with transient cerebral ischemia. *Journal of the Neurological Sciences*, **64**, 45–53.

45. Committee on Health Care Issues (1987). Does carotid endarterectomy de-

crease stroke and death in patients with transient ischemic attacks?. *Annals of Neurology*, **22**, 72–6.

46. Brott, T. and Thalinger, K. (1984). the practice of carotid endarterectomy in a large metropolitan area. *Stroke*, **15**, 950–5.
47. Whisnant, J. P., Sandok, B. A., and Sundt, T. M. (1983). Carotid endarterectomy for unilateral carotid system transient cerebral ischemia. *Mayo Clinic Proceedings*, **58**, 171–5.
48. Browse, N. L., Ross-Russel, R. (1984). Carotid endarterectomy and the Javid shunt; The early results of 215 consecutive operations for transient ischemic attacks. *British Journal of Surgery*, **71**, 53–7.
49. Easton, J. D. and Sherman, D. G. (1977). Stroke and mortality rate in carotid endarterectomy: 228 consecutive operations. *Stroke*, **8**, 565–8.
50. Ojemann, R. G. and Heros, R. C. (1983). Spontaneous brain hemorrhage. *Stroke*, **14**, 468–75.
51. Kase, C. S., Williams, D. A., Wyatt, D. A. *et al.* (1982). Lobar intracerebral hematomas: clinical and CT analysis of 22 cases. *Neurology*, **32**, 1146–50.
52. Matsumoto, K. and Hondo, H. (1984). CT-guided stereotaxic evacuation of hypertensive intracerebral hematomas. *Journal of Neurosurgery*, **61**, 440–8.

Prevention

1. Hatano, S. (1976). Experience from a multicentre stroke register, a preliminary report. *Bulletin of World Health Organization*, **54**, 541–53.
2. Oxfordshire Community Stroke Project (1983). Incidence of stroke in Oxfordshire: first year's experience of community stroke register. *British Medical Journal*, **287**, 713–17.
3. A. E. Doyle (1983). Vascular complications of hypertension. In *Handbook of hypertension, Vol 1: Clinical Aspects of essential hypertension* (ed. Robertson, J. I. S.) pp. 365–77 Elsevier Science Publishers, Amsterdam.
4. Stephens, W. E. (1972). Pathology of the cerebral blood vessels. In *Handbook of hypertension, Vol 1: Clinical aspects of essential hypertension*, (ed. Robertson J. I. S.) p. 196 Elsevier Science Publishers, Amsterdam.
5. Brice, J. G., Dowsett, D. J., and Lowe R. D. (1964). Haemodynamic effect of carotid artery stenosis. *British Medical Journal*, **2**, 1363.
6. Graham D. I. *et al.* (1983). Hypertension and the intracranial and ocular circulations: effects of antihypertensive treatment. In *Handbook of hypertension, Vol 1: Clinical aspects of essential hypertension*, (ed. Robertson, J. I. S.) pp. 174–201, Elsevier Science Publishers, Amsterdam).
7. Mohr, J. P., Caplan, L. R., and Melski, J. (1978). The Harvard Co-operative Stroke Registry; a prospective registry. *Neurology*, **28**, 754–62.
8. Adams, R. D. and Risher, C. M. (1961). Pathology of cerebral arterial occlusion. In *Pathogenesis and treatment of cerebrovascular disease* Field, W. S., (ed.) p. 126 Charles C. Thomas, Springfield, IL.
9. Adams, R. D., (1957). Pathology of cerebral vascular disease. B. Cranial cerebral lesions. In *Princeton conferences on cerebrovascular disease*, (ed. Millikan, C. H.) (2nd edn) p. 23 Grune and Stratton, New York.
10. Leishman, R. (1957). The eye in general vascular disease: hypertension and arteriosclerosis. *British Journal of Ophthalmology*, **41**, 641.
11. Harnish, A. and Pearce, M. L. (1973). Evolution of hypertensive retinal

vascular disease: Correlation between clinical and post-mortem observations. *Medicine (Baltimore)*, **52**, 483.

12. Fisher, C. H. (1965) Lacunes, small deep cerebral infacts. *Neurology*, **15**, 774–84.
13. Caplan, L. R. and Stein, R. W. (1986). Small vessel disease. In *Stroke a clinical approach*, pp. 167–77 Butterworths, London.
14. Charcot, J. M. and Bouchard, C. (1868) Nouvelles recherches sur la pathogénie de l'hemorragie cérébrale. *Archives de Physiologie Normale et Pathologique (Paris)*, **1**, 110–25.
15. Russell, R. W. R. (1963) Observations on intracerebral aneurysms. *Brain*, **86**, 425–35.
16. Marie, P. (1901) Des foyers lacunaires de desintégration. *Revues Médicales*, **21**, 281–96.
17. Hachinski, V. C., Lassen, N. A., and Marshall, J. (1974). Multi-infarct dementia: A cause of mental deterioration in the elderly, *Lancet*, **2** 207.
18. Toole, J. F., Janeway, R., Choi, K. *et al.* (1975). Transient ischaemic attacks due to atherosclerosis. *Archives of Neurology*, **32**, 5.
19. Strandgaard, S., Olesen, J., Skinhoj, E., and Lassen N. A. (1973). Autoregulation of brain circulation in severe arterial hypertension. *British Medical Journal*, **1**, 507.
20. Crawford, T. (1959). Some observations on the pathogenesis and natural history of intracranial aneurysms. *Journal of Neurology, Neurosurgery and Psychiatry*, **22**, 259.
21. Du Boulay, G. H. (1965). Some observations on the natural history of intracranial aneurysms. *British Journal of Radiology*, **38**, 721.
22. Cole, F. M. and Yates, P. O. (1968). Comparative incidence of cerebrovascular lesions in normotensive and hypertensive patients. *Neurology*, **18**, 255.
23. Baker, A. B., Resch, J. A., and Loewenson, R. B. (1969). Hypertension and cerebral atherosclerosis. *Circulation*, **39**, 701.
24. Fisher, C. M., Gore, I., Okabe, N., and White, P. D. (1965). Atherosclerosis of the carotid and vertebral arteries: extracranial and intracranial. *Journal of Neuropathology and Experimental Neurology*, **24**, 455.
25. McCormick, W. F., and Schmalstieg, E. J. (1977). The relationship of arterial hypertension to intracranial aneurysms. *Archives of Neurology*, **34**, 285.
26. Levy, R. I. (1979). Stroke decline: implications and prospects. *New England Journal of Medicine*, **300**, 490–1.
27. Bonita, R. and Beaglehole, R. (1982). Trends in cerebrovascular disease mortality in New Zealand. *New Zealand Medical Journal*, **95**, 411-13,
28. Haberman, S., Capildeo, R. and Rose F. C. (1978). The changing mortality of cerebrovascular disease. *Quarterly Journal of Medicine*, **47**, 71–88.
29. Friedman, G. D. (1979). Decline of hospitalization for coronary heart disease and stroke: the Kaiser-Permanente experience in Northern California 1971–1977. In *National Institutes of Health Publication*, No. 79–610, Bethesda MD.
30. Spence, J. D. (1986). Antihypertensive drugs and prevention of atherosclerotic stroke. *Stroke*, **17**, 808–10.
31. Kannel, W. B. *et al.* (1975). An evaluation of the epidemiology of atherothrombotic brain infarction. *Milbank Memorial Fund Quarterly*, **53**, 405–48.
32. Acheson, R. M. and Fairbairn, A. S. (1970). Burden of cerebrovascular disease in the Oxford area in 1963 and 1964. *British Medical Journal*, **i**, 621–6.

33. Garraway, W. M., Whisnant, J. P., Furlan, A. J., Phillip II, L. H. *et al.* (1979). The declining incidence of stroke. *New England Journal of Medicine*, **300**, 449–52.
34. Bulpitt, C. J. (1987). Does lowering blood pressure in hypertensive patients reduce the risk of death from coronary heart disease? Netherlands Journal of Medicine, **30**, 228–34.
35. Joossens, J. V., Kesteloot, H., and Amery, A. (1979). Salt intake and mortality from stroke. *Lancet*, **ii**, 1396.
36. Royal College of Physicians (1974). *Report of the Geriatrics Committee Working Group on Strokes*. Royal College of Physicians of London, London.
37. Harris, A. I., Cox, E., and Smith, C. R. W. (1971). *Handicapped and impaired in Great Britain, Part 1*. Office of Population Censuses and Surveys, HMSO, London.
38. Gill, J. S., Shipley, M. J, Tsementzis, S. A. *et al.* (1988). Cigarette smoking is a risk factor for haemorrhagic and non-haemorrhagic stroke. *Clinical Science*, **74**, Supplement 18, 5p–6p.
39. Klatsky, A. L. (1985). Blood pressure and alcohol consumption. In *Handbook of hypertension, Vol. 6, Epidemiology of hypertension*. (ed. Bulpitt, C. J.) pp. 159–74, Elsevier, Amsterdam.
40. Bulpitt, C. J., Shipley, M. J., and Semmence, A. (1987). The contribution of a moderate intake of alcohol to the prevalence of hypertension. *Journal of Hypertension*, **5**, 95–1.
41. Gill, J. S., Shipley, M. J., Tsementzis, S. A. *et al.* (1988). The pattern of risk from alcohol consumption does not differ in haemorrhagic and non-haemorrhagic stroke. *Clinical Science*, **74**, Supplement 18, 21p–22p.
42. Bulpitt, C. J. (1989). Definition, prevalence and incidence of hypertension in the elderly. In *Handbook of Hypertension. Vol. 12 Hypertension in the elderly* (ed. Amery, A. and J. Staessen) pp. 153–69, Elsevier, Amsterdam.
43. Bauer, G. E., Hunyor, S. N., and Stokes, G. (1985). Advertising and the treatment of hypertension. In *Handbook of hypertension, Vol. 6, Epidemiology of hypertension*. (ed. Bulpitt, C. J.), pp. 497–508. Elsevier, Amsterdam
44. Penfold, D., Styles, W. and Bulpitt, C. (1983). North Hammersmith stroke prevention project. *Journal of Epidemiology and Community Health*, **37**, 310–14.
45. Cartmel, B., Penfold, D., Styles, W. M., and Bulpitt, C. J. (1987). The North Hammersmith Stroke Prevention Project: changes in stroke mortality in the London health districts. *Bibliotheca Cardiologica*. **42**, 32–40
46. Miall, W. E. and Chinn, S. (1973). Blood pressure and ageing; results of a 15–17 year follow-up study in South Wales. *Clinical Science and Molecular Medicine*, **45**, 235.
47. Alderman, M. H. and Stanback, M. E. (1985). Hypertension detection and management through the worksite in the United States. In *Handbook of hypertension, Vol. 6, Epidemiology of hypertension* (ed. Bulpitt, C. J.), pp. 371–86. Elsevier, Amsterdam.
48. Tuomilehto, J., Nissinen, A., Puska, P., and Salonen, J. (1985). Community control of hypertension in Finland. In *Handbook of hypertension, Vol. 6, Epidemiology of hypertension* (ed. Bulpitt C. J.), pp. 387-411. Elsevier, Amsterdam.
49. Adelman, S. M. (1981). National survey of stroke: economic impact. *Stroke*, **12** (Suppl. 1), 69–87.

50. Hartunian, N. S., Smart, C. N., and Thompson, M. S. (1980). The incidence and economic costs of cancer, motor vehicle injuries, coronary heart disease and stroke: a comparative analysis. *American Journal of Public Health*, **70**, 1249–59.

51. Black, D. A. K. and Pole, J. D. (1975). Priorities in biomedical research in indices of burden. *British Journal of Social and Preventive Medicine*, **29**, 222–7.

52. Drummond, M. F. and Ward, G. H. (1986). The financial burden of stroke and the economic evaluation of treatment alternatives. In *Stroke: epidemiological, therapeutic and socio-economic aspects* (ed. Rose F. C.), Royal Soc. Med. Services. Int. Congress and Symposium Series No. 99, London pp.147–62.

53. Ruchlin, H. S., Melcher, L. A., and Alderman, M. H. (1984). A comparative economic analysis of work-related hypertension care programs. *Journal of Occupational Medicine*, **26**, 45–9.

54. Waaler, H. T. Helgeland, A. Hjort, P. F. *et al.* (1978) Quoted in Wilhelmsen, L. Cost effectiveness. In *Handbook of hypertension, Vol. 6, Epidemiology of hypertension*, (ed. Bulpitt C. J.), pp. 487–96. Elsevier, Amsterdam.

55. Mattila, K., Haavisto, M., Rajala, S., and Heikinheimo, R. (1988). Blood pressure and five year survival in the very old. *British Medical Journal*, **296**, 887–9.

56. Report by the Management Committee (1981). Treatment of mild hypertension in the elderly. *Medical Journal of Australia*, **68**, 398–42.

57. Amery, A., Birkenhager, W., Brixko, P., Bulpitt, C. *et al.* (1985). Mortality and morbidity results from the European Working Party on High Blood Pressure in the Elderly trial. *Lancet*, **i**, 1349.

58. Coope, J. and Warrender, T. S. (1986). Randomised trial of treatment of hypertension in elderly patients in primary care. *British Medical Journal*, **293**, 1145.

59. Medical Research Council Working Party (1985). MRC trial of treatment of mild hypertension: principal results. *British Medical Journal*, **291**, 97.

60. Maynard, A. (1987). Logic in medicine: an economic perspective. *British Medical Journal* **295**, 1537–41.

61. Fletcher, A. E. and Bulpitt, C. J. (1986). Quality of life after a stroke. In *Stroke: epidemiological, therapeutic and socio-economic aspects*, (ed. Rose, F. C.). Royal Soc. Med. Services. Int. Congress and Symposium Series No. 99, London pp. 115–121.

62. Weinstein, M. C. and Stason, W. B. (1976). *Hypertension. A policy perspective*. Harvard University Press, Cambridge, MS.

13

Drugs and old people: recent advances in geriatric pharmacology

L. OFFERHAUS

INTRODUCTION

Practically every clinician has at one time or another had the experience that the request to an elderly patient to have his medicines brought from home will produce a great number of old boxes, pots, and bottles. One wonders whether all these drugs were really necessary and how it was ever possible that no apparent adverse events were caused by this overload. If after reducing the drug intake to the essentials the patient's health and appetite slowly improve, and he (or she) appears less drowsy and confused, the conclusion that some doctors do more harm than good with drugs seems justified.

Fortunately the last decade has brought great improvements. The interest of the general practitioner, the geriatrician, and the clinical pharmacologist in pharmacotherapeutic problems in the elderly has definitely increased, though there is certainly still room for further improvement.

These problems have many different causes. Not unexpectedly, the elderly require a disproportionate share in health care, including drugs. Often much lower drug doses could have been given than those officially recommended for the same use in young adults. For the same reasons adverse reactions to drugs tend to be much more frequent in the elderly, and the symptoms of such adverse events may mistakenly be diagnosed as symptoms of senility.[1,2] Multiple pathology is the rule rather than the exception, and often the elderly patient is treated at the same time by a number of physicians who hardly communicate and may have potentially conflicting prescribing habits. In many cases the general practitioner is not optimally informed by his colleagues, and very few pharmacists are either physically or psychologically and scientifically well enough equipped to function as co-ordinator. The results are overprescribing, leading to failing compliance, failing confidence in the doctor[3], and finally the patient may take refuge in alternative medicine.

The use of drugs by elderly patients is marked by a number of well-defined problem areas. Some are of a *psychosocial* nature: patient-related problems are low compliance, misunderstanding, poor eyesight, and failing memory;[4] those that are doctor related include excessive prescribing, inadequate clinical assessment before instituting drug therapy, insufficient supervision of maintenance treatment and dosages, increased working pressure on geriatric wards[5] and hospitals,[6] and last but not least both the patient's and the doctor's exaggerated expectations of the achievements of any drug therapy.[7-11] There are also *pharmacokinetic* problems, such as decreased binding of drugs to serum proteins, changed volume of distribution (related to changes in body composition), tissue perfusion and penetration of the drug into the central nervous system, decreased metabolic capacity of the liver, and the physiological decline of kidney function with age.[12-15] *Pharmacodynamic* problems include increased sensitivity of the cerebral receptors to psychotropic drugs,[1] exaggerated reactions to hypotensive drugs caused by changed cardiovascular reflexes, hypoglycaemia induced by oral antidiabetic drugs, and decreased synthesis of coagulation factors in the liver.[16-18] Last but not least is the inappropriate use of what may be called '*problem drugs*'.

Though clinical pharmacological studies of drugs in the elderly have in recent years produced many new and unexpected results, the conclusions drawn from such studies still have to be tested in daily practice. Prescribing rules based purely on pharmacokinetic principles have on the whole proved disappointing. It seems therefore more pragmatic to look at several groups of problematic drugs which have proved difficult to handle in geriatric practice or seem to cause a disproportionate share of the incidence of side-effects. Such an approach means that one has to investigate: (a) which drugs are particularly prescribed for elderly patients, (b) which drugs are particularly prone to cause unnecessary and avoidable problems, and (c) why those drugs cause problems.

In this way it should be possible to restrict the discussion of problems of geriatric drug use to a number of specific drugs or groups of drugs which cause striking or well-defined efficacy or safety problems in elderly patients. A number of these problem areas will be discussed below (p. 216–22); these are *mere examples* of such problems, and many more—anticholinergic drugs, 'geriatric' drugs, corticosteroids—could come to mind.

PSYCHOLOGICAL AND SOCIAL PROBLEMS CONNECTED WITH THE USE OF DRUGS IN THE ELDERLY

Since the Second World War the percentage of the population over the age of 65 has gradually increased to approximately 15 per cent in northwestern Europe and 12 per cent in the USA. However, this section of the population is responsible for 25 per cent of all pharmaceutical expenses in the USA and between 30 and 50 per cent of all drug costs in Europe.[19, 20] This is to be expected, because the incidence of diseases like osteoarthritis, myocardial infarction, cardiac failure, cerebrovascular accidents, parkinsonism, and psychomotor disturbances due to cerebral atherosclerosis and senile dementia sharply increases with age, and such disorders often occur together in the same patient.[21] In countries with effective social insurance systems, prescription drugs are relatively easy to obtain, and in addition the consumption of over-the-counter drugs and alternative and herbal medicines is more widespread among the elderly. On the whole, modern drugs have become more potent and inherently more dangerous. It is often easier for the overworked general practitioner to take his prescription pad and give a drug rather than to explain his refusal to issue a prescription. Even if a strict medical indication is absent, the patient will, particularly in countries of central and southern Europe, put pressure on his doctor to obtain his (or her) favourite drug.[22] Specialist advice is asked for at an earlier stage than in the past, and it is not rare than on admission to a hospital the patient appears to have been using two beta blockers or benzodiazepines simultaneously. Elderly patients using drugs often have difficulties with the prescription regimen. More than half do not know the purpose of their drugs, why they were prescribed at all, and how much and at what times over the day they should be taken. Compliance is no better than an average of 40 per cent, and 60 per cent of patient make one or more mistakes.[21, 23] Moreover, between 10 and 20 per cent of all prescriptions are not filled at all, though the doctor lives under the illusion that the favourable effects he observes are due to his drug.[24] Often the elderly patient has not properly understood what the doctor has told him; sometimes he cannot read the label on the bottle, or is unable to open screw tops or so-called 'child-proof' lids.[25] He cherishes the particular colour of his pills, and becomes confused if prescribed white unidentifiable generics.[26] Some of the main errors are summarized in Table 13.1.

Too little attention is paid to instructing the patient or his relatives on how and when to take his drugs in order to obtain the best effects.[13] In particular, the elderly patient with chronic asymptomatic disorders such as high blood-pressure or diabetes will make mistakes; moreover, automatic repetitions of prescriptions are often left unfilled. It is therefore not surprising that drug-induced adverse events particularly befall the older age groups;[16, 17, 27] that such complications not infrequently necessitate admission to hospital,[28, 29] and that fatal complications, especially due to inappropriate prescribing or use of cardiovascular and antirheumatic drugs, can occur.

Despite the recent profusion of publications on geriatric drug use and on the specific clinical-pharmacological and pharmacokinetic problems

Table 13.1 Types of error made by out-patients aged over 60 years.[3]

Type of error	Number
Omission	126
Self-medication	47
Incorrect dosage	26
Improper timing sequence	15
Inaccurate knowledge	55
Total	269

in this age group, qualitative and quantitative data on drug consumption patterns tend to be rare, and even less is known about the reasons why particular drugs are especially favoured and/or overprescribed. A number of international discrepancies are known. In the UK diuretics and cardiac glycosides comprise more than 50 per cent; antidepressants and tranquillizers are together approximately 20 per cent, and analgesic and antirheumatic drugs (NSAIDs) are also around 20 per cent. In the United States and Canada diuretics (especially frusemide) are extremely popular (4.5 times the average in the age group 64–74 and even up to 13 times more in patients over 85). Despite the scientific uncertainty about the long-term effects of treatment of hypertension in the elderly, hypotensive drugs are grossly overprescribed, as are tranquillizers (particularly benzodiazepines) and laxatives. The average elderly patient uses three different drugs, but patients taking 10 or more are no exception.[28] The number of drugs taken correlates closely with the incidence of adverse reactions though in clinical practice, despite the alarming amount of information on potential interactions, only a few are due to such drug–drug interaction mechanisms. 'Forgotten' maintenance therapies such as coumarin anticoagulants, oral hypoglycaemic agents, and cardiac glycosides carry particular risk.

DRUG-INDUCED DISEASE IN THE ELDERLY CAUSED BY PHARMACOKINETIC PROBLEMS

The kinetic behaviour of a drug in the body is determined by four factors: *absorption*, *distribution*, *metabolism* and *excretion* (ADME). The evidence that deficient absorption (A) of drugs is of importance in geriatric clinical pharmacology is meagre and the incidental abnormal findings are of little or no clinical relevance.[14] The distribution (D) of a drug in body fluids and tissues is determined by body composition; body weight tends to decrease with age, old people 'dry up' (mainly at the expense of extracellular fluid), the quantity of striated muscle tissue decreases, and body fat increases proportionally. Serum albumin concentration decreases with age on the average by 25 per cent, and the drug-binding capacity of red cells falls off as well. The free, pharmacologically active fraction of the drug, which is not bound to proteins or cellular blood components, may show a relative increase. Many drugs are subjected to hepatic metabolism (M) and broken down by microsomal enzyme systems in the liver cells where (mainly through oxidative processes) better water-soluble and pharmacologically less- or even in-active metabolites, which the kidney can excrete, are formed. Liver blood flow decreases with age. In parallel the activity of the metabolizing enzymes falls off, thereby slowing down the metabolic breakdown of drugs which are exclusively excreted along this pathway. The increased elimination half-life causes longer residence times and higher serum levels (accumulation). Fortunately many drugs are inactivated by binding to glucuronic acid or sulphuric acid (conjugation); these conjugates lose their pharmacological activity and are rapidly excreted by the kidney. This process is independent of age. However, pharmacokinetic rules state that accumulation is not solely determined by the half-life, but by the *clearance*, which depends on the volume of distribution of the drug as well. Isolated observations on increases in drug half-life in elderly patients are therefore relatively meaningless if distribution data or data on the clinical duration of action of the drug are lacking.

Most drugs and their metabolites are excreted (E) by the kidney, but some (ampicillin, rifampicin, digitoxin) to a not inconsiderable extent via the bile (a process which is generally independent of age). Renal function, as determined by the inulin or the endogenous creatinine clearance, gradually deteriorates after the age of 40, but the inter-individual variation tends to be very large. For drugs which wholly or almost completely undergo renal elimination, such as most antibiotics, lithium salts, and digoxin, adjustment of dose to kidney function is the most important procedure in preventing overdosage and eventual intoxication symptoms.

Some pharmacokinetic problems in the elderly are more complex, because more than one determinant has undergone an age-dependent change. Typical examples will be described below (p. 216–22).

Despite greatly increased knowledge of altered pharmacokinetics in old people the new data are disappointingly little used in clinical practice, mainly because the drugs studied so far either have a large therapeutic index,[14] or serum level monitoring is applied regardless of age;[30] the case of digoxin is particularly illustrative (see p. 216).

Some pharmacokinetic changes observed in an elderly patient population may have clinical relevance as predictors of side-effects, though inter-individual variability may be so extreme that such knowledge is of no help in daily practice.[31]

CHANGES IN SENSITIVITY TO DRUGS IN THE ELDERLY DUE TO CHANGED PHARMACODYNAMICS

The clinical effect of a drug is determined by its concentration at the end organ (i.e. the 'receptor'). While the concentration is determined by the pharmacokinetic behaviour of the drug, the reaction of the body is also determined by the *quantity* of the receptors and their *sensitivity* to the drug or its metabolites; there is little hard evidence that old age causes any striking changes, and the evidence which is published is mainly of an anecdotal nature.[32] With increasing age the sensitivity to the effects of beta adrenergic blocking agents falls off, though the cause of this change is far from clear;[33] synthesis of clotting factors in the liver is also impaired, and the desired therapeutic effect is reached with lower doses of coumarin anticoagulants. Sensitivity to tranquillizers, sedatives, and anaesthetic agents also increases, and CNS side-effects induced by such agents are more frequent. Hypoglycaemic reactions to sulphonylurea compounds are more common, possibly because more endogenous insulin is set free. Blood-pressure-lowering drugs may cause exaggerated and postural or exertional hypotension with organ perfusion problems such as declining renal function, myocardial infarction, increased anginal or claudication complaints, syncope,[34, 35] and even stroke.[18, 36, 37] Nevertheless decreased sensitivity to drug effects seems to have little relevance for drug use and dosage in the normal recommended range, but more in regard to the development of adverse reactions. On the whole, insufficient effort has been devoted to the study of the effects of age on drug sensitivity[33] and too much emphasis has been placed on pharmacokinetics.

PROBLEM DRUGS

Cardiovascular drugs

Cardiac glycosides

Digitalis glycosides, whether or not in combination with diuretics, may cause serious side-effects in elderly people; in a geriatric population as many as 10 per cent may experience adverse reactions. Often the symptoms are atypical, and they may mimic neuropsychiatric disease: [2, 38] confusion, nightmares, pseudohallucinations, nervousness, excitability, tiredness, loss of appetite, cachexia, visual disturbances, and abnormal colour vision ('yellow vision' is an extreme form).[39] Many factors contribute to the typical clinical picture: accumulation of the drug in some parts of the brain and inhibition of cerebrospinal fluid formation,[40] decreased tissue binding and kidney function,[41] lack of exercise, dietary changes, and possibly also altered smoking and drinking habits.[42, 43] Loading and maintenance doses of digoxin in the elderly should be approximately 50 per cent lower than in young adults. With renal function and clinical effect as a guide—if possible also the serum digoxin concentration (SDC)[44]—the dose should be gradually adjusted upwards. Many old people do not need chronic digoxin therapy at all; in the majority treatment can safely be stopped once the acute phase of the illness or arrhythmia is over.[45] Recent negative results with digoxin in double-blind controlled trials in a number of 'classical' indications such as heart failure and acute rapid atrial fibrillation[46–8] imply that the use of cardiac glyscosides, particularly in old people, should be the exception rather than the rule. Digoxin seems to be on its way from a commonly used panacaea to a superspecialist drug for unusual occasions and indications.

Diuretics

Because many elderly patients suffer from high blood-pressure or cardiac failure, diuretics are widely used in geriatric medicine. For a number of reasons loop diuretics (e.g. frusemide) should be avoided except in emergencies.[36] There is considerable experience with the use of thiazide diuretics in the elderly in a number of recent large-scale trials of antihypertensive treatment in old people with high blood-pressure.[49] There is still controversy about the interpretation of the results,[45, 50] but the risks of long-term treatment—hyperuricaemia (mostly asymptomatic,[51] and very rarely leading to clinical gout), hyperglycaemia,[52] and deterioration of renal function—are negligible if the lowest possible dose is given. The relatively high incidence of impotence in elderly males reported in the UK Medical Research Council trial still remains unexplained, but dosages in that trial were unusually large.

Other drugs for high blood-pressure

Complications of hypertensive disease such as cardiac failure and stroke are much more frequent in elderly than in younger hypertensives. Despite the still marginal improvement in mortality reported in the trials (especially from stroke in females and myocardial infarction in males), antihypertensive drugs tend to be overprescribed. In most cases a simple (and cheap) thiazide diuretic will do. However, evidence is accumulating that very low doses of the ACE-inhibitor captopril can be effective and safe in elderly hypertensive patients as a second or additional choice,[53] as well as in old people with cardiac failure.[54] Though methyldopa has for many years been considered a relatively safe, cheap, and effective hypotensive drug, especially for old people, both efficacy and safety have been seriously questioned recently (sudden falls, depression, haemolytic anaemia, hepatitis, and drug fever have been noted). If possible it should be avoided. A similar controversy surrounds the use of beta blockers as hypotensive drugs in the elderly. Though their side-effects can be annoying,[17, 55] but not necessarily worse or more frequent than those experienced by younger patients,[56] they seem to be just as effective as antihypertensives in the elderly as low dosages of a thiazide diuretic.[57] However, elderly patients with peripheral vascular disease, broncho-spasm, low cardiac output or overt cardiac failure, and/or pre-existent hyperlipidaemia should preferably not be given beta blockers for hyper-tension.

Though undoubtedly no less effective in elderly hypertensives than in young patients,[58] experience with the so-called calcium antagonists (nife-dipine and analogues, diltiazem, and verapamil) is still too limited, and considerable caution is still advised.[59] The first choice in the elderly remains limitation of dietary salt intake, and subsequently a low dose of a thiazide diuretic; if necessary this should be supplemented with a cardio-selective beta blocker with or without an additional vasodilator. Preven-tion of hypokalemia with low doses of a potassium-sparing agent (amilor-ide or spironolactone) is rarely necessary, and mainly in digitalized patients.[60]

Other drugs used for disturbances of cardiac rhythm

There have been very few specific and systematic pharmacokinetic or pharmacodynamic studies of anti-arrhythmic drugs in the elderly. Age is a reason for lowering the intravenous dose of lidocaine by approximately 50 per cent, especially in the treatment or prophylaxis of ventricular arrhyth-mias accompanying acute myocardial infarction,[61, 62] and disopyramide dose should be approximately 30 per cent lower.[63] Reports on problems caused by the use of most other anti-arrhythmic drugs in the elderly are mainly anecdotal in nature.[17]

Oral anticoagulant drugs

Vitamin K deficiency and decreased synthesis of clotting factors in the liver, as well as decreased binding of coumarin-type drugs to serum proteins, are reasons to give considerably lower dosages in the elderly; in patients over 70 years of age warfarin doses are approximately 40 per cent lower than in the 40–50-year age group,[33] and similar results have been obtained with acenocoumarol.[64] Particularly dangerous changes in pro-thrombin levels and resulting haemorrhage can occur after accidental combination of coumarin-type drugs with aspirin or other non-steroidal anti-inflammatory drugs. In nursing homes this has been shown to be the only clinically relevant drug-drug interaction. Patients on chronic anticoagulant treatment in The Netherlands are specifically warned *not to use* aspirin (over 3 g), azapropazone, diflunisal, or phenylbutazone.[65]

Psychotropic drugs

Sedatives, tranquillizers, and hypnotics

Though benzodiazepines are useful drugs in situations in which insomnia or anxiety make life temporarily miserable, the indications for supplying them are often poor and the dosages, especially in the elderly, far too high. Chronic treatment with benzodiazepine hypnotics in old people is rarely necessary, and tolerance often makes such treatment futile after a few weeks. Many drugs of this type are extremely slowly eliminated with resulting accumulation and carry-over effects (if not a typical 'hangover') over the day,[66] resulting in 'sudden falls' and confusion.[67] Elderly patients suffer twice as often from paradoxical side-effects such as ataxia, irritability, hallucinations, and nightmares.[17] Therefore, if prescription of benzodiazepines is considered, preference should be given to those which, like oxazepam or temazepam, do not accumulate in the elderly and have an intermediate duration of action.[68, 69] Even so, they should be given in half the adult dose, and not continued indefinitely; abrupt discontinuation, however, may provoke serious withdrawal insomnia and even more threatening 'rebound' symptoms.

Though, in comparison with other drugs from the same group, temazepam seems to be a relatively safe hypnotic,[70] one of the alternatives which can be considered in patients who cannot tolerate benzodiazepines is the short-acting thiamine derivative chlormethiazole, a drug with hypnotic and anticonvulsant properties;[71] for this indication it seems to be reasonably safe.[72] Though quite popular in the UK where benzodiazepines are generally eschewed by geriatricians, it is not widely used elsewhere because of fears about abuse potential and dangerous interaction with alcohol.[73] The other old-fashioned alternative of chloral hydrate in a night-time dose of 500 to 1000 mg is quite safe, but the use has been largely abandoned because of its foul taste and smell.[74] Moreover, its therapeutic margin seems to be rather small.[71] Antihistamines (promethazine, diphenhydramine) are best avoided for this purpose because of their long duration of action, day-time after-effects, and close relationship with the neuroleptic drugs.

Antidepressants

Old people often suffer from mild forms of depression, which may be difficult to recognize; in many cases the symptoms are masked as hypochondriasis or pseudodementia,[75, 76] or they are drug-induced.[1] Experience with the use of tricyclic antidepressant drugs in old people is limited, but these drugs can be very effective and relatively safe if low doses are used;[77] under proper supervision the danger of adverse effects on the heart is limited.[78]

Nevertheless, there is a lack of properly controlled comparative studies of old against new antidepressants in elderly patients. Whereas the dangers of the tricyclics are real and well known (cardiac failure, rhythm and other disturbances, blood-pressure falls in the standing position, and anticholinergic side-effects like dry mouth and urinary retention), the efficacy of the 'second' generation antidepressants in this age group seems still insufficiently studied.[79] The long-term risks which some of the newer antidepressants carry have either been too great (as in the case of the recently withdrawn drugs zimelidine and nomifensine) or they are still largely unknown.[80–2] Nevertheless, if elderly patients are treated with tricyclic antidepressants, close clinical and pharmacokinetic monitoring seem essential.[75]

Neuroleptics (antipsychotics)

Phenothiazines, particularly thioridazine and haloperidol, are often used as alternatives for ordinary sedatives. Recent years have shown a considerable change in the attitude towards these drugs, particularly because of the increasing realization that disturbing involuntary movements (dyskinesias) caused by such compounds, including parkinsonism and akathisia, can become a permanent and untreatable handicap. Tardive dyskinesia, the worst side of the spectrum, can only be symptomatically treated by reinstituting the same neuroleptic drug or by giving a closely related one; the prognosis is extremely poor and a frequent reason for hospital admission.[29, 83–5] Moreover, the popular drug thioridazine may cause dangerous cardiac arrythmias.[86]

Other problem drugs

Oral antidiabetic drugs

The value of oral antidiabetic drugs of the sulphonylurea type in old people is quite limited, and there is consensus that they do not favourably influence long-term morbidity or mortality. Nevertheless they are of some value in those elderly patients who cannot use insulin, cannot keep to a diet, and have high blood sugar values and recurrent infections (particularly of the skin like candidiasis, intertrigo, impetigo, etc.). Those with a long half-life, such as chlorpropamide, should be avoided because of the danger of very low blood sugar values during the night, which can cause permanent brain damage. Moreover, it is one of the drugs known to cause the syndrome of inappropriate ADH secretion (SIADH), which may manifest itself in 4–16 per cent of the patients taking this drug as a combination of water intoxication and hyponatraemia.[87] Unfortunately the biguanide metformin, though not as prone as the now-banned drug phenformin to cause often fatal lactic acidosis in the elderly, is again being promoted as first-line antidiabetic; the history of adverse reactions often has to repeat itself a number of times before drastic action is taken.

Non-steroidal anti-inflammatory drugs (NSAIDs)

Ulcerogenic properties. A number of recent British studies have shown that the so-called NSAIDs are unsafe in elderly people, and that the incidence of gastric haemorrhage and perforation increases sharply with age.[88–90] Moreover, the fatality of such complications is high.

These findings have been traced to two different causes: one is massive overprescribing of NSAIDs to elderly people (mainly as analgesics for osteoarthristis); another lies in the specific properties of the NSAIDs preferred for such treatment.

Long-acting NSAIDs have acquired a bad reputation since oxyphenbutazone and benoxaprofen were taken off the market after a number of fatal accidents, mainly in elderly people. The safety of a similar drug, piroxicam, has also been questioned.[91] Nevertheless, some NSAIDs seem to be safer than others (Table 13.2), and some guidance can be given on the basis of pharmacokinetic data and experience with side-effects in rheumatological practice; it seems that NSAIDs with short half-lives which mainly undergo metabolic breakdown in the liver and do not accumulate in elderly patients are marginally safer than others.[92] Errors in dosage in old people seem more likely if the optimal dose is age-dependent.

Antirheumatic drugs and kidney damage. All NSAIDs are potentially damaging for the kidney[95] with the possible exception of low-dose aspirin

Table 13.2 Dose adjustment of NSAID in the elderly[92–4]

Adjustment necessary	Adjustment not necessary
Salicylates	Diclofenac
Azapropazone	Flurbiprofen
Ketoprofen	Ibuprofen
Tiaprofenic acid	Indomethacin
Naproxen	Pirprofen
Ketoprofen	Sulindac
Phenylbutazone	
Piroxicam	
Tiaprofenic acid	

as sole drug. The clinical experience in the last decade shows two different and distinct clinical syndromes. One is mainly characterized by irreversible renal damage, and sometimes papillary necrosis, and the histological picture of acute interstitial nephritis, with proteinuria and oliguria. The other is non-oliguric, often with massive oedema and high serum potassium, in the majority of cases reversible and without appreciable proteinuria, and sometimes precipitated by concomitant use of thiazide or other diuretics (especially triamterene) and/or the presence of gout.[96] This has mainly been observed in elderly people using indomethacin,[97] but no single NSAID seems exempt. Fortunately, in most patients, permanent kidney damage seems to be rare and largely preventable.

SUMMARY

Pharmacotherapeutic problems frequently encountered in geriatric care seem to be mainly limited to some drugs which are widely used in the aged but which nevertheless, because of their pharmacokinetic properties, their potency, or their side-effects profile, can be seen as 'problem drugs'. Though drug consumption patterns differ form country to country and are, among other things, influenced by the degree of institutionalization of geriatric care and the number of drugs on the market and available under social insurance schemes, some common patterns emerge.

First, digoxin and similar drugs seem to be a rather common cause of iatrogenic illness in the elderly. Recent studies have shown that long-term treatment with such drugs is rarely necessary, and that the indications can be curtailed.

Second, blood-pressure treatment should be far more selective; proper guidance on what to prescribe and under which circumstances is given by the results of a number of recent trials of antihypertensive drugs in the elderly.

Third, from the ivory tower of academic clinical pharmacology it is easy to criticize overprescribing or psychotropic drugs, but in the present unfavourable climate in geriatric institutional care, where budgets are increasingly restricted, 'drugging' patients is often the only practical alternative. Nevertheless recent advances in our knowledge should lead to a more selective and intermittent drug use in psychiatry. Iatrogenic pseudodementia and tardive dyskinesia may be just as bad as Alzheimer's and Parkinson's diseases.

Finally, along the same lines, more critical use of oral hypoglycaemic agents and NSAIDs could prevent many accidents.

The recent upsurge in scientific interest and knowledge in geriatric clinical pharmacology means that it is no longer possible for doctors in geriatric practice to hide themselves in a cloak of ignorance. Though clinical pharmacology, just like geriatrics, has been a neglected science for many years (and still is in many countries), both disciplines can help each other in the promotion of good pharmacotherapeutic habits in the care of the elderly.

THE WORLD HEALTH ORGANIZATION AND THE PHARMACOTHERAPEUTIC CARE OF THE ELDERLY

In 1980 a WHO technical group on use of medicaments by the elderly was convened in Geneva.[98] It is intriguing to analyse how much has been achieved since this committee formulated its recommendations. It would be too optimistic to state that drug consumption has fallen to scientifically acceptable levels, but the understanding of the process of drug action in the aged human body has made great strides forwards. The knowledge of the causes and the prevention of side-effects has also considerably improved, but in the mean time drugs have become more potent and patients seem to accept the disadvantages of drug use more easily. Unfortunately physician education has not kept pace with these developments, therefore our optimism should remain guarded.

Stricter drug regulation has regrettably only had limited effects in this domain. Looking back at the report of the WHO technical group it is obvious that improved scientific insights have superseded many of the 'problem drugs' of 1980 (Table 13.3); however, a similar list containing different drugs could certainly be drafted in 1989.

Table 13.3 Drugs with potentially severe or unusual side-effects in the elderly; their fate in 1987[98]

Barbiturates	Being phased out in most countries
Bethanidine	Considered obsolete
Benzhexol	Considered obsolete
Carbenoxolone	Superseded by H$_2$blockers
Chlorpropamide	Considered obsolete
Debrisoquine	Obsolete as antihypertensive
Ethacrynic acid	Superseded by loop diuretics
Guanethidine	Considered obsolete
Methyldopa	Superseded by better-tolerated drugs
Oestrogens	High dosages obsolete
Phenylbutazone	Use severely curtailed
Tetracyclines	Obsolete but for local applications

The report also formulated 12 recommendations. A few of these were successful. For instance, the quantity and the quality of research in geriatric clinical pharmacology have greatly improved. Drug regulatory agencies have formulated guidelines for the study of drugs in a geriatric population and in future they may require dosage recommendations of new drugs for elderly people to be based upon specific studies in such patients. However, the goals of the other, more practically oriented, recommendations seem to be just as far removed from their aims as in 1980.

For this reason, WHO Europe has attempted to record simple recommendations for drug use in old people as a book. Unfortunately, reaching a consensus of opinion has not been easy and the resultant publication[99] has not met with universal acceptance. Again, national problems have dominated other efforts like the input of WHO in initiating efforts for the formulation of guidelines for drug regulation; whereas problems caused by 'normal' drugs predominate in America, Britain, and Scandinavia, those drugs purporting to endow eternal youth seem to preoccupy the authorities in central and southern Europe[100] to a far greater extent.

Efforts should therefore be redirected to the original recommendations and use should be made of the tremendous progress made in this area since 1980.

ACKNOWLEDGEMENTS

With grateful thanks to COBIDOC, the Online Information Centre of the Dutch Ministry of Education, the Institute of Scientific Information, Philadelphia, and the editors of the *Dutch Medical Journal* (*Nederlands Tijdschrift voor Geneeskunde*), without whose material and immaterial help this article could never have been written.

References

1. Hollister, L. E. (1979). Psychotherapeutic drugs. In (*Neuropsychiatric side-effects of drugs in the elderly. Aging, Vol. 9* (ed. Levenson, A. J.), pp. 79–88 Raven Press, New York.
2. Wamboldt, F. S., Jefferson, J. W., and Wamboldt, M. Z. (1986). Digitalis intoxication misdiagnosed as depression by primary care physicians. *American Journal of Psychiatry*, **143**, 219–21.
3. MacLennan, W. J., Shepherd, A. N., and Stevenson, I. H. (1984). Practical problems—multiple pathology, polypharmacy and drug compliance. In *The elderly*. Treatment in clinical medicine, No. 3 (ed. Reid, J. L.), Ch. 2. Springer, Berlin.
4. Conrad, K. A. (1982). Compliance with drug therapy. In *Drug therapy for*

the elderly (ed. Conrad, K. A. and R. Bressler), Ch. 4, pp. 86–8. C. V. Mosby Cy., St Louis.

5. Razenberg, T. P. (1987). Neuroleptica — en laxantiagebruik in een psychogeriatrisch verpleeghuis. *Medisch Contact*, **42**, 304–6.
6. Gosney, M. and Tallis, R. (1984). Prescription of contraindicated and interacting drugs in elderly patients admitted to hospital. *Lancet*, **ii**, 564–6.
7. Petersen, D. M., Whittington, F. J., and Payne, B. P. (1979). *Drugs and the elderly—social and pharmacological issues*. Thomas, Springfield.
8. Royal College of Physicians (1984). Medication for the elderly. *Journal of the Royal College of Physicians of London*, **18**, 7–17.
9. Edwards, M. and Pathy, M. S. J. (1984). Drug counselling in the elderly and predicting compliance. *Practitioner*, **228**, 291–300.
10. Klein, L. E., German, P. S., Levine, D. M., Feroli, E. R., and Ardery, J. (1984). Medication problems among outpatients—a study with emphasis on the elderly. *Archives of Internal Medicine*, **144**, 1185–8.
11. Freer, C. B. (1985). Study of medicines prescribing for elderly patients. *British Medical Journal* **290**, 1113–4.
12. Jarvik, L. F., Greenblatt, D. J., and Harman, D. *Clinical pharmacology and the age patient. Aging, Vol. 16.* Raven Press, New York.
13. Bochner, F., Carruthers, G., Kampmann, J., and steiner, J. (1983). *Handbook of clinical pharmacology* (2nd edn). Little, Brown & Cy., Boston.
14. Cusack, B., Denham, M. J. and Kelly, J. G. (1984). Aspects of drug disposition. In *Clinical pharmacology and drug treatment in the elderly*, (ed. O'Malley, K.) pp. 18–38. Churchill-Livingstone, Edinburgh.
15. Schmucker, D. L. (1985). Aging and drug disposition: an update. *Pharmacol Review*, **37**, 133–48.
16. Lavarenne, J., Dumas, R., and Cayrol, C. (1983). Effets indésirables des medicaments chez les personnes agées. Bilan des observations receuillies pendant un an par l'Association Francaise des Centres de Pharmacovigilance. *Therapie*, **38**, 485–93.
17. Caird, F. I. and Scott, P. J. (1986). *Drug-induced diseases in the elderly*. Drug-induced disorders, Vol. 2. Elsevier, Amsterdam.
18. Jansen, P. A. F., Schulte, B. P. M., and Gribnau, F. W. J. (1987). Cerebral ischaemia and stroke as side effects of antihypertensive treatment; Special danger in the elderly. Review of the cases reported in the literature. *Netherlands Journal of Medicine*, **30**, 193–201.
19. Lamy, P. P. (1981). *Prescribing for the elderly* (2nd edn). PSG Publ. Cy., Littleton MA.
20. Helfand, W. H. (1984). Recent international demographic changes. In *The aging process—Therapeutic implications MEDAC symposium No. 5* (ed. Butler, R. N. and A. G. Bearn), pp. 83–91. Raven Press, New York.
21. Lamy, P. P. (1985). Patterns of prescribing and drug use. In *The aging process—therapeutic implications MEDAC Symposium No. 5* (ed. Butler, R. N. and A. G. Bearn) pp. 53–82. Raven Press, New York.
22. Nemitz, E. and van Melle, G. (1983). Les médicaments en médecine générale. Etude des profils de prescription et de la demande des malades. *Schweiz Medizinische Wochenschrift*, **113**, 1719–26.
23. Dunnell, K. and Cartwright, A. (1972). *Medicine takers, prescribers and hoarders*. Routledge & Kegan Paul, London.

24. Stuart, I. (1985). Audit report—do patients cash prescriptions? *British Medical Journal*, **291**, 1246–7

25. Davison, W. (1984). Practicalities of drug treatment. In *Geriatric pharmacology and therapeutics*. (ed. Brocklehurst, J. C.) pp. 27–40. Blackwell, Oxford.

26. Hurd, P. D. and Blevins, J. (1984). Aging and the color of pills. *New England Journal of Medicine*, **310**, 202.

27. Committee on the Safety of Medicines (1985). CSM update: drugs and the elderly. *British Medical Journal*, **290**, 1345.

28. Williamson, J. (1979). Adverse reactions to prescribed drugs in the elderly. In *Drugs and the elderly—perspectives in geriatric clinical pharmacology* (ed. Crooks, J. and I. H. Stevenson) pp. 239–46. MacMillan, London.

29. Hermesh, H., Shalev, A., and Munitz, H. (1985). Contribution of adverse drug reaction to admission rates in an acute psychiatric ward. *Acta Psychiatrica Scandinavica*, **72**, 104–10.

30. Triggs, E. J., Hooper, W. D., and Dickinson, R. G. (1984). The influence of age on drug metabolism—implications for drug dosage. *Medical Journal of Australia*, **141**, 823–7.

31. Cheymol, G. and Biour, M. (1983). Effets indésirables médicamenteux chez les personnes âgées. Bases pharmacocinétiques des effets indésirables médicamenteux chez le sujet âgé. *Therapie*, **38** 475–84.

32. Macdonald, E. T. and Macdonald, J. B. (1982). *Drug treatment in the elderly*. Wiley, Chichester.

33. Wood, A. J. J., and Feely, J. (1984). Effect of age on sensitivity to drugs. In *Clinical pharmacology and drug treatment in the elderly* (ed. O'Malley, K.), pp. 39–51. Churchill-Livingstone, Edinburgh.

34. Stegman, M. R. (1983). Falls among elderly hypertensives—are they iatrogenic? *Gerontology*, **29**, 399–406.

35. Lipsitz, L. A., Wei, J. Y., and Rowe, J. W. (1985). Syncope in the elderly, institutionalised population: Prevalence, incidence, and associated risk. *Quarterly Journal of Medicine*, **55**, 45–54.

36. Jansen, P. A. F., Gribnau, F. W. J., Schulte, B. P. M., and Poels, E. F. J. (1986). Contribution of inappropriate treatment for hypertension to pathogenesis of stroke in the elderly. *British Medical Journal*, **293**, 914–16.

37. Hankey, G. J. and Gubbay, S. S. (1987). Focal cerebral ischaemia and infarction due to antihypertensive therapy. *Medical Journal of Australia*, **146**, 412–14.

38. Boman, K. (1983). Digitalis intoxication in geriatric inpatients—a prospective clinical study of the value of serum digitalis concentration measurement. *Acta Medica Scandinavica*, **214**, 345–51.

39. Doherty, J., Soyza, N., Kane, J. J., Murphy, M. L., Scovil, J., and Watson, J. (1979). Cardiac glycosides. In *Neuropsychiatric side-effects of drugs in the elderly. Aging, Vol. 9* (ed. Levenson, A. J.), pp. 39–48. Raven Press, New York.

40. Krakauer, R. and Steiness, E. (1978). Digoxin concentration in chorioid plexus, brain, and myocardium in old age. *Clinical Pharmacology and Therapeutics*, **24**, 454–8.

41. Cusack, B., Kelly, J., O'Malley, K., Noel, J., Lavan, J., and Horgan, J. (1979). Digoxin in the elderly: pharmacokinetic considerations of old age.

Clinical Pharmacology and Therapeutics, **25**, 772–6.

42. Sonnenblick, M., and Abraham, A. S. (1985). Digoxin treatment and control in the elderly. *Israel Journal of Medical Science*, **21**, 276–8.

43. Marsh, J. D. and Smith, T. W. (1986). Miscellaneous uses of cardiac glycosides. In *Digitalis glycosides* (ed. Smith, T. W.), pp. 115–26. Grune & Stratton, Orlando FL.

44. Whiting, B., Wandless, I., Sumner, D. J., and Goldberg, A. (1978). Computer-assisted review of digoxin therapy in the elderly. *British Heart Journal*, **40**, 8–13.

45. Anonymous (1985). Needless digoxin. *Lancet*, **ii**, 1048.

46. Fleg, J. L. and Lakatta, E. G. (1984). How useful is digitalis in patients with congestive heart failure and sinus rhythm? *International Journal of Cardiology*, **6**, 295–305.

47. Mulrow, C. D., Feussner, J. R., and Velez, R. (1984). Reevaluation of digitalis efficacy—New light on an old leaf. *Annals of Internal Medicine*, **101**, 113–17.

48. Falk, R. H., Knowlton, A. A., Bernard, S. A., Gotlieb, N. E., and Battinelli, N. J. (1987). Digoxin for converting recent-onset atrial fibrillation to sinus rhythm—a randomized, double-blinded trial. *Annals of Internal Medicine*, **106**, 503–6.

49. European Working Party on High Blood Pressure in the Elderly (1986). Efficacy of antihypertensive treatment according to age, sex, blood pressure, and previous cardiovascular disease in patients over the age of 60. *Lancet*, **ii**, 589–91.

50. Bulpitt, C. J. (1986). Mortality and morbidity results from the European Working Party on High Blood Pressure in the Elderly trial. *Drugs*, **31** (Suppl. 1), 29–39.

51. Langford, H. G., Blaufox, M. D., Borhani, N. O. *et al.* (1987). Is thiazide-produced uric acid elevation harmful? Analysis of data from the hypertension detection and follow-up program. *Archives of Internal Medicine*, **147**, 645–9.

52. Vardan, S., Mehrotra, K. G., Mookherjee, S., Willsey, G. A., Gens, J. D., and Green, D. E. (1987). Efficacy and reduced metabolic side effects of a 15-mg chlorthalidone formulation in the treatment of hypertension. A multicenter study. *Journal of the American Medical Association*, **258**, 484–8.

53. Jenkins, A. C., Knili, J. R., and Dreslinski, G. R. (1985). Captopril in the treatment of the elderly hypertensive patient. *Archives of Internal Medicine*, **145**, 2029–31.

54. Murphy, P. J., Cammen, T. A. van der, and Malone, L. J. (1986). Captopril in elderly patients with heart fialure. *British Medical Journal*, **293**, 239–40.

55. Vandenburg, M. J., Cooper, W. D., Woollard, M. L., Currie, W. J. C., and Bowker, C. H. (1984). Reduced peripheral vascular symptoms in elderly patients treated with alpha-methyldopa—a comparison with propranolol. *European Journal of Clinical Pharmacology*, **26**, 325–30.

56. Herlitz, J., Hjalmarsson, A., and Holmberg, S. (1985). Tolerability to treatment with metoprolol in acute myocardial infarction in relation to age. *Acta Medica Scandinavica*, **217**, 293–8.

57. Wikstrand, J., Westergren, G., Berglund, G. *et al.* (1986). Antihypertensive treatment with metoprolol or hydrochlorothiazide in patients aged 60 to 75

years. Report from a double-blind international multicenter study. *Journal of the American Medical Association*, **255**, 1304–10.

58. Landmark, K. and Dale, J. and Antihypertensive, haemodynamic and metabolic effects of nifedipine slow-release tablets in elderly patients. *Acta Medica Scandinavica*, **218**, 389–96.

59. Abernethy, D. R., Schwartz, J. B., Todd, E. L., Luchi, R., and Snow, E. (1986). Verapamil pharmacodynamics and disposition in young and elderly hypertensive patients. Altered electrocardiographic and hypotensive responses. *Annals of Internal Medicine*, **105**, 329–36.

60. National Board of Health and Welfare—Drug Information Committee, Sweden (1983). *Treatment of hypertension in the elderly*. Workshop No. 4. Socialstyrelsens Läkemedelsavdelning, Uppsala.

61. Abernethy, D. R. and Greenblatt, D. J. (1983) Impairment of lidocain clearance in elderly male subjects. *Journal of Cardiovascular Pharmacology*, **5**, 1093–6.

62. Cusson, S., Nattel, S., Matthews, C., Talajic, M., and Lawand, S. (1985). Age-dependent lidocaine disposition in patients with acute myocardial infarction. *Clinical Pharmacology and Therapeutics*, 37, 381–6.

63. Bonde, J., Pedersen, L. E., Bodtker, S., Angelo, H. R., Svendsen, T. L., and Kampmann, J. P. (1985). The influence of age and smoking on the elimination of disopyramide. *British Journal of Clinical Pharmacology*, **20**, 453–8.

64. Arboix, M., Laporte, J. R., Frati, M., and Ruttlan, M. (1984). Effect of age and sex on acenocoumarol requirements. *British Journal of Clinical Pharmacology*, **18**, 475–80.

65. Federatie van Nederlandse Thrombosediensten (1987). *Vademecum voor poliklinische behandeling met orale anticoagulantia*. Bureau van de Federatie van Nederlandse Thrombosediensten, Den Haag. p/a Rode Kruis Ziekenhuis.

66. Greenblatt, D. J., Divoll, M., Abernethy, D. R., Ochs, H. R., and Shader, R. I. (1983). Benzodiazepine kinetics: Implications for therapeutics and pharmacogeriatrics. *Drug Metabolism Review*, **14**, 251–92.

67. Foy, A., Drinkwater, N., March, S., and Mearrick, P. (1986). Confusion after admission to hospital in elderly patients using benzodiazepines. *British Medical Journal*, **293**, 1072.

68. Ghabrial, H., Desmond, P. V., Watson, K. J. R. *et al.* (1986). The effects of age and chronic liver disease on the elimination of temazepam. *European Journal of Clinical Pharmacology*, **30**, 93–8.

69. Klem, K., Murray, G. R., and Laake, K. (1986). Pharmacokinetics of temazepam in geriatric patients. *European Journal of Clinical Pharmacology*, **30**, 745–7.

70. Bixler, E. O., Kales, A., Brubaker, B. H., and Kales, J. D. (1987). Adverse reactions to benzodiazepine hypnotics: spontaneous reporting system. *Pharmacology*, **35**, 286–300.

71. Hyams, D. E. (1984). Central nervous system—anxiolytics and hypnotics. In *Geriatric pharmacology and therapeutics* (ed. Brocklehurst, J. C.), pp. 131–42. Blackwell, Oxford.

72. Bayer, A. J., Bayer, E. M., Pathy, M. S. J., and Stoker, M. J. (1986). A double-blind controlled study of chlormethiazole and triazolam as hypnotics

in the elderly. *Acta Psychiatrica Scandinavica*, **73** (Suppl. 329), 104–11.
73. McInnes, G. T. (1987). Chlormethiazole and alcohol: a lethal cocktail. (Leading article) *British Medical Journal*, **294**, 592.
74. Vestal, R. E. (1984) *Drug treatment in the elderly*. ADIS Health Science Press, Sydney.
75. Montgomery, S. A. (1982) Treatment of depression in old age. In *Psychopharmacology of old age* (ed. Wheatley, D.), British Association for Psychopharmacology, Monograph No. 3. pp. 165–72. Oxford University Press, Oxford.
76. Balant-Gorgia, A. E., Balant, L., and Garrone, G. (1986). Lés états dépressifs de la personne agée et leur traitement. *Schweizerische Medizinische Wochenschrift*, **116**, 314–22.
77. Schnyder, C., Baumann, P., Jonzier-Perey, M., Koeb, L., and Wertheimer, J. (1985). Utilisation de l'amitriptyline a faible dose en psychogeriatrie. Une etude clinique, pharmacocinetique et pharmacogenetique. *Schweize Medizinisde Wochenschrift*, **115**, 1128–34.
78. Roose, S. P., Glassman, A. H., Giardina, E. G. V., Walsh, B. T., Woodring, S., and Bigger, J. T. (1987). Tricyclic antidepressants in depressed patients with cardiac conduction disease. *Archives of General Psychiatry*, **44**, 273–5.
79. Wakelin, S. (1986). Fluvoxamine in the treatment of the older depressed patient; double-blind, placebo-controlled data. *International Clinical Psychopharmacology*, **1**, 221–30.
80. Moeller, M., Thayssen, P., Kragh-Soerensen, P. *et al.* (1984). Mianserin: cardiovascular effects in elderly patients. *Psychopharmacology*, **80**, 174–7.
81. Dawling, S., Ford, S., Ariyanayagam, P., O'Neal, H., and Lewis, P. R. (1987). Plasma concentrations of mianserin after single dose and at steady-state in depressed elderly patients. *Clinical Pharmacokinetics*, **12**, 73–8.
82. Roeser, H. P. (1987). Drug-bone marrow interactions. *Medical Journal of Australia*, **146**, 145–8.
83. Stephen, P. and Williamson, J. (1984) Hospital practice—drug-induced parkinsonism in the elderly. *Lancet*, **ii**, 1082–3.
84. Schelling, J. L. (1985). Médicaments psychotropes chez les personnes âgées. *Schweizerische Medizinische Wochenschrift*, **115**, 1808–14.
85. Wilson, J. A., Primrose, W. R., and Smith, R. G. (1987). Prognosis of drug-induced Parkinson's disease. *Lancet*, **i**, 443–4.
86. Kiriike, N., Maeda, Y., Nishiwaki, S. *et al.* (1987). Iatrogenic torsade de pointes induced by thioridazine. *Biological Psychiatry*, **22**, 99–103.
87. Brass, E. P. and Thompson, W. L. (1982). Drug-induced electrolyte abnormalities. *Drugs*, **24**, 207–28.
88. Somerville, K., Faulkner, G., and Langman, M. J. M. (1986). Non-steroidal anti-inflammatory drugs and bleeding peptic ulcer. *Lancet*, **i**, 462–3.
89. Anonymous (1986). Non-steroidal anti-inflammatory drugs and serious gastrointestinal adverse reactions. I. British Medical Journal, **292**, 614.
90. Walt, R., Katschinski, B., Logan, R., Ashley, J., and Langman, M. J. M. (1986). Occasional survey: Rising frequency of ulcer perforation in elderly people in the United Kingdom. *Lancet*, **i**, 489–91.
91. Beermann, B. (1985). Peptic ulcers induced by piroxicam. *British Medical Journal*, **290**, 789.

92. Jansen, P. A. F., Ginneken, C. A. M. van, and Gribnau, F. W. J. (1987). Is dose adjustment on non-steroidal anti-inflammatory drugs necessary in the elderly? A review of the pharmacokinetics of NSAID in the aged. *Netherlands Journal of Medicine*, **30**, 248–58.

93. O'Brien, J. D. and Burnham, W. R. (1985). Bleeding from peptic ulcers and use of non-steroidal anti-inflammatory drugs in the Romford area. *British Medical Journal*, **291**, 1609–10.

94. Richardson, C. J., Blocka, K. L. N., Ross. S. G., and Verbeeck, R. K. (1987). Piroxicam and 5'-hydroxypiroxicam kinetics following multiple dose administration of piroxicam. *European Journal of Clinical Pharmacology*, **32**, 89–92.

95. Reeves, W. B., Foley, R. J., and Weinman, E. J. (1984). Renal dysfunction from nonsteroidal anti-inflammatory drugs. *Archives of Internal Medicine*, **144**, 1943–4.

96. Adams, D. H., Howie, A. J., Michael, J., McConkey, B., Bacon, P. A., and Adu, D. (1986). Non-steroidal anti-inflammatory drugs and renal failure. *Lancet*, **i**, 57–9.

97. Blackshear, J. L., Davidman, M., and Stillman, T. (1983). Identification of risk for renal insufficiency from non-steroidal anti-inflammatory drugs. *Archives of Internal Medicine*, **143**, 1130–4.

98. World Health organization (1981). Health care in the elderly: report of the technical group on use of medicaments by the elderly. *Drugs*, **22**, 279–94.

99. World Health Organization (1985). *Drugs for the elderly*. World Health Organization, Regional Office for Europe, Copenhagen.

100. World Health Organization, Regional Office for Europe (1981). *The control of drugs for the elderly*. Report on the ninth European Symposium on Clinical Pharmacological Evaluation in Drug Control. Schlangenbad, 18–21 November 1980. World Health Organization, Copenhagen.

14

Iatrogenic disorders

F. I. CAIRD

There is no doubt that adverse reactions to prescribed drugs are the most important single disorder in the elderly which is directly due to the activities of doctors; these are discussed elsewhere (p. 211). However, there are also many other important disorders which doctors and those caring for the elderly may cause by mechanisms over which the doctors have at least some control. These may therefore legitimately be said to be iatrogenic.

The mechanisms include: (1) the incorrect medicalization of conditions not truly medical at all, (2) attempting to answer the wrong question about the patient, (3) under- and over-investigation and under- and over-enthusiastic diagnostic effort, (4) ignorance of normal values for common diagnostic tests in old age, (5) failure to explain the purpose and likely outcome of investigations or treatment to relatives, (6) the preventable complications of hospitalization, and finally (7) the employment of inappropriate rehabilitative effort and procedures.

A simple example of the medicalization of non-medical problems is the tendency to diagnose manifestations of justifiable unhappiness on the part of patients about their situation as a depressive illness. What is required is not antidepressants, with all their hazards, but counselling and the deployment of appropriate social services.

Doctors may fail to address the main problems facing the patient as he himself would define them. The failure to take a full and detailed history and find out what is really troubling the patient may lead to inappropriate medical and nursing effort. If this continues, the patient may well leave medical care with his original problems as he sees them unameliorated by all the impositions of the doctors and all the effort (and money) that has been spent.

The purpose of an investigation is to achieve as accurate a diagnosis as is possible, since this has always been and remains the cornerstone of appropriate management at any age, and to assist in assessing the patient's progress. It follows that inadequate diagnostic effort is likely to lead to inappropriate management. This all too often results from the misconception, still too prevalent, that an accurate diagnosis is neither necessary nor possible in elderly patients. One of the main successes of geriatric medicine over the past 30 years has been to show the fallacy of this view.

A definite diagnosis must be pursued by all appropriate means. These may include modern and sophisticated non-invasive tests when indicated. Such tests are in general well tolerated by the elderly, especially those that require minimum patient co-operation. Considerations of cost alone should never be allowed to outweigh the importance of diagnostically necessary investigations in any elderly patient.

The opposite error, of overenthusiastic diagnostic and investigative effort, can be equally damaging to an elderly patient, since invasive procedures in particular carry increased risks in the elderly. In these circumstances it is essential to be certain, before the investigation is carried out, that there is a substantial chance that the patient or carer will benefit from the diagnostic or prognostic knowledge gained from it.

Although severe cardiac or respiratory illness may influence decisions about diagnostic effort, the limiting factor in deciding on the appropriateness or otherwise of many complex investigations is most often the patient's mental state. It must also be said however, that identification of the cause of mental disturbance of recent onset is one of the most important diagnostic tasks facing doctors working with the elderly.

The entire clinical situation must be taken into account. It is often for instance unlikely to be of practical benefit to attempt to diagnose (e.g. by endoscopy or barium meal examination) a possible carcinoma of the stomach in an elderly patient with anorexia and weight loss who also suffers from established severe dementia. Most symptoms the suspected neoplasm may eventually produce will not override those of dementia in affecting either the life expectancy of the patient or the practical problems which care may present. The only reason for pursuing investigations of this type in this situation is to give a better idea of prognosis, and perhaps also to satisfy relatives that all that can be done has been done. The latter by itself is a motive that must sometimes be viewed with caution, as relatives may press for more than is necessary because of their own feelings of guilt rather than out of any true understanding of what is best for the patient.

A further reason for investigation is *bona fide* research, which must always involve the patient's consent if he is capable of giving it, but if not then that of a responsible relative. The latter circumstance arises relatively infrequently, and can only really be justified in the setting of a major planned study of mental illness. There is much to be said for the researcher having the investigations carried out upon himself before he begins the study. If he is unable to tolerate them easily, it is unlikely that his elderly patients will.

A further problem with diagnostic tests arises from ignorance of the normal or common values for investigations in the elderly. Some haematological and biochemical tests give values that are different from those in younger people (Table 14.1). This may lead to either of two errors. The doctor may ignore what are in truth abnormalities in the elderly patient on the false premise that they are 'normal in old age', and thus may fail to diagnose a possibly remediable condition. Or he may fall into the opposite error of conducting potentially damaging and unnecessary over-investigation of the patient, where he has failed to realize that results which differ from those conventionally accepted and taught as normal in younger adults may be normal results for the elderly.

It is important that doctors explain to patients' relatives, as needed, the purpose and likely outcome of investigations and treatment, and also that they repeat the explanation as necessary if the situation changes (and often also if it does not). An optimistic attitude towards a patient's return home should always be maintained when this is appropriate. Failure in this important activity may lead to relatives refusing to take a patient home when this is a possible outcome. This problem may be less common in some settings than that of relatives who take home a patient whom it would be entirely rational for them to leave in hospital.

The complications of hospitalization are also important. The consequences of bed rest are the most obvious (Table 14.2), but lack of physical activity can affect hospitalized patients even when they are not bed-bound, and institutionalization is the most insidious and perhaps the most intractable of situations. All can be considered iatrogenic in so far as they

Table 14.1 Normal values which differ in the older patient from those in the young[1]

Haematological:	
	White cell count
	lymphocyte count
	Erythrocyte sedimentation rate
	Serum folate
Biochemical:	
	Urea
	Creatinine
	Cholesterol
	Calcium
	Phosphate
	Alkaline phosphatase
	Uric acid

Table 14.2 Complications of the bedfast state[2]

Psychological:	*Musculoskeletal*:
Confusion	Muscle wasting
Reduced motivation	Contractures
Dependency	Foot drop
Depression	
Nutritional and gastrointestinal:	*Cutaneous*:
Dehydration	Pressure sores
Poor nutrition	
Constipation, faecal impaction	
Incontinence	
Cardiorespiratory:	
Thromboembolism	
Postural hypotension	
Hypostatic pneumonia	

are preventable and under medical control. Bed rest is dealt with later. Physical inactivity may be a result of the short distances that have to be walked, and a pattern of ward activites which involve late rising, an afternoon nap, and early putting to bed—all three deviations from the patient's normal daily routine being often imposed by staff more for their own convenience than for any better reason. Institutionalization results from longer-lasting or more frequent hospitalization, but its insidious onset leads to its being often overlooked by the less than vigilant. It has many manifestations, all unrelated to the condition leading to admission:

(1) apathy, lack of interest (including in personal appearance);

(2) submissiveness, loss of responsibility and ability to make decisions;

(3) boredom, idleness, inactivity;

(4) withdrawal.

A number of factors contribute to its development:

(1) loss of contact with the outside world;

(2) loss of personal identity: loss of friends, possessions, events;

(3) loss of prospects;

(4) attitudes of staff;

(5) ward atmosphere.

Many of the issues are dealt with by Denham.[3] It may be difficult to prevent in a ward population with a high prevalence of severe dementia, but a number of active measures can be taken to avoid the contributory factors. By far the most important are the attitudes of ward staff, and the activities they permit or stimulate. It must not be forgotten that staff as well as patients may become institutionalized, and unvarying routine and lack of contact with others may both contribute to this.

Another, and perhaps the most difficult to assess, of the dangers to which elderly patients are subjected by their doctors, results from inappropriate rehabilitative effort. Again, there are two opposite errors. Most of the complications of too-late mobilization are those of bed rest (Table 14.2). They operate to prolong the bed rest still further and thus compound the situation. This may be especially the case with pressure sores, where a few hours of failure of prevention can lead to many weeks of expense and suffering. The early mobilization of the elderly has probably been responsible for the reduction that is apparent to clinicians in the frequency of pulmonary embolism. This is now virtually confined to patients with advanced malignant disease or cardiac failure—both patient groups frequently immobilized in bed for considerable periods. Muscle wasting and contractures are preventable by a vigorous policy of physiotherapy, and foot drop by the use of bed cradles. It is important to realize that the worst nutrition is in those elderly patients whose difficulties in feeding have not been recognized; this obviously applies to the ambulant as well as to the bed-bound. Hypostatic pneumonia may be the consequence of aspiration in patients with unrecognized difficulty in swallowing.

Bed rest should, therefore, never be of greater duration than the absolute minimum necessary in the very many cases in the elderly where a policy of early ambulation is justifiable. It is particularly important that elderly patients with infections, fractures, and stroke should be at least out of bed as soon as feasible, even if standing and walking are impossible at that time.

The contrary error of too-early mobilization is also possible, though much less common. It may result for instance in the development of cardiac failure following a myocardial infarct, perhaps because its severity has been underestimated, and is obviously also to be avoided. However, if this particular situation occurs it can be rectified relatively easily.

The more difficult decisions concern the risks which it is permissible to take during active rehabilitation. For instance, a patient whose mobility is beginning to improve with rehabilitation but whose balance is as yet imperfect risks falling. This risk cannot be removed entirely, though it may be substantially reduced, by judicious supervision. A fall in hospital carries with it a small but definite chance of a potentially dangerous fracture (e.g. of the femur).[4] Such risks have however, to be weighed against those resulting from a failure to attempt to improve the patient's mobility, or doing so over a more prolonged period of time. These are undoubtedly much greater, though they cannot be quantified precisely. The dividing line between the two errors may be a matter of considerable judgement and experience; in consequence it is very difficult to give any definite guidelines for individual cases.

ACKNOWLEDGEMENT

I am grateful to Miss B. Sharp, SRN, for her contribution.

References

1. Caird, F. I. (1985). Problems of interpretation of laboratory findings in the old. In *Medicine in old age* pp. 116–24. British Medical Association, London.
2. Caird, F. I., Kennedy, R. D., and Williams, B. O. (1983). *Practical rehabilitation of the elderly*. pp. 85–91. Pitman, London.
3. Denham M. J. (ed.) (1983). *Care of the long-stay elderly patient*. Croom Helm, London.
4. Gryfe, C. I., Amies, A., and Ashley, M. J. (1977). A longitudinal study of falls in an elderly population: I Incidence and morbidity. *Age and Ageing*, **6**, 201–10.

15

Hearing disorders of aging: identification and management

DOUGLAS NOFFSINGER, JAMES P. MARTIN, and
SHERALYN HEAD LEWIS

The problems in defining and describing the effects of aging on hearing are many because inevitably mixed with the effects due solely to the passage of time in a person's life are those effects that are inextricably interwoven with the passage of time but are not truly aging effects. Hawkins[1] has discussed this issue clearly. Among contributors to hearing loss in older people are the various causes of noise to which people voluntarily or involuntarily subject themselves and the medication and drugs with which people are healed of disease and/or poison themselves. If to this list are added the possible complications posed by heredity, disease, diet, race, environmental complexity, and pollutants, then the difficulties in defining the effects of aging *per se* on hearing and the hearing system become apparent.

The best solution to dealing with the intertangled causes of hearing loss in elderly people is to recognize the obvious. Many older people have hearing loss. Such loss has many manifestations which range from loss of sensitivity to certain types of sounds to the more subtle, a failure of the auditory nervous system to do the unique kinds of analysis and processing which allow human beings to be remarkably agile communicative creatures. The task, therefore, is to use tools and approaches which will allow the sorting of people into categories which are as diagnostically and functionally distinct as is possible. This will enable strategies to be adopted that will maximize the ability of the older human to remain viable in societies based on communication. The solution will sometimes be as simple as using devices to amplify sound; usually, however, it will necessitate a programme of rehabilitation, environmental modification, and behavioural structuring, especially if one of the goals of the process is the maintenance of an individual's dignity and satisfaction with life as a communicator.

Hearing loss in the elderly population can provoke misconceptions about an elderly individual's basic functional abilities. Misguided compensation for hearing loss prompted by a person's denial or repression of a progressive problem can mislead an observer into the belief that the apparent inappropriate responses of an old person are the result of decreased cognitive function. This conclusion may arise from an un-awareness that aged, hearing-impaired listeners will often answer a question erroneously or give a response that is inappropriate simply because they did not hear a question or statement clearly, but yielded to a need for social interaction. It is possible for such faulty communication due to hearing loss to result in judgements of low mental status in both formal and informal evaluations. This misjudgement can affect subsequent decisions about the management and lives of elderly patients.

Presbyacusis (or presbycusis) is the result of degenerative processes that affect the physical structures, metabolic activity, and electrical properties of the hearing mechanism. Schuknecht[2] described, from an oto-pathological and functional framework, four types of presbyacusis: (1) In *sensory* presbyacusis the hair cells in the cochlea atrophy, resulting in a progressive high-frequency hearing loss. Clinical experience suggests that this type of presbyacusis, usually symmetrical in the two ears, is the most common. Generally, this variety of hearing loss reduces a listener's ability to hear both high-pitched tones and the higher-frequency portions of speech and contributes to a decreased word recognition ability. This is particularly true in noisy situatioins in which the listener requires those sounds to understand speech. (2) *Neural* presbyacusis occurs primarily at the cochlea—VIIIth nerve interface and at the auditory section of the VIIIth cranial nerve proper; it is the result of depopulation of nerve fibres. This degenerative change does not usually cause loss of hearing sensitivity until late in life, but can affect the quality of neural transmission of sound to the brainstem with consequent distortion of the signal involved. Neural presbyacusis is likely to be the culprit when an old person states that he can hear speech, but cannot understand what is being said. (3) *Metabolic* presbyacusis describes a condition that occurs when the source of blood supply providing nutrients to the inner ear atrophies. Stria vascularis abnormality is a major cause. The result of such dysfunction is hearing loss that affects all frequencies and progresses slowly with age. (4) *Mechanical* presbyacusis involves a stiffening or hardening of the normally pliable tissues of the middle and inner ear structures. The result is a slowly progressive hearing loss that is greater for high-pitched sounds. Mechanical presbyacusis, in combination with other forms of presbyacusis, can result in hearing problems that not only decrease the loudness or volume of speech and other sounds, but also inflict upon listeners (when they do hear) a distorted or unclear message. A fifth type of presbyacusis due to vascular changes in the cochlea has also been described.[1]

The remainder of this chapter is concerned with the hearing mechanism *per se*, including functional characteristics of the system, the effects of aging on performance, and the practical considerations which should be borne in mind in constructing a reasonable management approach to the hearing-impaired, elderly individual. In particular, the areas of concern are the following:

1. A review of the major parts of the auditory system, all of which to one extent or another are subject to changes associated with aging and other influences which occur over a lifetime.

2. A survey of some auditory tests which have been found to be useful in evaluating the functional integrity of the hearing mechanism both peripherally and centrally. These tests are necessary to sort people into performance groups for which rehabilitative and assistive approaches may be quite different.

3. A summary of the known effects of aging on hearing performance, including those that manifest themselves as losses of hearing sensitivity and those that are revealed in more subtle disturbances of brainstem and brain function.

4. A review in some detail of certain practical considerations in managing elderly people with hearing loss. Emphasis will be placed on the prescription and use of amplification and other assistive devices, the value of an organized aural rehabilitation programme, and the modification of acoustic environments with the goal of minimizing unnecessary distortion of sound in places where the elderly communicate.

Hearing problems are common in the elderly. This is particularly true in highly industrialized, increasingly noisy environments in which more and more of the world's population resides. Although one of the problems in the field of geriatrics and hearing loss is inadequate census of the dimensions of the problem, in an industrialized country such as the United States, it is estimated that as many as 13 million people have a disabling hearing loss,[3] and that half of these are aged 65 years or older.

Most often, the hearing loss found in the elderly patient is sensorineural hearing loss, that is, hearing loss due to damage to the cochlea, the sense organ of hearing, and/or to the peripheral nervous system and the central auditory nervous system which support the auditory system. These kinds of age-related hearing problems are usually not amenable to medical or surgical intervention. This combination of pathology and circumstances leaves prosthetic and assistive devices, rehabilitation, and common-sense understanding and patience as the major avenues of remediation for the aged, hearing-impaired individual.

COMPONENT PARTS OF THE AUDITORY SYSTEM

Peripheral hearing system

This system has the following parts:

1. The outer, visible ear called the *auricle*, or pinna.

2. The *eardrum* or tympanic membrane, the membrane which separates the ear canal from the middle ear.

3. The series of tiny bones occupying the middle ear called the *ossicular chain*. These bones, the malleus, incus, and stapes, serve as an intricate mechanical transfer bridge between the tympanic membrane and the inner ear.

4. The *Eustachian tube*, a ventilating tube allowing the maintenance of atmospheric pressure in the middle ear by furnishing a passage connecting it with the outside world.

5. The inner ear called the *cochlea*. This is the sense organ of hearing, and the place in the peripheral auditory system producing the most obvious kind of presbyacusis—a loss of sensitivity to sound often accompanied by imperfect understanding of speech.

6. The *cochlear nerve*, a portion of the VIIIth cranial nerve. This neural pathway is the conduit for transmission of signals from the inner ear to the central nervous system.

Functionally, the primary contribution of the peripheral hearing system is transmission of signals arriving at the external ear to the first way-station of the central auditory nervous system in the brainstem. If such transmission is inefficient or destroyed, serious hearing loss and poor communication result. The peripheral hearing mechanism is quite complex and vulnerable. It involves molecular motion in the ear canal, mechanical vibration of the eardrum and the ossicular chain in the middle ear, and hydromechanical and electrical events in the inner ear. The process includes translation of an acoustic signal into its neurally coded equivalent, which then traverses the cochlear portion of the VIIIth nerve to the brainstem. All of this elegant network must work efficiently in co-ordination for normal hearing to occur. When it is slowed or incoordinated by aging, compounded by any of the other influences mentioned earlier, problems occur and communication suffers.

Auditory brainstem

From the point of synaptic termination of the auditory VIIIth nerve up to the areas of the brain known to have responsibilities for hearing there lies an enormously complicated yet tremendously compact assemblage of neural networks and nuclei which make up the auditory brainstem. The parts of most importance to hearing are:

1. The entrance point of the auditory nerve to the brainstem, an area usually called the *cerebello-pontine angle* in reference to the structures forming it.

2. The *cochlear nucleus*—the first nuclear centre concerned with hearing in the brainstem and the termination point of the auditory nerve. From this point, some fibres cross to the opposite side of the brainstem and begin their ascent toward the brain proper. Others make their way upward on the same side as their entrance to the brainstem.

3. The *superior olivary complex*—a nuclear group of particular importance in the auditory system. It is the first nuclear centre to receive input from both ears and thus is physiologically the first point where binaural (two-ear) interaction is possible.

4. The *lateral lemniscus*—the major ascending fibre tract through the brainstem. It has nuclei of its own and other nuclear groups form way-stations along its course.

5. The *inferior colliculus*—another nuclear group along the auditory pathways of the brainstem. It is higher in the brainstem than those nuclei previously listed. Although this is a site of another major crossing of some fibres from one side of the brainstem to the other, the functional significance of the decussation is unclear.

6. The *medial geniculate*—the last nuclear centre before the auditory tracts move into the brain.

7. The *auditory radiations*—the neural fibre tract that carries information from the top of the brainstem to auditory areas in the brain (i.e. a brainstem-to-brain tract).

The auditory brainstem is not merely a simple transmission system, although it does serve to transport electrical events from the peripheral hearing mechanism to the auditory brain. The auditory areas of the brainstem have several other important responsibilities: they serve as the first area where binaural processing takes place; they also control certain auditory reflexes which occur in response to loud sounds amongst other stimuli. The binaural or two-ear interactions are probably dependent on complicated time and phase correlation. These interactions make possible such elementary but critical discriminations as sound localization and lateralization—abilities of great importance to survival. Binaural correlation/cancellation events are also capable of enhancing the intelligibility of a signal, such as speech, in an unfavourable background of noise. Unlike the case when damage is done to the peripheral hearing mechanism, damage to the brainstem itself usually does not manifest itself in hearing loss *per se*. It may lead to difficulty in locating a sound source or in perception of auditory signals in an unfavourable noise background. Thus, whereas the primary function of the peripheral hearing mechanism is to provide initial coding and transmission of auditory signals, the brainstem has unique functional capabilities concerned with the interaction of signals from both ears.

Auditory brain

Certain areas of the brain have special responsibility for processing auditory input.[4,5] Since these areas are in many respects instrumental in characteristics that make humans unique, such as language function, they are critical areas indeed. Since cerebrovascular accidents can damage these areas in elderly people, they are of special interest. The regions of greatest importance in the brain relating to hearing are:

1. The *anterior temporal lobe*, which is thought to be responsible for at least some basic preliminary processing of incoming auditory information.

2. The *posterior temporal lobe*—a particularly important area of the brain in terms of hearing. It is thought to house centres responsible for the final processing of speech information, particularly in the left half of the brain.

3. The *parietal lobe*, particularly the areas immediately adjacent to the posterior temporal lobe.

4. The *corpus callosum*—a large tract of fibres that allows each half of the brain to communicate with its counterpart on the other side. This inter-hemispheric communication is important in the auditory system for a number of reasons, but particularly with regard to the manner in which the brain processes certain configurations of speech signals.[5]

The auditory brain is the final repository and processing centre of the hearing mechanism. Each hemisphere of the brain seems to be dominant in the processing of certain categories of signals,[6] even though signals to each ear are doubtlessly channelled to both halves of the brain. In humans the left hemisphere (specifically the left temportal-parietal lobe area) is dominant in the perception of speech. At a minimum, the auditory area of the brain is responsible for the conscious perception of sound, for the interpretation of speech, and for the initiation of responses to sound. Similar responsibilities are exercised by other areas of the brain in the spatial and musical domains. Damage to hearing areas of the brain does not produce loss of sensitivity to sound; however, it can interfere devastatingly with speech processing and language. Severe aphasia and extremely faulty auditory processing abilities are often so intertwined as to make the exact contribution of each to poor communication capabilities impossible to sort out.

USEFUL TASKS IN ASSESSING HEARING FUNCTION

There are three major kinds of hearing tests that are useful in assessing elderly subjects. Standard hearing tests are useful in assessing the peripheral auditory system. Binaural tests which involve two ear interaction are useful in examining the status of the auditory brainstem. Difficult speech tasks are prominent in the evaluation of cortical (brain) function. These tasks vary considerably in complexity, ranging from relatively easy standard procedures which examine sensitivity to the presence of sound, to difficult speech tests which measure the ability of the auditory system to handle speech signals in complicated listening situations.

Standard auditory tests

The standard tests are those typically included in a basic hearing evaluation. Their aim is to measure hearing loss either as a loss of sensitivity to the presence of sound or as a loss of ability to recognize speech signals accurately. The hearing loss producing such disabilities is usually caused by damage to, or dysfunction of, parts of the peripheral hearing system, and most importantly to the cochlea or the auditory VIIIth cranial nerve. This kind of hearing loss is the most well recognized and perhaps the most common problem encountered by the elderly person. The procedures used to define the dimensions of this type of hearing problem include:

1. Measures of sensitivity for tones of various pitches and for speech. These are called *threshold measures* and their goal is simply to discover

how loud the tonal or speech signals need to be before a listener recognizes they are present. The test of tone thresholds can be done as a function of the frequency (pitch) of the tones, and thus indicates whereabouts a particular lack of sensitivity occurs in the range of pitches which are audible to humans.

2. Measures of speech discrimination or understanding. These procedures are designed to examine how well a person can understand speech when it is loud enough to be heard easily. The typical procedure is to measure, in a noise-free environment, how many words can be correctly repeated from a list of words that is chosen to include all of the sounds of a language.

3. Measures of the mobility of the tympanic membrane and the ossicular chain. Although presbyacusis due primarily to faulty transmission of sound through the middle ear system is relatively rare, it can nevertheless occur. More frequently, it is a component of hearing loss due to mixed causes. Special test procedures, tympanometry and acoustic reflex measures, allow definition of such mechanisms.

Binaural test measures

These tests determine whether the brainstem can correlate or otherwise manipulate signals arriving from both ears. Such manipulation allows normal listeners to lateralize or localize sound sources and can also separate a sound source like speech from an unfavourable background of noise to make the speech easier to hear and understand. A common complaint of people who are old is that, in a situation in which there are many talkers or television/radio background noise, they have extreme difficulty not only in figuring out where a message is coming from, but also in understanding the message against the background babble from other sources.

To find out whether an individual is having such problems, the following tests help:

1. Studies of lateralization ability. These are typically procedures which examine the ability of the auditory system to fuse signals from the two ears into a single sound image—the 'stereophonic effect', and to localize in space or lateralize in the head the location of that image.[7] A common task is to present identical tones to the two ears and determine whether the resultant behavioural experience is a fused image located somewhere in space (if, for example, the sound sources are loud speakers) or somewhere in the head (earphone or ear-insert sources). If a fused

image is the perception, further exploration is made of how the image moves as the intensities of the two or many sound sources are made different. For a normal listener, the fused image aroused by more than one sound source presenting identical or nearly identical signals will seem to be located in the direction of the more intense source. Breakdown of the ability of the brainstem to perform such analysis and to locate the source of sound can occur with aging and can put the elderly individual in a confusing and sometimes dangerous situation when confronted with a complicated acoustic environment.

2. Studies of signal recognition in noise. The measures alluded to here are those that examine the ability of an individual to listen with both ears to a target signal in the presence of noise also arriving at both ears. The tests are referred to as 'masking level difference tasks'[8] and they study how well a signal delivered to both ears can be recognized in the presence of noise delivered to both ears as a function of the phase of the signals. It is known that, for a normal auditory system, a binaural signal is more intelligible to a listener in the presence of binaural noise when the signal is out of phase. In an oversimplified but perhaps useful explanation, out of phase means that the brainstem is receiving signals that are different in their timing although having the same frequency and intensity characteristics. For reasons that are imperfectly understood, the hearing system finds signals which are different in this way more recognizable in the presence of noise than it does signals which are identical in every way including phase.[9]

Difficult speech tests

These procedures involve speech signals—some meaningful, some not— which have been made difficult to understand by deliberate distortion. This distortion is accomplished in many ways. Some of the procedures examine one ear's performance at a time (monotic tests) and some force the listener to attend to both ears at the same time (dichotic tests). All are based on the assumption that abnormal performance by areas of the brain responsible for processing speech signals will result in breakdown in performance on such hard-to-understand speech materials. Typically, breakdown in speech understanding is seen in the ear opposite to the side of the brain that is functioning poorly, although damage to the left side of the brain in the temporal–parietal lobe area can be devastating to auditory processing of signals from both ears and be part of an overall reduction or destruction of language and communication ability. Since elderly persons are a high-risk group for stroke, use of difficult speech tests can reveal important information about communication difficulties, including central hearing problems secondary to cerebrovascular accident. Common tasks used in seeking such problems include:

1. Degraded monotic speech tests. These procedures examine the ability of an individual to understand one or more signals delivered to one ear at a time. Ways of degrading the speech are numerous, but two general methods exist. The first makes the speech difficult to understand by mixing it with a second kind of sound which may be speech, noise, or some other sound. The second method makes the speech hard to decipher by changing its characteristics. Common ways of doing this include altering the frequency characteristics of the speech by filtering it, changing the rate at which the speech is delivered, and many others. Aged individuals without obvious focal brain lesions often have difficulty with such monotic materials when delivered to either ear. Those with known or silent vascular damage to the brain affecting auditory areas will usually show breakdown on difficult speech materials when these are delivered to the ear on the side opposite that of the brain damage.

2. Dichotic speech tests. These include procedures which force an individual to listen to speech messages delivered to both ears, usually in a roughly or precisely simultaneous fashion, and to respond in some manner to one or both of them. These tests range from the quite simple to the frustratingly difficult for even normal listeners. They are very useful, however, in studying the functional integrity of auditory areas of the brain. With proper use of difficult dichotic speech tasks, information can be gleaned from the results about hemispheric dominance in the brain for speech and about localization of damage to auditory areas of the brain in both hemispheres, and in tracts which connect them such as the corpus callosum.

PERFORMANCE OF OLD SUBJECTS

Elderly individuals can have problems associated with the aging process at each of the three major functional areas of the auditory system. At the level of the peripheral hearing mechanism, old people typically have losses of sensitivity to tones of various pitches, usually in the high frequencies, and to speech. They also often have difficulty in understanding what they hear—that is, they have classic hearing loss. They need sound to be made louder in order to be heard, and often have discrimination problems when they do hear. People with primarily brainstem aging effects usually do not have problems in hearing sound, but they often complain of difficulty in locating a sound in space or in understanding speech in a noisy background situation. People with problems affecting auditory regions of the brain may have difficulty in understanding speech compounded with language problems, especially if age effects include stroke.

Some of the documented effects of aging on the hearing system are:[1-3, 10]

(1) atrophy and disappearance of cells in the inner ear;

(2) angiosclerosis of tissue and blood cells in the inner ear;

(3) calcification of membranes in the inner ear;

(4) bioelectric and biomechanical imbalance in the inner ear;

(5) degeneration and loss of ganglion cells and their fibres in the VIIIth cranial nerve;

(6) VIIIth nerve canal collapse with consequent destruction of nerve fibres;

(7) atrophy and cell loss at all auditory centres in the brainstem;

(8) reduction of cells in auditory areas of the brain;

(9) changes in cytoplasm consistent with cortical anemia.

That these kinds of deterioration can and probably do occur in many aged people in simultaneous or sequential fashion makes the challenge and dimension of managing their hearing needs apparent.

Although accurate worldwide epidemiological information about hearing is lacking, the situation in a highly industrialized country such as the United States is revealing. Thirty-five to fifty per cent of people over 65 years of age have hearing loss and half of these are over 75 years of age. More revealing is the finding that these numbers are derived from studies which used as a standard the results of the most basic of hearing tests, (i.e. tests of sensitivity to sound and basic speech discrimination). Thus it does not include those persons who have problems relating to aging attacks on functions unique to the auditory brainstem and brain. The National Academy of Sciences of the United States estimates that, by the year 2000, 31.8 million citizens of that country will be over 65 years of age. Further, prevalence of hearing loss in long-term care facilities for the older individual is thought to exceed 50 per cent.[3, 11, 12]

HEARING AIDS AND ASSISTIVE LISTENING DEVICES

With the advent of presbyacusis, efforts have to be made to compensate for progressive hearing deficit. Since there is usually no medical or surgical treatment for presbyacusis, the appropriate recommendation is usually amplification.[13] Hearing aids attempt to restore lost hearing by electronically amplifying environmental sounds. A hearing evaluation can determine the need for amplification and, with appropriate medical approval, a hearing aid is prescribed that is designed to meet the specific needs of the user. Often two hearing aids are necessary. Technological advances have improved the quality of amplification in order to resolve or lessen some of the problems that are associated with age-related hearing loss. If the appropriate amplification is chosen and the user receives appropriate counselling on the use, care, and maintenance of the device, then amplification can provide a benefit that can be easily incorporated into the routine of everyday living for the geriatric patient. One inaccurate but surprisingly tenacious myth is that hearing aids will not help people with 'nerve' deafness. On the contrary, millions of people world-wide with sensorineural hearing loss use hearing aids very successfully.

Hearing aids

The fundamental design of a hearing aid is not complicated. The basic components include a microphone, which picks up environmental sound, the body of the hearing aid containing the electronic components that amplify the received sounds, which can be adjusted depending on the type and amount of hearing loss, a volume control, which allows the user to adjust the level of amplification or loudness of the sound, a battery compartment that contains the power source, and a coupler or earphone that delivers the amplified sound to the ear. If a fresh battery is correctly placed in the battery compartment, and the hearing aid is properly placed in the ear, hearing aid use is simply a matter of setting the volume control to the appropriate loudness level.

There are four types of hearing aids that are commonly dispensed once a hearing evaluation has determined that amplification is appropriate. The most frequently dispensed type is the 'all-in-the-ear' device. This is made to fit directly into the ear canal in order to deliver the amplified sound. An audiologist or hearing aid specialist takes a moulded impression of the ear(s) to be fitted and sends it, along with specific audiological test results, to a hearing aid manufacturer. The hearing aid manufacturer then custom shapes the hearing aid to fit into the user's ear, and the hearing aid is assembled to meet the specified sound production needs of that user. The all-in-the-ear type of hearing aid is often preferred for its simple operation and visual obscurity. The second type of commonly used hearing aid is the 'postauricular' or 'behind-the-ear' aid. The behind-the-ear aid is coupled by tubing to an earmould, and the custom-made earmould delivers sound to the listener's ear. The behind-the-ear type of hearing aid is usually not manufactured for a specific user, but is chosen from a selection of hearing aids with different amplification characteristics. Adjustments are then made by the dispenser in order to meet the specific amplification needs of the user. The third type of hearing aid, the 'body-level' aid, is usually selected for individuals with severe hearing loss or for the patient who cannot manipulate the smaller controls on the all-in-the-ear or behind-the-ear aids. This aid is usually worn clipped into a shirt pocket or in a specially designed harness that affixes the aid to the user's body. A wire from the casing leads to a coupler, which converts the electrical impulses to amplified sound. This is directly attached to an earmould that delivers the amplified sound to the listener's ear. A fourth type of hearing aid, the 'eyeglass' aid, is less common. In this aid, the electronics are built into the stem or temple of a pair of eyeglasses. Tubing from the stem of the glasses carries the sound to an earmould, which then delivers the amplified sound to the listener's ear. The eyeglass aid is not commonly dispensed because of the problems involved in combining two prosthetic devices.

Once the appropriate type of amplification is chosen, a hearing aid evaluation is performed. This is a two-part process. The first part involves a series of procedures to determine whether the hearing aid chosen is appropriate. If it is suitable, physical adjustments are made to ensure a comfortable fit and to fine tune the acoustic characteristics of the hearing aid in order to meet the sound production needs of the user. The second part of the hearing aid evaluation is necessary to ensure appropriate use. Hearing aid orientation is an important part of the evaluation and it is helpful if the spouse or a primary care person can be involved in the counselling session in order to help the user become familiar with the function and care of the device. During this session the recipient is taught how to place the hearing aid in the ear, how to manipulate the controls, how to change the battery, and how to care for and maintain the aid. Follow-up sessions are planned to ensure appropriate use and to lessen the chance of rejection. The follow-up sessions are a good opportunity to determine how well the user is managing with the hearing aid and to provide additional training as necessary. At this time, care and maintenance can also be reviewed.

The care and maintenance of hearing aids are responsibilities that should be shared by the user as well as by family and the support personnel in, for example, the long-term care setting. The geriatric patient, however, often lacks in visual acuity and manual dexterity necessary to maintain the appropriate function of the hearing aid. In-service training for support personnel, including hands-on exposure to the four types of hearing aids that may be encountered, can provide skills that are necessary to assist the hearing aid user. Such personnel and/or family should also be familiarized with the specific needs and use recommendations for each patient. The following is a list of care and maintenance suggestions that will help maintain a hearing aid:

1. Do not drop the hearing aid. Its delicate electronics or casing may be damaged. If possible, when fitting the hearing aid stand over a soft surface such as a rug or sit on a sofa or bed.

2. Do not expose the hearing aid to moisture. It should be removed while washing, bathing, or when exposed to adverse weather conditions such as rain.

3. Remove the hearing aid at night and store it in a safe place.

4. When the aid is not in use, remove the battery. This will avoid unnecessary battery drain and will protect the battery compartment from leakage if the hearing aid is not used for prolonged periods of time.

5. Keep the hearing aid and earmould clean. With everyday use, the accumulation of cerumen (earwax) can block the bore that delivers the amplified sound. If this does occur, for the behind-the-ear type remove the earmould from the hearing aid and try to extract the cerumen by gently washing the earmould. After making certain that the tubing or earmould do not have residual water, re-affix the tubing to the hearing aid. With an all-in-the-ear type aid, carefully remove the cerumen from the bore, but do not wash the aid. Wipe it clean with a soft cloth or tissue.

6. Follow the manufacturer's instructions when replacing the battery. Replacing it incorrectly could damage the delicate battery compartment.

7. Have the aid checked regularly by a hearing aid sepcialist.

With everyday use, problems may occur that can affect the output of the hearing aid. Often the problems require only basic troubleshooting strategies by the user or care assistant in order to restore the amplification. Learning these strategies could avoid the debilitating loss of hearing that results if a hearing aid specialist is not immediately available for help.

There are three basic problems common to hearing aid use. The first is a dead hearing aid. Here the hearing aid provides no amplification to the user. The second is feedback. This is caused by a hearing aid picking up and re-amplifying its own output. This results in a loud, high-pitched whistling or squealing sound. The third problem is weak or intermittent hearing aid performance. For all three types of problems, if the user or person assisting the user is familiar with the basic function of the hearing aid then running through the Hearing Aid Troubleshooting Guide (Appendix A) may provide the necessary solution. If a review of this checklist does not resolve the problem, *do not* take the hearing aid apart or tamper with the electronic components. The hearing aid should be returned to the dispenser or manufacturer, with a basic explanation of the problem for repair.

ASSISTIVE LISTENING DEVICES

In addition to hearing aids there are assistive listening devices in production that are designed to meet some of the more specific needs of the hearing-impaired geriatric patient. The following are some of the more useful and commonly used devices:

1. Direct audio input (DAI)—this is a special option that can be ordered on some hearing aids. It incorporates a special socket on the hearing aid that allows hardwire input from auxillary sound sources, such as a television or radio, to be plugged in if a compatible connector is available. This device allows the listener to take advantage of the hearing aid's custom amplification.

2. Telephone amplifiers—special amplifiers can be affixed or incorporated into the telephone that will increase the loudness of the signal or message. Many of the more severely hearing-impaired geriatric patients cannot use a telephone without this help. For more information about the types and availability of telephone amplifiers, contact the nearest agency responsible for telephone service or a hearing aid specialist.

3. Telecommunication device for the deaf (TDD)—the telecommunication device for the deaf is actually a portable typewriter that can be coupled to a telephone receiver. The telephone conversation appears as a visual readout above the keyboard. The device can send and receive messages but is restricted by its ability to communicate only with other TDDs. It is, however, a very effective means of communication for an individual with a severe or profound hearing loss or for individuals with very poor word recognition ability who cannot use the conventional telephone, particularly in an emergency situation.

4. Telecaptioning decoder—this is a visual aid that provides a television programmes audio dialogue to the television viewer in the form of

text running across the bottom of the television screen. The decoder is easy to install and an increasing number of television and videocassette programmes now incorporate this system for the hard-of-hearing viewer.

5. Personal FM system—this comprises an extension microphone that requires no connecting cable. The transmitter broadcasts an FM signal to a receiver that is worn or carried by the listener. The receiver has no speaker so the signal is delivered to the listener through an earphone, DIA, or conduction couplers. This system is particularly valuable for initial medical assessment, a mental status interview, or patient placement or management situations in which the patient has not yet received appropriate amplification. In the authors' experience, remarkable improvements in personal interaction attitudes of patients using personal FM systems are frequently observed and at least one unit should be considered as essential equipment for all long-term care facilities. This system is also gaining greater popularity in cinemas and auditoriums where multiple receivers are used. They can be set to the same frequency for the hearing-impaired members of the audience.

6. Alerting devices—a variety of such devices have been developed to provide the hearing impaired with visual and tactile signals in situations where conventional alerting signals, such as door bells, fire alarms, or smoke detectors, cannot be heard. The devices are strategically placed to signal the user and available in a variety of forms, such as flashing lights, movement devices, and bed vibrators.

With the growth of technology, advances are expected in the development of even more sophisticated assistive listening devices than these basic types. It is important that the professional who is responsible for the long-term care of the geriatric patient be aware of these technological advances as they are sure to lead to greater availability, reduced costs, and improved design efficiency. For more information about the types and availability of these devices contact the appropriate Department for Public Health. Also see Appendix B for suggestions.

AURAL REHABILITATION

Hearing loss often adversely affects the communication process and puts stress on interpersonal relationships. For the elderly individual, a loss of hearing may affect the quality of life. Many hard-of-hearing people who undergo an aural rehabilitation program experience significant improvement in communication skills and have a better understanding of their disability. The goal of aural rehabilitation is to help each hearing-impaired person reach his/her optimal level of communication by max-imizing the use of residual hearing, visual information, and communica-tion strategies or coping techniques.[14] The hearing-impaired person may need to learn new skills as well as new behaviours to cope effectively with hearing loss. Aural rehabilitation may be provided by any hearing health professional (HHP) with a background in audiology, speech pathology, or education of the hearing-impaired.

Aural rehabilitation techniques

Aural rehabilitation therapy may consist of one or more of the following:

Counselling
The hearing health professional (HHP) may provide information about the hearing loss in order to promote a better understanding of the disability. This involves explaining the test results and the effects of the person's own hearing loss on everyday situations including home, voca-tion, and social activities and answering all questions that the hearing-impaired individual may have. The HHP may seek to motivate the client to take both responsibility for the disability and whatever actions are necessary to resolve communication problems that arise (e.g. using a hearing aid if recommended). It is imperative that the hard-of-hearing person develop a positive attitude of acceptance toward hearing loss so that new coping behaviours may be acquired. It is often necessary to counsel significant contacts also (i.e. family members, friends) as well as staff in a long-term care facility. Specific instructions can be given to help the elderly client and others to adjust to hearing loss and alleviate problems directly resulting from it.

Hearing aid orientation
Once a hearing aid is issued to the hearing-impaired client, the HHP may instruct him/her in its use and care. The geriatric client—depending on his/her mental/medical status—may require extensive counselling, prac-tice, and repetition to adjust to the new prosthetic device. The HHP's goal is for the elderly individual to be as independent as possible in the operation of the hearing aid. In order to reach this goal, the duration of aural rehabilitation may extend anywhere from 2 days to 2 months.

Selection and use of assistive listening devices
The hearing health professional may help the hearing-impaired client choose from a variety of assistive listening devices available. Instruction in their use may also be provided. See the previous section of this chapter.

Auditory training

Instruction in the development of improved listening skills and in the recognition, discrimination, and comprehension of speech is an important part of the aural rehabilitation process. The person's need for auditory training is dependent on the degree of hearing loss and use of residual hearing for communication. For the elderly patient, the emphasis should be on adjusting to amplification and comprehension of conversational speech in quiet and poor listening environments. The elderly client must develop realistic expectations and accept the limitations that may be imposed by the hearing impairment.

Instruction in speech reading (lip reading) and use of visual cues

Speech reading helps the hard-of-hearing person to compensate partially for hearing loss, particularly in difficult listening situations. The client is taught to recognize speech patterns on the lips, use non-verbal information, and apply visual cues (i.e. gestures, facial expressions) in the environment in order to comprehend conversational speech. The elderly client will require instruction and drill in basic principles of speech reading and discrimination of gross visual patterns of words, phrases, and sentences that are generally applicable to daily communication needs and living environment. The HHP should be careful to provide opportunities for success at all times throughout instruction in order to prevent discouragement. Auditory and visual modes of communication may be combined for speech-reading practice to reduce the difficulty of tasks presented.

Communication techniques and coping strategies

The HHP can provide insight and instruction in ways to reduce communication problems that occur as a result of hearing loss. Specific suggestions such as 'watch the speaker', 'ask others to speak more slowly or clearly when necessary without shouting', 'ask others to repeat or rephrase when there is a misunderstanding', 'ask questions to get specific information that is missed', 'stay within 1 to 2 metres from the speaker when in conversation', may be offered as strategies to improve communication and cope with hearing loss. The use of audio-visual materials such as brochures and videotapes on hearing loss and coping strategies in addition to discussion and role playing can help to reinforce concepts and behaviors taught. The long-term care geriatric patient may require extensive repetition and practice.

Peer support groups

Aural rehabilitation classes and groups are instrumental in disseminating information, providing emotional support, sharing common problems, feelings, and experiences, and reinforcing new communication strategies. Aural rehabilitation groups are cost effective as well as beneficial to the hearing-impaired client. A homogeneous group of hearing-impaired people who are grossly compatible, with similar hearing losses and interests, can be grouped for discussion or support groups and classes in speech reading, hearing aid orientation, and coping strategies. Such groups should be structured so that they provide a positive communication experience and successful learning experience. An effort should be made to make the groups fun, motivating, and beneficial to the elderly client's daily communication needs whether he/she lives in a long-term care facility or at home.

Sample aural rehabilitation programme

Although the tendency is to view hearing-impaired elderly people as a homogeneous group, it is important to realize that they are a diversified group made up of individuals with different health problems, interests, personalities, and ages (often ranging from age 60 to over 100 years), and they should be viewed as individuals when therapy plans are written. An aural rehabilitation programme should meet the client's communication needs, providing both individualized and group aural rehabilitation therapy. A simple questionaire or evaluation of communicative function may aid the HHP in determining the client's specific rehabilitative needs.[15] The following describes a sample aural rehabilitation approach and programme for elderly patients.

1. Identify the patient with hearing loss.
2. Counsel patient about hearing loss and steps for remediation.
3. Perform hearing aid evaluation and provide instruction in hearing aid usage.
4. Evaluate (subjectively) the aural rehabilitation needs (i.e. informal interview, hearing handicap questionnaire).
5. Determine patient's goals and behavioural objectives.
6. Provide aural rehabilitation therapy individually or in group.
7. Provide counselling session following the aural rehabilitation group to determine further needs for rehabilitation.
8. Continue aural rehabilitation if necessary.

9. Make medical referrals if needed (i.e. otolaryngologist, psycho-social worker, etc.).

10. Make community referrals to groups, organizations, or centres for the hearing impaired.

The hearing-impaired elderly individual in a long-term care (LTC) facility may require extensive follow-up and repetition because of memory deficits. Efforts should be made to identify residents with hearing loss and all professional staff, including physicians, therapists, and nurses should be notified of those persons. A simple way to do this is to mark medical charts and place notices in the patient's room. The information and coping strategies presented to the LTC patient should be simple, practical, and applicable to his/her living situation. The HHP should attempt to make the client as independent as possible in hearing aid usage, although realistic goals must be established. In the LTC facility, aural rehabilitation may be limited to the appropriate and consistent usage of hearing aids for some patients. It may be necessary to instruct LTC staff (i.e. primary care nurses) in the care and usage of hearing aids (see Appendix A) so that they may assist the patient on a daily basis. Frequent monitoring of hearing aid use is necessary to promote good communication between patient and staff and to reduce loss and damage of hearing aids. The HHP has the responsibility of making the LTC staff aware of each patient's communication needs and must suggest ways to help the patient achieve adequate communication with or without a hearing aid.

ROOM ACOUSTICS

Environmental considerations are very important in a discussion of living and long-term care facilities for geriatric individuals. Undesirable room acoustics can amplify noise and make communication difficult for the hearing-impaired resident. Large recreation areas or dining rooms are usually the focus of this problem. For the hearing-impaired resident, there are many sources of unwanted noise in the LTC setting that can interfere with the perception of speech. Uncontrolled background noise present within a dining room or recreation area may include kitchen activity, heating or air conditioning, recreational activities, normal furniture movement, competing speech, and the normal daily activities of the residents. Reverberation contributes to the overall noise level and has a severe effect on the speech discrimination (recognition) ability of hearing-impaired residents, many of whom listen through hearing aids that compound the problem by adding their own distortion products.

This situation can be greatly improved by applying sound-absorbent materials to 20–50 per cent of the boundary surfaces of the room. Modification of these surfaces can be achieved with the use of materials such as carpeting, drapes and acoustic ceiling tiles. Recent extensive study of a large dining/recreation area at a Veterans Administion Medical Center (Los Angeles) Nursing Home Care Unit was made to determine the noise reduction capability generated by replacing a hard-surfaced, sound-reflective type of ceiling tile with one chosen for its noise reduction acoustic characteristics.[16] The sound level measurements made before and after acoustic modification of the room indicated that decreasing reverberation times by acoustically modifying the ceiling and adding acoustically designed wall panels reduced the level of background noise and hence dramatically improved the listening environment for the hearing-impaired residents. Previous studies suggested that the 12 dB noise level reduction that was achieved in the dining/recreation area of the nursing home in question were capable of improving word recognition abilities of similar subjects by more than 30 per cent.[17]

Since dining rooms and recreation areas are meant to be the focal point of socialization and communication for LTC residents, it is imperative that the optimum acoustic environment be achieved. Failure to do so leads to a situation that will ensure avoidance of these areas by residents who would prefer the relative quiet and isolation of their rooms, which is hardly conducive to achieving the goal of making the LTC facility a comfortable home.

SUMMARY

Half of the persons who are sufficiently hearing impaired to be considered disabled, comprising some 7–8 per cent of the world's population, are aged 65 years or older.[11] It is clear that aged individuals who spend significant amounts of time in LTC facilities are more likely than not to have disabling communicative disorders, including hearing loss. These prevalence figures can only increase with the gradually increasing average age of the world's population.

All parts of the hearing mechanism, both peripheral and central, are subject to damage over a lifetime. How much of that damage is an inevitability of a programmed aging process and how much is created or compounded by other influences like noise and drugs is difficult to determine. The central fact remains: hearing disorders are a major problem for great numbers of elderly individuals.

Many avenues should be used to help the elderly retain lives of some meaning when hearing begins to fail. Failure to do so guarantees frustration, withdrawal, and the curtailment of an individual as a communicating being.

Several approaches are suggested in this chapter. They include taking advantage of rapidly improving hearing aid technology, the use of various assistive devices to improve communication, the provision of aural rehabilitation programs to teach the hearing-impaired person to use every available modality and strategy, and the modification of acoustic environments, particularly in LTC facilities, to ensure that the quality of sound and acoustic surroundings will maximize rather than penalize efficient communication. Taking such steps and making such efforts are sensible, economically practical, and humane.

References

1. Hawkins, J. E. and Johnsson, L.-G. (1985). Otopathological changes associated with presbyacusis. *Seminars in Hearing*, **6**, 115–33.
2. Schucknecht, H. F. (1974)). *Pathology of the ear*. Harvard University Press, Cambridge, MA.
3. Hayes, D. (1985). Aging and speech understanding. *Seminars in Hearing*, **6**, 147–59.
4. Benson, D. F. and Zaidel, E. (1985). *The dual brain: hemispheric specialization in humans*. Guilford, New York.
5. Sparks, R, Goodglass, H. and Nickel, B. (1970). Ipsilateral versus contralateral extinction in dichotic listening resulting from hemisphere lesions. *Cortex*, **6**, 249–60.
6. Noffsinger, D. (1985). Dichotic-listening techniques in the study of hemispheric asymmetries. In *The dual brain: hemispheric specialization in humans*, (ed. Benson, D. F. and E. Zaider) *E*, pp. 127–41. Guilford, New York.
7. Jerger, J. and Harford, E. R. (1960). Alternate and simultaneous balancing (ed. Benson, D. F. and E. Zaidel) pp. 127–41. Guilford, New York.
8. Olsen, W. O., Noffsinger, D. and Carhart, R. (1976). Masking level differences encountered in clinical populations. *Audiology*, **15**, 287–301.
9. Durlach, N. L. and Colburn, H. S. (1978). Binaural phenomena. In *Handbook of perception: hearing, Vol. 4*. pp. 365–466. (ed. Carterette, E. C. and M. P. Friedman), Academic, New York.
10. Roush, J. (1985). Aging and binaural auditory processing. *Seminars in Hearing*, **6**, 135–46.
11. Tower, D. B. and Ward, P. H. (1979). *Report of the panel on communication disorders*. pp. 3–144. National Institute of Health, Washington DC.
12. Stockford, D. D. (1983). *Speech pathology: communicative disorders among patients in VA medical facilities: part 1, 2*. Veterans Administration, Washington DC.
13. Hull, R. H. (1985). Hearing aids for the older adult: Considerations for fitting and dispensing. *Seminars in Hearing*, **6**, 181–91.
14. Bate, H. L. (1985). Aural rehabilitation of the older adult. *Seminars in Hearing*, **6**, 193–205.

15. Alpiner, J. (ed.) (1978). *Handbook of adult rehabilitative audiology*, pp. 30–66. Williams and Wilkins Co., Baltimore.
16. Martin, J. P. (1988). Acoustic modification of dining/recreation areas. Unpublished report. pp.1–32. Veterans Administration, Los Angeles.
17. Finitzo-Hieber, T. and Tillman, T. W. (1978). Room acoustics effects on monosyllabic word discrimination ability for normal and hearing-impaired children. *Journal of Speech and Hearing Research,* **21**, 440–58.

APPENDIX A: HEARING AID TROUBLE-SHOOTING GUIDE

Problem	Possible cause (checklist)	Solution
1. Hearing aid 'dead'	1. a. Earwax occluding earmould	1. a. Remove earmould from hearing aid and clean earmould (bore)
	b. Switches not appropriately set	b. Set O-T-M switch to 'M'; set volume control to half-on position.
	c. Battery dead	c. Replace battery
	d. Tubing twisted or bent	d. Re-insert earmould
	e. Battery is reversed in compartment	e. Match '+' on battery to '+' mark on the battery compartment
	f. Cord plugs not firmly inserted in receptacles (body aids)	f. Push in firmly; if necessary tape in place
	g. Hearing aid broken or cannot determine problem	g. Refer problem to the hearing aid dispenser or manufacturer
2. Feedback (hearing aid whistling or squealing)	2. a. Wax occluding external ear canal	2. a. Request or perform otoscopic examination of ear canal
	b. Earmould inserted improperly	b. Re-insert earmould.
	c. Volume control set too high	c. Set volume control to comfortable level or half on
	d. Hearing aid too close to another object (pillow, wall, etc.)	d. Clear area around aid or reposition head
	e. O-T-M switch in wrong position	e. For normal use keep on 'M' position
	f. Physical problem (broken stem, damaged tubing, or can't determine problem)	f. Refer problem to the hearing aid dispenser or manufacturer
3. Complaint of weak or intermittent hearing aid performance	3. a. Weak battery	3. a. Replace battery
	b. Earmould not properly positioned in ear	b. Re-insert earmould
	c. Tubing twisted or bent	c. Re-insert earmould
	d. Body-level aid — cord plugs not firmly inserted in receptacles — microphone is facing the body	d. Body-level aid — push in firmly; if necessary tape in place — face microphone away from body
	e. Cannot determine problem	e. Refer problem to the hearing aid dispenser or manufacturer

APPENDIX B: USEFUL CONTACT INFORMATION

1. The most complete directory of manufacturers and dispensers of every kind of hearing instrument available, including hearing aids, assistive devices, acoustic environment modifiers, amplifiers, artificial ears and mastoids, attenuators, calibration equipment, audiometers, test rooms and booths, batteries, earmoulds, ear protectors, etc., is published in a United States professional journal. Importantly, in addition to an exhaustive listing of companies in the USA, there is extensive coverage of organizations, manufacturers, and distributors of information and products for 58 nations of the world. Names, addresses, phone numbers, and contact people are given.

   The journal is: *Hearing Instruments*, 1 East First Street, Duluth, Minnesota 55802, USA.

   The latest international directory is contained in the May 1988 issue. It can be purchased separate from a subscription by sending $13 (US) to the address given above. (Be sure to ask for the May 1988 directory issue.)

2. Three USA organizations publish complete lists of their members who reside in countries other than the USA. The Acoustical Society of America has members in some 60 other nations. The American Speech–Language–Hearing Association and the American Academy of Otolaryngology–Head and Neck Surgery each have members in some 30 nations. These organizations can be contacted for such directories at the following addresses. Request information and cost.

   Secretary,
   Acoustical Society of America, 500 Sunnyside Boulevard, Woodbury, New York 11797, USA.

   American Speech-Language-Hearing Association, 10801 Rockville Pike, Rockville, Maryland 20852, USA

   American Academy of Otolaryngology, 1101 Vermont Avenue NW, Suite 302, Washington, DC, 20005 USA

3. The following organizational publications contain useful information about aural rehabilitation. They are published on a regular basis.

   Self Help for Hard of Hearing People (SHHH), 4848 Battery Lane, Suite 100, Bethesda, Maryland 20814, USA

   Journal of Academy of Rehabilitative Audiology, c/o Hugo L. Beykerch, Business Manager, Communicative Disorders, Communication Arts Center 229, University of Northern Iowa, Cedar Falls, Iowa 50614, USA.

5. Useful reference books for aural rehabilitation:

   Jeffers, J. and Barley, M. (1971). *Speechreading*, Charles C. Thomas, Springfield, Illinois, USA

   Alpiner, J. (ed). (1978). *Handbook of adult rehabilitative audiology*, Williams and Wilkins, Baltimore, Maryland, USA.

16

The effectiveness of intervention for the mental health of the elderly

BARRY J. GURLAND, RICHARD MAYEUX,
and BARNETT S. MEYERS

OVERVIEW

The effectiveness of an intervention is strictly speaking to be judged by the gains it brings over the natural outcome of a condition. However, this perspective alone does not indicate the desirability of treatment; that depends also on how bad the outcome is likely to be without intervention, the risks and discomforts of treatment, and the optimum outcome that can be achieved if the benefits of nature and intervention are summated. Therefore, we will not limit this discussion to effectiveness in the strict sense.

Probably the main misconception regarding the effectiveness of interventions for mental health of the elderly has to do with underestimating the good outcomes that can be obtained with most mental conditions, even relative to those obtained with younger patients. For example, the schizophrenic-like states which begin in old age (the paraphrenias) are less likely to show progressive deterioration of emotions, inability to express thoughts coherently, or loss of initiative than is typical in younger schizophrenics.[1] The response of the elderly paraphrenic's condition to pharmacological treatment is good if the compliance of the patient is maintained.[2]

The success of intervention in the elderly may sometimes be obscured and overlooked because of the complexity of adequate treatment and the care required in its administration. This is seen in the depressions that coexist with age-related changes in the pharmacodynamics of antidepressant medications or which are intermingled with the chronic physical disorders of old age.[3] Despite the added difficulties of treating depressions in old age, the frequency of recovery from distressing and disabling symptoms can be comparable with the outcomes reported in younger patients.[4, 5]

It is useful for the discussion of the effectiveness of intervention to draw a distinction between the so-called functional or non-organic mental conditions of old age, such as depression, anxiety and paraphrenia, and the organic mental conditions such as the dementias.[6] Although there are points of overlap, on the whole the functional disorders are more responsive to treatment and have better outcomes than the organic disorders. This point is made to underline the similarity of outcomes of the functional mental conditions of the elderly to those that occur in younger patients, but also to focus attention on the wide range of outcomes that can be affected by intervention even in the organic conditions.

Interventions aimed at the crucial pathophysiology of the primary degenerative dementias (Alzheimer's disease is the most common type) are now at a promising but still experimental stage. For the present, these conditions tend to be progressive. Nevertheless, there are a subset of treatable and reversible organic disorders which may have distinctive clinical symptoms (the deliria or acute confusional states) or may resemble the picture of a primary dementia but be distinguished by suitable clinical and laboratory investigations. Moreover, much can be done to give relief from the symptoms of a primary dementia to both the patient and caregivers, even if the ultimate course of the illness is downhill. The value of a treatment which achieves partial improvement, slows an inevitable decline, or modulates the most troublesome symptoms should not be underestimated.

DEPRESSION

The clearest statements on the outcomes of depression in the elderly can be made about those conditions which have marked symptoms, a relatively clear onset, and also characteristic somatic (vegetative) features. These are variously known as major depressions, affective disorders, or endogenous depressions. The great majority of these cases (around 70 per cent or more) should be relieved by treatment within 3 to 6 weeks.[7] Without proper treatment probably less than half would improve to the same degree or within the same time period. There is no doubt that appropriate intervention is desirable and effective and that the immediate outcome is good. For this condition, appropriate intervention is primarily antidepressant medication or electroshock therapy.

To be effective, treatment should be in skilled hands since it must be sufficiently cautious to avoid toxicity or adverse drug interactions, yet determined enough to achieve adequate dosage levels. Moreover, effective treatment involves a continuing management plan for the patient since a substantial majority of the recovered patients will relapse[8, 9] With maintenance treatment (with either antidepressants or lithium carbonate) where indicated, relapses can be avoided in over half of the recovered patients (again similar to the outcomes reported for adult patients by

Prein *et al.*[10]) and early detection of incipient relapse can allow timely intervention and truncation of the episode of depression.

Intervention is less effective if delayed. Depressions lasting over 2 years are particularly difficult to treat. The condition is also more likely to resist treatment at a later age of onset or occurrence, where the patient has been chronically maladjusted, or in the absence of a family history of depression.

There is little to choose between the types of antidepresesants in terms of their effectiveness for severe depression. The selection of a particular antidepressant may be guided by the response of a patient to a particular antidepressant in a previous episode if any, or be aimed at minimizing the risk of potential interactions with other medications the patient may be taking, and especially at avoiding a clash between an antidepressant's side-effect profile and the elderly patient's vulnerabilities.[11] Although antidepressants (such as the tricyclics) are of proved value in the elderly, they nonetheless have side-effects which can at times limit their efficacy; these include apathy, unsteadiness and inco-ordination that can result from excessive sedation, heart failure from disruption of the normal rhythms of the heart-beat, fainting and falling from lowering of blood-pressure that may occur on standing up, and confusion, urinary retention or raised intraocular pressure from inhibition of cholinergic neurotransmitters.

Episodes of elevated mood or mania during the course of bipolar depression or manic-depressive disorder can be kept under control by lithium carbonate, with added neuroleptics in an emergency.

The effectiveness of electroshock therapy for severe depressions in the elderly tends to be overlooked because it is often misconceived as a traumatic treatment. In fact it is remarkably safe and effective; there are few contraindications and it often succeeds where other treatments have failed.[5] Moreover, it may be the intervention of first choice where the depressive symptoms have reached dangerous proportions with rapid progression, severe loss of weight, or imminent risk of suicide. Fears about the effects of this treatment on memory have been exaggerated; any such disturbance is temporary and short-lived and is negligible in any case where the current is applied only to the same side of the head as the non-dominant hemisphere of the brain.

Even where interventions for depression do not at first succeed, persistence, addition or substitution of interventions may prevail.[7] Thus, antidepressants of a different type may be tried, or electroshock therapy introduced, and in some cases lithium or neuroleptic medications may be added. Psychotherapy is often an effective adjuvant when symptoms are not too severe.

Depressions which are of a clinical level of severity but do not meet criteria for a major disorder also may respond to the physical treatments described above but are less certain to do so. For these less severe depressions, psychotherapy and cognitive therapy have proved to be of value.[12]

DEMENTIA

Approaches to the diagnosis and classification of the dementias are summarized in the Appendix (p. 683). We consider here three topics; Alzheimer's disease and related disorders, multi-infarct dementia and the dementia syndrome resulting from depression.

Alzheimer's disease and related disorders (ADRD)

The effectiveness of interventions should first be considered in terms of what can be done for the patient who presents with symptoms that might be due to ADRD. From this angle, the most beneficial intervention is to search for conditions whose symptoms resemble those of ADRD but which are more responsive to treatment.

In some clinical settings up to 20 per cent of cases investigated for suspected ADRD have been found to have a potentially reversible condition[13] though this proportion is much lower where cases have been properly screened before referral. Potentially reversible conditions may be indicated by a distinctive clinical picture as in a delirium or acute confusional state, or in depression (depressive pseudodementia), but may be indistinguishable from ADRD until investigation exposes a reversible cause. Effective intervention is then aimed at the underlying condition such as an intracranial mass, accumulation of cerebrospinal fluid, or disorder arising elsewhere in the body but affecting brain function (e.g. pernicious anemia, thyroid dysfunction).

The appropriate treatment of a potentially reversible dementia is to treat the underlying condition; adequate treatment is usually successful in returning the patient's mental function to normality. Conversely, if neglected, these underlying conditions may in some instances be fatal or lead to permanent brain damage. In addition to a full clinical examination of a suspected case of ADRD it is advisable to employ a battery of laboratory and special investigations because this will allow the detection of most reversible causes of the symptoms of dementia; even if only a small proportion of cases turn out to be reversible this would be economically and ethically worth while. The battery should extend beyond standard blood and serum analysis to include at least tests of B_{12}, folate levels and thyroid function, and brain imaging (usually CAT scan with a contrast medium).

New interventions intended to redress the neurotransmitter abnormalities involved in the intellectual deficits of Alzheimer's disease are being intensively generated and evaluated. They have displaced interest in the earlier treatments, which are now regarded as lacking a specific rationale and being either misdirected (e.g. vasodilators or oxygenating techniques), weak at best (e.g. hydergine) or useful only for reducing disturbing behaviours.

The current generation of specific interventions for Alzheimer's disease (by far the most common form of primary dementia) is concentrated on restoring the functioning of the cholinergic neurotransmitter pathways which mediate memory and certain other intellectural capacities. The strategies adopted attempt to influence each step in the production, flow, enhancement, and breakdown of the neurotransmitter acetylcholine. Dietary supplements of choline (a precursor of acetylcholine) such as lecithin (phosphatidylcholine) or deanol have been tried in an effort to promote production of acetylcholine. Inhibitors of enzymes which breakdown acetylcholine at the synapse (nerve ending) have been administered in order to preserve what little acetylcholine is secreted; the anticholinesterase physostigmine has produced improvement in some aspects of memory but is quite short acting[14] while newer drugs such as tetrahydroaminoacridine (THA) are longer acting and therefore theoretically more promising. Acetylcholine agonists (i.e. surrogates) such as arecoline, oxotremorine, or bethanechol are used on the grounds that they might stimulate the next nerve in the chain, through the postsynaptic receptor site which is known to be unimpaired by the disease; however, there is some doubt that these agonists can enhance the precise and infinitely varying patterns of release of neurotransmitters that is required for transmission of useful neural messages.[15] A class of drugs called nootropics (e.g. piracetam, aniracetam) are being tested because they stimulate memory and learning (at least in animals), possibly by increasing the rate at which neurones fire and secrete their message-laden distinctive neurotransmitter sequences. Some substances such as hydergine (dihydroergotoxine) are extensively used for the milder symptoms of dementia on the grounds that they seem to boost cerebral metabolism in a non-specific manner; their benefit probably stems from improving the mood and motivation of the patient.[16]

Some of these neurotransmitter-oriented interventions, alone or in combination, appear to be effective to a measurable but variable and modest degree, for a limited period of time, at an early stage of the disease, and in certain patients. In some cases the useful improvement in the patient's functioning has impressed the clinician and family members. However, the most that can be concluded with confidence for the present is that these interventions may be keyed to important aspects of the pathophysiology of dementia and should be evaluated on a larger scale. Furthermore, it is unlikely that they will halt the progressive degeneration of the neural structures caused by the disease.

A sampling of studies gives a flavour of the wide-ranging and stringent efforts to exploit the therapeutic potential of the cholinergic deficit in Alzheimer's disease. Numerous controlled studies have demonstrated little significant benefit from acetylcholine precursor administration,[17] though slight improvement has been found on combining these drugs with a nootropic.[18] The anticholinesterases have given erratic results but in some studies have been distinctly encouraging,[14,19] not only for mental function but also for performance of the daily tasks of self-care; here also the addition of a nootropic has improved the therapeutic effect.[17] The cholinergic agonists have also produced definite improvements in mental function and social behaviour but these have so far been slight.[20] Some of the conflict between the results of studies on the effectiveness of specific treatments for dementia of the Alzheimer type can be attributed to differences in methodology but also to variability in dosage and absorption of the medications (e.g. physostigmine).

Imbalances in non-cholinergic neurotransmitter systems and other agents influencing neuroactivity may also be involved in producing the symptoms of Alzheimer's disease; correspondingly, the experimental treatments must be that much more complicated. In this direction, studies are proceeding on the effect of noradrenaline, vasopressin (as the synthetic analogue DDAVP), and naloxone.

The nature and causes of multi-infarct dementia are still controversial and the benefits of intervention are unclear. Prevention and treatment of hypertension and stroke are for many other reasons desirable and may also reduce the incidence of multi-infarct dementia. Removal of plaques in the external carotid arteries has also been tried but its effectiveness is not convincingly documented.

General treatments

There are other interventions which are less in the limelight but more useful in the contemporary treatment of the symptoms of dementia. Although there is a lack of properly controlled studies in support of this assertion, it is apparent that temporary resort to sedative or neuroleptic medication can be effective in managing the restlessness, agitation, or resistiveness that can exhaust both patient and caregivers; in the longer run, these symptoms can best be abated by careful restructuring of the patient's environment and daily routines to engage the patient's interest and reinforce a sense of mastery. These general principles have sometimes been formalized into detailed techniques such as orientation therapy; controlled evaluations of the effectiveness of such technical approaches have not yielded conclusive or striking results.

In communities which are well organized and rich in services there should be a network of agencies able to arrange for homecare, daycare, respite care, and the organization of self-help groups to shore up the efforts of the family to keep the ADRD patient at home for as long as is reasonable. Clinical experience, client satisfaction, and demand for these services attest to their efficacy. However, there are few studies which have objectively demonstrated the advantages of these interventions with respect to reducing admission to nursing homes, alleviating distress among caregivers, or improving the patient's morale and functioning. Similar remarks apply to the use of psychotherapy, remotivation therapy, or other means of helping the patient to adapt to the advance of the disease.

It is also widely accepted without necessity of formal proof that good medical and nursing care can forestall or postpone the secondary complications of dementia and thereby prolong the ADRD patient's active life. It is not likely that this will become the subject matter of controlled evaluation of effectiveness, but it does raise ethical issues on the value of interventions.

Dementia syndrome resulting from depression

Symptoms resembling dementia may arise during the course of an episode of depression and resolve when the depression recedes; this syndrome has been called 'pseudodementia'. Its history offers a cautionary note on the hazards of judging the effectiveness of interventions for the mental health of the elderly.

Several studies found that the treatment of the underlying depression in pseudodementia restored the intellectual performance of the patient and that the long-range prognosis was that of depression, not dementia.[21] However, recently it has been recognized that 20–50 per cent of these cases may retain the symptoms of dementia.[22] Moreover, in one study with a lengthy follow-up,[23] after initially improving, the vast majority of cases eventually developed a progressive dementia.

It thus appears that the treatment of the pseudodementias is effective in the short term but less effective for the longer term.

ANXIETY

Generalized anxiety, phobic anxiety, and panic attacks are as effectively treated in the elderly as in younger patients. The preferred approach involves non-pharmacological interventions such as supportive psycho-therapy and involvement in supervised social group activities. If this does not dispel the symptoms then medications will be required, or behaviour therapy for phobic anxiety. Panic disorders respond to tricyclic antidepressants and monoamine oxidase inhibitors. Where depression is a significant additional feature the tricyclic antidepressants are the preferred treatment.[24]

The benzodiazepines are fairly safe and helpful in generalized anxiety at the minimum dosage level required for therapeutic effect;[25] as with the other tranquilizers they are only an interim solution until the non-pharmacological interventions take effect. If given for sustained periods, accumulation and toxicity may occur with uncoordination, confusion, and alteration of sleep patterns.

SCHIZOPHRENIA AND RELATED CONDITIONS

Early onset schizophrenics who age

As schizophrenic patients grow older under good clinical care, there is a tendency for their symptoms to become less intense and less frequent.[26] In about 66 per cent of these cases, the vivid psychotic features abate either completely or considerably, although the aging patients may become more withdrawn and blunted in affect. About one third recover virtually completely with respect to both symptoms and social adjustment. These aged schizophrenics often no longer require medication to control their symptoms, or can get by with lowered dosage. Thus it seems that advancing age increases the chances of a favourable outcome for early onset schizophrenics.[27] There is no evidence of any increased risk of dementia.

Neuroleptics with high potency such as fluphenazine or haloperidol are effective in the aging schizophrenic and if given cautiously have fewer dangerous side-effects (drop in blood-pressure on standing, urinary retention, and confusion) than the less potent drugs such as thioridazine or chlorpromazine.[28] Nevertheless, the effectiveness of these interventions is limited by the risk of neurological side-effects (parkinsonism or tardive dyskinesia) and the less serious drug-induced discomforts which undermine the co-operation of the patient.

Late onset schizophrenics

Paraphrenia, a syndrome resembling schizophrenia and probably related to it, can begin in old age. The persecutory symptoms that characterize this condition can be very troublesome to the patient and others, and the need for intervention is usually pressing. Paraphrenia does not show the deterioration of thinking, emotional range, and intiative that is seen with some early onset cases. On the other hand, the chances of spontaneous recovery without therapeutic intervention are slight. Indeed, the most powerful predictors of improvement in one series[2] centred around the context of treatment—compliance with treatment, maintaining medications over time, and a good relationship with the treating physician. More effective results are also obtained where the patient has been reasonably well socialized and adjusted throughout life, is older at the onset of the illness, and evinces symptoms which come on relatively suddenly and have a depressive admixture.[29]

Prior to the widespread use of neuroleptic medication virtually all paraphrenics remained disturbed or soon relapsed.[1] In contrast, the use of phenothiazines for acute episodes and its maintenance thereafter can lead to complete recovery in as many as 50 per cent of cases; there is sufficient improvement, despite continuing symptoms, to allow return to the community in most of the remaining patients.[2] About one-third of cases can be kept free of relapses.

Haloperidol can be given by injection for rapid action where urgently required but phenothiazines orally are the standard medication. The minimum effective dose for maintenance is found by adjusting medications downwards and observing symptom levels. Injecting intramuscular depots of a long-lasting neuroleptic (e.g. fluphenazine enanthate) is sometimes more effective than an oral phenothiazine, possibly because it ensures that the medication is actually taken.[27]

Here, as in other interventions for mental health conditions of the elderly, more space is devoted to describing the effectiveness of pharmacological agents than that of psychosocial interventions. This reflects the relative amount of available information on systematic evaluation of effectiveness and is not intended to distract from the great importance of psychosocial interventions in clinical practice. In addition to compliance with medication regimens, the paraphrenic patient can benefit from social activities and retraining in interpersonal skills, from attention to hearing impairments[30] which may be adding to a sense of isolation, or from relocation to a sheltered environment.

CONCLUSION

There is no reason to be complacent about the effectiveness of interventions for mental health of the elderly. Intensive research is urgently needed to document the details and context of effectiveness, to improve the outcomes currently enjoyed, to increase the safety and reduce the side-effects of treatments, and to carry forward the momentum of treatments for the refractory mental conditions. Nevertheless, for the majority of mental health conditions of the elderly, the goals of intervention should be as high as for younger patients.

References

1. Kay, D. W. K. (1963). Late paraphrenia and its bearing on the aetiology of schizophrenia. *Acta Psychiatrica Scandinavica*, **39**, 159–69.
2. Post, F. (1984). Schizophrenic and paranoid psychoses. In *Handbook of studies on psychiatry and old age* (ed. Kay, D. W. K. and G. D. Burrows), pp. 291–302. Elsevier Science Publishers BV, New York.
3. Ouslander, J. G. (1982). Physical illness and depression in the elderly. *Journal of the American Geriatrics Society*, **30**, 593–9.
4. Georgotas, A., McCue, R. E., Hapworth, W. *et al.* (1986). Comparative efficacy and safety of MAOI's versus TCA's in treating depression in the elderly. *Biological Psychiatry*, **21**, 1155–66.
5. Godber, C., Rosenvinge, H., Wilkinson, D., and Smithies, J. (1987). Depression in old age: prognosis after ECT. *International Journal of Geriatric Psychiatry*, **2**, 19–24.
6. Roth, M. (1955). The natural history of mental disorder in old age. *Journal of Mental Science*, **101**, 281.
7. Meyers, B. S., Greenberg, R., and Mei-Tai, V. (1985). Delusional depression in the elderly. In *Treatment of affective disorders in the elderly* (ed. Schamoian, C. A.), pp. 17–28. American Psychiatric Press, Inc., Washington, DC.
8. Murphy, E. (1983). The prognosis of depression in old age. *British Journal of Psychiatry* **142**, 111–9.
9. Post, F. (1984). Affective psychoses. In *Handbook of studies on psychiatry and old age* (ed. Kay, D. W. K. and G. D. Burrows), pp. 227–8 Elsevier Science Publishers BV, New York.
10. Prien, R. F., Kupfer, D. J., Mansky, P. A. *et al.* (1984). Drug therapy in the prevention of recurrences in unipolar and bipolar affective disordeus. *Archives of General Psychiatry* **41**, 1096–104.
11. Neshkes, R. E. and Jarvik, L. F. (1986). Depression in the elderly: Current management concepts. *Geriatrics*, **41**, 51–8.
12. Borson, S. and Raskind, R. (1986). Antidepressant-resistant depression in the elderly. *Journal of the American Geriatrics Society*, **34**, 245–7.
13. Cummings, J. L. (1983). Treatable dementias. *Advances in Neurology*, **38**, 165–83.
14. Thal, L. J., Fuld, P. A., Masur, D. M., and Sharpless, N. S. (1983). Oral physostigmine and lecithin improve memory in Alzheimer's disease. *Annals of Neurology*, **13**, 491–6.
15. Davies, P. (1981). Theoretical treatment possibilities for dementia of the alzheimer's type: the cholinergic hypothesis. In *Strategies further development of an effective treatment for senile dementia* (ed. Crook, T. and S. Gershon), Mark Powley Associates, New Canaan, CT.
16. Crook, T. (1985). Geriatric Psychopathology; An overview of the ailments

and current therapies. *Drug Development Research*, **5**, 5–23.

17. Bartus, R. T., Dean, R. L., Beer, B., and Lippa, A. S. (1982). The cholinergic hypothesis of geriatric memory dysfunction. *Science*, **217**, 408–17.

18. Smith, R. C., Uroalis, G., Johnson, R., and Morgan, R. (1984). Comparison of therapeutic response to long-term treatment with lecithin versus piracetam plus lecithin in patients with Alzheimer's disease. *Psychopharmacological Bulletin*, **20**, 542–5.

19. Summers, W. K., Viesselman, J. O., Marsh, G. M., and Candelora, K. (1981). Use of THA in the treatment of Alzheimer-like dementia; pilot study in twelve patients. *Biological Psychiatry*, **16**, 145–53.

20. Wettstein, A. and Spiegel, R. (1984). Clinical trials with the cholinergic drug RS86 in Alzheimer's disease (AD) and senile dementia of the Alzheimer type (SDAT) *Psychopharmacology*, **84**, 572–3.

21. Mahendıa, B. (1985). Depression and dementia: The multi-faceted relationship. *Psychological Medicine*, **15**, 227–36.

22. Rabins, P. V. (1984). The reversible dementias. In *Recent advances in psychogeriatrics* (ed. Arie, T.), pp. 99–102. Churchill Livingstone, London.

23. Kral, V. (1983). The relationship between senile dementia (Alzheimer type) and depression. *Canadian Journal of Psychiatry*, **28**, 304–6.

24. Crook, T. (1982). Diagnosis and treatment of mixed anxiety-depression in the elderly. *Journal of Clinical Psychiatry*, **43**, 35–43.

25. Allen, R. (1986). Tranquilizers and sedative/hypnotics: Appropriate use in the elderly. *Geriatrics*, **41**, 75–88.

26. Ciompi, L. (1985). Aging and schizophrenic psychosis. *Acta Psychiatrica Scandinavica*, Suppl. **319**, 93–105.

27. Raskind, M. A. and Risse, S. C. (1986). Antipsychotic drugs and the elderly. *Journal of Clinical Psychiatry*, **47** (5) Suppl, 17–22.

28. Branchey, M. H., Lee, J. H., Amin, R. and Simpson, G. M. (1978). High- and low-potency neuroleptics in elderly psychiatric patients. *Journal of American Medical Association*, **239**, 1860–2.

29. Retterstol, N. (1966). *Paranoid and paranoiac psychoses*. Charles C. Thomas, Springfield, Illinois.

30. Eastwood, R., Corbin, S., and Reed, M. (1981). Hearing impairment and paraphrenia. *Journal of Otolaryngology*, **10**, 306.

31. Lauter; H. (1985). What do we know about Alzheimer's today? *Danish Medical Bulletin*, **32**, 1–21.

17

The efficacy of continence treatment

J. G. OUSLANDER

INTRODUCTION

Urinary incontinence, defined as the involuntary loss of urine, is a prevalent, disruptive, and costly health problem among elderly people. As many as one-third of community-dwelling elderly people admit to some degree of incontinence. Prevalence rates and the frequency of incontinence episodes are greater among elderly patients in long-term care institutions.[1-5]

Despite the high prevalence of incontinence, its adverse effects on the well-being of those affected,[6-8] its potential role in the decision to enter a long-term care institution,[9] and its cost,[10-11] many elderly incontinent people do not undergo a diagnostic evaluation for this condition.[4, 12-15] This may be related to the embarrassing nature of incontinence and the belief that it is an inevitable and untreatable consequence of growing older; agism and lack of understanding of the diagnosis and treatment of incontinence on the part of health professionals may also contribute. Since there is a growing evidence that a variety of therapeutic interventions may be effective in curing or substantially ameliorating incontinence even among the elderly, it is important to change existing attitudes towards this condition.

TYPES AND CAUSES OF GERIATRIC URINARY INCONTINENCE

The maintenance of continence requires: (1) adequate function of the lower urinary tract to store and empty urine, (2) adequate cognitive function to recognize the need to urinate and find the appropriate place, (3) adequate physical mobility and dexterity to get to a toilet or toilet substitute and to manage clothing, (4) motivation to be continent, and (5) absence of environmental or iatrogenic barriers to continence. Among the elderly, especially those in acute care and long-term care institutions, one or more of the above factors often plays an important role in the pathogenesis of incontinence. These factors must be identified and addressed in order for treatment to be successful.

Incontinence generally presents in two basic forms: acute incontinence, which is often reversible with appropriate management of an underlying condition, and persistent or established incontinence. The causes of acute, reversible forms of incontinence can be remembered by the acronym 'DRIP': *d*elirium, *r*estricted mobility, *i*nfection or *i*nflammation of the lower urinary tract and faecal *i*mpaction, and *p*olyuria and *p*harmaceuticals.[16–17] There are four basic types of persistent urinary incontinence commonly encountered in the elderly. Table 17.1 includes a description of these types and examples of underlying causes for each.

Table 17.1 Basic types and causes of persistent geriatric urinary incontinence

Type	Definition	Common causes
Stress	Involuntary loss of urine (usually small amounts) with increases in intra-abdminal pressure (e.g. cough, laugh, exercise)	Weakness and laxity of pelvic floor musculature Bladder outlet or urethral sphincter weakness
Urge	Leakage of urine (usually larger volumes) because of inability to delay voiding after sensation of bladder fullness is perceived	Unstable bladder, isolated or associated with the following: Local genitourinary condition such as cystitis, urethritis, tumours, stones, diverticula, and mild outflow obstruction Central nervous system disorders such as stroke, dementia, parkinsonism, spinal cord injury
Overflow	Leakage of urine (usually small amounts) resulting from mechanical forces on an overdistended bladder	Anatomic obstruction by prostate, stricture, cystocoele Acontractile bladder due to diabetes, spinal cord injury
Functional	Urinary leakage associated with inability (because of impairment of cognitive or physical functioning), psychological unwillingness, or environmental barriers to use a toilet or toilet substitute	Severe dementia and other neurological disorders Psychological conditions such as depression, regression, anger, hostility Inaccessible toilets or toilet substitutes Unavailable caregivers

Elderly incontinent patients often have more than one of these types simultaneously. Table 17.1 therefore represents a clinical rather than a physiological or urodynamic classification of incontinence; other classifications based on neurourological abnormalities are also available.[17-20]

APPROACHES TO DIAGNOSIS

A history, focused physical examination, postvoid residual determination, urinalysis, and urine culture will identify the conditions which can cause or contribute to acute and reversible forms of incontinence (Table 17.2). Bladder records or incontinence charts can be helpful adjuncts to the history provided by patients or caregivers in identifying the frequency, amount, and factors associated with episodes of incontinence.[16,21,22] The physical examination should focus on mental status and mobility as they relate to toileting skills, lumbosacral innervation, abdominal and rectal examinations, and, in women, vaginal examination. Detailed descriptions of the clinical assessment of incontinent elderly patients are available.[16,17,23]

A postvoiding residual determination, performed by sterile 'in-and-out' catheterization within 5–10 minutes of the patient's voiding, is a helpful diagnostic procedure for two reasons: it accurately determines the degree of bladder emptying, and it provides an uncontaminated specimen of bladder urine for analysis and culture. The risk of initiating bacteriuria from a single sterile 'in-and-out' catheterization is probably less than 5

Table 17.2 Basic components of the diagnostic evaluation of urinary incontinence

---

All patients
History
Physical examination
Postvoid residual determination
Urinalysis and culture

Selected patients
Urological or gynaecological evaluation:
  cystourethroscopy
  voiding cystourethrography (VCUG)

Urodynamic tests:
  cystometrogram (CMG)
  urine flowmetry
  pressure flow study
  urethral pressure profilometry (UPP)
  sphincter electromyography (EMG)

---

per cent.[24, 25] Ultrasound offers a less invasive method of determining residual urine volume,[26-8] but small portable ultrasound devices that would be useful in clinic and nursing home settings cost $2000-3500, and in some instances are difficult to interpret. With improved technology these devices might play a helpful role in following the results of treatment for incontinence with drugs that can potentially precipitate urinary retention in (see section on pharmacological treatment).

Some incontinent patients benefit from further diagnostic procedures (Table 17.2). The appropriate roles of cystourethroscopy, radiographic, and other urodynamic tests are controversial. On the one hand, these tests can help to define treatable anatomical and physiological abnormalities which are associated with incontinence—even among elderly outpatients and very old institutionalized patients.[29-34] Many investigators suggest, however, that they should play a limited role in the routine evaluation of incontinence in the elderly.[8, 17, 23, 29, 35-40] Numerous factors contribute to the controversy including the following: (1) the tests are relatively expensive—in the US the charges for a full urodynamic evaluation (not including cystoscopy) could be over $600;[10] (2) the tests can be uncomfortable and may cause bacteriuria in a substantial proportion of patients in whom antibiotics are not used prophylactically;[41] (3) the tests are generally available only in selected medical centres and urologists' or gynaecologists' offices; they therefore require a separate visit to a location with the equipment and personnel trained in its use and the interpretation of the results; (4) until recently there has been little standardization of the testing methods,[42] and even less is known about the test–retest reliability of the results;[43-6] (5) there is a substantial prevalence of what are generally considered 'abnormal' urodynamic tests results in elderly without incontinence, thus complicating the interpretation of these findings in elderly incontinent patients;[29, 47-53] (6) urodynamic findings often do not correlate well with either presenting symptoms or changes in symptoms with treatment;[29, 54-7] and, probably most important,[7] it is not clear that documention of urodynamic abnormalities is an essential prerequisite for making appropriate decisions about initial treatment plans.[35-40]

Several algorithms have been described which attempt to make a diagnosis and treatment plan for the majority of patients who have persistent forms of urinary incontinence without the need for formal urodynamic testing, and to identify patients who would benefit from further evaluation.[23, 29, 35, 38, 39] These diagnostic strategies have been tested prospectively in only small selected samples of incontinent elderly people, mostly women.[35, 35, 38-40] In both clinic and institutional settings, appropriate treatment plans could be developed in the majority of patients without formal urodynamic testing. Further studies are needed to determine the generalizability of these results and the sensitivity of the algorithms for identifying conditions which require more invasive testing and surgical treatment. Until further studies can define more precisely the optimal strategies for diagnostic evaluation, a conservative approach such as that outlined in Table 17.3 will enable primary health care professionals to develop an appropriate initial treatment plan for many elderly incontinent patients, and to identify the vast majority of those who will benefit from further evaluation.

Table 17.3 A conservative approach to the initial evaluation of incontinent elderly patients

---

1. Perform history, focused physical examination, postvoid residual determination, urinalysis, and urine culture.
2. Identify and treat potentially reversible causes and contributing factors.
3. Refer patients for further urological, gynaecological, and/or urodynamic evaluation if:
   (a) there are prominent complaints of voiding dysfunction, such as severe urinary hesitancy, interrupted stream, impaired sensation of bladder filling or emptying;
   (b) symptoms of stress incontinence or constant leakage occur in man who has previous transurethral surgery;
   (c) anatomical abnormalities, such as marked pelvic prolapse (uterine or bladder), or pelvic or prostatic masses are present;
   (d) there is difficulty passing a 12 or 14 French catheter;
   (e) the postvoid residual is greater than 100 ml;
   (f) haematuria is present (in the absence of infection).
4. In *women*:
   (a) base initial behavioural and/or pharmacological therapeutic approaches on the patient's predominant symptom when possible (many elderly women have mixed symptoms which may require a combination of treatment approaches);
   (b) refer for further evaluation if bothersome symptoms persist despite an adequate therapeutic trial.
5. In *men* with urge incontinence and other irritative voiding symptoms (i.e. frequency, nocturia, urgency) the decision to refer for urologic evaluation must be individualized:
   (a) since symptoms, physical signs and residual urine volume are not predictive of urodynamic obstruction, and most men improve symptomatically after prostatectomy, referring all patients who have bothersome enough symptoms and who are candidates for consideration for surgery is a reasonable approach;
   (b) non-surgical approaches (behavioural and pharmacological) may be effective; bladder relaxant drugs must be used carefully because of the risk of precipitating urinary retention.

TREATMENT

Acute, reversible forms of incontinence

Management of acute forms of incontinence involves identifying and treating the potentially reversible contributing factor(s). Treatment and resolution of acute illness, with improvements in mental function and mobility, will generally lead to resolution of incontinence associated with delirium and restricted mobility. Urinary frequency and urge incontinence at night may be caused or worsened by several reversible conditions which lead to increased urine production at night, such as intake of coffee, tea, or alcohol in the evening hours, and mobilization of lower extremity oedema from venous insufficiency or congestive heart failure. Modifying fluid intake patterns and treating the oedema during the day (when the patient may have better access to the toilet) can reduce nocturnal incontinence, and also eliminate the risk of falls on the way to the bathroom in the middle of the night.

Inflammation related to atrophic vaginitis and urethritis can cause urinary frequency, urgency, dysuria, and urge incontinence, and can be treated with oestrogen. Although the optimal route of administration, dosage, and duration of oestrogen therapy for these conditions are not known, a common approach would be to prescribe a 4–8-week course of vaginal cream, or 0.625 mg daily of oral conjugated oestrogen for women who are unwilling or unable to use the cream. For patients whose symptoms improve and subsequently relapse, repeat courses of therapy could be instituted. Acute bacterial cystitis can precipitate urge incontinence which will resolve with antimicrobial therapy. Far more common, however, is the elderly incontinent patient with otherwise 'asymptomatic bacteriuria'. This condition is found in 10–20 per cent of community-dwelling elderly people and 30–50 per cent of elderly nursing home patients, many of whom are also incontinent. The bacteriuria frequently resolves spontaneously without treatment and may recur; thus, its role in the pathogenesis of incontinence and other symptoms, as well as its association with overall morbidity and mortality, is controversial.[58–64] Most studies suggest that incontinence does not generally resolve when otherwise asymptomatic bacteriuria is treated, although symptoms may improve in some patients.[65–7] Thus, a reasonable approach remains to attempt to eradicate bacteriuria if present on the initial evaluation of an incontinent elderly patient; if incontinence persists, which it often will, further evaluation and treatment should be undertaken.

A variety of pharmacological agents can affect continence through their effects on mental status and mobility (e.g. psychotropic drugs), on the volume of urine flow (diuretics), on the contractility of the bladder (anticholinergics, narcotics), and on tone in the bladder outlet and urethra (alpha adrenergic agonists and blockers). Eliminating these types of drugs whenever possible or altering the drug regimen can also play an important role in improving or resolving incontinence.

Persistent incontinence

Numerous treatment modalities are available for the management of persistent forms of incontinence. Table 17.4 lists the primary treatment

Table 17.4 Treatment modalities used for persistent forms of urinary incontinence

Behaviourally oriented therapies (see Table 6):
Patient-dependent procedures
   biofeedback
   pelvic floor (Kegel) exercises
   bladder retraining (habit retraining, bladder drill)
   behavioural therapy
Caregiver-dependent procedures
   habit training
   prompted voiding
   scheduled toileting

Pharmacological:
Drugs which inhibit bladder contraction
   anticholinergics
   smooth muscle relaxants
   calcium antagonists
   other
Drugs which increase outlet resistance
   alpha adrenergic agonists
   oestrogen
Drugs which facilitate bladder emptying
   cholinergics
   alpha adrenergic antagonists

Surgical:
Bladder neck suspension procedures
Removal of obstructing or pathological lesions

Devices:
Catheters
   continuous indwelling
   intermittent catheterization
   external
Electrical stimulation (intravaginal, anal)
Artificial urinary sphincter

modalities used in the elderly, based on the basic types of persistent incontinence (see Table 17.1 and 17.6). Before reviewing existing evidence on the effectiveness of specific treatments, those organizations and programmes which have developed an interest in incontinence and non-specific interventions helpful in managing incontinent people will be briefly discussed.

Supportive organizations, programmes, and non-specific interventions

Organizations.   Both lay and professional organizations in the US and Europe have begun to address the problem of incontinence in the elderly. In the US two lay organizations—Help for Incontinent People ('HIP') and the Simon Foundation—publish regular newsletters for incontinent people. The latter has produced a book and videotape for such people.[8] Several private foundations have supported research and education on incontinence in the elderly. One foundation has developed educational materials on incontinence for licensed nurses and nurses' aides working in long-term care and home health settings.[68] The National Institute on Aging has recently funded several investigations on the epidemiology, pathophysiology, diagnostic evaluation, and treatment of incontinent elderly Americans. In Great Britain, continence advisors serve as public health nurses dedicated to managing incontinent patients, providing direct care, educating, and participating in research.[69] The Association of Continence Advisors publishes a newsletter and engages in many educational and research activities relating to the elderly. The International Continence Society is a relatively new and growing multidisciplinary scientific organization whose annual meeting provides an opportunity for researchers on incontinence to share their findings. An increasing number of abstract submissions relate to geriatric incontinence.[70]

Incontinence (or continence) clinics.   Specialized clinics for the evaluation and treatment of incontinence have existed in Great Britain for several years. These are frequently run by geriatricians and continence nurse advisors, as well as urologists and gynaecologists. An increasing number of similar clinics are being established in the US.[71] An interdisciplinary approach involving nurses, geriatricians, urologists, gynaecologists, and behavioural psychologists can offer a unique and broad array of assessment and treatment strategies. Although the functioning and cost-effectiveness of such programmes have not been evaluated, they should certainly help encourage health professionals to pay more attention to the problem of incontinence and provide effective treatment for many elderly incontinent people.

Environmental manipulations.   Numerous factors in the design of home and institutional bathroom facilities for the elderly can foster the maintenance of continence. Facilities which are appropriately located, accessible, and safe for physically impaired elderly are relatively easy to plan. The optimal design and use of toilet substitutes, such as urinals, bedpans, and bedside commodes, will enhance the management of incontinence among the dependent elderly. A detailed review of such environmental support techniques is availalbe elsewhere.[72]

Undergarments and padding. A variety of specially designed undergarments and pads have been developed and are being actively marketed in the US and Europe. Many are launderable and re-usable, others are completely disposable, and some are launderable with disposable inserts. Some are available without prescription in pharmacies in the US, and some are advertised on television. Highly absorbent polymers make these products very effective in maintaining dryness. Evaluation studies, usually sponsored by the manufacturers, suggest that the products are comfortable and save labour and laundry costs in long-term care institutions.[73,74] While these products are probably safe and helpful in the management of many elderly incontinent people, they should generally not be used as a first-line solution to the problem of incontinence. There should be an assessment which excludes serious underlying conditions and types of incontinence which might be treated effectively with more specific modalities before garments and pads are used as primary treatment. If used inappropriately, these products could foster dependence and diminish the incentive to become continent.[68, 69, 73] Except in the most severely impaired or acutely ill elderly incontinent people, garments and pads are probably best used as adjuncts to other forms of treatment in optimizing comfort. More specific treatment modalities may cure the incontinence, or improve it so that extra garments and pads are not necessary for comfort and hygiene in many of the more functional elderly incontinent people.

Specific interventions

Behavioural therapies. A heterogeneous group of techniques have been classified under the general heading of 'behavioural'. The taxonomy and effectiveness of these types of therapies have recently been reviewed in detail.[75, 76] Table 17.5 presents a classification of several of these techniques based on their primary focus either on the incontinent individual (therefore requiring adequate cognitive and physical functioning and motivation) or on caregivers such as nursing home staff or family.

Biofeedback has been used successfully to treat both stress and urge incontinence among elderly outpatients; it reduces the frequency of episodes of incontinence by 80–90 per cent.[77, 78] It may be more effective than pelvic floor exercises alone for stress incontinence in many younger women;[79] similar studies are now being carried out among elderly women

Table 17.5 Examples of behaviourally oriented procedures for the management of geriatric urinary incontinence[a]

Procedure	Description	Use(s)	Comments
I. Patient-dependent:			
Pelvic floor (Kegel) exercises	Repetitive contractions of pelvic floor muscles	Stress incontinence	Requires adequate cognitive and physical function and motivation May be done in conjunction with biofeedback
Biofeedback	Use of bladder, rectal, and/or vaginal pressure or electrical recordings in teaching patients to contract pelvic floor muscles and relax bladder	Stress and urge incontinence	Requires equipment and trained personnel Relatively invasive Requires adequate cognitive and physical function and motivation
Bladder retraining	Progressive lengthening or shortening of intervoiding interval, with adjunctive techniques— intermittent catheterization used in patients recovering from overdistention injuries with persistent urinary retention	Acute incontinence e.g. post-indwelling catheterization, stroke, or overdistention of bladder	Goal is to restore normal pattern of voiding and continence Requires adequate cognitive and physical function and motivation

Table 17.5 (*cont.*)

Procedure	Description	Use(s)	Comments
II. Caregiver-dependent:			
Habit training	Variable toileting schedule with positive reinforcement and adjunctive techniques[b]	Urge and functional incontinence	Goal is to prevent wetting episodes Can be used in patients with impaired cognitive and physical function Requires staff/caregiver availability and motivation
Scheduled toileting	Fixed toileting schedule with prompted voiding; some adjunctive techniques may also be used	Urge and functional incontinence	Goal is to prevent wetting episodes Can be used in patients with impaired cognitive and physical function Requires staff/caregiver availability and motivation

[a] The taxonomy of these and other similar procedures is discussed further in the text.
[b] Examples includes techniques to trigger voiding (running water, stroking thigh, suprapubic tapping), completely empty bladder (bending forward, suprapubic pressure), and alterations of fluid and/or diuretic intake patterns.

in the US but the results are not yet available. One study reported that the educational component of biofeedback may be just as effective as education with biofeedback for urge and mixed stress/urge incontinence among elderly women;[78] in it there was a mean reduction of incontinence episodes of close to 85 per cent. The results of the studies carried out in elderly patients are comparable to those in younger populations, which have generally reported short-term success (cure or improvement) rates of 70–90 per cent.[75–6, 80] The data for the elderly are promising, because behavioural therapies do not involve the use of drugs or surgery.

Much has been written about 'bladder training' and related techniques for functionally disabled elderly institutionalized incontinent patients, but few controlled studies of these interventions have been reported.[5, 75, 76] Two small studies, neither of them controlled, reported that fixed toileting schedules cured or improved incontinence in 50 and 85 per cent respectively.[81, 82] One controlled study of a prompted voiding programme with behavioural reinforcement techniques reduced the frequency of incontinence by 49 per cent, with no improvement seen in controls.[83] Two controlled studies in which forms of scheduled toileting were combined with bladder relaxant drugs in functionally disabled elderly people in institutional settings showed no substantial clinical improvement in the frequency of incontinence.[37, 67] No study of behavioural interventions for functionally disabled incontinent people living at home has been reported. The National Institute on Aging is currently supporting several large studies of behaviourally oriented interventions for incontinence in nursing home patients. The results of these will be important in determining whether these interventions are practical in nursing home settings, whether they are effective, which types of patients are most likely to benefit, and whether reductions in the frequency of incontinence lead to concomitant reductions in morbidity and the costs of care.

Pharmacological therapy. Drug treatment is primarily used for urge and stress incontinence (Table 17.6). Well-designed studies of drug treatment

Table 17.6 Primary treatments for different types of persistent geriatric urinary incontinence

Type of incontinence	Primary treatments
Stress	Behavioural e.g. pelvic floor exercises biofeedback (see Table 17.5) Pharmacological e.g. alpha adrenergic agonists, oestrogen Surgical e.g. bladder neck suspension
Urge	Behavioural e.g. bladder retraining (see Table 17.5) Pharmacological e.g. bladder relaxant drugs Surgical e.g. removal of obstructing or irritating lesions
Overflow	Surgical e.g. removal of obstruction lesions Catheterization e.g. intermittent chronic indwelling
Functional	Behavioural e.g. habit training, scheduled toileting (See Table 17.5) External collection devices Undergarments or pads

for incontinence are difficult to carry out. Thus, many studies in the literature have methodological limitations including: imprecise definitions of subjects and their symptoms, lack of placebo control groups, a focus on changes in urodynamic measurements rather than on the frequency of incontinence and associated symptoms, and the explicit or inadvertent addition of behavioural interventions which make the effects of the drugs alone impossible to evaluate.[73, 84, 85]

Pharmacological management of urge incontinence generally involves anticholinergic agents such as propantheline, dicyclomine, flavoxate, oxybutinin, imipramine, and terodiline. Several of these agents have other pharmacological actions which include direct smooth muscle relaxation (oxybutinin, flavoxate), alpha adrenergic agonism (imipramine), and calcium channel blocking (terodiline; not available in the US). The anticholinergic side-effects of these drugs can be troublesome; they include dryness of the mouth, blurred vision, and constipation. Such drugs can also precipitate urinary retention and must be used especially carefully in men who may have bladder outflow obstruction due to an enlarged prostate. In several studies which have involved at least some elderly subjects, this class of drugs has led to cure or substantial amelioration of the incontinence in from 40 to 100 per cent of cases.[73, 84, 85] However, many of the studies were not placebo controlled, and included some type of concomitant behavioural intervention (e.g. scheduled toileting). Emepromium, an anticholinergic drug which has been the subject of several studies in the United Kingdom, has generally been shown to be no more effective than placebo. A few recent studies have indicated that drug treatment of urge incontinence among elderly patients with functional disabilities may not be very effective, even when combined with a toileting programme.[37, 67, 86, 87]

Pharmacological treatment for stress incontinence in women involves the use of an alpha adrenergic agonist to increase sphincter resistance, together with oestrogen—several of whose effects can, in theory, increase resistance in the bladder outlet and urethra. However, published placebo-controlled studies of these agents, alone or in combination, have involved only very small numbers of elderly women, and most have not reported high cure rates.[73, 85] Conversely, uncontrolled studies of oestrogen have reported symptomatic improvement in many patients.[85] Although hard data are lacking, these drugs offer a reasonable approach for women with stress incontinence who do not respond to behavioural interventions alone (or who are unable or unwilling to co-operate with them) before surgery is considered. Alpha adrenergic agonists must be used carefully in patients with hypertension and cardiovascular disease, and prolonged administration of oestrogen should be accompanied by a progestogen[88] in women who have not had a hysterectomy. Many elderly women have a combination of stress and urge incontinence.[3, 35, 52, 57] Imipramine, because it has both anticholinergic and alpha agonist properties, is in theory an appropriate choice for women with this mixed form of incontinence. However, this drug has a number of potential cardiovascular side-effects and must be used carefully in the elderly.

Other pharmacological approaches to incontinence include drugs which stimulate bladder contraction (e.g. the cholinergic agonist bethanechol) for patients with overflow incontinence, and alpha antagonists for patients with incontinence or other symptoms related to bladder outflow obstruction. The effectiveness of the former approach is controversial, and cholinergic agents are probably not useful in elderly patients with persistent overflow incontinence on either an obstructive or a neurogenic basis.[89, 90] Alpha adrenergic blockers such as phenoxybenzamine and prazosin have been used in patients with neurological lesions, as well as in men with prostate enlargement. In the latter, alpha-adrenergically-mediated contractions of the smooth muscle of the prostatic urethra and capsule may play a role in the pathogenesis of symptoms, and some studies indicate that drug therapy can be effective.[91] The same symptoms respond well to prostatic resection (see below). Thus, this type of pharmacological approach may be of benefit to elderly patients with bothersome symptoms in whom prostate surgery is either contraindicated or unwanted.

Surgery.   Bladder neck suspension for stress incontinence in women and prostatic resection for urge and overflow incontinence in men are the surgical procedures used most commonly in the management of incontinence in the elderly. Several different bladder suspension techniques are used, and there is no consensus among gynaecological and urological surgeons on which is most effective. Certain procedures may be indicated when specific types of anatomical abnormalities are present.[92] Newer techniques can be done quickly and thus minimize the anaesthetic time required.[93] There is some controversy over the effectiveness of surgery for stress incontinence when detrusor instability is present. This occurs in as many as one-third of older women.[34, 52, 57, 94, 95] Some studies suggest it adversely effects surgical outcome, while the largest series indicates that surgery is highly effective even when the instability is present.[94] Most reported surgical series, even those involving elderly women, report very high cure rates in the range of 80–90 per cent.[92–4, 96, 97] Thus, in properly selected elderly women with stress incontinence that remains very troublesome after attempts at behavioural and/or pharmacological management, surgery offers a highly effective alternative.

Transurethral resection of the prostate (TURP) is generally a safe and effective surgical procedure for elderly men with symptoms of prostatism

—which can include urge incontinence and postvoiding dribbling.[98–103] Half to two-thirds of men with irritative voiding symptoms associated with prostatic obstruction have detrusor instability; this generally resolves after TURP.[100] However, symptoms may persist in some men after surgery and they can be managed with bladder relaxant drugs. Despite the low morbidity and high effectiveness of TURP, there is controversy about the role and timing of surgery, and wide variation in the frequency with which this procedure is performed in mildly to moderately symptomatic men who are not in urinary retention.[98, 104, 105] Some studies suggest that symptoms may not be progressive and acute urinary retention may not occur in many men over several years of follow-up.[104–5] A large prospective randomized study of TURP versus medical follow-up for moderately symptomatic prostatism has recently been initiated in the US Veterans Administration Cooperative Studies Program.

Several other surgical procedures, including removal of lesions such as tumors and stones and bladder augmentation are also used to manage incontinence in patients with incontinence associated with specific types of pathology. These will not be reviewed in any detail in this report.

Devices. Catheters, electrical stimulators, and artificial sphincters are examples of devices used in the management of incontinence. Catheters are used in three ways: external, intermittent, and chronic indwelling. External condom-type catheters are frequently used to manage incontinence in functionally disabled elderly men.[5] Several styles are available which vary in their methods of application. Problems may be encountered when the catheters fall off frequently or twist and cause penile skin irritation.[106, 107] External catheter use is associated with the development of urinary tract infection (UTI), but no cause-and-effect relationship has been documented [107–9] These devices should not be used in men with urinary retention, or merely as a matter of convenience; they are, however, appropriate for the elderly man with severe functional disabilities whose incontinence cannot be adequately managed with behavioural or other more specific techniques.

Clean intermittent catheterization has become popular in the management of young patients with overflow incontinence secondary to spinal cord injuries and other neurological disorders because it is associated with less morbidity than chronic indwelling catheterization.[110] While one study indicates that this technique can be used effectively for incontinence associated with urinary retention in elderly women in an ambulatory clinic setting,[111] many elderly people are unable or unwilling to catheterize themselves and do not have a caregiver available to do it for them. Repeated catheterization may be difficult and uncomfortable for elderly men with prostatic enlargement. In nursing homes where infection control procedures may not be well developed, repeated catheterizations without the use of sterile catheters would pose a substantial risk of serious nosocomial infections, and using sterile catheters for each catheterization would be very expensive. Thus, the favourable experience with this technique in younger people is not readily applicable to the elderly.

Continuous indwelling catheterization is probably used more often than is necessary in the management of incontinence in nursing homes especially.[4, 5, 112–15] All patients with indwelling catheters for longer than 2–3 weeks develop significant bacteriuria, and there is a substantial incidence of symptomatic UTI among nursing home patients, especially males, managed with these devices.[116–18] Because of the potential morbidity from UTI and other complications, the use of continuous indwelling catheterization for incontinence in the elderly should be reserved for patients in whom: (1) accurate monitoring of urine output is necessary during an acute illness, (2) urinary retention is present which cannot be managed by other methods and is of sufficient degree to cause complications such as infections and kidney damage, (3) the healing of skin wounds is being impaired by the leaking urine, or (4) severe or terminal illness makes managing the incontinence by undergarments or pads distressing or uncomfortable. Sound catheter care guidelines and infection control policies in institutional settings,[5, 116, 117, 119, 120] and the involvement of visiting nurses in home settings, will help prevent complications. Antimicrobials given orally, instilled into the bladder or drainage system, or applied topically to the urethra have not been shown to be of value in reducing infectious complications.[116, 117, 120, 121]

Electrical stimulation has been used to treat both stress and urge incontinence in women. This technique involves placing an electrical stimulator in the vagina or rectum for variable periods of time. No controlled studies have been reported although several clinical series have been published by European authors.[73, 122–4] In the most recent and systemic study of 35 patients, 25 improved and another 8 were cured.[124] Patients with urge or mixed urge and stress incontinence did better than patients with pure or genuine stress incontinence. This and other similar studies involved very few elderly people. Thus, although this may be a promising technique, its acceptability and effectiveness in elderly patients is still to be determined.

Artificial sphincters can be used very effectively to treat refractory incontinence in carefully selected patients. Their use requires surgical implantation, and the patient must be able to manipulate the device or have someone available to do it for them. The device probably has a limited role in the management of incontinence in elderly people. Perhaps its most useful and effective application is in elderly men who have had sphincter damage related to previous transurethral surgery.[73]

References

1. Mohide, E. A. (1986). The prevalence and scope of urinary incontinence. *Clinics in Geriatric Medicine*, **2**, 639–55.
2. Harris, T. (1986). *Aging in the eighties: prevalence and impact of urinary problems in individuals age 65 years and over.* National Center for Health Statistics, Advance Data No. 121 Bethesda MD.
3. Diokno, A. C., Brock, B. M., Brown, M. B., and Herzog, A. R. (1986). Prevalence of urinary incontinence and other urological symptoms in the non-institutionalized elderly. *Journal of Urology*, **136**, 1022–5.
4. Ouslander, J. G., Kane, R. L., and Abrass, I. B. (1982). Urinary incontinence in elderly nursing home patients. *Journal American Medical Association*, **248**, 1194–8.
5. Ouslander, J. G. and Fowler, E. (1985). Incontinence in VA Nursing Home Care Units. *Journal of the American Geriatrics Society*, **33**, 33–40.
6. Ory, M. G., Wyman, J. F., and Yu, L. (1986). Psychosocial factors in urinary incontinence. *Clinics in Geriatric Medicine*, **2**, 657–72.
7. Noelker, L. S. (1987). Incontinence in aged cared for by family. *Gerontologist*, **27**, 194–200.
8. Gartley, C. B. (ed.) (1985). *Managing incontinence: a guide to living with loss of bladder control.* Jameson Books, Ottawa, Illinois.
9. Smallegan, M. (1985). There was nothing else to do: needs for care before nursing home admission. *Gerontologist*, **25**, 364–9.
10. Ouslander, J. G. and Kane, R. L. (1984). The costs of urinary incontinence in nursing homes. *Medical Care*, **22**, 69–79.
11. Hu, T-W. (1986). The economic impact of urinary incontinence. *Clinics in Geriatric Medicine*, **2**, 673–87.
12. Starer, P. and Libow, L. S. (1985). Obscuring urinary incontinence: diapering the elderly. *Journal American Geriatrics Society*, **12**, 842–46.
13. Mitteness, L. S. (1987). The management of urinary incontinence by community-living elderly. *Gerontologist*, **27**, 185–93.
14. Thomas, T. M. Plymat, F. R. Blannin, J. *et al.* (1980). Prevalence of urinary incontinence. *British Medical Journal*, **281**, 1243–5.
15. Everett, D., Learman, L., and Avorn, J. (1985). Incontinence: related claims in an elderly population. *Gerontologist*, **25** (Special Issue), 246–7.
16. Kane, R. L., Ouslander, J. G., and Abrass, I. B. (1989). *Essentials of clinical geriatrics*, McGraw Hill, New York.
17. Resnick, N. M. and Yalla, S. V. (1985). Management of urinary incontinence in the elderly. *New England Journal of Medicine*, **313**, 800–5.
18. Williams, M. E. and Pannill, P. C. (1982). Urinary incontinence in the elderly. *Annals of Internal Medicine*, **97**, 895–907.
19. Blaivas, J. G. (1981). The Neurophysiology of micturition: a clinical study of 550 patients. *Journal of Urology*, **127**, 958–63.
20. Wein, A. J. (1981). Classification of neurogenic voiding dysfunction. *Journal of Urology.* **125**, 605–9.
21. Ouslander, J. G., Uman, G. C., and Urman, H. N. (1986). Development and testing of an incontinence monitoring record. *Journal of the American Geriatrics Society*, **34**, 83–90.
22. Autry, D., Luazon, F., and Holliday, P. (1984). The voiding record, an aid

in decreasing incontinence. *Geriatric Nursing*, January/February, 22–5.

23. Ouslander, J. G. (1986). Diagnostic evaluation of geriatric urinary incontinence. *Clinics in Geriatric Medicine*, **2**, 715–30.

24. Walter, S. and Vejlsgaard, R. (1978). Diagnostic catheterization and bacteriuria in the female with urinary incontinence. *British Journal of Urology*, **50**, 106–8.

25. Kunin, C. M. (1987). *Detection, prevention and management of urinary tract infections*, Lee and Febeiger, Philadelphia.

26. Widder, B., Kornhuber, H. H., and Rewner, A. (1983). Residual urine measurement with a small ultrasound apparatus in outpatients. *Deutsche Medizinische Wochenschrift*, **108**, 1552–5.

27. Ravichandran, G. and Fellows, G. J. (1983). The accuracy of a hand-held real time ultrasound scanner for estimating bladder volume. *British Journal of Urology*, **55**, 25–7.

28. Beacock, C. J. M., Roberts, E. E., Rees, R. W. M., and Buck, A. C. Ultrasound assessment of residual urine—a quantitative method. *British Journal of Urology*, **57**, 410–13.

29. Abrams, P., Feneley, R., and Torrens, M. (1983). *Urodynamics*, Springer-Verlag, New York.

30. Blaivas, J. G., Awad, S. A., Bissada, N. *et al.* (1982). Urodynamic procedures: recommendations of the urodynamic society I. Procedures that should be available for routine urologic practice. *Neurology and Urodynamics*, **1**, 51.

31. Blaivas, J. G. (1983). Urodynamic testing. In *Female urology*, (ed. Raz, S.) pp. 79–103. Saunders, Philadelphia.

32. Leach, G. E. and Yip, C.-M. (1986). Urologic and urodynamic evaluation of the elderly population. *Clinics in Geriatric Medicine*, **2**, 731–55.

33. Castleden, C. M., Duffin, H. M., and Asher, M. J. (1981). Clinical and urodynamic studies in 100 elderly incontinent patients. *British Medical Journal*, **282**, 1103–5.

34. Resnick, N. M., Yalla, S. V., and Laurino, E. (1989). The pathophysiology of urinary incontinence among institutionalized elderly persons. *New England Journal of Medicine*, **320**, 1–7.

35. Hilton, P. and Stanton, S. L. (1981). Algorithmic method for assessing urinary incontinence in elderly women. *British Medical Journal*, **282**, 940–2.

36. Eastwood, H. D. H. and Warrell, R. (1984). Urinary incontinence in the elderly female: prediction in diagnosis and outcome of management. *Age and Ageing*, **13**, 230–4.

37. Tobin, G. W. and Brocklehurst, J. C. (1986). The management of urinary incontinence in local authority residential homes for the elderly. *Age and Ageing*, **15**, 292–8.

38. Ouslander, J. C., Staskin, D. S., Orzeck, S., Blaustein, J. (1986). Diagnostic tests for geriatric incontinence. *World Journal of Urology*, **4**, 16–21.

39. Resnick, N. M., Yalla, S. V., and Laurino, E. (1986). An algorithmic approach to urinary incontinence in the elderly. *Clinical Research*, **34** 832A.

40. Ouslander, J., Orzeck, S., Raz, S., Blaustein, J. *et al.* (1986). Assessment of geriatric incontinence using an algorithm and simplified diagnostic tests. *Clinical Research*, **34**, 830A.

41. Sabanathan, K., Duffin, H. M., and Castleden, C. M. (1985). Urinary tract

infection after cystometry. *Age and Ageing*, **14**, 291–5.

42. Abrams, P., Blairas, J. G., Stanton, S. L., and Anderson, J. T. (1988). Standardisation of terminology of lower urinary tract function. *Neurourology and Urodynamics*, **7**, 403–27.
43. Wein, A. J., Hanno, P. M., Dixon, D. O., Raezer, x.x. and Benson, G. A. The reproducibility and interpretation of carbon dioxide cystometry. *Journal of Urology*, **120**, 205–6.
44. Ramsden, P. D., Smith, J. G., Pierce, J. M., and Ardran, G. M. (1977). The unstable bladder—fact or artefact? *British Journal of Urology*, **49**, 633–9.
45. Bhatia, N. N., Bradley, W. E., and Haldeman, S. (1982). Urodynamics; continuous monitoring. *Journal of Urology*, **128**, 963–8.
46. Jensen, D. (1981). Pharmacological studies of the uninhibited neurogenic bladder. *Acta Neurologica Scandinavica*, **64**, 145–74.
47. Brocklehurst, J. C. and Dillane, J. B. (1966). Studies of the female bladder in old age. I. Cystometrograms in non-incontinent women. *Gerontology Clinics*, **8**, 285–305.
48. Andersen, J. T., Jacobsen, O., Worm-Petersen, J. *et al.* (1978). Bladder function in healthy elderly males. *Scandinavian Journal of Urology and Nephrology*, **12**, 123–7.
49. Jorgensen, J. B., Jensen, K. M.-E., Bille-Brahe, N. E., and Mogensen, P. (1986). Uroflowmetry in asymptomatic elderly males. *British Journal of Urology*, **58**, 390–5.
50. Rud, T. (1980). Urethral pressure profile in continent women from childhood to old age. *Acta Obstetrica et Gynecologica Scandinavica*, **59**, 331–5.
51. Jones, K. W. and Schoenberg, H. W. (1985). Comparison of the incidence of bladder hyper-reflexia in patients with benign prostatic hypertrophy and a ge-matched female controls. *Journal of Urology*, **133**, 425–6.
52. Ouslander, J. G., Raz, S., Hepps, K., and Su, H. L. (1986). Genitourinary dysfunction in a geriatric outpatient population. *Journal American Geriatrics Society*, **34**, 507–14.
53. Jensen, K. M.-E., Bruskewitz, R. C., and Madsen, P. O. Urodynamic findings in elderly males without prostatic complaints. *Urology*, **24**, 211–13.
54. Drutz, H. P. and Mandel, F. (1979). Urodynamic analysis of urinary incontinence symptoms in women. *American Journal of Obstetrics and Gynecology*, **13**, 789–92.
55. Frimont-Moller, P. C., Jensen, K. M., Iversen, P. *et al.* (1984). Analyses of presenting symptoms in prostatism. *Journal of Urology*, **132**, 272–6.
56. Ouslander, J. G. (1989). Lower urinary tract disorders in the elderly female. In *Female urology*, (ed. Raz, S.) Philadelphia, Saunders.
57. Ouslander, J. G., Staskin, D., Raz, S., Hepps, K., and Su, H. L. (1987). Clinical versus urodynamic diagnosis in an incontinent geriatric female population. *Journal of Urology*, **137**, 68–71.
58. Brocklehurst, J. C., Dillane, J. b., Griffiths, L. *et al.* (1968). The prevalence and symptomology of urinary infection in an aged population. *Gerontology Clinics*, **10**, 242–53.
59. Sourander, L. B. and Kasanen, A. (1972). A 5 year follow-up of bacteriuria in the aged. *Gerontology Clinics*, **14**, 274–81.
60. Dontas, A. S., Kashi-Charvati, P., Papanayiotou, P. C. *et al.* (1981). Bacter-

iuria and survival in old age. *New England Journal of Medicine*, **304**, 939–43.

61. Nordenstam, G. R., Brandberg, C. A., Oden, A. S., Svandborg-Eden, C. M., and Svandborg, A. (1986). Bacteriuria and mortality in an elderly population. *New England Journal of Medicine*, **314**, 1152–6.

62. Nicolle, L. E., Bjornson, J., Harding, G. M. K. *et al.* (1983). Bacteriuria in elderly institutionalized men. *New England Journal of Medicine*, **309**, 1420–5.

63. Norman, D. C., Yamamura, R., and Yoshikawa, T. T. (1986). Pyuria; its predictive value of asymptomatic bacteriuria in ambulatory elderly men. *Journal of Urology*, **135**, 520–2.

64. Boscia, J. A., Kobasa, W. D., Knight, R. A., Abrutyn, E., Levison, M. E., and Kaye, D. (1986). Epidemiology of bacteriuria in an elderly ambulatory population. *American Journal of Medicine*, **80**, 208–14.

65. Fossberg, E., Sander, S., and Beisland, H. (1981). Urinary incontinence in the elderly: a pilot study. *Scandinavian Journal of Urology and Nephrology*, Suppl., **60**, 51–3.

66. Boscia, J. A., Kobasa, W. D., Levison, M. E., Kaplan, J. E., and Kaye, D. (1986). Lack of association between bacteriuria and symptoms in the elderly. *American Journal of Medicine*, **81**, 979–82.

67. Ouslander, J., Blaustein, J., and Connor, A. (1987). Habit training and oxybutinin for incontinence in nursing home patients: a placebo controlled trial. *Journal of the American Geriatrics Society*, **36**, 40–6.

68. Wendland, C. J. and Ouslander, J. G. (1986). *A rehabilitative approach to urinary incontinence in long-term care: monograph for nurses*. The Beverly Foundation, Pasadena, CA.

69. Duffin, H. M. and Castleden, C. M. (1986). The continence nurse adviser's role in the British health care system. *Clinics in Geriatric Medicine*, **2**, 841–55.

70. International Continence Society (1987). Proceedings of the International Continence Society, *Neurourology and Urodynamics*, **6(3)**.

71. Ouslander, J. G. (1984). Incontinence clinics. *Generations*, **8**, 18–19.

72. Brink, C. A. and Wells, T. J. (1986). Environmental support for geriatric incontinence: Toilets, toilet supplements and external equipment. *Clinics in Geriatric Medicine*, **2**, 829–40.

73. Ouslander, J. G., Kane, R. L., Vollmer, S., and Menzes, M. (1985). *Technologies for managing incontinence* (Health Technology Case Study 33), OTA–HCS–33, July. Washington DC. US Congress, Office of Technology Assessment.

74. Smith, B. M. T. (1985). A comparative trial of urinary incontinence aides. *British Journal of Clinical Practice*, 311–24.

75. Hadley, E. (1986). Bladder training and related therapies for urinary incontinence in older people. *Journal of the American Medical Association*, **256** (3), 372–9.

76. Burgio, K. L. and Burgio, L. D. (1986). Behaviour therapies for urinary incontinence in the elderly. *Clinics in Geriatric Medicine*, **2**, 809–27.

77. Burgio, K. L., Whitehead, W. E., and Engel, B. T. (1985). Urinary incontinence in elderly—bladder–sphincter biofeedback and toilet skills training. *Annals of Internal Medicine*, **104**, 507–15.

78. Burton, J. R., Pearace, K. L., Burgio, K. L., Engel, B. T., and Whitehead, W. E. (1986). Comparison of biofeedback to a program of education self-management as treatment for urinary incontinence in elderly ambulatory ptaients. *Proceedings of the 3rd Joint Meeting of the International Continence and Urodynamic Societies*, Boston, MA.
79. Burgio, K. L., Robinson, J. C., and Engel, B. T. (1986). The role of biofeedback in Kegel exercise training for stress urinary incontinence. *American Journal of Obstetrics and Gynecology*, **154**(1), 58–64.
80. Cardozo, L., Stanton, S. L., Hafner, J. *et al.* (1978). Biofeedback in the treatment of detrusor instability. *British Journal of Urology*, **50**, 250–4.
81. Spangler, P. F., Risley, T. R., and Bilyew, D. D. (1984). The management of dehydration and incontinence in nonambulatory geriatric patients. *Journal Applied Behaviour Analysis*, **17**, 397–401.
82. Sogbein, S. and Awad, S. A. (1982). Behavioral treatment of urinary incontinence in geriatric patients. *Californian Medical Association Journal*, **127**, 863–4.
83. Schnelle, J. E., Traughber, B., Norgan, D. B. *et al.* (1983). Management of geriatric incontinence in nursing homes. *Journal of Applied Behavioral Analyses*, **16**, 235–41.
84. Wein, A. J. (1986). Physiology of micturition. *Clinics in Geriatric Medicine*, **2**, 689–99.
85. Ouslander, J. G. and Sier, H. C. (1986). Drug therapy for geriatric incontinence. *Clinics in Geriatric Medicine*, **2**, 789–807.
86. Castleden, C. M., Duffin, H. M., Asher, M. J., and Yeomason, C. W. (1985). Factors influencing outcome in elderly patients with urinary incontinence and detrusor instability. *Age and Ageing*, **14**, 303–7.
87. Zorzitto, M. L., Jewett, M. A. S., Fernie, G. R., Holliday, P. J., and Bartlett, S. (1986). Effectiveness of propantheline bromide in the treatment of geriatric patients with detrusor instability. *Neurourology and Urodynamics*, **5**, 133–40.
88. Judd, U. L., Clearly, R. E., Creasman, W. I. *et al.* (1981). Estrogen replacement therapy. *Obstetrics and Gynecology*, **58**, 267–75.
89. Downie, J. W. (1984). Bethanechol chloride in urology—a discussion of issues. *Neurourology and Urodynamics*, **2**, 211–22.
90. Finkbeiner, A. E. (1985). Is bethanechol chloride clinically effective in promoting bladder emptying? A literature review. *Journal of Urology*, **134**, 443–449.
91. Caine, M. (1986). The present role of alpha-adrenergic blockers in the treatment of benign prostatic hypertrophy. *Journal of Urology*, **136**, 1–4.
92. Schmidbauer, C. P., Chiang, H., and Raz, S. (1986). Surgical treatment for female geriatric incontinence. *Clinics in Geriatric Medicine*, **2**, 759–76.
93. Raz, S. (1981). Modified bladder neck suspension for female stress incontinence. *Urology*, **17**, 82–5.
94. McGuire, E. J. and Savastano, J. A. (1985). Stress incontinence and detrusor instability/urge incontinence. *Neurourology and Urodynamics*, **4**, 313–16.
95. Diokno, A., Wells, T., and Brink, C. (1989). Urinary incontinence in elderly women: Urodynamic evaluation. *Journal American Geriatrics Society*, **35**, 940–6.

96. Stanton, S. I. and Cardoza, (1980). L. D. Surgical treatment of incontinence in elderly women. *Surgery, Gynaecology and Obstetrics*, **150**, 555–7.
97. Pow–Sang, J. M., Lockhart, J. G., Suarez, A., Lansman, H., and Politano, V. A. (1986). Female urinary incontinence: preoperative selection, surgical complications and results. *Journal of Urology*, **136**, 831–3.
98. Hinman, F. (ed.) (1983). *Benign prostatic hypertrophy*. Springer-Verlag, New York.
99. Dorflinger, T., Frimodt-Moller, P. C., Bruskewitz, R. C., Jensen, K. M.-E., Iversen, P., and Madsen, P. O. (1985). The significance of uninhibited detrusor contractions in prostatism. *Journal of Urology*, **135**, 819–21.
100. Abrams, P. (1985). Detrusor instability and bladder outlet obstruction. *Neurourology and Urodynamics*, **4**, 317–38.
101. Meyhoff, H. H. and Nordling, J. (1986). Long term results of transurethral and transvesical prostatectomy. *Scandinavian Journal of Urology and Nephrology*, **20**, 27–33.
102. Ball, A. J., Feneley, R. C. L., and Abrams, P. H. (1981). The natural history of untreated 'prostatism'. *British Journal of Urology*, **53**, 613–16.
103. Blaivas, J. G. and Berger, Y. (1986). Surgical treatment for male geriatric incontinence. *Clinics in Geriatric Medicine*, **2**, 777–87.
104. Schlossberg, S. M., Lubin-Finkel, M., Darracott-Vaughan, E., Jensen, D., Riehle, R. A., and McCarthy, E. C. (1984). Second opinion for urologic surgery. *Journal of Urology*, **131**, 209–12.
105. McPherson, K., Wennberg, J. E., Hovind, O. B., and Clifford, P. (1982). Small-area variations in the use of common surgical procedures: an international comparison of New England, England and Norway. *New England Journal of Medicine*, **307**, 1310–14.
106. Jayachandran, S., Morran, U. M., and Kin, H. (1985). Complications from external (condom) urinary drainage devices. *Urology*, **25**, 31–4.
107. Johnson, E. T. (1983). The condom catheter urinary tract infection and other complications. *Southern Medical Journal*, **76**, 579–82.
108. Hirsh, D. D., Fainstein, V., and Musher, D. M. (1979). Do condom catheter collecting systems cause urinary tract infection? *Journal of the American Medical Association*, **242**, 340–1.
109. Ouslander, J. G., Greengold, B. A., and Chen, S. (1987). External catheter use and urinary tract infection among incontinent male nursing home patients. *Journal of the American Geriatrics Society*, **35**, 1063–70.
110. Lapides, J. and Diokno, A. C. (1983). Clean, intermittent self-catheterization. In *Female urology* (ed. Raz, S.), pp 344–8 Saunders, Philadelphia.
111. Bennett, C. J. and Diokno, A. C. (1984). Clean intermittent self-catheterization in the elderly. *Urology*, **24**, 43–5.
112. Marron, K. R., Fillit, H., Peskowitz, M. *et al.* (1983). The nonuse of urethral catheterization in the management of urinary incontinence in the teaching nursing home. *Journal of the American Geriatrics Society*, **31**, 278–81.
113. Kunin, C. M. (1983). The incontinent patient and the catheter. *Journal of the American Geriatrics Society*, **31**, 259–60.
114. Ribeiro, B. J. and Smith, S. R. (1985). Evaluation of urinary catheterization and incontinence in a general nursing home population. *Journal of the American Geriatrics Society*, **33**, 479–82.

115. Gleckman, R. A. (1985). The chronically catheterized elderly patient. *Journal of the American Geriatrics Society*, **33**, 489–91.
116. Warren, J. W., Muncie, H. L., Berquist, E. J. *et al.* (1981). Sequelae and management of urinary infection in the patient requiring chronic catheterization. *Journal of Urology*, **125**, 1–7.
117. Kunin, C. M. (1984). Gentourinary Infections in the patient at risk: Extrinsic Risk Factors. *American Journal of Medicine*, **76**, (Suppl. 5), 131–9.
118. Ouslander, J. G., Greengold, B. A., and Chen, S. (1987). Incidence of symptomatic urinary tract infection among male nursing home patients with chronic indwelling catheters. *Journal of Urology*, **138**, 1191–5.
119. Wong, E. S. and Hooton, T. M. (1981). Guidelines for prevention of catheter-associated urinary tract infections. *Infection Control*, **2**, 125–30.
120. Warren, J. W. (1986). Catheters and catheter care. *Clinics in Geriatric Medicine*, **2**, 857–71.
121. Thompson, R. L., Haley, E. C., Searcy, M. A. *et al.* (1984). Catheter-associated bacteriuria: Failure to reduce attack rates using periodic instillations of a disinfectant into urinary drainage systems. *Journal of the American Medical Association*, **251**, 747–51.
122. Fall, M. (1984). Does electrostimulation cure urinary incontinence? *Journal of Urology*, **131**, 664–7.
123. Suhel, P. and Kralj, B. (1983). Treatment of urinary incontinence using functional electrical stimulation. In *Female urology* (ed. Raz, S.), pp. 189–228 Saunders, Philadelphia.
124. Fall, M., Ahlstrom, K., Carlsson, C.-A., Ek, A., Erlandson, B.-E., Frankenberg, S., and Mattiasson, A. (1986). Contelle: pelvic floor stimulator for female stress-urge incontinence. *Urology*, **27**, 282–7.

18

Falls in later life

MARY JO GIBSON

Falls are the most frequent and serious home accident involving the elderly. Everyone involved with older people is familiar with their fear of falling and of the serious consequences which may result from a fall. The consequences range from the indignity and embarrassment of sprawling on the ground with torn clothes, a split shopping bag and a bruised face, to the need for prolonged hospitalization following a fracture of the femur. From the perspective of the older person, falls are painful and frightening, and may lead to loss of confidence, restrictions in mobility, depression, and death. Even if the fall does not result in physical injury, elderly victims of falls may lose confidence in their ability to engage in routine physical and social activities, resulting in isolation and withdrawal. Their families may feel guilty that they did not prevent the fall and attempt to impose limitations on their loved one's independence.

Although for older persons and their families, falling is a serious condition, there is no rubric for 'falls' in the medical diagnostic indices. It is common for physicians to overlook the need to question the elderly patients about their experience of falls. Falls are part of common experience throughout life and that may be why their full significance for elderly people is often not grasped.

Older people's fears of suffering a serious injury from a fall are real. In the United States, there are 172 000 hip fractures per year among persons aged 65 and older.[1] The incidence of hip fracture increases steeply after age 50, and is highest among the very elderly.[2] Among those who live to 90 years of age, 32 per cent of women and 17 per cent of men will suffer a hip fracture.[3]

Falls among the elderly carry high societal as well as individual costs because they result in heavy demands on both short-stay and long-term health care. In the US, it has been estimated that the economic cost of all hip fractures is in the neighbourhood of $7 billion per year.[4] In both the United Kingdom and France, falls without fracture are among the most common causes of admission of the elderly to geriatric hospitals, residential homes, and nursing homes. The toll taken in older people's loss of mobility and independence cannot be quantified.

It is important to emphasize that the great majority of older people do not sustain serious physical injuries from falls. Despite this fact, high proportions of the elderly report a fear of falling. In a recent study of persons aged 75 and over in a community in the US, over one-third (36 per cent) of people who had never fallen admitted to this fear, as did 50 per cent of those who had fallen previously.[5] In the light of such data, there is a clear need to put falls into perspective by providing accurate information about their causes and prevention.

Older persons and their families, and even some health care professionals, often erroneously attribute falling to 'old age itself'. Such fatalistic attitudes need to be countered, since falls are not a normal part of the aging process. Rather, they are due to underlying physical illnesses, medications, environmental hazards, and social factors, often in interaction.

Falls have been defined as 'events which lead to the conscious subject coming to rest inadvertently on the ground'. It is the nature of the event which is the key to the variation in the significance of falls. At one extreme, a resolute but imprudent elderly man ascends a shaky ladder, extends his head backwards, reaches an arm out to change an electric bulb, and the ladder moves, pitching him to the ground. He may or may not suffer serious injury as a consequence, but he is essentially a fit person and his health is not likely to suffer seriously. At the other extreme, a weak, malnourished, ill old person walks slowly across the room, her legs give way, and 'down she goes'. She may sustain little injury, but be so shocked and weakened by the experience that she is unable to rise, lies on the floor for hours until rescued, and becomes gravely ill.

In between the extremes, falls involving many diverse circumstances occur to people with a wide range of physical and medical characteristics. The causes and consequences of falls, as well as their methods of treatment and prevention, vary greatly. Hence, it is important to distinguish clearly between different kinds of falls in different groups of older people. Such distinctions are central to developing effective intervention programmes.

Health care and other professionals, as well as older people themselves and their families, can benefit from increased awareness about the causes and methods of preventing falls. Although considerable efforts have been directed toward preventing accidents by the young, the prevention of falls by older people has received relatively little attention. The successful experiences of many nations in preventing home and traffic accidents in general, however, suggest that similar approaches may be effective in developing fall prevention programmes for the elderly.

DEFINITIONS OF FALLING

Everyone 'knows' what a fall is, yet every scientific paper on the subject opens with a different definition. Common to all are the concepts of change of position of the body and lack of intention to do so. Researchers differ in how they treat, for example, a fall into a chair, a fall out of a chair, a fall which results from loss of consciousness or the onset of a stroke or an epileptic attack, a fall resulting from a violent blow, or simply the situation in which a person is found lying on the ground and unable to explain how he got there. The causes and consequences of falls in such different circumstances vary greatly. It is important not so much to strive after a form of words which covers every situation, but rather for each researcher to declare which of these circumstances he has included in his definition and which he has excluded. Readers are then in a position to estimate the significance of the report findings.

We recommend that, in reporting studies of the clinical significance and correlates of falls in old age, research workers might agree to the use of the following definition, or, if they prefer a different one, to state the deviations from our proposal which they have adopted and their reasons for doing so.

Proposed definition of a fall

A fall is an event which results in a person coming to rest inadvertently on the ground or other lower level and other than as a consequence of the following:

—— sustaining a violent blow;

—— loss of consciousness;

—— sudden onset of paralysis, as in a stroke;

—— an epileptic seizure.

THE POPULATION AT RISK OF FALLING AND BEING SERIOUSLY INJURED: AN OVERVIEW

How frequently do falls occur?

The magnitude of the problem is difficult to determine. Epidemiological data on falls by the elderly are limited, and studies of older persons living in the community usually rely upon the subject's recall, leading to a probable underreporting of the actual prevalence of falls. However, the prevalence in the home appears to involve roughly one-third of persons aged 65 and over.[6] A major study of falls conducted in New Zealand, for example, indicated that about one-third of the population aged 65 and over had experienced one or more falls in the preceding year; this figure rose to almost one-half of persons aged 80 and over.[7] Other studies in the

UK show comparable rates.[8,9] Similarly, in France it is estimated that 20–45 per cent of persons aged 65 over have one or more falls each year.[10]

Many of the studies on falls have been conducted in institutional settings, where the frequency of falls is reported to be considerably higher than that among those living in their own homes.[6,11] Residents in institutional care facilities are typically in poorer health and have more mobility impairments which increase the likelihood of a fall. In addition, institutional care facilities are not always designed to minimize the occurrence of falls, and residents must adjust to unfamiliar environments.

How frequently do falls result in serious physical injury?

The great majority of falls by the elderly do not result in serious physical injury. In France,[10] reports that only 6 per cent of falls by older persons result in a fracture, and another 10 per cent in injuries without fracture. Similarly, Gryfe and colleagues[12] report that 6 per cent of falls by elderly Canadians living in residential accommodations result in fractures, of which 1 per cent are fractures of the proximal femur (hip). In Great Britain also it has been estimated that less than 1 per cent of all falls among those aged 65 and over result in hip fractures.[13]

Although the proportion of falls with fracture is low the absolute number of those who experience fractures is high. Although the literature is contradictory, several European studies also indicate that there has been a steady increase in the incidence of hip fractures in recent years.[14] In Nottingham, for example, the numbers of older people admitted to orthopaedic units with fractures of the proximal femur (hip) increased at an annual rate of 6–10 per cent between 1971 and 1980, while the population aged 65 and over increased at a rate of only 2 per cent.[15] Finally, falls can result in injuries other than fractures. Even those falls which result in no physical injury often have serious social and psychological consequences.

Who is at greatest risk of falling?

A broad body of research indicates that advanced age is associated with an increased risk of falling, and that both the risk of falling and that of suffering serious physical injury increase substantially up to the eighth decade of life.[16]

The data suggest that most falls occur among older women. Of course, there are far more women than men within the general older population in most nations, and particularly among the very old. However, even when age adjustments are made, older women experience significantly more falls than do older men.[9] The former are also more likely to be single (e.g. widowed or separated and living alone). Research results on whether marital status *per se* is associated with higher rates of falling have been contradictory;[16] however, researchers in both New Zealand and France report that elderly women living alone are at significantly greater risk of falling and being injured.[7, 10]

The many risk factors for falls are not yet known, and some older people who experience multiple falls have the same functional capability as those who have not fallen. However, a number of characteristics have been found to be associated with the risk of falling. These include poor health status, especially chronic illness, impaired mobility and postural stability, and a history of prior falls. Ill people also tend to be on treatment with multiple medications, which may add to their difficulties in sustaining balance. Among the diseases common in this high-risk group are arthritis in the lower limbs, structural diseases of the feet, and visual impairments. Not only are these factors individually associated with the risk of falling, but the greater the number of disabilities, the greater is the risk of falling.[17]

Hence, the risk becomes a serious problem when multiple disabilities, involving multiple functions, interfere with the person's ability to compensate.

Falls occur when a person undertakes an activity which requires correction of an unexpected displacement, and lacks the capacity to correct the displacement in the available time. Therefore those who might be at risk of falling were they to continue in their former activities generally slow down and reduce the risks they might otherwise take. Nonetheless, they remain vulnerable to small irregularities in their environment since, as balance function becomes impaired, there is a tendency for falls to occur with less and less provocation. Among active individuals, a high proportion of falls occurs outdoors or at points of hazard. Among the severely disabled, a high proportion occurs indoors and in less hazardous surroundings.

Who is at greatest risk of serious physical injury?

It is generally agreed that women of advanced age (75 years and over) are most likely to suffer serious physical injury from a fall. In the United Kingdom, women aged 75 and over, who represent about one-quarter of the population aged 65 and over, account for over half of the hospital-treated falls among the elderly population.[18]

Many types of serious fractures are characterized by incidence rates that rise with age and are greater among older women than older men. This general pattern is observed for each of the following fracture sites:

proximal femur (hip), distal forearm (wrist), proximal humerus (upper arm), and pelvis.[19] In the USA, UK and Scandanavia, female hip fracture patients aged 75 and over outnumber males by approximately two to three to one.[20, 21] The increase in the incidence of hip fractures among white females begins around age 40 and doubles with each 5 to 6 years of life thereafter in an exponential curve.[22]

Osteoporosis, which is more common among women than men, appears to be an important contributing factor to the higher incidence of fractures among women.[2] Men also experience age-related increases in osteoporosis and fractures. Recent national hospital data from the USA are now showing fractures of the hip and other bones to be a significant problem among males aged 75 and over as well as females.[1]

In addition to the fact that bone loss predisposes to fractures, another important part of the problem may be age-related reductions in protective responses to falls, such as extending a hand to break the impact.[23] The incidence of Colles (wrist) fractures peaks among women in the mid seventies, after which it plateaus or declines;[24, 25, 26] this has been attributed to a loss in protective responses to falling. After the age of 70, there is a steep increase in the incidence of hip fractures, possibly as a consequence of unprotected falls.[20, 27, 28]

Evidence that fractures may be the result of violent, unprotected falls comes from Great Britain and France. In recent studies in both countries, older people who suffered fractures were more active and more likely to have fallen outside on to the hard ground. Those who were less active and fell more slowly inside their homes did not sustain fractures, but were more prone to further falls.[29, 30]

What are the major consequences of falls?

Falls may result in a number of physical injuries, including:

—— soft-tissue damage (bruising and lacerations);

—— fractures (of the hip, wrist, and other bones);

—— trauma to the nervous system (rare, but very serious);

—— hypothermia, dehydration, and pneumonia after a 'long lie'.

Both hip fractures and what has been termed the 'long lie' (remaining on the ground or floor for more than an hour after a fall) are associated with high mortality rates among the elderly. The mortality rate of those who have suffered a fractured hip may be between 12 and 20 per cent higher than that of persons of similar age and sex who have not, with most of these deaths occurring in the first 4 months following the fractures.[2]

Hip fractures also are a leading cause of disability among the elderly; roughly half of the survivors never recover normal functioning.[2] In the USA, the average length of stay for hip fracture patients in acute care hospitals is 3 weeks—longer than for any other diagnosis.[1]

The 'long lie' is a marker of weakness, illness, and social isolation. A British study suggested that half of those who lie on the floor for an hour or longer die within 6 months, even if there is no direct physical injury from the fall.[31, 32] Complications associated with the long lie include hypothermia, bronchopneumonia, and dehydration, all of which can lead to death.[33] Data from France suggest that long lies are not uncommon. In Toulouse, 10 of 48 elderly patients hospitalized for falls had been on the ground for 1 hour or more, and one had been there for 3 days.[10]

It is important to emphasize that, even if a fall does not result in physical injury, it can lead to other serious consequences. The shock of falling may generate the fear of falling again, which may lead to anxiety, loss of confidence, social withdrawal, and restriction in daily activities. In a study conducted in a US community, in which high proportions of older persons reported fears of falling, 40 per cent of those with this fear said it had led them to restrict their basic daily activities.[5] In a French study, slightly more older people who fell in their homes were found at 6-month follow-up to have restricted their activities compared with a control group of those who had not fallen. In the institutionalized sample, the falls were associated with behavioural disorders, such as agitation be and mood disturbances among 13 per cent of those followed.[34]

Not only older people themselves but also their families often respond with anxiety to falls. It is not uncommon for families to become 'overprotective' and attempt to restrict their older relative's autonomy.[35] In some cases, the family's reaction may even lead to unnecessary institutionalization. In Toulouse, France, a shocking 39 per cent of 295 persons aged 70 and over who had fallen but suffered no serious physical injury were institutionalized upon their family's request.[36]

THE REASONS OLDER PEOPLE FALL: AN OVERVIEW

When physicians ask older people who have fallen to explain why they fell, some typical responses are:

'I just fell.'
'I must have tripped.'
'My legs gave way under me.'
'The floor came up and hit me.'
'I lost my balance.'
'Something came over me.'

Such comments illustrate the difficulties physicians, other health care professionals, and research workers confront in interpreting the causes of falls based on the reports of the victims, who may be fatigued, frightened, forgetful, or ill.

Another problem is that circumstances surrounding the falls are often not specified in record-keeping systems within institutions. It is, however, very important to attempt to establish what the person was doing at the time of the fall. For example, the cause of a fall which challenges balance control (such as standing on a step-ladder) is quite different from that of one which occurs during slow and habitual movement (such as transferring from a chair). The latter implies much greater impairment in the balance mechanisms.

Many investigators have recognized various types of falls due to differing causes and have adopted distinguishing terms to describe these events. Campbell and his colleagues,[7] for example, have distinguished between 'pattern' or recurrent falls and 'occasional' falls among the elderly. 'Pattern' falls were assessed as being caused primarily by disorders in postural stability or balance rather than external influences; they occurred more commonly among persons aged 80 and over who had more functional disabilities and more impairments in mobility. 'Occasional' falls generally occurred in younger people who were in better health and more active, and hence exposed to more environmental hazards. They fell in circumstances which would make most fit persons liable to fall. Similar characteristics have been used in identifying groups of older people who are at high and low risks for falls.[37]

In essence, such categories are efforts to discriminate between two ends of a continuum in which intrinsic and extrinsic factors play greater and lesser roles in causing falls by older people. They are clearly not intended to describe the wide range of falls experienced by older people, in which both intrinsic and extrinsic factors usually interact. As these categories suggest, the causes of falls are very different for people of varying ages, health status, and levels of mobility. It is also true that the same person may fall at different times for different reasons.

One common thread linking many studies is the strong association of poor health status and mobility problems with the frequency of falls in the elderly.[6] Many studies also have indicated that older persons taking certain types of medications are at much higher risk of falling. Environmental hazards contribute to falls by some older people, especially those who are younger and more active. For those elderly persons with impaired balance who tend to avoid the challenging environment of the outside world and may become confined to their homes or institutions, minor but unexpected irregularities in the environment become hazardous. For the purposes of prevention, it is important to consider factors associated with both the person and the environment, often in interaction.

While the multiple reasons why older people fall are not yet well understood, it is clear that impairments in balance and gait are not normal aspects of aging. The sequence of events in a fall sometimes follows the following pattern:

1. A movement such as walking is planned and initiated.
2. An unexpected or unperceived hazard is encountered and distorts the pattern of movement.
3. The body is displaced beyond its support base.
4. The corrective mechanism is delayed or inaccurate.
5. The point of no return has passed and the patient falls.

Balance, the ability to prevent falls upon displacement, relies upon the proper functioning of a number of anatomical structures. It can be impaired by disease or age-related changes in any one of these structures, by drugs which reduce their efficient functioning, and by environmental factors. Each of these three challenges to balance form the subject matter of this section.

Diseases and conditions

Three primary systems govern normal postural balance: vision, vestibular function, and proprioception. These systems all provide important sensory information about orientation in space. Diseases in these systems, as well as other conditions which contribute to impairments in balance among the elderly, are discussed below.

Visual system

Visual problems are obvious and important contributors to falls among the elderly. There is an increasing incidence in later life of structural diseases of the eye (such as cataract, glaucoma, and retinopathy), and such visual disorders can impair the ability to judge an imminent fall and to take appropriate and speedy corrective action.

Misinterpretation of spatial information, such as the nature of ground surfaces or misjudgement of distance, are not always the result of eye diseases. The use of visual information also can be impaired by age-related deficits in visual acuity, restriction of the visual field, increased susceptibility to glare, and poorer depth perception.[38]

In addition, there may be an age-related deficit in gaze stability, which can result in visual disorientation.[39]

In a community-based study of older adults in the United States, Tobis and his colleagues,[40] found significant impairments in the visual perceptual abilities of fall victims. Compared with those who had not fallen, fall victims showed a larger error in establishing the true vertical and horizontal; those who suffered the worst falls showed the largest error. The authors postulate that the relatively greater dependence on visual sources among the elderly generally, and some fallers specifically, may develop in response to impairment of feedback on posture and gait from the kinaesthetic and vestibular systems as a result of age and chronic health problems. This greater dependence upon environmental cues in maintaining posture and gait suggests that ambiguous or misleading environmental information can predispose older adults to falling.

It even has been hypothesized that part of the explanation of the large sex differences in the frequency of falls may be related to a difference in receptivity to optical information (e.g. women may take longer to detect body sway).[41] Similarly, Overstall[42] observes that, when visual and postural information conflict, women are more 'field dependent'— that is, they rely more heavily on the spatial framework provided by vision.

Vestibular system

Vestibular disorders, particularly when asymmetrical, may be common and troublesome to the elderly. Although age-related changes affecting vestibular function have not been widely studied, they may be important since the vestibular apparatus helps to keep the head and neck in vertical position and affects the corrective mechanisms needed to do so.[38]

Propriceptive disorders

Loss of proprioceptors in cervical joints may give misleading information about the position and movement of the head in space. Diseases in weight-bearing joints in the lower limbs may contribute to error in foot placement. Distorted or painful feet and poorly fitting shoes may give misleading information on the nature of ground contact and produce errors during the swing phase.

In a recent study of falls by older people in intermediate care facilities in the USA, Tinetti and colleagues[43] found that decreased knee strength and symptoms during a neck examination were associated with falling. Subjects with sensations of staggering or imbalance during neck 'range-of-motion' testing were eight times more likely to fall than those without such symptoms. (The frequent finding of decreased knee strength also lends to support to the comment often made by people after a fall that their 'knees gave out'.)

As of yet there are little data on age-related deficits in proprioception. there is however, some evidence that, while these are not apparent if the movement in question is preselected by the subject, problems can occur if the movements are unexpected or forced.[38]

Functional disruption of central processing

Even when there is no disorder in end-organ function there can be problems in the central processing of information from peripheral structures. Vision, vestibular sensation, and proprioception all interact centrally. These interactions can be disrupted by aging or disease, resulting in balance control deficits. Disruptions in vestibulo-ocular reflexes, vestibulospinal function, and balance performance have been well documented for patients with peripheral and/or central lesions.[44] Adaptive protocols which require changes in sensorimotor organization may prove to be most useful for deciphering central postural control dysfunction.[45]

Disorders of perfusion

Momentary disturbances of perfusion, especially of the hindbrain and upper cord, may suffice to impair muscle tone long enough for a fall to occur. Reduced perfusion, when effort is exerted, may result from constrictive lesions reducing cardiac output. Impaired baroreceptor function may reduce perfusion when there is a postural change.

Transient hypotension due to impaired regulation of systemic blood-pressure is one common process thought to cause falls by the elderly. With advancing age, there is progressive decline in homeostatic capacity, which means that seemingly minor changes, such as changes in posture as well as acute illness, or a new medication, may threaten blood pressure stability and precipitate a fall.[46]

In the United Kingdom, large fluctuations in blood-pressure without any symptoms during a 24-hour period have been found among both older and younger people with previously unexplained falls.[37] A key issue seems to be the speed of the change in blood-pressure and the ability of cerebral perfusion to adapt. This, however, is very difficult to measure.

Structural changes

Changes in the cerebral cortex exert relatively slight effects on balance. Pyramidal tract disorders affect the patterning of gait and may weaken supporting limbs. Extrapyramidal disorders gravely alter the sequencing of pacing and may also impair the speed of correction after displacement. Cerebellar disorders create grossly abnormal stepping patterns and impair corrective mechanisms. Weakness and wasting of muscles disturb the stability of support and delay the effectivenss of corrective messages.

Effects of medications and alcohol

It is not clear whether the falls that have been associated with some medications are due to the medications themselves or to the illnesses for which they have been prescribed. Research results on the relationship between medications and falls among the elderly have been somewhat contradictory. It does appear, however, that some types of drugs increase the frequency of falls among the elderly. Older persons taking multiple medication are at particular risk.[47]

Those drugs which reduce mental alertness and the speed of transmission within the central nervous system in particular have been implicated as contributors to falls. For example, in a British study of older people at home, fallers were more likely than controls to have taken hypnotics, tranquillizers, and sedatives.[32] Some studies also have shown a link between tricyclic antidepressants and falls.[48] Antihypertensive drugs and diuretics are probably also important contributors to falls.[9, 47] Knowledge about variations from drug to drug within major drug groups, however, is far adequate.

Clinicians may see patients where alcohol appears to have been a contributing factor. In a study of falls by older people in the United States which resulted in injury, 8 per cent were attributed to alcohol use.[49] However, one study in Great Britain found no such association between alcohol and falls.[9]

Environmental factors

Hazards in both the external environment and the home precipitate many falls in older people. While dangers in the external environment appear to be more important causes of falls by active and healthy older people, those in the home assume increasing importance for those in advanced age and ill health who tend to restrict their activities in the outside world.

Few would deny that the external environment, with its fast-moving vehicles, irregular ground surfaces, blinking lights, and the like, is often unsafe for the general population and especially for the elderly. In a British study of 100 healthy people aged 65–74, most of the falls which occurred over a 1-year period were due to encounters with external environmental hazards, and imprudence or errors in perception.[50]

However, it is the familiar but often very dangerous home environment where most older people, and particularly the very old and those in poor health, spend most of their time. Loose rugs, unstable furniture, poor lighting, unsafe stairs, and the like all pose significant risks to the unwary. Moreover, what once was not an environmental hazard to a healthy person of relatively young age may become so in advanced age and ill health. For example, elderly people often fail to appreciate a small but critical decline in their ability to prevent a fall, and continue to perform familiar but now more difficult tasks. Standing on steps to change a light bulb, which involves an unstable position and loss of eye contact with the ground, is a good example, and underlines the importance of considering the reciprocal relationship between the faller and the environment.

Of the many environmental factors which predispose the elderly to falls, problems in foot–ground contact appear to be especially important. Such problems arise from improperly fitting shoes, irregular ground surfaces, and low slip resistance between the foot and surface. In a study of falls by the elderly in a rural northern climate in the USA, for example, one-third of the treated falls involved icy or wet surface or rough ground; many occurred on public streets or pavements.[51] Faulty footwear, such as slippers, also has been implicated in several British studies as a major cause of falls by older people.[50, 52]

Falls by the elderly, particularly those of advanced age, frequently occur during such simple and familiar daily activities as arising from a chair or getting out of bed. Improperly designed chairs which slope or are too high or low may be contributing factors, as are beds which are too high, low, or soft.

Stair accidents have been found to be more common among the young elderly (65–74) than those of advanced age,[18] who are less likely to use stairs or to do so very cautiously. Although the elderly have fewer accidents than those in other age groups because of less frequent use, those accidents which do occur are much more serious. In the USA, 85 per cent of all deaths attributed to stair accidents are among persons aged 60 and older.[53] Most of the serious accidents occur on descent, and visual impairments have been implicated as a cause. Older people, for example, may have difficulty judging the size of the tread below. It has been observed that stair accidents are often not simply due to human imprudence, but rather to 'architecturally triggered human error'.[53]

While older people also use escalators less frequently than do the young, they are disproportionately involved in escalator fall accidents. Some of these falls may be due to jostling by other riders. However, repeating optical patterns on escalator treads can cause a visual depth illusion, resulting in disorientation.[54] Such optokinetic patterns, which also occur on tile and floor surfaces, may be important contributors to falls among the elderly.

A note on social and behavioural factors

There is very little information available on the social and behavioural factors which may predispose the elderly to falls. Some investigators, however, have observed that mental and emotional status may influence mobility, including gait, balance, and awareness of and desire to manoeuvre in the environment.[43] Since mobility limitations have been found to be important predictors of falls,[31, 43] mental and emotional status may be at least indirectly associated with falls.

There is some empirical evidence that the fear of falling is common among both the elderly who have experienced falls and those who have not, and that this fear often leads to restrictions in daily activities.[5] It is probable that for some individuals, the reduced mobility in turn precipitates other falls.

An interesting example of the interaction between social and physical factors in causing falls comes from a study of institutionalized women with dementia.[55] Those women who showed the least decline in their social relationships and made more efforts to maintain communication were found to fall the most frequently. Since these women had also experienced abrupt declines in their physical vigour, it is possible their attempts to maintain social interaction presented them with more opportunities to fall. Such data point to the need for a delicate balance between protecting the institutionalized elderly who are vulnerable to falls and fostering their sense of mastery and independence.

THE METHODS OF PREVENTING FALLS

As the above review of some of the known and postulated causes of falls attests, it is clearly not possible to prevent all falls by the elderly. In the face of our limited empirical knowledge about the causes of falls, *ad hoc* measures have sometimes been developed which are now suspected of resulting in more falls. For example, efforts to prevent falls in institutional settings through the use of physical and chemical restraints often result in both reduced mobility and loss of personal autonomy. The attempt by some families to limit an older relative's activities is another example of a well-meaning but misguided effort to prevent falls.

Both research evidence and common sense, however, suggest that it is possible to prevent falls by the elderly through methods which do not undermine mobility or autonomy. Several different groups, including health care professionals, older people and their families, and planners and architects, are all appropriate audiences for information on the steps that can be taken to prevent falls in later life.

It is important to bear in mind that older people of varying ages, health, status, and mobility levels fall for different reasons. Although there are few data evaluating the efficacy of various preventive approaches with different subgroups of older people, it may be useful to distinguish between those methods which may prove to be more effective with two broad groups of the elderly: older people who are at high or at low risk of falling. The high-risk group includes individuals with impaired mobility and stability, multiple pathologies, and histories of prior falls. They are usually but not always aged 75 or older. For this group, a particularly useful approach may be through action by health care professionals. Physicians, for example, need to identify and treat reversible medical conditions that have contributed to falls, identify impairments in gait and balance, and help to improve balance through activity programmes, better nutrition, and good general care. Older persons who are at low risk of falling are those who are active, generally healthy, and usually but not always under the age of 75. Since this group experience approximately one-half of all fractures of the femur, small improvements in their balance could be very effective in reducing the total number of fall-related injuries. For this group, exercise and activity programmes, programmes to improve balance, and education regarding environmental hazards in the home seem particularly appropriate.

It is important to educate all elderly people, including the younger and more healthy, to recognize that a fall may be an early sign of illness which should be reported to their physicians for identification and treatment. At the same time, it is necessary to encourage them all, including the very old and chronically disabled, to remove home hazards and to remain as active as possible. Distinguishing between those preventive approaches likely to be most effective with groups which are at high or at low risk for falls is not intended to promote 'either/or' approaches, but simply to suggest where greater emphasis may need to be placed.

RESEARCH ISSUES

Although in recent years growing research attention has been devoted to falls among the elderly, neither their causes nor the most effective methods of preventing them are yet well understood. Epidemiological research on falls among the elderly is also at an embryonic level. Research on falls is hampered because falls are not recorded as a disease entity in medical indices such as the *Index medicus* or the *International statistical classification of disease*. This problem should be remedied.

One major barrier to research on falls have been the lack of a clear definition of falls, which covers many disparate events (see pp. 298–302 for a proposed definition). In addition, there is a need for a system of classifying different types of falls in order to make research findings more comparable.

The methodological problems in research on falls are many. Community-based samples have largely relied upon retrospective data and result in misreporting and underreporting of fall events. (Prospective studies are costly unless based on unrepresentative samples.) Very few community-based studies have used representative population-based samples, which limits their generalizability. Studies comparing the characteristics of those who have fallen with matched samples of those who have not fallen are rare. It also is not clear whether age and sex would have independent effects upon the risk of falling if health status and mobility were controlled. Since most studies have utilized cross-sectional designs, little is known about the changes over time in the risk factors for falling, and the effects of age cannot be assessed. The problem of selective attrition, common in longitudinal studies of older people, may be especially pronounced in studies on falls.

Finally, some important issues related to falls among the elderly remain uncharted research territory, including the effectiveness of various fall prevention strategies, and the social/emotional precipitants and consequences of falls.

Because of these limitations in our knowledge base about falls among the elderly, there is a need to:

1. Develop a terminology of falls.

2. Develop a more comprehensive and uniform system for data collection which fulfils the requirements for epidemiological studies. The already existing systems for recording accidents leading to injuries could be expanded by adding a few more questions related to falls.

3. Add questions on falls to other investigations of older people, including both longitudinal studies and other clinical research programmes.

4. Conduct longitudinal studies to identify risk factors for falls in both community and institutional settings.

5. Evaluate fall prevention and fall rehabilitation programme for different subgroups of the older population, such as those who are at high or low risk of falling.

6. Investigate the possible role of social and emotional factors in the aetiology of falls, about which very little is known.

7. Identify both the behavioural and the psychological consequences of falling, even if no injury has resulted, on mobility and morale.

8. Determine the behaviour of administrators and other staff in institutional care facilities with respect to falls.

9. Most importantly, elucidate the physiological mechanisms of and impairments in gait and balance among the elderly, whether or not they are related to falls. There is also a need to investigate the biomecha-

nics of the gait of elderly people, the ergonomics of their footwear, the nature of floor surfaces, and their interaction.

ACKNOWLEDGEMENTS

This chapter is an edited extract from a Report of the Kellogg International work Group on the Prevention of Falls by the Elderly, published as 'The prevention of falls in later life' in the *Danish Medical Bulletin* (1987), Volume 34, Supplement No. 4. The report was written by Mary Jo Gibson (International Federation on Aging, Washington DC, USA) in co-operation with Robert O. Andres Ph.D. (Department of Exercise Science, University of Massachusetts, USA) Bernard Isaacs MD (Charles Hayward Professor of Geriatric Medicine, University of Birmingham, England), Teresa Radebaugh MD (Natural Institute of Aging, Bethesda, USA), and Jorgen Worm-Petersen MD (Chief, University Department of Neurology, Gentofte Hospital, Hellerup, Denmark). Reproduced with permission of the author and publisher.

References

1. Baker, S. P. and Harvey, A. H. (1985). Fall injuries in the elderly. In *Clinics in Geriatric Medicine*, Vol. 1, No. 3 (ed. Radebaugh, T. S. *et al.*) pp. 501–12 W. B. Saunders Company, Philadelphia.
2. Cummings, S. R., Kelsey, J., Nevitt, M., and Dowd, K. (1985). Epidemiology of osteoporosis and osteoporotic fractures. *Epidemiologic Reviews*, **7**, 178–208.
3. NIH Consensus Development Conference on Osteoporosis (1984). *Journal of the American Medical Association*, **252**, 799–802.
4. American Institute of Architects Foundation (1986). *Design for aging: an architects guide*. AIA Press, Washington DC.
5. Tinetti, M. E. (1986). Personal communication.
6. Perry, B. C. (1982). Falls among the elderly: a review of methods and conclusions of epidemiologic studies. *Journal of the American Geriatrics Society*, **30**, 367–7.
7. Campbell, A. J., Reinken, J., Allan, B. C., and Martinez, G. S. (1981). Falls in old age: a study of frequency and related clinical factors. *Age and Ageing*, **10**, 264–70.
8. Exton–Smith, A. N. (1977). Functional consequences of aging: clinical manifestations. In *Care of the elderly: meeting the challenge of dependency*. (ed. Exton-Smith AN and J. Grimley Evans) pp. 41–53 Academic Press, London.
9. Prudham, D. and Evans, J. G. (1981). Factors associated with falls in the elderly: a community study. *Age and Ageing*, **10**, 141–6.
10. Vellas, B. (1985). *La chute chez la personne âgée*. IPSEN, Paris.
11. Berry, G., Fisher, R. H., and Lang, S. (1981). 'Detrimental incidents, including falls, in an elderly institutional population.' *Journal of the American Geriatrics Society*, **29**, 322–4.

12. Gryfe, C. I., Amies, A., and Ashley, M. J. (1977). A longitudinal study of falls in an elderly population: I. Incidence and morbidity. *Age and Ageing*, **6**, 201–10.
13. Baker, L. (1985). The preventability of falls. In *Prevention of disease in the elderly* (ed. Muir Gray, J. A.) pp. 114–24 Churchill Livingstone, London.
14. Johnell, D., Nilsson, B., Obrant, K. *et al.* (1984). Age and sex patterns of hip fractures: changes in 30 years. *Acta Orthopaedica Scandinavica*, **55**, 290–2.
15. Wallace, W. A. (1983). The increasing incidence of fractures of the proximal femur: An orthopaedic epidemic. *Lancet*, **i**, 1413–14.
16. Mossey, J. M. (1985). Social and psychologic factors related to falls among the elderly. In *Clinics in Geriatric Medicine*, Vol. 1, No. 3 (ed. Radebaugh, T. S. *et al.*) pp. 541–54 W. B. Saunders Company, Philadelphia.
17. Tinetti, M. E. (1986). A performance-oriented assessment of mobility problems in elderly patients. *Journal of the American Geriatrics Society*, **34**, 119–26.
18. Abrams, M. (1984). Falls by the elderly, England and Wales. Unpublished paper.
19. Melton, L. J. and Riggs, B. L. (1985). Risk factors for injury after a fall. In *Clinics in Geriatric Medicine*, Vol. 1, No. 3 (ed. Radebaugh, T. S. *et al.*) pp. 525–40 W. B. Saunders Company, Philadelphia.
20. Evans, J. G., Prudham, D. A., and Wandless, I. (1979). A prospective study of fractured proximal femur: Incidence and outcome. *Public Health (London)*, **93**, 235–41.
21. Kreutzfeld, J., Haim, M., and Bach, E. (1984). Hip fracture among the elderly in a mixed urban and rural population. *Age and Ageing*, **13**, 111–19.
22. Brody, J. A., Farmer, M. E., and White, L. R. (1984). Absence of menopausal effect on hip fracture occurrence in white females. *American Journal of Public Health*, **74**, 1397–8.
23. Evans, J. G. (1982). Epidemiology of proximal femoral fracture. In *Recent Advances in Geriatric Medicine 2* (ed. Isaacs, B.) pp. 201–14. Churchill Livingstone, Edinburgh.
24. Falch, J. (1983). Epidemiology of fractures of the distal forearm in Oslo. *Acta Orthopaedica Scandinavica*, **54**, 291–5.
25. Jensen, G. F., Christiansen, C., Boesen, J., Hegedus, V., and Transbol, I. (1982). Epidemiology of post-menopausal spinal and long bone fractures: a unifying approach to post-menopausal osteoporosis. *Clinical Orthopaedics*, **166**, 75–81.
26. Miller, S. W. M. and Evans, J. G. (1985). Fractures of the distal forearm in Newcastle: an epidemiological survey. *Age and Ageing*, **14**, 155–8.
27. Garraway, W. M., Stauffer, R. N., Kurland, L. T., and O'Fallon, W. M. (1979). Limb fracture in a defined population. 1–Frequency and distribution. *Mayo Clinic Proceedings*, **54**, 701–7.
28. Benton, K. G. F. and Strouthidis, T. M. (1985). After a fall. In *Fits, faints and falls in old age*, (ed. Kataria, Mohan S) pp. 109–32 MTP Press Ltd. Lancaster.
29. Allen–Narker, R. C., Isaacs, B., and Nayak, U.S.L. (1986). Prognostic factors in fractures of the wrist in patients aged 65 and over. Unpublished paper.
30. Ficat, J. J., Vellas, B., and Albarede, J. L. (1986). Mechanism and prevention of falls with hip fracture in the elderly. Communication to the Kellogg International Work Group on the Prevention of Falls by the Elderly, Geneva.

31. Wild, D., Nayak, U. L., and Isaacs, B. (1981). How dangerous are falls in old people at home? *British Medical Journal*, **282**, 266–8.
32. Wild, D., Nayak, U.S.L., and Isaacs, B. (1981). Prognosis of falls in old people at home. *Journal Epidemiology and Community Health*, **35**, 200–4.
33. Mitchell, R. G. (1984). Falls in the elderly. *Nursing Times*, January 11–17, 51–3.
34. Vellas, B., de Penille, F., Cayla, F., Bocquet, H., Pous, J., and Albarede, J. L. (1985). *Prospective study of restriction of activity in old people after falls.* Communication at meeting of the Société Française de Gerontologie, Paris, 14 novembre.
35. Yong, Lim Chan (1985). Physiological changes and medical problems in old people. *Singapore Elders*, **8**, (1 and 2).
36. Albarede, J. L. and Vellas, B. (1985). *Restriction d'activités après la chute chez la personne âgée.* Rapport a l'OMS, Centre International de Gerontologie Sociale, Versailles.
37. Isaacs, B. (1985). Clinical and laboratory studies of falls in old people: prospects for prevention. In *Clinics in Geriatric Medicine*, Vol. 1, No. 3 (ed. Radebaugh, T. S. *et al.*) pp. 513–24 W. B. Saunders Company, Philadelphia.
38. Stelmach, C. E. and Worringham, C. J. (1985). Sensorimotor deficits related to postural stability: implications for falling in the elderly. In *Clinics in Geriatric Medicine*, Vol. 1, No. 3 (ed. Radebaugh, T. S. *et al.*) pp. 679–94 W. B. Saunders Company, Philadelphia.
39. Leibowitz, H. W. and Shupert, C. L. (1985). Spatial orientation mechanisms and their implications for falls. In *Clinics in Geriatric Medicine*, Vol. 1, No. 3. (ed. Radebaugh, T. S. *et al.*), pp. 571–80. W. B. Saunders Company, Philadelphia.
40. Tobis, J. S., Reinsch, S., Swanson, J. M., Byrd, M., and T. Scharf. (1985). Visual perception dominance of fallers among community-dwelling adults. *Journal of the American Geriatrics Society*, **33**, 330–1.
41. Owen, D. H. (1985). Maintaining posture and avoiding tripping: optical information for detecting and controlling orientation and locomotion. In *Clinics in Geriatric Medicine*, Vol. 1, No. 3 (ed. Radebaugh, T. S. *et al.*) W. B. Saunders Company, Philadelphia, pp. 581–600.
42. Overstall, P. W. (1985). Epidemiology and pathophysiology of falls. In *Fits, faints and falls in old age.* (ed. Kataria, S. M.) pp. 15–26. MTP, Lancaster.
43. Tinetti, M. E., Williams, T. F., and Mayewski, R. (1986). A fall risk index for elderly patients based on number of chronic disabilities. *American Journal of Medicine*, **80**, 429–34.
44. Honrubia, V. and Brazier, M. (ed.) (1982). *Nystagmus and vertigo: clinical approaches to the patient with dizziness.* Academic Press, New York.
45. Nashner, L. M. (1977). Fixed patterns of rapid postural responses among the muscles during stance. *Experimental Brain Research*, **30**, 13–24.
46. Lipsitz, L. (1985). Abnormalities in blood pressure homeostosis that contribute to falls in the elderly. In *Clinics in Geriatric Medicine.* Vol. 1, No. 3 (ed. Radebaugh, T. S. *et al.*) pp. 637–48 W. B. Saunders Company, Philadelphia.
47. Davie, J. W., Blumenthal, M. D., and Robinson–Hawkins, S. (1981). A model of risk of falling for psychogeriatric patients. *Archives of General Psychiatry*, **38**, 463–7.

48. Macdonald, J. B. (1985). The role of drugs in falls in the elderly. In *Clinics in Geriatric Medicine*, Vol. 1, No. 3 (ed. Radebaugh, T. S. *et al.*), pp. 621–36 W. B. Saunders Company, Philadelphia.
49. Waller, J. A. (1974). Injury in the aged: clinical and epidemiological implications. *New York State Journal of Medicine*, **74**, 2200–8.
50. Gabell, A., Nayak, U.S.L., and Isaacs, B. Gait, balance and falls in healthy old people. In preparation.
51. Kinsman, R. (1983). Falls in the elderly. Unpublished audit. Barnet Health Authority, London.
52. Waller, J. A. (1978). Falls among the elderly—human and environmental factors. *Accident Analysis and Prevention*, **10**.
53. Cohn, T. E. and Lasley, D. J. (1985). Visual depth illusion and falls in the elderly. In *Clinics in Geriatric Medicine*. Vol. 1, No. 3 (ed. Radebaugh, T. S. *et al.*), pp 601–20 W. B. Saunders Company, Philadelphia.
54. Archea, J. C. (1985). Environmental factors associated with stair accidents by the elderly. In *Clinics in Geriatric Medicine*. Vol. 1, No. 3 (ed. Radebaugh, T. S. *et al.*), pp. 555–70 W. B. Saunders Company, Philadelphia.
55. Brody, E. M., Kleban, M. H., Moss, M. S., and Kleban, F. (1984). Predictors of falls among institutionalized women with Alzheimer's Disease. *Journal of the American Geriatrics Society*, **32**, 877–82.

19

Prevention in the aging

A. M. DAVIES

INTRODUCTION

This review is based on the premise that the objective of care of the elderly 'is to help old people remain as independent as possible for as long as possible and to offer them as much control over their lives as possible'.[1] Preventive activities therefore must address themselves to pathological processes and to the normal frailties of old age, as well as to the social and physical environment which could enhance or ameliorate their effects. The distinction between prevention and cure becomes academic.

At ages 70 to 80, classical approaches to prevention must be modified. The possibilities for primary prevention are very few and the distinctions between secondary prevention (early diagnosis to stop the progress of disease) and tertiary prevention (adequate treatment of established disease to diminish disability) become blurred.[2] The end point prevention must be defined if it is to be monitored.[3] Delay of death, limitation of disability, and maintenance of well-being, for instance, are among the desired results of early intervention. Discussing these and other outcomes, the WHO Scientific Group,[4] in a search for a global end point for epidemiological use, proposed maintenance of autonomy as the basic requirement of the elderly, and prevention of its loss as the objective of intervention programmes. The concept has been amplified by Grimley Evans in a stimulating article,[5] but its practical application requires the development of standard definitions and measurements. A wide range of more specific objectives has been used in the literature, from the prevention of influenza to delay in admission to a nursing home. The vast majority of them, however, can only be achieved using multiple routes of intervention. Much of this intervention requires social support, public changes of attitude, and manipulation of the environment, in addition to the activities directed to the individual—that is, the holistic approach to prevention embodied in the new 'health promotion'.[6] For most elderly individuals, the objective is not prevention of a specific disease—it is often too late for that—but prevention of progression of the disease to disability, handicap, or death.[7] To put it another way: what strategy should be employed to maintain autonomy as long as possible in spite of the presence of disease?

THE PREVENTABLE CONDITIONS

This section considers the conditions due to disease, the health services, and the environment common in old age that have potential for prevention.

Cardiovascular disease

Heart disease and stroke increase in incidence with age, and are by far the most commonly certified causes of death in the elderly,[8] being over half the causes of death in the statistics of developed countries.[9] Circulatory diseases account for a third of hospital admissions over the age of 65, and more than a quarter of visits to the doctor.

The same risk factors that predict mortality in middle age, such as hypertension, smoking, and blood lipids, continue to operate in old age, but the degree of their association is much reduced. Current opinion on their importance is based on associations in a few longitudinal observations, as most population studies stop at age 55 or 59. It is not known whether changes in the risk factor at higher ages will still affect mortality, nor even whether the factor can be manipulated. apart from the European study of the treatment of hypertension in the elderly,[10] there are as yet no data from controlled clinical trials or attempts to reduce any of the risk factors in the seventh and eighth decades.

The European trial was able to demonstrate differences in cardiovascular mortality between treated and untreated groups of hypertensives aged 60 and over. The benefits of treatment were independent of level of blood-pressure at entry, and were significantly related to systolic (but not diastolic) pressure achieved. The effect of treatment decreases with age and little or no benefit could be demonstrated in patients, mainly women, over the age of 80.[11]

A consensus conference of the US National Heart, Lung and Blood Institute recently reviewed the evidence for the continued effect of risk factors and the efficacy of preventive measures.[12] It withheld judgement on the effect on cardiovascular diseases of the treatment of systolic hypertension, and underlined the current lack of knowledge on the effect of stopping cigarette smoking, blood lipid reduction, weight reduction, or physical activity in the elderly. It did, however, point out other benefits of reduction of obesity and of physical activity.

On the other hand, there may be some survival value in being overweight; in some studies, fat hypertensives seem to be at lesser risk for cardiovascular outcomes.[13] Much depends on the population studied and whether the end point measured is cardiovascular disease or cardiovascular-associated 'other events'. For instance, in a 6-year follow-up of 1223 elderly persons, Branch and Jette[14] found significant association between the risk of dying and health behaviour, including physical activity, regularity of meals, cigarette smoking, and use of alcohol. They did not report specifically on cardiovascular deaths; however, in a longitudinal study of 2674 individuals aged 65–74 Jajich *et al.*[15] showed a decrease in deaths from coronary heart in those who stopped smoking cigarettes, compared with smokers. There is a clear need for controlled intervention studies in representative samples of elderly with clearly defined outcomes.

A recent consultation of the World Health Organization again reviewed the evidence and underlined the uncertainty of specific preventive interventions. However, some general recommendations for the prevention of cardiovascular diseases have implications for general well-being and the prevention of other conditions.[13] These include a prudent diet, reduction of gross obesity, stopping smoking, exercise, and social activities.

Death from cancers

There is a considerable increase in incidence and mortality from cancer of specific sites with age; cancers are the second most common cause of death up to age 85 and the third thereafter. For males aged 75 and over, the three leading cancer sites are lung, prostate, and colorectum; for females they are colorectum, breast, and lung.[9, 16] The rules for early detection are the same as in the middle aged: tests for occult blood, breast examination, cervical smears, and investigation of persons with specific symptoms. However, little is known of the benefits, risks, and feasibility of cancer screening in the elderly, although some experts recommend annual examination for colorectal cancer in both sexes, and breast and cervical examinations in women.[17, 18] As Kennie[19] points out, a finding of even a trace of blood in the stool, which could be due to several causes, mandates an extensive work-up, such as sigmoidoscopy, colonoscopy, and barium enemas, which, with the attendant bowel preparation, can be traumatic for the elderly. Elderly women are likely to be lifelong non-users or under-users of screening for cancer of the cervix, even in areas where the cervical smear is accepted and freely available.[20] Women at the highest risk of cervical cancer are least likely (in the USA) to have been screened.[21] They are also less likely to have had a routine breast examination by a physician or to perform self examination of the breasts, or even to have been instructed in its method, compared with the middle aged.[22] They are also unlikely to respond to an invitation to come to a screening examination, particularly if it does not come from their own doctor (see below).

Thus, breast examination at the time of a patient-initiated consultation can be recommended, as can a careful history, to detect suspicious signs and symptoms of any cancer. However, the efficacy, benefit, and cost-effectiveness of routine screening procedures do not justify their use in the elderly, or at any rate in the oldest old.

Osteoporosis

Osteopososis—diminution of bone tissue mass to the extent that fractures can occur with minimal trauma—is a heterogenous disease with multiple causes.[23] Fractures from osteoporosis are eight times more common in women than in men, the main problem being fracture of the hip, which causes considerable morbidity, mortality, and cost to the health care system.

The major risk factors in women include age, race (white more than black in the United States and in South Africa), thinness, premature menopause, low calcium intake, inactivity, smoking, and excessive alcohol intake.[23, 24]

Preventive activities have centred around calcium replacement, with or without supplementary oestrogens, and exercise. Calcium is important for the young skeleton and for those with low intake and negative calcium balance, but its effectiveness in reducing bone loss after menopause is slight or nil.[25] The NIH consensus conference[26] recommended that the daily calcium intake of premenopausal women should be 1.0 g, and of postmenopausal women at least 1.5 g, but there has been no support for this from subsequent studies.[26, 27] The most recent Danish randomized trial showed that bone mineral content in postmenopausal women fell significantly over 2 years in those given either 2g calcium or placebo daily.[28] However, evidence is accumulating on the importance of the precise formulation of the calcium supplement: calcium citrate is better absorbed than calcium carbonate in individuals with hypochlorhydria, and calcium with glucose is better than calcium with sorbitol. Much remains to be done in clarifying mechanisms of calcium absorption and metabolism in the elderly. In the Danish study, administration of 17-beta-oestradiol prevented bone loss, confirming earlier studies that oestrogens prevent osteoporosis and fractures.[23, 25]

A further reason to give oestrogens to postmenopausal women is the hope that cardiovascular disease will be reduced,[27] although there is a small but definite risk of endometrial cancer and, perhaps, venous thrombosis.[25] Complications are dose-related and it is possible that the dose can be reduced if combined with exercise—itself another therapeutic strategy that is logical, recommended, and unproved. Here, too, the type and formulation of the oestrogen could be important. Other preventive strategies—calcitonin, fluoride, and vitamin D metabolites—have advocates, but as yet there are no definitive answers from controlled clinical trials.

Attention should be paid to prophylaxis in high-risk categories, and calcium from milk products could be better absorbed than that from other types of supplement. However, large-scale bone mineral screening to detect individuals at special risk is still expensive, inaccurate, and a poor predictor of fractures.[29, 30]

Accidents, falls, and fractures

In the United States, injuries are the sixth most common cause of death in adults aged 75 and over, with falls the leading source of such deaths.[31] Measurement of the frequency of falls is very difficult, but one estimate is an annual incidence of 140 per 1000 aged 65–75, and an increase with age.[32] Eighty to ninety per cent of fatal home accidents in the elderly result directly from falls. Another detailed review of falls in later life reports that 20–45 per cent of those aged 65 and over in different countries report at least one fall in the past year, as do 50 per cent aged 80 and over.[33] It is estimated that 1–6 per cent of falls produce fractures—in old women mainly of the neck of the femur; however, if many falls are unreported this proportion may be lower. Statistics are not very good and vary greatly from country to country. It is generally accepted that, in the elderly, fatal accidents increase with age, that 20–25 per cent are traffic accidents and the rest take place elsewhere, mainly in the home.[34, 35]

Road accident statistics are better, and the oldest drivers have a higher accident rate than any other age group over 25, especially if this is calculated on the basis of distance travelled. Most are attributable to errors in perception and judgement, rather than to speed or alcohol.[36] The high rate of accidents in elderly pedestrians is similarly attributed to slowness in walking and reaction time, and such environmental hazards as too-short road-crossing times.[33, 36, 37]

Most accidents are not fatal, take place in the home, and are due to falls. Those at special risk are women over 75 years of age, living alone, and having a history of previous falls. Falling is associated with chronic illness, particularly arthritis and foot problems, and environmental hazards, such as poor lighting, frayed carpets, and lack of hand-holds. Falls and their consequences are particularly common in residents of institutions (perhaps the recording is better), and many of the episodes are attributed, as in the home, to mental confusion due to sleeping tablets and other drugs. Prevention programmes are directed both to the individual and to the environment.[33, 35, 38]

For the frequent faller, there must be clinical evaluation of causes, tests of balance and gait, and exercises to improve them. Advice on shoes and spectacles is part of rehabilitation. In institutions, design of the environment to prevent falls is important, with staff awareness and proper dressing of residents. In and out of institutions, attention must be paid to those people receiving medications which reduce alertness.[38] Environmental hazards can be reduced by adequate lighting, particularly during the night, aids to mobility and safety, such as rails and canes with non-skid tips, non-skid mats on the floor and in the bath, and raised toilet seats with handholds.

Outside the home, there is need to increase pedestrian crossways, with central islands to protect the slow where roads are wide. Better lighting, steps on buses, improvement of pavement surfaces, clearer signs, and colours easier of interpretation have all been proposed. Note that measures to reduce traffic accidents in the elderly benefit all ages.[32, 36]

While these measures are logical, it must be pointed out that there is no objective evidence that exercises to improve gait actually reduce the frequency of falls, nor have there been any carefully evaluated community intervention programmes for the prevention of falls and fractures. The cost-effectiveness of different procedures is thus unknown.

Deficiencies in sight, hearing, and chewing

The most common accompaniments of old age, these deficiencies are the most neglected. They are conditions where early intervention is often simple and can greatly improve the quality of life.

Sight

The problems of vision changes with age are dealt with elsewhere in the volume. Reference is made here to the normal changes with age, including presbyopia and changing hyperopic or myopic status, causing a quarter to a half of the elderly in different surveys to report difficulty in seeing to read.[4] There is thus need to check whether spectacles are worn, and if so whether they are currently suitable and kept clean. It is also important to detect other underlying pathology, thus raising the question of the desirability of periodic routine ophthalmological examinations.

Hearing

One-third to a half of those interviewed in the WHO Eleven Country Study reported difficulty in hearing what a single speaker says, and more

had difficulty with group conversations.[39] The proportion of those needing elevated levels of speech is 50 per cent at ages 75–79, and 60 per cent
at 85–89. In Denmark, where counselling and hearing aids have been
freely available for many years, 15–20 per cent of those aged 70 and over
have hearing aids, with no change over time.[40]

There are no agreed standards for the definition of hearing handicap,
and the difference between self-rating and measured impairment is great.
This may contribute to the delay, often of several years, between suspi-
cion of need and the fitting of a hearing aid.

For some hard-of-hearing people there is no reduction in daily activity
(watching television, mobility, and personal and family contacts), although they report greater handicap.[40] There are, however, individuals
who are particularly affected by hearing loss and who gain special relief
from hearing aids.[41] Many so handicapped tend to withdraw from social
contact and can become depressed, so that there is a need for social and
psychological counselling of the hard of hearing. In addition to treatment of the individual, the hard of hearing of all ages can be assisted by
environmental aids, louder telephone and door bells, telephone amplifiers, and availability of augmented headphones in cinemas and other
public places. Sympathetic professional and public opinion are essential
elements of prevention.[40, 41]

Chewing

Twelve to 60 per cent in the Eleven Country Study reported difficulty in
chewing, while the proportion with dentures increased with age to 87 per
cent in the highest age groups of both sexes.[39] Although an increasing
proportion of elderly do have their own teeth,[43] the main problems
are those of the edentate. A high proportion have ill-fitting dentures or
dentures in need of repair, and most of the elderly examined in one
typical study were in need of urgent dental attention.[42] Bone involution
of the jaw is common in old age and dentures several years old do not fit
snugly and may need modifying. If uncomfortable, the elder may remove
them to eat and modify the diet accordingly. If extremely uncomfortable,
they may not be worn at all, and the sufferer, usually a woman, shuns
company and seeks isolation with its attendant dangers.

Therefore an oral examination of the state of the oral mucosa and of
the remaining teeth, as well as the good fit of the denture, is an essential
part of the clinical assessment of the elderly.[43] Early intervention can
prevent much misery.

Infections

Deterioration in immunological defences against infections, and a lowering of the humoral response to immunization, are characteristics of nor-

mal aging.[44] The importance of influenza and pneumonia as causes of death of the old provides an opportunity—the only opportunity—for the practice of primary prevention in this age group. Immunization against these two diseases has been widely recommended,[1, 16, 19] although the proportion of the population accepting immunization is low both in and out of long-term care institutions.

There is clear evidence of the efficacy of influenza vaccine in the elderly in nursing homes in the face of an epidemic—provided, of course, that the vaccine is of appropriate strain—with protection against clinical disease, hospitalization, and death.[45] The newer purified vaccines may be better, but there is still need for evaluation of their efficacy in the community.[46]

Pneumonia due to *Streptococcus pneumoniae* infection has a high fatality in hospitalized elderly,[47] but the severity and case fatality is probably much lower in the general population.[48] Trials of a vaccine, which contains the 14 pneumococcal polysaccharide antigens responsible for over 70 per cent of cases, have proved disappointing, with a protective efficacy 'very low to zero'.[44, 49] Moreover side-effects, though mild, are common, and these facts do not justify pressing for immunization against pneumococcal infection as a routine procedure.

Iatrogenic disease and physician neglect

Kane *et al.* point out that 'iatrogenic illnesses are probably the most common preventable disease in old age'.[16] These include drug reactions, enthusiastic medical investigation, neglect of 'minor' functional problems, and, in institutions, nosocomial infections, loss of mobility, and dependency.[16, 19] The sins are both of omission and of commission. Many conditions of the elderly are missed by physicians due to lack of interest or skills (see below), or may not be reported by the elderly through not being seen as relevant to the scope of medical care.[1] Physicians are likely not to look at hearing, vision, teeth or feet, and thus miss many opportunities for preventive care. Most independent surveys of the elderly reveal new, treatable conditions unknown to their physicians.[1, 19, 49, 50, 51]

In the United Kingdom, the United States, and Israel the elderly are more likely to receive drugs than younger patients,[16, 52] and to buy more drugs over the counter. In some patients these will have side-effects, such as confusion and blurred vision, as well as organ-specific effects, and in turn they can potentiate falls, depression, and isolation.[16, 33] Better education in appropriate prescribing behaviour, smaller doses, and frequent symptom review are some of the strategies that have been proposed to overcome this problem.

Physicians may tend to see the elderly as stereotypes and view work with old patients as uninteresting and unrewarding even in the United

Kingdom, which has pioneered good clinical geriatrics.[1, 52] Doctors over 40 are unlikely to have had any formal training in the care of the elderly, and thus to be exposed to the new knowledge, attitudes, and practice incorporated in good geriatric medicine (see below). But the situation in long-term care facilities may not be much better, and problems relating to eyes, teeth, feet, hearing, and mental state may go undiagnosed.[16, 53]

Admission to an institution

For many frail elderly, admission to a nursing home offers the best, sometimes the only, solution. And if the care offered is of a high standard, so much the better. But admission to an institution is frequently neither desirable from the elder's point of view, nor the best solution professionally—and so, wherever possible, it becomes a potentially preventable state.

The disadvantages of institutional care are lack of autonomy and loneliness, together with an increased risk of nosocomial infections, enforced immobility, falls, and confusion.[19, 53, 54] On the other hand, keeping an old person at home requires appropriate space and facilities, social support, and the availability of professional services of different kinds. The groups at greatest risk for admission in one study were the very old, those living alone, those recently discharged from hospital, the divorced or separated, and those who had recently moved.[55] Age, female sex, poverty, and lack of social support also characterize those admitted in other settings.[16] Longitudinal studies following up cohorts of elderly people to measure risks of admission prospectively are rare, and the availability and accessibility of long-term care facilities within the health care system are additional variables which will need to be taken into account.[56]

Improvements of home care services with preventive visiting have been shown to reduce the need for admission to hospital in Denmark and Britain.[57, 58, 59] These experiments were organized within the framework of prepaid primary care services with doctor–nurse teams and close collaboration with social support services. Frequent home visits by health personnel led to increased confidence, distribution of aids, modifications to homes, and more home help. In the Danish study, the savings in bed-days were twice the additional cost of the intervention.

THE ROLES OF SERVICE PROVIDERS

The approach to the care of the elderly, and thus to prevention, is ideally a combination of the contributions of several professionals, including the doctor, nurse, social worker, dentist, pharmacist, physiotherapist, occupational therapist, and chiropodist, supported by homemakers, family, neighbours, and volunteers, and backed up where necessary by medical and surgical specialists.

It is beyond the scope of this review to detail the role of each in preventing disease and further disability, other than to emphasize the need for a team approach. Mobilization of support for the old person will require both an understanding of the role of each provider of service and of the organized structure of the health and social service frameworks in which they operate. Traditionally, the physician has assumed the role of leader of the team, but this is by no means essential; other professionals, particularly social workers and nurses, have taken the lead in different service models. In particular, in the Netherlands and Denmark nurses play a prominent role in health visiting, in comprehensive appraisal of the needs of elderly people, and in the introduction of preventive regimens.

'Good geriatric medicine'

The physician practising geriatric medicine is different from his physician colleagues; he 'must endeavour to treat the physical, mental and social illnesses of his patients' and must take a leading role in a multidisciplinary care team.[60] His training must thus be different to provide him with the necessary skills, and the organization of the health and social services must be such as to facilitate mobilization of the resources. The point has been made above that doctors over 40 are unlikely to have received formal training in care of the elderly, and several generations will be in need of postgraduate training.

The preventive nature of good geriatric practice is emphasized in modern texts, as is the need to assess functional loss, not only pathology, and to strive for health maintenance.[1, 19, 54, 61, 62] Given such an holistic approach to the care of the elderly, it is impossible to separate preventive activities, particularly secondary and tertiary prevention, from the traditional practice of medicine, so that preventive care is dependent on good curative care.

All agree that examples of good geriatric medicine are uncommon, and examples of physician neglect have been given earlier. Factors militating against the practice of good medicine can be identified in the doctor, in the patient, and in the system.

The traditional curative doctor sees patients only when called. Unless trained, he does not know how to diagnose and treat the elderly, and may not be particularly interested in an aspect of medicine that is 'unrewarding'. Moreover, he does not handle 'non-medical' aspects of practice, but may, if aware of the need, refer else where. There is thus an attitude and belief system that is difficult to change.[1, 52]

The old person is often fatalistic with a belief system that leads him or her to expect aches, pains, and disabling conditions as the price of aging. Certain conditions such as cardiac and respiratory symptoms or acute pains are recognized as being within the compass of medical care, and these are reported to the doctor. Others, such as locomotor, sensory, and sphincter problems, are frequently unreported,[1, 4, 39] and unless sought by the doctor will be neglected. The system of health care and constraints on physician's time often diminish the chances of meaningful doctor–patient contact. A shortage of nurses will lessen the chances of home assessment and supervised preventive regimens, while the separation of health and welfare agencies causes additional bureaucratic barriers.

Many models of health care for the elderly have been developed in different countries, usually by enthusiasts, to overcome these problems, but they are still models and most of the world's elderly are badly served. The application of new knowledge and the preventive approach will require changes both in professional attitudes and in the organization of services for the elderly.

Screening and case finding

Any population of elderly will have much undetected treatable disease awaiting discovery, and many different approaches have been proposed to bring it to light.

Rogers *et al.*[63] have recently refined the health goals of Breslow and Somers[64] into proposed criteria for a health-screening programme. Such a programme would determine the presence or absence of prevalent problems, detect previously unknown or untreated conditions, and facilitate development of a comprehensive plan to maximize the quality of life. The concepts are reasonable, but only 7 per cent of 5000 Blue Cross subscribers who were invited actually participated in the scheme, which was organized independently of the normal channels of medical care.

In Britain and Northern Europe, screening has been performed by the general practitioner or by a nurse attached to the practice. The main thrust has been the development of a cost-effective approach, conserving the time of the physician, and the response rate has been high.[1, 65, 66] In the United States, population screening has been offered as a research project with a much lower response rate.[63, 67, 68] Organization and success of screening activities depend very much on the organizational pattern of health care.

As already stated, the distinction between screening and case finding in the elderly is irrelevant. One doctor's case finding is another's good medicine, but outside the interest or competence of a third. In Britain, 90 per cent of those over 75 visit their doctor at least annually, and the rest are probably well, so that screening can be left to opportunistic case detection at the next visit.[66] In the United States and much of Europe, up to 30 per cent of the elderly may not see the doctor each year,[4, 39] and if screening is desirable then these must be reached.

There are no comparative studies as to the validity, efficacy, and cost-effectiveness of different screening methods, nor a consensus as to the content of such an examination.[69] The questions asked and the tests done vary greatly, from the identification in individuals at risk of break-down to disease diagnosis packages.[65, 70]

The strategy of screening

This is dependent on the health care system and varies widely. Barber[65] sent a letter to the elderly in his practice with nine questions requiring a 'yes' or 'no' answer. The questions were: do you live alone? are you without a relative who could be called for help? are you dependent on someone for regular help? are there days without a hot meal? are you confined to the house due to ill health? is there concern or difficulty with your health? is there difficulty with your vision? is there difficulty with your hearing? and have you been hospitalized during past year? The response was excellent, and a positive answer to any question indicated a patient at risk and in need of assessment. Follow-up was by a health visitor, who in that practice needed 11 hours weekly for updating and surveillance. This is excessive, considering the constraints on British general practice;[52, 66] the burden could be reduced by confining the prog-ramme to those aged 80 or 85 and over. For the others, a high-risk profile might suffice, identifying the elderly with the following characteristics: lives alone, widowed within past 2 years, hospitalized during past year, housebound, registered blind, or has major physical difficulties.

Other strategies involved home visits by public health nurses, solicited and not,[51] inviting patients to see the doctor, and telephoned surveys.[22] Rubenstein *et al.*[67] followed up elderly clients who had come to a com-munity centre for a check-up; 54 per cent had been referred to their physicians for advice or intervention, but only 70 per cent of these went, and 38 per cent (15 per cent of the entire group) received treatment. One approach to save professional time now being tested is the use of a new WHO minimal screening questionnaire by lay volunteers with built-in 'alarms' so that a positive answer to defined questions would trigger a visit and assessment by nurse or social worker.

The criteria for screening

These include validity of the detection manoeuvre, the existence of an intervention of proved efficacy in the elderly, and benefit to the patient rather than merely to an intermediate end point.[19] Williamson[1] gives a checklist of items for detection and action by a nurse observer which include social and environmental conditions and checks of health problems. Others, following Barber,[65] propose undefined medical work-ups to those in high-risk groups, although the selection of the subset is not sensitive or specific.[66] The consensus in Britain and Canada tends toward opportunistic case finding by the general practitioner. On the content of screening programmes, the Canadian Task Force defined 128 potentially preventable conditions, of which only 16 were considered to be screenable; for only 6 of these there was sufficient evidence of efficacy to include them. These six were dental caries, hypertension, and various immunizations.[71]

In summary, therefore, there is insufficient evidence to justify mass screening of the elderly for the detection of disease and disability. There is full agreement on the need for maintaining the health of the elderly by the health team, but no suggestions as to what might be done for those whose access to health care is limited.

MAINTENANCE OF PERSONAL HEALTH

While, ideally, promotion of health and the establishment of healthy lifestyles should start in infancy and continue throughout life, there is already abundant evidence that it is never too late to promote health or to delay disability. Much of this evidence, however, is based more on tradition than on scientific inquiry, although a good deal is suggested by clinical experience.

Healthy lifestyles

If changes in lifestyle make people feel better and do no harm, there would seem to be no advantage in waiting until their effect has been demonstrated objectively before recommending them. The main guidelines to a healthy lifestyle include:

A prudent diet

Diet should be sufficient to maintain normal weight and avoid obesity, and include plenty of vegetables and fruit. Fat consumption should be restricted and preference given to vegetable oils. Salt intake should probably be limited to no more than 5 g a day, while an increased intake of calcium-containing foods (preferably milk products) is recommended.[8, 72] Education in the choice of desirable foods may be called for, and guidance in the selection of prepared, convenience foods.

Weight control

Gross overweight limits mobility, strains cardiac function, and increases the risk of hypertension and premature death. For the very fat, therefore, efforts should be made to lose weight by diet and exercise. Group activities hold most promise of success (see below).

Exercise

This should be exercise started earlier in life, and should be continued as long as possible for its beneficial effects on self-esteem, mobility, car-diovascular function, osteoporosis, and longevity.[2, 8, 23, 73, 74] For the wholly sedentary, it is never too late to start gentle exercise, while the health, age, and lifestyle of the individual will determine how strenuous it can become.

Smoking cigarettes

Smoking is harmful at any age, and every effort should be made to give up the habit, or at the very least to reduce it considerably. Even at ages over 70, continued smoking is a risk factor for heart and respiratory disease and for osteoporosis.[8, 13, 75]

Social life and social contacts

These improve the quality of life and stimulate mental and physical activity. The kinds of activity where the elderly meet each other and engage in pleasurable and educational activities can provide peer pressure and support for changes in health behaviour.

Other good health habits

Often recommended are adequate sleep, eating of breakfast and regular meals, mental stimulation, hobbies, and keeping of pets.

Use of medicaments and alcohol

The elderly are enthusiastic consumers of medicines, both prescribed and purchased over the counter, and often need education and support in reducing their intake. Professional guidance is important in good pre-scribing and in advice concerning bowel habits and sleep.[16]

Alcohol abuse by the elderly may be misdiagnosed as senility and be a cause of serious accidents. Its frequency may be increasing in elderly population in the United States and Sweden, but there is evidence that elderly alcoholics respond to treatment better than do young patients.[76, 77, 78]

Control of the immediate environment

In every country the old, more than others, tend to live in poor-quality, run-down housing with diminished protection from heat, cold, or damp, and increased risk of accidents. Suitable domicile is particularly important to the elderly, who often live alone and spend most of their time there. Adaptations to the house, weather-proofing, the provision of practical domestic aids to daily living, and appropriately designed equipment can make life much easier for those with restricted mobility. Of particular importance are non-skid surfaces, adequate lighting, uncluttered rooms, and, where necessary, hand holds, raised toilets, and the possibility of preparing food sitting down.[33, 79, 80, 81] Modification of dwellings is an important goal for volunteer support groups.

Support groups—the self-care movement

'Self care activities in the elderly have potential, not only for treatment of disease, but even more for prevention and treatment of disability and dysfunction'.[82] The world-wide trend toward associations of individuals for mutual help includes the elderly, and such groups can play an important role in social support, particulary of those who live alone. Self-care groups take many forms, from those organized with professional direction for prevention or treatment of defined conditions, to purely voluntary fraternities for social intercourse. While their programme goals differ widely, such groups can play an important educational and supportive role in the changing of health behaviour and provide consumer pressure in such areas as improving the quality of goods and the standard of medical care available to the old.[83, 84, 85]

HEALTH PROMOTION IN THE COMMUNITY

Public concern for the rights and welfare of the elderly is an essential precondition for the mobilization of resources for their care, and for the facilitation of preventive measures.

Rights of the elderly

Butler has cogently described the existence and consequences of negative stereotypes of the elderly.[86] To improve their status and well-being, all societies must adopt active measures to counter 'agism' and accept that aged persons form a heterogeneous group each entitled to equity in their own right.[74, 87, 88] The first step is, therefore, a change in the attitudes and behaviour of society, for the sentiments can be pervasive and detrimental.[89] In recent years the realization that institutional life is not necessarily the only or the best solution for the frail elderly and that there are desirable alternatives in the form of services in the community has led to a change in thinking of ways to organize support for the elderly in their own homes. Emerging models of professional, local, and voluntary services are being extended to include the support of the independent elderly in the community.

Social support

Support of the elderly, an essential component of prevention, requires measures to foster independence, of which retirement pensions, arrangements for continued employment, and flexible retirement ages are but the beginning. Descriptions of the many forms of social and community support which have been proposed and tested form a growing literature. They include social centres, home help, assistance with shopping and cooking, help with housing repairs, and a wide range of voluntary activities, all designed to help elders to stay in their own homes as long and as independently as possible. Such help also includes the services offered by the various formal agencies and the informal support network of family, neighbours, and friends.[90] Facilities for continued education ('university of the third age') both for groups and for individuals at home are powerful aids to continued mental activity.

Special facilities

Special facilities for the elderly that are important for the maintenance of autonomy include physical arrangements to permit their full participation in social activities, and subsidies to help them. Examples are barrier-free access to public transport (steps on buses) and public buildings (ramps and elevators), maintenance of pavement surfaces, lighted streets, clear signposting, adequate pedestrian crossings, and so on. Many countries offer cheap transport at certain hours, and entrance to places of public entertainment at reduced cost.

These physical helps to the mobility of the elderly also help the handicapped of all ages and, in the long run, the whole community.

SUMMARY

Prevention in old age requires a multifaceted, multisectorial approach which includes social support and environmental changes, as well as the pursuit of a healthy lifestyle by the individual and the care of health professionals.

There is evidence that a prudent diet, reduction of gross obesity, stopping cigarette smoking, active exercise, and participation in social activities will improve the general standard of health, and may reduce mortality from cardiovascular disease and the severity of osteoporosis. The fact that controlled clinical trials have not yet been undertaken in the prevention of most of the detriments of age means that there is little scientific justification for many recommended procedures. However, early treatment for the common afflictions of mobility, sight, hearing, and chewing will prevent much misery, and good medical care will include many elements of prevention and early diagnosis.

Scientific study of the efficacy of prevention by different forms of intervention will require operational definitions of autonomy and other desirable 'end points' and standardization of their measurement. But whatever specific preventive measures are found to be efficacious, promotion of the health of the elderly will require fulfilment of three cardinal conditions. The first is the recognition by society of the rights of the old to equity, and a willingness to provide the basic financial, housing, social, and environmental conditions essential for their well-being. The second is the willingness of members of the healing professions to learn and practice good geriatric medicine, which is inseparable from prevention. And the third is an administrative organization which facilitates optimal mobilization of resources for the best combination of prevention and care.

References

1. Williamson, J. (1985). Preventive medicine and old age. In *Textbook of geriatric medicine and gerontology* (ed. Brocklehurst, J. C.) (3rd ed), pp. 1011–20. Churchill-Livingstone, Edinburgh, London.
2. Morris, J. N. (1975). *Uses of epidemiology*, (3rd ed). Churchill Livingstone, Edinburgh, London.
3. Kane, R. L. (1988). Empiric approaches to prevention in the elderly: are we promoting too much? In *Health promotion and disease prevention in the elderly* (ed. Chernoft, R. and D. A. Lipschitz). Raven, New York, NY.
4. World Health Organization (1984). *The uses of epidemiology in the study of the elderly*. Technical Report Series, **706** Report of a WHO Scientific Group, Geneva.
5. Grimley Evans, J. (1984). Prevention of age-associated loss of autonomy: epidemiological approaches. *Journal of Chronic Diseases*, **37**, 353–63.
6. Kickbusch, I. (1986). Health promotion, a global perspective. *Canadian Journal of Public Health*, **77**, 321–6.
7. World Health Organization (1980). *International classification of impairments, disabilities and handicaps*. WHO, Geneva.
8. Strasser, T. (ed.) (1987). *Cardiovascular care of the elderly*. World Health Organization, Geneva.

9. Lopez, A. D. and Hanada, K. (1982). Mortality patterns and trends among the elderly in developed countries. *World Health Statistics Quarterly*, **35**, 203–24.

10. European Working Party on High Blood Pressure in the Elderly (1985). An international trial of antihypertensive therapy in elderly patients. Objectives, protocol and organization. *Archives International Pharmacodynamie Therapie*, **275**, 300–85.

11. Amery, A., Brixxo, R., Clement, D. *et al.* (1986). Efficacy of antihypertensive drug treatment according to age, sex, blood pressure and previous cardiovascular disease in patients over the age of 60. *Lancet*, **ii**, 589–92.

12. Chesney, M. A. (1986). Primary and secondary prevention of coronary heart disease in the elderly: Report of working group II. In *Coronary heart disease in the elderly* (ed. Wegner, N. K., C. D. Furberg, and E. Pitt), pp. 211–29. Elsevier, New York.

13. World Health Organization (1987). *CVD/AGE meeting on prevention of cardiovascular diseases among the elderly*. March, Geneva.

14. Branch, L. G. and Jette, A. M. (1984). Personal health practices and mortality among the elderly. *American Journal of Public Health*, **74**, 1126–9.

15. Jajich, C. L., Ostfeld, A. M., and Freeman, D. H. (1984). Smoking and coronary heart disease mortality in the elderly. *Journal of the American Medical Association*, **252**, 2831–4.

16. Kane, R. L., Kane, R. A., and Arnold, S. B. (1985). Prevention in the elderly: risk factors. *Health Services Research*, **19**, 945–1006.

17. Stults, B. M. (1986). Preventive cancer care for the elderly. *Frontiers of Radiology Therapy in Oncology*, **20**, 182–91.

18. Banta, H. D. and Luce, B. R. (1983). Assessing the cost effectiveness of prevention. *Journal of Community Health*, **9**, 145–65.

19. Kennie, D. C. (1986). Health maintenance of the elderly. *Clinics in Geriatric Medicine*, **2**, 53–83.

20. Mandelblatt, J., Gopail, I., and Wistreich, M. (1986). Gynecological care of elderly women. Another look at Papanicolaou smear testing. *Journal of the American Medical Association*, **256**, 367–71.

21. Kleinman, J. C. and Kopstein, A. (1981). Who is being screened for cervical cancer? *American Journal of Public Health*, **71**, 73–6.

22. Celentano, D. D., Shapiro, S., and Weisman, C. S. (1982). Cancer preventive screening behaviour among elderly women. *Preventive Medicine*, **11**, 454–63.

23. Riggs, B. L. and Melton III, L. J. (1986). Involutional osteoporosis. *New England Journal of Medicine*, **314**, 1676–86.

24. Lindsay, R. (1985). Prevention of osteoporosis. In *Prevention of disease in the elderly* (ed. Muir Gray, J. A.) pp. 95–113. Churchill Livingstone, Edinburgh London.

25. Smith, R. (1987). Osteoporosis: cause and management. *British Medical Journal*, **294**, 329–32.

26. National Institutes of Health (1984). Osteoporosis: consensus conference. *Journal of the American Medical Association*, **252**, 799–802.

27. Culliton, B. (1987). Osteoporosis reexamined: complexity of bone biology is a challenge. *Science*, **235**, 833–4.

28. Riis, B., Thomsen, K., and Christiansen, C. (1987). Does calcium supplementation prevent postmenopausal bone loss? *New England Journal of Medi-*

cine, **316**, 173–7.
29. Hall, F. M., Davis, M. A., and Baran, D. T. (1987). Bone mineral screening for osteoporosis. *New England Journal of Medicine*, **316**, 212–14.
30. Ott, S. (1986). Should women get screening bone mass measurements? *Annals of Internal Medicine*, **104**, 874–6.
31. Baker, S. P. and Harvey, A. J. (1985). Fall injuries in the elderly. *Clinics in Geriatric Medicine*, **1**, 501–8.
32. Baker, S. L. (1985). The preventability of falls. In *Prevention of disease in the elderly* (ed. Muir Gray, J. A.), pp. 114–29. Churchill Livingstone, Edinburgh-London.
33. Gibson, M. J. *et al.* (1987). The prevention of falls in later life. *Danish Medical Bulletin*, **34**, Suppl. 4.
34. International Center of Social Gerontology (1983). *Medical and social aspects of accidents among the elderly*. Report of a WHO working group in cooperation with ICSG, Paris.
35. World Health Organization (1981). *The epidemiology of accident trauma and resulting disabilities*. Report on a WHO symposium. EURO Reports and Studies **57**. WHO Regional Office for Europe, Copenhagen.
36. Hogue, C. C. (1982). Injury in late life. Part II: Prevention. *Journal of the American Geriatrics Society*, **30**, 276–80.
37. Svanborg, A. (1982). *Epidemiological studies on social and medical conditions of the elderly*. EURO Reports and Studies **62**. WHO Regional Office for Europe, Copenhagen.
38. Kataria, M. S. (ed.) (1985). *Fits, faints and falls in old age*. MTP Press Ltd. Lancaster.
39. Heikkinen, E., Waters, W. E., and Brzezinski, Z. J. *The elderly in eleven countries*. Public Health in Europe, **21**. World Health Organization, Copenhagen.
40. Salomon, G. (1986). Hearing problems and the elderly. *Danish Medical Bulletin*, **33**, Suppl. 3.
41. Herbst, K. R. G. (1982). Deafness, depression, dementia. In *The psychopharmacology of old age* (ed. Wheatley, D.), Oxford University Press, London.
42. Fleishman, R., Peles, D., and Pisanti, S. (1985). Epidemiological study of oral health among the elderly of Baka, a Jerusalem neighborhood. *Israel Journal of Medical Science*, **21**, 270–5.
43. Gordon, S. R. and Jahnigen, D. W. (1986). Oral assessment of the dentulous elderly patient. *Journal of the American Geriatrics Society*, **34**, 276–81.
44. Fox, R. A. (1985). Immunology of aging. In *Textbook of geriatric medicine and gerontology* (ed. Brocklehurst, J. C.), (3rd ed.), pp. 82–104. Churchill Livingstone, Edinburgh, London.
45. Patriarca, P. A., Weber, J. A., Parker, R. A. *et al.* (1985). Efficacy of influenza vaccine in nursing homes. *Journal of the American Medical Association*, **253**, 1136–9.
46. Ruben, F. L. (1985). Prevention of influenza in the elderly. *Journal of the American Geriatrics Society*, **30**, 577.
47. Marrie, T. J., Haldane, E. V., Faulkner, R. S. *et al.* (1985). Community-acquired pneumonia requiring hospitalization. Is it different in the elderly? *Journal of the American Geriatrics Society*, **33**, 671–80.

48. Hirschmann, J. Y. and Lipsky, B. A. (1981). Pneumoccocal vaccine in the United States. *Journal of the American Medical Association*, **246**, 1428.
49. Williamson, J., Stokoe, I. H., Gray, S. *et al.* (1964). Old people at home. Their unreported needs. *Lancet*, **i**, 1117–20.
50. Rubinstein, L. Z., Rhee, L., and Kane, R. L. (1982). The role of geriatric assessment units in caring for the elderly: an analytic review. *Journal of Gerontology*, **37**, 513–21.
51. Harrison, S., Rous, S., Martin, E., and Wilson, S. (1985). Assessing the needs of the elderly using unsolicited visits by health visitors. *Journal of the Royal Society of Medicine*, **78**, 557–61.
52. Thompson, M. K. (1981). Primary care. In *The impending crisis of old age* (ed. Shegog, R. F. A.) pp. 115–25. Oxford University Press London.
53. Tomer, A., Fleishman, R., and Schwartz, R. (1986). *The quality of institutional care: psychosocial aspects*. Discussion paper D–137 Brookdale Institute of Gerontology, Jerusalem.
54. Kane, R. L., Ouslander, J. G., and Abrass, I. B. (1984). *Essentials of clinical geriatrics*. McGraw Hill, New York.
55. Taylor, R., Ford, G., and Barber, H. (1983). *The elderly at risk: A critical review of problems and progress in screening and case finding*. Research perspectives on aging No. 6. Age Concern Research Unit, Mitcham.
56. Beland, F. (1987). Identifying profiles of service requirements in a non-institutionalized elderly population. *Journal Chronic Diseases*, **40**, 51–64.
57. Hendricksen, C., Lund, E., and Strøngård, E. (1984). Consequences of assessment and intervention among elderly people: a three year randomized controlled trial. *British Medical Journal*, **289**, 1522–4.
58. Vetter, N. J., Jones, D. A., and Victor, C. R. (1984). Effect of health visitors working with elderly patients in general practice: a randomized controlled trial. *British Medical Journal*, **288**, 369–72.
59. Tulloch, A. J. and Moore, V. (1979). A randomized controlled trial of geriatric screening and surveillance in general practice. *Journal of the Royal College of General Practitioners*, **29**, 733–42.
60. Anderson, W. F. (1985). An historical overview of geriatric medicine: definition and aims. In *Principles and practice of geriatric medicine* (ed. Pathy, M. S. J.) pp. 7–13. Wiley, Chichester.
61. Pathy, M. S. J. (ed.) (1985). *Principles and practice of geriatric medicine*. Wiley, Chichester.
62. Almind, G., Freer, C., Muir Gray, J. A., and Warshaw, G. (1985). The contribution of the primary care doctor to the medical care of the elderly in the community. *Danish Medical Bulletin*, **32**, Suppl. 2.
63. Rogers, J., Supino, P., and Grower, R. (1986). Proposed evaluation criteria for screening program for the elderly. *Gerontologist*, **26**, 564–70.
64. Breslow, L. and Somers, A. R. (1977). The lifetime health-monitoring program. *New England Journal of Medicine*, **296**, 601–8.
65. Barber, J. H. (1984). Screening and surveillance of the elderly at risk. *Practitioner*, **228**, 269–73.
66. Freer, C. B. (1985). Geriatric screening: a reappraisal of preventive strategies in the care of the elderly. *Journal of the Royal College of General Practitioners*, **35**, 288–90.
67. Rubenstein, L. Z., Josephson, K. R., Nichol Seamons, M., and Robbins, A.

S. (1986). Comprehensive health screenings of well elderly adults: an analysis of a community program. *Journal of Gerontology*, **41**, 342–52.

68. Williams, G. O. and Dueker, D. L. (1985). Non use of free health screening by rural elderly. *American Journal of Preventive Medicine*, **1**, 52–7.

69. World Health Organization (1986). The effectiveness of health promotion for the elderly. Summary report of a WHO Advisory Group, Hamilton, Ontario, Canada.

70. Brodsky, J., Haron, T., Katz, H. and Loval, N. O. (1986). *A look at screening content in preventive health examinations of elderly* Brookdale Institute of Gerontology, Jerusalem.

71. Canadian Task Force on the Periodic Health Examination (1979). The periodic health examination. *Canadian Medical Association Journal*, **121**, 1–45.

72. Schneider, E. L., Vining, E. M., Hadley, E. C., and Farnham, S. A. (1986). Recommended dietary allowance and the health of the elderly. *New England Journal of Medicine*, **314**, 157–60.

73. Muir Gray, J. A., Bassey, E. J., and Young, A. (1985). The risks of inactivity. In *Prevention of disease in the elderly*(ed. Muir Gray, J. A.), pp. 78–94. Churchill Livingstone, Edinburgh.

74. Paffenbarger, R. S., Hyde, R. T., Wing, A. L., and Hsieh, C. C. (1986). Physical activity, all-cause mortality and longevity of college alumni. *New England Journal of Medicine*, **314**, 605–13.

75. Mellström, D. and Svanborg, A. (1987). Tobacco smoking—a major cause of sex differences in health. *Comprehensive Gerontology A*, **1**, 34–9.

76. Hartford, J. T., and Samorajski, T. (1982). Alcoholism in the geriatric population. *Journal of the American Geriatrics Society*, **30**, 18–24.

77. Brody, J. A. (1982). Aging and alcohol abuse. *Journal of the American Geriatrics Society*, **30**, 123–6.

78. Svanborg, A. (1986). Strategies for disease prevention and disability postponement in the elderly. Findings from the longitudinal study. MS prepared for the WHO Advisory Group on the Effectiveness of Health Promotion for the Elderly. Hamilton, Ontario, Canada.

79. United Nations (1982). *Report on the World Assembly on Aging*. Vienna, 26 July to 6 August 1982, A/CONF 113/31. United Nations, New York.

80. Jay, P. (1984). *Coping with disability*, (2nd ed.). Disabled Living Foundation, London.

81. Gloag, D. (1985). Rehabilitation of the elderly. 1. Settings and services. 2. Mind and body. *British Medical Journal*, **290**, 455–7; 542–4.

82. Kane, R. A. and Kane, R. L. (1983). Self care and health care: inseparable but equal for the well being of the old. Paper prepared for the International Symposium on Health and Aging: *European and North American Perspectives on Health Behaviour and Self Care in Old Age*, May 18–20.

83. DeFriese, G. H. and Woomert, A. (1983). Self care among US elderly. Recent developments. *Research on Aging*, **5**, 3–23.

84. World Health Organization (1984). *Self health care and older people*. A manual for public policy and programme development. Unpublished manuscript. WHO Regional Office for Europe, Copenhagen.

85. EURAGE (1986). *Active aging: self help and mutual assistance*, Newsletter **46**. European Federation for the Welfare of the Elderly, Graz, Austria.

86. Butler, R. (1975). *Why survive? Being old in America*. Harper and Row, New York.
87. Birren, J. E., Munnichs, J. M. A., Thomae, H., and Marois, M. (ed.) (1983). *Aging: a challenge to science and society, Vol. 3, Behavioural sciences and conclusions*. Oxford University Press London.
88. Thomae, H. and Maddox, G. L. (ed.) (1983). *New perspectives on old age. A message to decision makers*. Springer, New York.
89. Lutsky, N. S. (1980). Attitudes toward old age and elderly persons. *Annual Review of Gerontology and Geriatrics*, **1**, 287–336.
90. Shuval, J. T., Fleishman, R., and Shmueli, A. (1982). *Informal support for the elderly. Social networks in a Jerusalem neighborhood*. Brookdale Institute of Gerontology, Jerusalem.

Part III

Health care

20

Introduction

R. L. KANE

Care for the elderly in different settings has in common the centrality of primary care and the family. With attention to the problems of those elderly persons with dependency needs, concerns are focused on the role of the informal support systems. For the most part, this informal care is provided by family. Changing patterns of family relationships precipitated by mobility and altered family structures raise special concerns about the future of this form of care. In developed countries, as women enter the labour force in greater numbers, they will be less available to provide such care. In developing countries, migration from rural to urban areas and changes in living and working arrangements threaten to leave the elderly with fewer family resources. However, it seems likely that the family will continue as the mainstay of long-term care for older persons.

In countries both with universal comprehensive health care insurance and without there is a reassuringly consistent finding that families continue to provide about 75–85 per cent of the total personal care received by the elderly. Betty Havens and colleagues have summarized numerous studies estimating the proportion of care given by informal support networks in Table 20.1. As can be seen from it, as pressures on women expand, they continue to provide the bulk of personal support for family members.

At the same time, not all elderly have family, especially spouses and children. Finding, training, and supporting new and existing sources of personnel to provide personal care services for dependent older persons will present one of the important challenges of the next decade.

Long-term care of the elderly represents a merging of medical and social care with housing and economics. Older persons tend to suffer problems in clusters. Indeed, the geriatric paradigm is the simultaneous presentation of multiple, interacting problems from a variety of domains, including physical, social, and psychological. Changes in one sphere are likely to affect performance in others. The patterns of care for the elderly will depend, for better or worse, on existing resources. Efforts to change the way care is delivered must recognize that the established care providers have a strong stake in what happens. Often they represent strong influences in setting standards for new forms of care and may exert a conservative influence. Planners in developing countries may look too expectantly toward the developed countries for models of care. In the case of long-term care, there has been an overly heavy reliance on

Table 20.1 Summary of research on informal care

Author(s)	Percentage of care received from informal support networks
Liu et al.[1] ⎫ Liu et al.[2] ⎭	75% solely informal
Bressler et al.[3]	80%
Shanas[4]	80%
Community Council of Greater NY[5]	77%
Rubin[6]	>75%
Comptroller General of US[7]	70–80%
Stone et al.[8]	nearly 75%
Brody[9]	80–90%
Wilson and Battino[10]	80%
Soldo[11]	≈75%
Senate Special Committee on Aging[12]	84%
Gurland et al.[13]	80%
National Center for Health Statistics[14]	80%
Morris et al.[15]	Nearly 90%
Tobin and Kulys[16]	Nearly 90%
Doty et al.[17]	60–85%
Morginstin[18]	86%
Chappell[19] Chappell and Havens[20] Chappell[21]	94%
Chappell and Powell[22]	78%
Chappell and Horne[23]	66% of hours of care
Executive Directors Report[24]	Nearly 75%
Kelman[25]	Nearly 75%
Doty[26]	Nearly 75%

Source: This table was prepared Dr Betty Havens, Manitoba provincial Gerontologist, and colleagues (Neena L. Chappell and Audrey A. Blandford from the Centre on Aging, University of Manitoba, and Analee E. Beisecker, National Extension Center of Gerontology, University of Missouri–Kansas City).

institutional forms of care. Although recent efforts have been directed toward emphasizing the importance of community-based care, the nursing home has emerged as the touchstone of care; all other forms seem to be irresistibly compared with it. Countries just beginning to cope with the demographic shift to an aging society have the opportunity to eschew dependence on institutional care and to establish a system with community care in its centre. In such an arrangement some institutional services may be needed but they are generally called upon only after community efforts have been attempted.

An ongoing issue with regard to the care of the elderly is the role of the specialty of geriatrics. Special training for physicians and other caregivers is becoming more accessible. Such persons have useful skills in merging the social and medical management of dependent elderly populations. They serve an important role as advocates and organizers of care for the elderly. However, even where such care is available, it is usually offered as an adjunct to primary care. The mainstay of care for older persons will continue to develop around primary care arrangements. These will take different forms depending on the availability of personnel and resources. In all cases, however, special training and techniques will make the care of older persons more effective.

Just as function is the common language of geriatrics, assessment lies at the heart of its practice. Special techniques that utilize comprehensive examinations of the multiple problems and their functional consequences offer a way to structure the approach to these often complicated dilemmas. Geriatric assessment has been tested in a variety of forms. The specifics seem to be less important than the very act of systematically approaching clients with the belief that improvement is possible.

Closely linked to assessment is the use of case managers to co-ordinate care across the several modalities and agencies that are often a part of long-term care. Case managers have played a variety of social and practice roles. Each represents an effort toward a slightly different goal. They may serve as co-ordinators or brokers of care provided by other persons. In so doing they will have different levels of authority over resource use. This can vary from persuasion to the power to purchase services. In other systems, they will be part of the care delivery process itself, with the attendant problems of potential conflicts of interest. In a related sense, case managers may be seen as the advocates of the clients, helping them to obtain all the services they are felt to need, or they may work as gate keepers, limiting access to care. Whatever the arrangement and expectation, the case manager can succeed only to the extent that there are services to manage. A system based in case management but bereft of services will not achieve much.

References

1. Liu, K., Manton, K., and Liu, B. M. (1985). Home care expenses for the disabled elderly. *Health Care Financing Review*, **7**, 51–8.
2. Liu, K., Manton, K., and Liu, B. M. (1986). Home care expenses for non-institutionalized elderly with activities of daily living and instrumental activities of daily living limitations. *Health Care Financing Review*, **8**, 241–5.
3. Bressler, D. S., Loewinsohn, R. J., and Baldwin, L. E. (1984). *Hand in hand: learning from and caring for older parents*, p. 2. American Association of Retired Persons, Washington DC.

4. Shanas, E. (1979). The family as a social support system in old age. *The Gerontologist*, **19**, 169–74.
5. Community Council of Greater New York (1978). *Dependency in the elderly of New York City*. Community Council of Greater New York, New York.
6. Rubin, S. S. (1986). *Family caregivers: the invisible network of long-term care*. Unitarian Universalist Service Committee, New York.
7. Comptroller General of the United States (1977). *The well-being of older people in Cleveland*. General Accounting Office, Washington DC.
8. Stone, J., Cafferata, G. L., and Sangl, J. (no date) *Caregivers of the frail elderly: a national profile*, DHHS, US Public Health Service, Washington DC.
9. Brody, E. M. (1985). Parent care as a normative family stress. *The Gerontologist*, **25**, 19–25.
10. Wilson, W. R. and Battino, R. (1987). Long term care alternatives: a project to develop informal caregivers for the elderly in the community. Paper presented at American Public Health Association meeting, New Orleans.
11. Soldo, B. (1983). *The elderly home care population: national prevvalence rates, selected characteristics and alternative sources of assistance*. Working Paper No. 1466–9. The Urban Institute, Washington DC.
12. Senate Special Committee on Aging with American Association of Retired Persons (1987–8). *Aging America: trends and projections*. Senate Special Committee on Aging, Washington, DC.
13. Gurland, B., Dean, L., Gurland R., and Cook, D. (1978). The dependent elderly in New York City. In *Dependency in the elderly of New York City*, Community Council of Greater New York. NY.
14. National Center for Health Statistics (1979). *Current estimates from the health interview survey, 1978*. Vital and health statistics series 13 No. 130. US Government Printing Office, Washington DC.
15. Morris, J. N., Morris, S., and Sherwood, S. (1984). Assessment of informal and formal support systems in high risk elderly populations. In *Functional assessment in rehabilitation medicine* (ed. Granger, C. V. and A. E. Gresham), pp. 223–53.Williams and Watkins, Baltimore.
16. Tobin, S. S. and Kulys, R. (1980). The family and services. *Annual Review of Gerontology and Geriatrics*, **1**, 370–99.
17. Doty, P., Liu, K., and Weiner, J. (1985). An overview of long-term care. *Health Care Financing Review*, **6**, 69–78.
18. Morginstin, B. (1987). Long-term care insurance in Israel. *Ageing International*, Winter, 10–12.
19. Chappell, N. L. (1985). Social support and the receipt of home care services. *The Gerontologist*, **25**, 47–54.
20. Chappell, N. L. and Havens, B. (1985). Who helps the elderly person: a discussion of informal and formal care, In *Social bonds in later life*, (ed. Peterson, W. and J. Quadagno), pp. 211–27. Sage Publications, Beverly Hills, CA.
21. Chappell, N. L. (1988). Long-term care in Canada. In *North American elders: United States and Canadian perspectives* (ed. Rathbone–McCuan, E. and B. Havens), pp. 73–88. Greenwood Press, Westport, CT.
22. Chappell, N. L. and Powell, C. (1989). Living arrangements and their relevance for informal and formal care of the elderly, (in preparation).

23. Chappell, N. L. and Horne, J. (1988). *Study of supportive housing among seniors*, Canada Mortgage and Housing Corporation, Ottawa.
24. *Executive Director's Report*, (1987). American Association of Retired Person's *News Bulletin*, December, p. 4.
25. Kelman, H. R. and Thoman, C. (1987). Social support and social policy. Paper presented at European Regional Meeting of International Association on Gerontology, Brighton, UK.
26. Doty, P. (1987). Health status and health services use among older women: an international perspective. *World Health Organization Statistics Quarterly*, **3**.

21

Role of primary health care for the elderly

GARY ANDREWS

PRIMARY HEALTH CARE AND PRIMARY CARE

Following the Alma-Ata declaration of 1978, primary health care as a concept has been increasingly proposed as a basis for review of the organization of comprehensive health services in both developed and developing countries. The Alma-Ata report described primary health care in the following terms:

'Primary health care is essential health care based on practical, scientifically sound and socially acceptable methods and technology made universally accessible to individuals and families in the community through their full participation and at a cost that the community and country can afford to maintain at every stage of their development in the spirit of self-reliance and self-determination. It forms an integral part both of the country's health system, of which it is the central function and main focus, and of the overall social and economic development of the community. It is the first level of contact of individuals, the family and community with the national health system bringing health care as close as possible to where people live and work, and constitutes the first element of a continuing health care process'.[1]

Expressed in these terms, primary health care is clearly very relevant to the conceptualizaton, planning, and delivery of health services for the elderly in a population. As the 'first level of contact' between a national health system and the individuals, families, and community which the system is organized to serve, primary care constitutes a critical point of entry to the health system. The sensitivity of health services at that point to the special characteristics of the elderly in need of care, the degree of accessibility, and the quality of services provided may constitute the major determinants in outcome resulting from an encounter between an elderly person and the system.

Primary health care is a broad concept which not only embraces aspects of traditional health services delivery but also includes elements of community education, community participation, and intersectoral considerations.[2] The question of the relevance of primary care in the health of the elderly has often been addressed from the more narrow perspective of the role of the primary care doctor.[3-6] Although this approach is legitimate enough in a medical care review, it fails to deal with the issue of how the primary care physician or family doctor relates in his/her role to the wider social, community, and economic environment in which the interaction between doctor and patient takes place. I intend therefore to explore the issues associated with this wider view of primary health care.

A commitment to a primary health care approach requires decision makers, planners, and practitioners to lend support at several levels. Although the nature and extent of support needed will vary in different circumstances, a basic classification of the kinds of support is possible and one review sets it out thus:

1. *Promotion of primary health care*:
—— establishment of policy and priorities;
—— mobilization of intersectoral support;
—— legislation;
—— mobilization of community support.

2. *Development of primary health care*:
—— planning and programming, including intersectoral coordination, choice of appropriate technology, community participation, evaluation, and appropriate research;
—— manpower development, including re-orientation of existing workers and training of new ones;
—— organization, including referral mechanisms;
—— provision of financing and facilities.

3. *Functioning of primary health care*:
—— management of resources, including finance, manpower, and information;
—— coordination of components, including both sectoral institutions and communities;
—— supportive supervision;
—— provision of equipment, supplies, and drugs.[7]

This framework calls for a fundamental re-orientation of the established health delivery systems and agencies at several levels. There has been a tendency in some settings to interpret such a strategy as a direct criticism of health professionals, services, and technologies that have generally operated in a principally diagnostic and curative mode. Those on either side of the resulting debate frequently express profoundly felt beliefs about the relative allocation of health care resources between established curative services and a kind of 'new deal' promising effective strategies to promote and maintain the health of individuals and communities rather than providing a sickness-oriented service. Such debates are more often reflections of professional bias and heartfelt zeal, rather than logically formulated analyses based upon some degree of rational and convincing evidence. In terms of the elderly and their health needs, what is now required is a systematic review of health service policies and programmes from a primary health care perspective. Strategies for strengthening primary health care within the overall health care delivery system to ensure improved health for the elderly in the populations can then be articulated in a manner relevant to the context of the health delivery system being considered.

At present there appears to be surprisingly little hard information beyond the widely expounded rhetoric in support of the concept of primary health care. Investment should now be made in the systematic collection of relevant and source information on primary care needs of the elderly. Well-designed and executed studies to evaluate alternative strategies for provision of primary care, workforce studies, and analyses designed to test effectiveness and measure costs should be encouraged and supported.

PRIMARY HEALTH CARE FOR THE ELDERLY

The elderly constitute an integral component of society. Their inherent vulnerabilities as a group are such that the concepts of primary health care with its wide scope of activity and influence appear particularly relevant to defining and meeting their health needs.[8] There has been growing recognition of the fact that the majority of elderly at any point in time are not dependent and disabled, but active and self-reliant. An effective health service will ensure the early identification of those at risk of medical or social decompensation, will facilitate their referral to appropriate assessment, and will ensure the provision of services needed to achieve the maximum possible restoration of their health and well-being and the continued maintenance to the highest degree possible of this status. At the same time, the ideal health service will accommodate a wider educational and promotional activity aimed at achieving maximum possible health status of all of the aging individuals it serves and will provide an appropriate degree of community input in the organization and the delivery of its services. In addition, the wider context in which the health service operates will be recognized so that the contribution of a health perspective to such questions as economic security, general education, housing, transport, recreation, labour policies, etc. will be acknowledged and acted upon. The notion of primary health care encompasses all of these essential elements.

In practice, the way in which primary health care is organized will vary greatly according to the structure of the health system in which it is based, the level of development of that system generally, and the broader socio-economic and cultural context in which it operates.

The basic operational notion of primary health care, or primary care, is that of the point of first contact with the health system. It is the portal of entry to the delivery system and embraces a whole range of provisions which are directed at assessment, support, care, and education which can be provided on self-referral without reference to more technical services provided at other levels. However, beyond provision of basic primary care services, the requirements of appropriate onward referral, of collaborative work with other components and levels of the system, including specialized services and continuity of care, are essential to the concept.

For the elderly in particular, the initial point of entry into programmes of care can occur over an extraordinarily diverse range of places and agencies. Thus a member of family, a neighbour, a voluntary agency, a family medical practitioner, a health care worker, a traditional health care practitioner, district nurse, local government worker or agency, hospital ambulatory care service, member of the police force, welfare worker or agency, or a number of other formal or informal referral mechanisms might be the initial key to the individual's entry to health care. A misjudgement at this point may delay appropriate action and ultimately cost the individual and the community dearly in view of a missed opportunity for appropriate early intervention and possible prevention. Anecdotes abound, and one particular occasion graphically illustrates the issue. In a comprehensive survey of the health and social circumstances of an elderly population served by a local health centre in Kilsyth, Scotland, an 85 year-old woman was included in a random sample of subjects. Her principal complaint was that she could no longer manage the walk from her home on a hill to the town centre for her weekly shopping and social expedition. The local welfare system assessed her as 'frail' and provided a home help to assist with housekeeping and to do the necessary shopping, so freeing the old lady both of her major source of social interaction and of enjoyable, and probably beneficial, physical activity. However, the physical examination and screening tests which were offered in accordance with the study protocol subsequently revealed the real source of her problem to be a severe degree of iron deficiency anaemia consequent upon a chronic bleeding peptic ulcer. A straightforward regimen of management of her anaemic condition and treatment of the peptic ulcer meant a rapid return to her former functional status and the home help was no longer necessary. No doubt the progression of her condition would have eventually brought her to direct medical attention but in her imposed sedentary state the already quite severe anaemia may have progressed by that stage to a more complicated, and indeed life-threatening, condition. On the other hand, there are circumstances where, for instance, an isolated, bereaved, and financially strained elderly woman might after a standard consultation with a medical practitioner be offered an antidepressant or tranquillizer for her 'condition' when what is actually required is counselling and local support.

A key to effective provision of primary health care lies in the idea of an appropriate formal and informal network of assessment to which the individual is exposed on entry and which is capable of maintaining itself, monitoring its own effectively, and imposing a regular review process to which its elements and operations are subject. Such a network might be established in some circumstances between a primary care worker in a rural village and the key local and community structures which influence the daily lives of the village inhabitants. At another level of organization and development a similar network might be institutionalized in the form of a multidisciplinary community centre incorporating health, welfare, legal, and general community elements. The objective in both instances is the same—to ensure that all of the relevant considerations can be taken into account in the assessment of an individual who presents for care. In addition, the potential is established for accumulation of collective information which is relevant to defining issues and needs generally, as well as for identifying potentially positive areas for preventive interventions.

An element essential to any primary care network is the supporting record system. This should be straightforward, as standardized as possible, and should be available with appropriate guarantees of privacy to all of the relevant personnel at primary care level. The record provides a vital tool which can contribute to continuity of care, quality assessment, and programme evaluation.

Teamwork, a communication network between professionals and agencies, and effective continuity of care are essential to the provision of high quality and appropriate services at the primary care level. Good communications between the health professionals involved in primary health care might be achieved in a number of ways in different settings. The solo practitioner, whether a community health worker providing services at a village level in a developing country, a trained health visitor, a family medical practitioner, or a district nurse or welfare worker, critically needs an understanding of the respective roles of various other members of the primary care system. The mere exposure to such knowledge is probably insufficient in itself and there is need to foster respect for the multidisciplinary practice. At present, such experience remains a fairly uncommon feature of health professional undergraduate training. There is a need (in my view) to find effective strategies for overcoming this lack of exposure of individual professionals to other disciplines during their training. At the operational level, the model of the multidisciplinary primary health care centre provides an opportunity for teamwork between a range of professionals but does not guarantee it.

At graduate level too there is a need to foster the development of good interprofessional understanding and relationships. There is a real risk in any multidisciplinary setting one professional group being over-dominant—a situation which inevitably leads to reduced effectiveness in delivery of primary care. Skills in leadership, teamwork, and group dynamics are not inherent: they need to be taught actively and fostered as an intrinsic component of professional development in the primary care setting.

Successful operationalization of the concepts of primary health care thus requires identification of the essential structural components within any particular setting, a definition of key interrelationships, a supporting record system, a defined communication process, an education programme, and a system of evaluation and review to which both professionals and the community contribute formally.

THE ORGANIZATION AND DELIVERY OF PRIMARY CARE FOR THE ELDERLY

The organization and delivery of comprehensive health services for the elderly has been the subject of extensive review in the past.[9] Although the basic requirements for health care of an aging population are generally agreed, the exact nature of the delivery system will vary according to the overall arrangements for health service delivery which apply. It is not the intention of this paper to attempt a restatement of the health care requirements for the elderly; rather, the issue to be addressed is: what constitutes an effective primary care programme for that group of the population and how should such a primary care service integrate with the other elements which comprise comprehensive health services? Furthermore, what is the appropriate way of interfacing primary care for the elderly with related wider social, economic, and public policy arenas?

There will be many views of the most appropriate organization of care and a variety of models have been described. At present the impression is of a rather *ad hoc* approach to policy formulation and programme development in this area. A selective annotated bibliography on 'The contribution of the primary care doctor to the medical care of the elderly in the community', published recently in the Danish literature,[10] was revealing in its wide range and diversity of perspectives on the question. A number of principles on which there seems to be consensus do emerge from the literature, however. Some of the more important are as follows:

—— Whatever the point of first contact is between an elderly individual and the health system, a teamwork approach is necessary to ensure that the appropriate professional skills and resources are applied to assessment and decisions about management.

—— The elderly person presenting to the health system should not be considered in isolation from their family, local, and community relationships.

—— The role of family care givers to the elderly should be recognized in any assessment process and account should be taken of the stresses applying to informal support arrangements.

—— Continuity of care is fundamental to the assurance of quality of care and an essential means of supporting continuity is a basic record system to which several primary care team members contribute.

—— A medical and social perspective is essential to ensure comprehensive assessment and management at the primary care level.

—— Primary care for the elderly should include a preventive component especially directed at the oldest of old people and those persons identified as at risk of medical/social breakdown.

—— Accountability of the primary caregivers should be clearly established to promote critical review of the quality of care provided and stimulate the development of improved health care delivery.

—— Appropriate referral mechanisms should be in place in order to ensure full access to more technical care, including specialized geriatric services when this becomes necessary.

The mere enunciation of principles underpinning a primary care programme is not of itself sufficient assurance of good quality of care. By its very nature the capacity of primary care to deal with complex medical and social problems will be limited. Primary care services for the elderly should be provided within the framework of a comprehensive health care programme for them which includes access to specialized services and ensures appropriate referral. Alternative care provisions, including day care programmes, institutional care, geriatric specialist assessment, rehabiliation, and long-term care, should be readily accessible. Within this framework, however, the basic tenets of primary health care should remain intact, thus ensuring accessibility, acceptability, and quality of care.

One of the most important requirements for good quality of care is effective teamwork. The roles of the various professionals who constitute the team, their arenas, obligations, and lines of accountability need to be clearly articulated in operational terms. In different settings teams can function effectively in a variety of ways, but only if the essentials of good communications and clear role relationships have been fully defined and agreed.

Many of the primary care scenarios that have been described assume the existence of one or another structural framework, for example a practice clinic, health centre, or day care facility upon which the primary care system under consideration is based. Such an approach has serious limitations as an exercise in setting out the basic principles and guidelines for primary care since the available infrastructure will vary widely according to the nature of the health care delivery system within which it is located. It is more appropriate to begin with a consideration of those characteristics of the elderly which govern their primary health care needs individually and collectively. From such an analysis it is possible to derive a series of operational implications which can then be used to identify the basic programme requirements. Identification of specific outcome measures and expected benefits will provide the basis of a structured evaluation and review mechanism.

Aging is essentially a universal experience and the physical, mental, and social accompaniments of the process are generally remarkably consistent between otherwise different populations in very different geographic and societal environs. While the context may vary greatly, and therefore the precise manifestations, the underlying processes seem remarkably constant.[11] Thus the elderly in any community will: exhibit a range of specific social, physical, psychological, and behavioural characteristics, be subject to certain defined vulnerabilities closely associated with aging, embody a set of aspirations and expectations which can be described broadly for various subgroups, and exhibit reasonably predictable outcomes as a population group according to age. While these defining qualities will show very substantial individual and subgroup variations, they are nonetheless sufficiently well defined in population terms to provide a sound basis for establishing the need for a range of support systems including those related to primary care.

The detail included in a framework such as that outlined in Table 21.1 can be developed for any given programme according to the defined characteristics of the target elderly population and the resources available in primary health care. The examples of key features and implications given here are not meant to be exhaustive, but only indicative of the approach.

In responding to the identified health care needs of the elderly in any population, resources outside the formal health care system should be considered. In many circumstances volunteers can contribute effectively within a primary care setting and there is a growing recognition of the importance of the concepts of self-help and self-care in relation to the health of the elderly.[12]

Table 21.1 Examples of population characteristics and programme links

Population characteristic	Operational implications	Programme requirements	Outcome measure
Non-reported illness	Early diagnosis of 'hidden' pathology	Screening programmes targeted to high-risk categories	Reduction in non-diagnosed illness in community Higher detection rates of common problems
Fatalistic acceptance of problem, disabilities and functional limitations (agism)	Education of community, the elderly, and care providers	Self-help and health promotion/ health education activities within primary care	Measurable improvement in attitude and knowledge regarding aging over time
Multiple drug usage multiple pathology	Regular assessment and review of diagnoses and treatment	Record linkage 'Recertification' of medication Diagnostic periodic review	Reduction in polypharmacy and adverse drug effects Improved diagnosis rates
Functional limitations due to chronic disabling illness	Identification and correction of remediable handicap	Multidisciplinary assessment—basic retraining	Improved functioning and reduced dependence
Increased prevalence of dementia	Early detection and support for dementing elderly and their families	Accurate screening and referral	Earlier identification of dementia within community
Accidents	Identification and correction of accident hazards and risk behaviour	Accident risk assessment and prevention programmes including education	Reduction in specific accident rates
Social isolation	Identification and referral of those at risk of social isolation	'At risk' registration	Reduction in prevalence of isolation as aggravating factor in illness

MODELS OF PRIMARY CARE FOR THE ELDERLY

The formal organization of primary care for the elderly is rarely the subject of critical professional review, especially in relation to developing country settings. When such programmes have been described it is usually in bureaucratic programme report form and rarely published in the professional literature. Though as noted previously an extensive literature now exists relating to the role of the primary medical care practitioner, there is a relative dearth of information on primary care for the elderly programmes in conceptual terms, either as formal programme descriptions or as the subject of evaluative review. A clear need exists for investment in this area of health care planning, review, and evaluation. The necessary processes of achieving some consensus regarding the conceptual framework, the identification of key programme elements and precise definition of measurable outcomes requires a defined commitment and the availability of appropriate resources to support such activities in various academic, professional, and bureaucratic settings. It will be necessary to draw upon a diverse range of skills including those of epidemiologists, health service researchers, health economists, social anthropologists, and others to contribute to this process if it is to be effective.

A recently developed programme providing community-based health care and support services for the elderly in Singapore illustrates some of the key elements in the formulation, implementation, and development of primary care services for the elderly.[13] Following a report on problems of the aged in Singapore which identified a need for community-based health care, the Home Nursing Foundation (HNF)—a voluntary organization providing nursing care to the non-ambulant and aged sick in their own homes—decided to establish Senior Citizens' Health Care Centres (SCHCCs) in the various housing estates of Singapore. Two pilot centres were established in the first instance with the following defined objectives:

(1) to provide supportive day care to the semidependant elderly who would otherwise remain alone at home;

(2) to provide rehabilitation (physiotherapy and occupational therapy) for those elderly who are discharged from hospitals and who require or will benefit from such service;

(3) to provide rehabilitation for the well elderly who will benefit from maintenance sessions;

(4) to provide social contacts and participation in social and recreational activities for the lonesome elderly;

(5) to provide free medical screening so that chronic diseases can be detected and treated early;

(6) to provide health education and health promotion to the elderly and their families.

The centres are meant to provide, for the non-institutionalized elderly of Singapore, a 'package' of programmes including day care, rehabilitation, health education, and health screening 'on their doorstep'.

The expected benefits of the project (for which planning was commenced in February 1985) were identified and include, improved quality of life for the individual elderly and their families, improved functional capacity and decreased dependency of the impaired elderly, stimulation of community support, improved opportunities for social interaction, maintenance of health and fitness, improved mental status, reduced costs associated with hospitalization, and reduction in requirements for long-term institutional care. An active programme of community liaison and involvement was embarked upon and consultation took place with appropriate ministries, local hospital staff, and general practitioners working in the areas where the centres were established. Funding has been raised entirely from donations from the public.

In the initial 5 months after commencement of the centres in May 1986, 119 clients attended for a total of 2096 occasions. The majority attended two to three times per week for a period of 1 to 5 months. The diagnostic categories of elderly attending the centres have been listed as poststroke clients, those suffering from a variety of chronic diseases, the frail elderly, and those suffering from early dementia.

Evaluation of the outcomes for 102 clients is said to have revealed improvement in health status of 77, or 75 per cent, while another 13 (13 per cent) were said to have been maintained at their original functional level and prevented from further deterioration or dependency.

The elderly attending the centres are seen periodically by medical staff of nearby geriatric clinics in the community health services, and voluntary sight and hearing screening services are provided. Close liaison is maintained with the elderly individuals' nominated general practitioner.

The value of these pilot programmes in Singapore—a city state of just over two and a half million people with 196 000 (1985 figures) persons aged 60 years and over living in the community (the majority in housing estates)—has been widely accepted and plans are currently being developed for a further eight centres in other locations in the city.

The programme as described encompasses several of the basic elements of primary care, including preventive services, health education, restorative care, and referral. A basic medical record system which is simple, well designed, meticulously maintained, and contributed to by all the involved professionals provides an essential underpinning element to the programme. Community involvement is maintained, continuity of care is ensured, and a form of ongoing evaluation has been built into the development.

The Singapore programme is an important pilot exercise, many of the essential features of good primary care are encapsulated in the project. Benefit would undoubtedly accrue from more formal and technical evaluation and detailed analysis of associated costs and benefits.

COSTS AND BENEFITS

Primary health care services for the elderly represent a significant cost in any comprehensive health care delivery system. The elderly are generally recognized as greater consumers of health services than the rest of the population. Economic considerations are difficult in a broad review such as this, since absolute and relative costs will be influenced by many factors and will vary greatly in different settings. It has been argued, however, that relatively modest investment on a *per capita* basis could greatly improve primary health care delivery in developing countries with consequent savings to the health delivery system in the longer term.[14] However, primary health care and community care are not always either the most economic or the most appropriate way to provide services to the elderly. It has been forcibly argued that the implementation of primary health care programmes will inevitably result in significantly increased costs, especially in developing country situations. One country's reply to a review of the implications of primary health care quoted in a WHO study read thus:

The indications are that primary health care will lead to an increase in the total health expenditure. The major factors responsible for the increase have been identified as follows:

—— cost of drugs;

—— logistic support for the storage and distribution of drugs;

—— expanded immunization and other control activities (particularly for malaria and diarrhoeal diseases);

—— training of primary health care workers;

—— supervision of primary health care workers;

—— development of training and reference manuals;

—— construction of clinics, dispensaries, etc.[15]

There can be little doubt that developing a more organized and comprehensive primary health care service for the elderly carries a significant price in any setting. The consequent expansion of the family practitioner's role and the development of a team approach, the institution of preventive and educational programmes, and creation of consultative process all imply some degree of investment which is unlikely to be recouped by any simplistic attempt at re-allocation of resources within existing health care systems. The information at present available is too limited for any worthwhile in-depth analysis of the costs and benefits of a significant move towards extension and development of primary health care for the elderly. There is a pressing need for well-designed cost–benefit and cost-effectiveness studies in this area and for clearer definitions of the detailed costs involved at all levels. Monitoring will be important and attention should be given to the identification of categories of health expenditure related to primary health care and to sources of financing. The contribution of the elderly in the population to these costs will be a critical consideration in setting future priorities and in the planning and implementation of primary health care strategies. Similarly, the often-expressed effectiveness and benefits of improved primary health care delivery to the elderly will need more than simple anecdotal evidence. The present emergence of longitudinal studies of aging and community level will provide a much-needed opportunity for testing a variety of interventions and may provide a more rational basis for choosing between various options at the primary care level in the future.

RECAPITULATION AND CODA

Primary health care policy, organization, and delivery will for several reasons be important considerations with respect to the health of the elderly. The vast majority of the elderly in all populations live in the wider community and their health status and health care needs are subjected to many influences outside the traditional health services area. Thus public policy decisions and programmes in education, housing, transport, environment and planning, the economy, and other broad areas which impact upon the community generally may be highly relevant ultimately to the health and well-being of the aging in a given population. In these diverse areas of public policy, the mobilization of intersectoral support and the achievement of intersectoral coordination will be important strategies in achieving health goals for an aging population. Prevention of illness and the promotion and maintenance of health within the aging population will likewise need to be underpinned by actions beyond the health system *per se* in legislation, community education, and in certain instances through broad community-based action. The structure and operational principles of primary health care can facilitate these initiatives through a process of legitimizing the health input into public policy formulation and into relevant areas of programme planning and implementation. The principal argument for a primary health care approach at this level is an *a priori* one and there is a case for a more systematic evaluation of the processes involved. Many health care systems around the world are now responding to a call for restructuring to accommodate the primary health care approach and an opportunity exists for critical review of the impact of these changes in practice.

Similarly it appears self-evident that the point of first contact with health care delivery, as represented by primary care, will be a major determinant of the appropriateness and quality of the response to an individual elderly person's needs. Again, the evidence is largely lacking for the effectiveness of primary health care in many settings. Thus while the structure and processes of primary care for the elderly have been the subject of wide descriptive review, very little is available which relates investment at that level to measurable outcomes in terms of the well-being and health status of the elderly population. Well-designed and well-conducted evaluation studies which address these issues would be very valuable for future planning.

Primary health care, no matter how well developed, cannot of its own ensure the delivery of comprehensive health care for the elderly. The appropriate initiation of referral and access to more technical assessment and care as needed is essential in a comprehensive approach. Judgement will need to be exercised by primary care workers and teams in defining the point at which referral beyond a primary care setting is warranted. Certainly referral should be made to the appropriate specialized services at any point at which an individual's health status or needs change to a degree which warrants an adjustment in service provision beyond 'fine tuning', especially when a temporary or long-term accommodation change is contemplated. There is certainly a need for operational studies which focus on the dynamics of decision making within primary care at the interface between primary care and specialized services. In this regard the issues related to communication between various levels in the health system and those which affect continuity of care deserve close attention.

There will be a great range of variations on the theme of primary care for the elderly. Current models of delivery need better cataloguing and review, especially in developing countries. There would be some value at this time in establishing an agreed basic framework encompassing primary care principles to provide a simple schema for planning, quality assurance, and evaluation criteria in place of the rather *ad hoc* approach which seems to be generally adopted at present.

While the primary care physician clearly has a central role to play as a member of any primary care team, there is a real risk of medical dominance in situations where medical practitioners enjoy a traditional place at the peak of the hierarchy of health professionals. At the primary care level in particular, presentation of a medical problem may be the vehicle for expression of more basic social, economic or psychological difficulties being experienced by the individual. In these circumstances the perspectives and contributions of other members of the primary care team may be more relevant in assessment and management. Within the primary care team, however constituted, knowledge of and respect for the contribution of all the members of the team by each is essential for effective teamwork. This has implications for health professional training at both undergraduate and graduate levels. Studies should be encouraged which identify the requirements in various settings for effective teamwork at the primary care level.

The scope for preventive action, health education, and health promotion within primary care is substantial. The primary care health worker enjoys an entry into the homes and lives of the elderly which provides an opportunity for influencing their knowledge, decisions, and actions in areas related to health. The sensitive exploitation of this within the social and cultural context of the individual circumstances seems appropriate. The identification of appropriate strategies in prevention and health promotion to be applied by primary health care workers should be undertaken systematically and the agreed approaches subject to critical evaluation in practice.

Primary health care for the elderly is principally about ensuring access to appropriate resources and the mobilization of those resources to achieve individual and collective health goals. Many other inputs, including those of a variety of specialized services, may be relevant to the final outcome; primary health care embodies the notion of integration of those inputs to ensure effective continuity of care and co-ordination at the level of the individual, the family and local community. It is here that the greatest risk of disjunction emerges: good communication and an effective basic record system become vital at this point. The processes of referral from and back to primary care need greater consideration than they appear to have been given in the past. More attention appears to be paid to the internal processes of primary care delivery and to the organization and delivery of various other forms and levels of care than to the linking arrangements which are so fundamental to an integrated system of comprehensive care.

While the approach of primary health care appears to have a great deal to offer, a clearer enunciation of the resource implications and workforce requirements in various settings is required. By linking these to projected outcomes and benefits, the basis for cost-effectiveness and cost–benefit analyses is established. Prospective studies of primary health care provision linked to outcome measures within the elderly community should now be instituted to achieve this.

To address the many issues and question both implied and enunciated above, a comprehensive research agenda is needed.

References

1. World Health Organization Alam-Ata (1978). *Primary health care report of the International Conference on Primary Health Care, Alma-Ata, USSR.* 'Health for All' Series, No. 1. WHO, Geneva.
2. Kleczkowski, B. M., Elling, R. H., and Smith, D. L. (1984). *Health system support for primary health care.* A study based on the technical discussions held during the thirty-fourth World Health Assembly, 1981. WHO, Geneva.
3. Anderson, N. A. (1978). The assessment of need for support services as seen by general practitioners and a geriatric population. *Australian Family Physician*, **7**, 304–12.
4. de Buda, Y. (1979). The care of the aged: a responsibility and challenge for the family physician. *Canadian Family Physician*, **25**, 1489–92.
5. Reichel, W. (1979). Family practice and care of the elderly. *American Family Physician*, **20**, 85–6.
6. Strong, J. R., Caine, N., and Acheson, R. M. (1983). Team care of elderly patients in general practice. *British Medical Journal*, **286**, 851–4.
7. Kleczkowski, B. M., Elling, R. H., and Smith, D. L. (1984). *Op. cit.*, pp. 10–11.
8. World Health Organization (1981). *Preventing disability in the elderly: report on a WHO working group.* EURO Reports and Studies 65. WHO, Copenhagen.
9. World Health Organization (1974). *Planning and organization of geriatric services: report of a WHO Expert Committee.* (Technical Report Series No. 548. WHO, Geneva.
10. Almind, G., Freer, C., Muir Gray, J. A., and Warshaw, G. (1985). The Contribution of the Primary Care Doctor to the Medical Care of the Elderly in the Community. *Danish Medical Bulletin*, **32** (special supplement series No. 2).
11. Andrews, G. R., Esterman, A. J., Brannack–Mayer, A., and Rungie, C. (1986). *Aging in the western Pacific—a four-country study.* WHO Western Pacific Regional Office, Manila.
12. Hickey, T. (1986). Health behaviour and self-care in late life: an introduction. In *Self-care and health in old age* (ed. Dean, K., T. Hickey, and B. E. Holstein), pp. 1–11. Croom Helm, London.
13. *Report of Project: Senior Citizens Health Care Centres at Kuo Chan and KG UBI, being Operated by Home Nursing Foundation since May 1986* (1987). Home Nursing Foundation, Singapore.
14. Evans, J. R. *et al.* (1981). Health care in the developing world: problems of scarcity and choice. *New England Journal of Medicine*, **305**, 1117–27.
15. Kleczkowski, B. M., Elling, R. H., and Smith, D. L. (1984). *Op. cit.*, pp. 55–6.

22

The role of the family in the care of the elderly in developing countries

NANA ARABA APT

INTRODUCTION

The global aging of nations is an inevitable consequence of development bringing about higher standards of living, better nutrition, and improved health care. There is, however, a wide range of negative situations and conditions confronting older persons in society today which are the by-products of such development processes. Conversely, the widespread achievement of old age in this century is historically acknowledged to have been the greatest human advancement.

One of the most remarkable features of this century has been the rapid fall in death rates in almost all parts of the developing world. Since the end of the Second World War, advances in medical technology and public health measures have continued. Much disease control, both preventive and curative, can now be carried out cheaply. The result has been a fall in the level of mortality at a rate far exceeding that experienced by the industrialized countries in the nineteenth century. The lowering of death rates and the resulting ability to guarantee a greater chance of survival into old age has become a reality in many developing countries today.

Although the world population of age 65 years and over is estimated to increase by approximately 140 million in the next 20 years, much of that increase will be in the developing areas of the world (Table 22.1). In the period from 1970 to 2000 in the less developed regions, the increase of those 60 years of age and over will be approximately 130 per cent (Table 22.2). The total number of persons 60 years and over in East Asia, for example, will increase more than 100 per cent during the 30 years period while, Latin America will experience a significant increase of 151 per cent in contrast to one of 119 per cent for all ages.

Furthermore it is those of more advanced age who are statistically increasing more rapidly over the whole world, these are technically speaking the most dependent older age group who require the greatest range and number of health and social care. Even though the rate of increase of this segment of the population is extremely high for all regions, it is particularly so for the developing regions—160 per cent in

Table 22.1 Total population and population 65 years and over: 1960, 1980, and 2000[1]

	Year	Total Population	Population 65 years & over	Percentage 65 & over	Percentage less than 15
World:	1960	3027	158	5.2	37.0
	1980	4415	258	5.8	35.0
	2000	6199	397	6.4	31.6
Developed countries:					
	1960	945	80	8.5	28.6
	1980	1131	129	11.4	23.0
	2000	1272	167	13.2	21.5
Third World:					
	1960	2082	78	3.7	40.9
	1980	3284	129	3.9	39.2
	2000	4927	229	4.6	34.2

Africa, 205 per cent in Latin America, 146 per cent in East Asia, and 158 per cent in South Asia.

This phenomenon of increased aging certainly has important implications for policy makers and planners of social and economic development, particularly in the developing regions. Indeed, not so long ago, the topic of old age was not an issue for discussion in most of the developing countries. As a rule only a small proportion of the population of these countries lived beyond the middle age, therefore those few that actually survived into old age were almost deified. Solidly entrenched within the various forms of extended family structures, the elderly of most of the traditional societies now in the threshold of development lived a fuller, more fulfilling life wielding a great deal of social, economic, and political power.

The generally held view on the aging situation of the developing countries, particularly in Africa, is founded on the traditional status and role of the elderly in these societies. For a long time the myths have prevailed that the extended family, with its structures and patterns of family solidarity and blood ties, would render virtually insignificant the problems of aging faced by the industrialized countries of the world.

The strengths of the extended family system in the context of trends to modernization and development in these countries are to a large extent untested and unproven. Also, although there is no substantial empirical evidence to the contrary about the situation of the elderly in the develop-

Table 22.2 Estimated and projected distribution of the total population of the major areas in the age group (Percentages, number, and percentage increase: percentage increase of population of all ages 1970–2000)[2]

	Percentage				Number (in thousands)			Total population
	1970	1980	1990	2000	Estimated 1970	Projected 2000	Increase (%)	(% increase)
World total	8.4	8.5	8.9	9.3	304 341	581 431	91	73
More developed regions	14.2	14.8	16.2	17.2	153 424	233 851	52	25
Less developed regions	6.0	6.1	6.5	7.1	150 917	347 579	130	94
Africa	4.7	4.7	4.9	5.2	16 704	42 135	152	131
Latin America	5.8	6.1	6.4	6.7	16 483	41 528	151	119
Northern America	13.8	14.9	15.2	14.5	31 276	42 965	37	31
East Asia	8.5	9.1	10.2	11.5	78 333	157 770	101	48
South Asia	4.9	5.0	5.4	6.1	53 997	137 443	154	106
Europe	16.7	16.7	17.9	18.5	76 450	99 947	30	18
Oceania	10.8	11.1	11.5	11.1	2 081	3 631	74	69
USSR	12.0	13.1	15.6	17.8	29 018	56 007	93	30

ing countries, observers indicate irreversible social and economic trends taking place which, if not seriously studied, analysed, and programmed for, could have detrimental effects on the aging situation in many developing countries. For instance in many of these countries today it is known that the extended family system, the mainstay of the elderly, is being weakened by social change. It is necessary therefore to re-examine the place of older persons and their social roles in these societies in the light of present development trends and socio-economic realities as a means to offset the drastic consequences of social change.

AGING: ROLE OF THE TRADITIONAL FAMILY

The importance of family life for the well-being of the elderly is universally acknowledged. Consequently, in discussing the traditional family's role in the care of the aged, it is necessary to review that role in shaping attitudes towards the elderly; after all, it is through the family that the individual is socialized in the cultural patterns of a society.

The social significance of attitudes has prompted a great deal of theory and research by social psychologists and one of the major conclusions drawn is that attitudes play an essential role in determining people's behaviour towards others. Lambert and Lambert[3] define attitude as 'an organized and consistent manner of thinking, feeling and reacting with regard to people, groups, social issues, or more generally an event in one's environment'. They analyse its essential components as being 'thoughts and beliefs, feelings or emotions and tendencies to react'.

Since attitudes are commonly learned through transfer in essentially the same way that we learn meanings of words and concepts through instruction, the family role in shaping attitudes towards the elderly becomes very significant. Through the family, the desired and expected behaviour towards the elderly is standardized for transmission into the next generation.

The extended family

In the developing countries, the existence of an extended kin network in which parents, children, uncles, aunts, and other relatives are in regular and frequent contact with one another is a fundamental part of the traditional welfare system. The term 'extended family' is usually and widely applied to the family system commonly found in the developing countries 'in which the ideal of the society is that several generations should live under one roof'.[4]

Historically, in Africa the living conditions in the forest or savannah evolved for centuries a family pattern consistent with the environment and survival. The African 'family'—the centre of all life and survival efforts—extended over several generations and exercised authority and division of duties among its members. The African family pattern comprised, in its widest interpretations, all of the father's and mother's dependents down to the youngest offspring, so that there were generally at least three generations in one compound, which was naturally supplemented by second-degree relatives. This family structure finds its expression in circular architectual designs all over Africa that are commonly known in West Africa as the 'compound house'. In the Philippines, the concept of the family embraces the *Kama-anak*—that is, the circle of relations from both the mother's and father's sides. These extensions of the family are formed through consanguineous relationships through affinity of marriage relations.[5] Like the African model, the traditional Philippine family can extend to three generations in the direct line and collaterally can include brothers and sisters, their spouses, and children.

The Indian joint family, often referred to as extended, is made up of *co-parceners*—that is 'persons who have a right to the products of the family property'.[4] Thus brothers in the first generation with their sons in the second and third generations in direct line all form part of the family unit. The Hindu tradition, which gives the male child a right to the family property, places this emphasis on brothers and brother's sons. The Chinese system, like that of the Arabs, is equally extended, comprising parents living with their married sons and their families, and with unmarried sons and daughters and their grand-children or great grandchildren in the patrilineal line.

The extended family system traditionally practised in many African, Arab, Asian, and Latin American societies, whether patrilineal in structure (that is, tracing kin through father's blood line) or matrilineal (through the mother's) and whether polygamous or monogamous, has common distinctive features differentiating it from the Western conjugal or nuclear-type family. These features are given prominence in the cultural values of such societies. One major common feature responsive to the care and security of the elderly in these societies is the family's collective responsibility towards all household members great and small, strong or weak. Like a modern social security scheme, caring for the elderly, the handicapped, and the young is an accepted and shared responsibility of all family members.

Perhaps the most important attribute of the extended family which gives credence to this collective responsibility is to be found in its inner dynamics, namely the social relations and interaction among members and the roles and responsibilities assigned to different age groups. The African example may be used to illustrate this collective dynamism.

In a typical multigenerational household are found adults, elderly per-

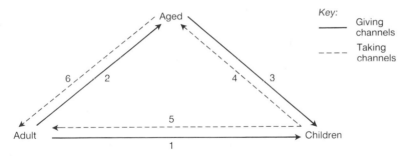

Fig. 22.1 Scheme of complementary interaction.[6]

sons, young people, and children. The traditional form of stratification and interactions recognizes both the help young people can give to the elderly and the experience to be gained from them. Thus, while adults provide livelihood, the provision of food and shelter, and general protection against the exigencies of life, the aged in turn give to the adults both advice and moral support and to their children they give child minding—a task which could be a constraint to adult productivity. Similarly, while children in a typical household do minor taskwork for the elderly and give companionship to both parents and grandparents, they in turn receive from such interaction an education in morals, skills, and folklore from the elderly.

This social arrangement enables the young and the old in the traditional African family system to engage in productive intercourse, and intergenerational experiences are shared; the young have something to learn from the old and the old person in turn is given a helping hand. This is illustrated by a proverb of the Akans of Ghana: 'The hand of the child cannot reach to shelf, nor can the hand of the elder get through the neck of the gourd on the shelf'. This daily encounter between generations places the elderly person in a strong position that is useful and challenging.

The domain of kinship network within which the elderly resides under tradition is illustrated in Fig. 22.1 and, as can be deduced from the diagram, the type of social relations and interactions among members of a household, old and young, induces a feeling of worthiness especially among the elderly in both an economic and a psychological sense. Line 1 is the most frequent line of interaction through which the adult population within the family provide the range of rearing, minding, and economic support to their children. The duration of the parent/children interaction varies, but in general the provision of basic needs lasts until children grow up to adulthood. Line 2 also proceeds from the adult population but this time the recipients are the older generation. The giving consists of livelihood, the provision of food, shelter, and general protection against the exigencies of life. Line 3 emphasizes the unique position of children, who receive from both the adults and the aged. The giving from the aged, however, is usually that of ideas rather than of material goods. Thus morals and skills are passed on to the children in such interactions. Lines 4 and 5 accord with the domination of receiving by children. They in turn do most of the giving back to parents and grandparents in the form of companionship. Depending on their ages and sex, however, they can give very substantial returns in terms of labour input in the family production system. Line 6 is the channel through which the aged are in communion with the adult population. Although the adults are the producers and the most energetic actors, the aged receive some degree of authority and relevance as the reservoir of collective wisdom in cultural, social, and practical realms.

Despite variations in the practice of extended and intergenerational living, it is certain that the African example of interdependency and co-operation between generations is equally valued and observed in other developing societies that place a high valuation on some form of extended family. From a national report of Argentina to the World Assembly on Aging [1], we deduce that traditionally there is an uninterrupted flow of care between generations, as adult children protect and sustain their aging parents and the parents in turn contribute to the subsistence of the family. The traditional Thai family, consisting of a well-integrated kinship group with a strong leadership role for the male head of the household, exhibits a highly developed sense of mutual responsibilities and obligations among family members. In the People's Republic of China the housekeeping work of the grandmother frees the daughter-in-law to assume greater role in the labour force, thus increasing family income. In Thailand, grandmothers take on the responsibilities of raising their grandchildren and thereby free the mothers to work in the rice fields. Similarly in Guatemala, Jamaica, and Panama, the primary role of elderly women in the extended family is to help with housework and provide care for children of working mothers. Besides, even when not living in their children's household, grandparents in parts of Africa and South America have been known to be obliged to live with and raise their grandchildren.

In particular, the sense of obligation which is of paramount importance in the socialization of children in these cultures is cultivated early through acts of dependency. In the Philippines, for example, although the child is often encouraged to assume responsibilities for others, he is also expected to reach out for help. Thus, 'the child seeks help even when he does not need it as a bridge for affection and attention...if the child rejects help that is proffered or help that is understood as available, the one who offered help is hurt and the pattern of responsibility of one for another is disturbed...from childhood, he learns to enjoy being taken care of and realizes that he can make others happy by being dependent on them.[17]

The process of social control is also of immense importance in the socialization of children in traditional families. Respect for the elder is greatly emphasized in these societies and so is the act of obedience. Elders' authority is manifested through their ritual power. Accordingly, they are placed in an advantageous position which commands awe, prestige, and honour.

The respect accorded to the elderly is highlighted in Bolivia's contribution to the World Assembly. The Bolivian report states that in rural areas the aged constitute principal figures within the family, responsible for maintaining family integration and giving guidance in work activities. The Guatemala report similarly refers to the authority of fathers and grandfathers in the traditional patriarchal society. This authority is expressed in their roles as advisors and transmitters of experience and knowledge. Thai society has traditionally accorded great respect to its elderly members. Outward manisfestation of this respect are to be seen in the traditional practices of bowing before one's elders and even kneeling when communicating with them. The same cultural manifestations are expressed in Africa by the Yorubas of Nigeria.

Due to the imminence of their death, elders in these societies are considered to be closest to the spiritual realm. The Yoruba of Nigeria, the Akans of Ghana, and many other African cultures practising ancestral religious worship regard the aged as a link between the departed ancesters, the living, and the unborn. In this position they officiate at ceremonies to do with birth, marriage, and death as well as pacification and purification rituals for wrong doing within the family. In consequence, the respect, honour, and care accorded to elderly persons by their families within the traditional societies is very specific.

This spiritual essence is well articulated in many of the World Assembly country reports of Asia, Latin America, and the Southern Pacific. Such respectful attitudes are instilled in the young in Asia mostly through religious teachings. For instance in Sri Lanka, Pakistan, India, and Thailand, the extended family system is strenthened by Buddhist and Hindu cultures and religions which give pride of place to elders in the family. In India the seventieth birthday is celebrated with particular pomp as the period of the merging of the human and the divine. In China, Confucius is said to have noted 70 as the age of wisdom: the age that one follows the dictates of the heart without disobeying the moral law. In fact, in all portrayals of the aged in the developing societies, there is an element of mysticism embodying both wisdom and authority and thereby making obedience of the authority of the aged all the more embracing. Their knowledge of herbs to heal family members, combined with their knowledge of traditional practices, skills, and religious rules, makes them the obvious choice for consultation by the young. This gives them enormous social and political power.

In summary, within the traditional extended family, the aged are respected because they never cease to be productive. They occupy an important place in the family system and are generally consulted by the young. The interaction which thus exists between generations gives the elderly confidence that life is worth living, and that every one is needed. Besides, traditional communities are small and therefore the aged can get along according to their capabilities and are better able to master their environment. They get along in a position of trust and this gives them a sense of belonging and social relevance. Social relevance can best be achieved within the framework of the extended family system—a family system within which the positions, roles, responsibilities, and rights of all age groups are sharply defined and monitored.

CHANGING FAMILY PATTERNS

Almost all the developing countries presently find themselves in a period of transition in which all the well-known symptoms of modernization are being exhibited, including the negative symptons of alienation and cultural disorientation. Goode[8] draws conclusions about the sub-Sahara African scene as follows: 'I believe that much of the African industrialized and ubanized population is living in a state of social disorganization'. This opinion is based on three observations: (1) that many Africans have accepted both the traditional and modern values but have little moral commitment to either, (2) that the present society itself gives insufficient means for achieving certain values, and (3) that the modern African is moving in two (or more) disparate cultures and has no legitimate place in either of them. It can be stated that in this respect the newly emerging African nations are merely following the path of many other developing countries. A crucial contribution in the above observations is made by the role strains and difficulties which the average individual in such emerging countries encounters in meeting his expected obligations to his kin—such a view projects the present role relation and indeed the whole social fabric of these societies to be functioning under considerable tension.

Nevertheless, and in spite of the cultural imbalance in modern times, observers of the developing world agree that the emotional ties and economic support among family members still remain relatively strong. Individuals continue to send money home to their families even when away from the kingroup and many continue to take as much part as they can in political and social events. The latter observation is particularly outstanding in the Africa region. In many parts of the continent the ideal for the urban worker is to retire comfortably in the home village. From studies involving 11 African countries, Peil and Sada[9] reported that the highest rates of intended return home (over 90 per cent) were recorded in Ghana, Zambia, and Kenya.

In Ghana, 'going to the home town' for Easter has become an accepted and expected norm for the urban worker. Similarly, in the Latin America region, in Jamaica, Dominican Republic, and in Costa Rica, the frequency of intergenerational contact is reported to be high even where family members live separately.[10]

While the manifestations of extended kin network are observable in a majority of the developing countries, the extended family as a traditional household unit is generally disintegrating in the face of modernization, industrialization, and urbanization, leaving the practice of extended living mostly in rural areas of these countries. For instance, in Costa Rica, almost 90 per cent of the rural elderly live with relatives. In Argentina rural families are still living three or more generations to one household, and in rural Panama and Jamaica the most common living arrangement is for the elder persons to live with their children and relatives. The African situation is similar.

In urban areas, however, the family structure is becoming increasingly more nuclear than extended. In the mainstream of modernization, the extended family is becoming remoulded into nuclear family units, mostly in living quarters which by their very narrow design are restrictive to the continuity and cohesion of former traditional living arrangements. Consequently, in the urban areas of the developing world for practical as well as economic reasons the family structure is becoming more nuclear than extended.

A few studies may be cited to illustrate this fact: for instance, as far back as 1920 the number of sons in urban Syria continuing to live jointly with their parents after marriage was diminishing.[8] By the 1950s the 'paternal' joint family was to be found only in small towns or among very conservative circles and 'the large houses which at the turn of the century sometimes contained thirty or forty family members...are divided into separate units for several conjugal families, or rented out as schools, institutes, etc'.[11] Similar trends are reported in Lebanon. In a Beirut survey of 1952 the average number of persons recorded per household was 4.04.[5]

Also, in India since 1911, colonial reports of the provinces express a growing tendency of the 'joint family' towards disintegration,[12] in 1951 the census data already confirmed this disintegration: 'The percentage of small households (three members or less) is larger in the urban than in the rural sectors, while correspondingly the percentage of large families (seven to nine members) is greater in rural than urban areas'.[12] In West Africa, the studies of Little,[13] Caldwell,[14] Oppong,[15] and Azu[16] give empirical support to the diminishing extended family and the increasing rate of nucleated units in urban areas.

We can deduce from the above discussions that migration has had drastic consequences on the traditional family structure. Even though the form of migration and the distances people travel have been changing over time, one feature remains central to the developing countries—that is, the young, educated, and ambitious are mostly the ones migrating from rural to urban centres in search of jobs. The importance and impact of migration and urbanization on social relations in these modernizing societies is to be found specifically in the possibilities afforded the individual for building his independent economic base outside the family circles for his own decisions; consequently there is a breakdown of traditional authority.

Modernization: effects on the elderly

Migration and urbanization have both separately and jointly underminded the traditional marriage structure and pattern and have in turn contributed to the destabilization of the values which in traditional times sustained the adults and elderly in a closely knit age-integrated society. Concern about the well-being of the elderly left behind in rural areas while the young and able bodied migrate is well emphasized in almost all national reports of developing country delegates to the World Assembly. It is reported that some older Africans find themselves deprived of their formal family-based resources of support as they become increasingly isolated in the rural areas. Zambia, which experienced large-scale rural shift in population (according to the 1963 and 1969 population censuses) identified the elderly as those most affected by the shift. According to their national report, the elderly are left behind in the rural areas to eke out a living from the land with very limited tools. The situation of the elderly left on their own in villages in Botswana is said to be worsened by periodic droughts that make subsistence farming even more difficult;[10] in Ghana in the first-ever survey of the aged undertaken in 1962, as much as 18 per cent of the rural households interviewed had 'come close to having lost contact with their educated offspring who migrated to the towns'.[17]

If the elderly should follow their offspring to the cities, UN studies[27] indicate that they live in slums and uncontrolled settlements. In fact, the ability of modern families in the developing countries to care for older relatives in an urban environment is, according to many observers seriously impaired by crowded housing, limited financial resources, and the increasing employment of women throughout the developing world.

As a result of economic crises in most of these countries, the average wage earner often lacks adequate resources to provide proper care and nutrition for parents and grandparents. Elderly parents have generally become economic appendages to their offspring's families instead of, as in the past, integrated members with economic activities revolving around them.

The decline in status of the aged in developing countries is another factor affecting their well-being. Through education, the young have taken over the power base of knowledge from the elderly and the communicational channels between the two is seemingly being hindered. Consequent to their acquired education and technological skill, the youth of such countries come to discover an economic-based power to which they have privileged access. They find that in their newly acquired urbanized positions they can make their own decisions as they no longer have to look to their elderly forebears for economic and social sustenance.

Rowe[18] finds in Asia that village gerontocracy has eroded as a result of Indian modernization. The young men find waged work in the cities and return home impatient with tradition. Furthermore they find themselves more affluent than their elder relations on their return from the cities, and this further corrodes the esteem of the aged. Press and Mckool[19] find a similar effect in the villages of Mayan Mexico where young men moving to work in factories outside the villages found they could buy their own land before their father was ready to surrender the family holdings to them.

The shift in power on the basis of economics has shown similar effects in Africa. In one of the few cross-cultural studies linking mental illness to loss of elderly prestige, Arth[20] found that young Ibos who acquire independent wealth from waged work no longer rely on their fathers for the authority bride wealth. In consequence, the father's prestige declines; the author concluded that 'psychosenility' has become prevalent among the elderly casualties of Ibo modernization. We can draw the conclusions that with modernization the traditional culture which stresses ritual access to power loses its meaning. Power becomes secularized; it is represented by cash by technological acquisitions (and even by the quality of acquired alcoholic drinks). Modernization has made the skills and knowledge of the elderly obsolete, thus further lowering their status and increasing the regard for those who are educated and the technologically skilled.

While beneficial changes for women have accompanied modernization in these countries (e.g. access to education and employment, accompanied by legal rights), the situation of older women appears to be particularly precarious. Research in eight resettlement colonies in Delhi in India indicates that more older women than men consider their status within the family to have deteriorated with age.[21] This is explained

Table 22.3 Age dependency ratios for selected regions (1975 and 2025)[26]

Region and year	Dependency ratio a/(per thousand)		
	Total	Age 0–14	Age 60 and over
Africa:			
1975	984	887	97
2025	688	576	112
East Asia:			
1975	784	637	147
2025	634	314	320

primarily as a consequence of widowhood and economic dependency on their families.[22] Azam Khan[23] observes that the values of city life are undermining the traditional norms of respect accorded by daughters-in-law to mothers-in-law in Pakistan. Similarly, in Turkey it is observed that migration of sons create serious problems for older women, especially widows who are dependent upon their sons for economic support.[24] In Nigeria among the Yoruba, Adeokun[25] reports that the number of elderly women living in isolation is increasing owing to the outward migration of children.

These and other concerns are being increasingly expressed and discussed at international meetings [2] by representatives and experts from developing countries. Listening to presentations and contributions from developing countries, one is immediately struck by the similarities in developmental issues and the rate at which the social and economic lives of the people are undergoing changes. There is an undertone of feeling among these representatives of the developing countries that their countries will soon, much sooner than expected, have to face the issue of elderly survivors and the problems of their welfare.

OLD AGE CARE: FUTURE STRATEGIES

The conclusion drawn from the trends in the developing countries discussed above (see Table 22.3) is that, unless family support channels in these countries are reviewed in the light of present socio-economic developments and where possible strengthened to advantage, creation of a new service infrastructure will be required in the coming decades as substitutes for or an addition to the traditional informal support systems. Given the current constraints on economic resources of the majority of these countries and the competing demands from a large youth population, the feasibility of creating new systems of care may well be questioned.

As is well publicized in the world media, the development problems faced by governments throughout the developing countries are many and complex. This paper need not delve into the causes of or reasons for their present predicaments. What is of consequence, however, is that the resulting very severe balance of payment problems coupled with the strains of monetary deficiency is rather hard-felt and acts an impediment for many of these governments. Action for the welfare of the elderly based on sophisticated welfare models of the developed world will no doubt require financial commitments which are currently far beyond the capacities of most governments of the developing countries.

In realization of this factor, developing country participants to the 1982 Hamburg Aging Symposium [3] made it quite explicit that there were no spectacular programmes to be expected from their governments although they themselves were firmly convinced of the need to begin concrete measures aimed towards the improvement of the situation of the elderly in their respective countries. Consequently, for socio-economic as well as humanitarian reasons, strengthening the resources of traditional carers and community self-help systems rather than creating new institutions was the central concern of the developing country delegates to the World Assembly.

In the Africa region, institutionalization of the aged is totally rejected. Policy makers are by and large placing primary emphasis on strengthening family resources and motivation for continuing their care-giving functions. As argued by the Malawi representative to the World Assembly, 'Viable communities still exist within the extended kin group which if equipped can take the strain of social change and improve the living conditions of the elderly'.[27] Thus, in Africa, policy alternatives so far considered include policies for financial support to families caring for elderly relatives. For instance, in Ethiopia, the Rehabilitation Agency for the Disabled provides assistance to some families who cannot take care for their aged due to financial constraints. In Kenya tax relief is being considered for families supporting elderly relatives. The 'Joot of Ahera' scheme which is in an experimental stage in Kenya contains a propelling concept: the strengthening of the integration of the aged through an intensification of the informal communication network of the family, neighbourhood, and community. The 'Harambe' scheme, also in Kenya, capitalizes on traditional mutual assistance concepts to achieve help for elderly people. In Botswana, Morocco, and Tunisia, granting of allowances, indemnities, or subsidies to families taking care of the elderly is also being reviewed for policy implementation.

Similarly, in Latin America, specific family-oriented policies proposed include financial subsidies to families caring for elderly relatives. In addition, there are proposals to subsidize design of housing units to accommodate multigenerational families. Promotions of 'foster families' for the elderly, provision of community-based social services for both elderly clients and their familes, and of special motivation programmes aimed at encouraging young people to take care of the elderly are all programme areas of great interest.

Naturally Asian countries, like their African and Latin American counterparts, are mostly inclined to channel aid through families rather than through state-run welfare institutions. Specific policies include direct financial assistance, provisions of grants for establishing family-based income-generating projects, assistance in the acquisition of multigenerational living units, and educational awareness campaigns stressing respect for and care for the elderly. In both India and Pakistan there are proposed plans for the establishment of 'day centres' to cater to the needs of most of the elderly persons. These will provide companionship, nutritional support, elementary medical care, recreational facilities, continuing education, and even employment opportunities. Thailand places emphasis on the development of programmes to promote the utilization of the occupational skills and talents of the elderly who may wish to support themselves as long as possible. At the same time, a programme providing free medical care to needy elderly people in selected hospitals throughout the country is being implemented. Since 1979 it has enlarged its welfare services to the elderly to strengthen existing family support structures in order to help the aged remain in their own homes. Service centres in communities provide ambulatory medical care, day care, family assistance, and counselling services. In addition, mobile units provide similar assistance in areas which are not within easy reach.

POLICY DIRECTIVES

As has been discussed above, in traditional societies the aged had a well-established place and role in the framework of the extended family system. This is to say that the day-to-day affiictions, calamities, suffering, and hardships encountered by the aged concerned the whole family group of which they formed an intergral part. Remedies, if available, were for the benefit of all who had fallen in similar circumstances and were not specifically designed for the aged. It is of considerable importance, therefore, that developing countries guard against aged-specific programme in their policy plans for the welfare of the aging. The overall socio-economic conditions prevailing in each country ought to come into focus so that any welfare programmes planned can, as far as possible, form an integral part of each country's development strategies from birth to old age. The need for individual national studies cannot be overemphasized. Integrated care has implications for the development and improvement of community health, housing, and environment, education for knowledge and upgrading of skills for modern living and improvement in community life and community self-help. Voluntary organization can play a crucial role. Developing countries must work at maintaining the strong links which still exist between generations within kin groups and the ways of traditional living with supportive measures using neighbourhood and community assistance to keep elderly members of the society active and useful.

Unless family support is strengthened then, given present socio-economic developments, new service infrastructures will be required. They will become substitutes for or expansions of the traditional informal support systems. Given the competing demands from a large youth population and the constrained economic resources, the feasibility of creating new systems of care for developing countries may be questioned.

Policy options being considered place primary emphasis on strengthening both family resources and the motivation to continue care to the elderly. These include policies for financial support in the form of allowances, indemnities, subsidies, and tax relief to families caring for the elderly. In some countries, provisions for establishing family-based, income-generating projects [4] and assistance in the acquisition of multigenerational housing units are being discussed, as are proposals for 'day centres' to provide companionship, institutional support, elementary medical care, recreational facilities, and continuing education.

In the developing countries emotional ties and economic support among primary family members remain very strong. These should be encouraged and strengthened by supportive services in the community.

Other types of benefits which could be supportive to families with elderly relatives are discounts in rent as well as in the prices of medicines and basic foods. There will always be some who need institutional care and their needs will have to be addressed. Voluntary organizations can play a crucial role. Developing countries should guard against age-specific programmes in plans for the welfare of the aging. The welfare programmes for the elderly ought to be an integral part of each country's development strategies from birth to old age. The need for individual national studies cannot be overemphasized.

CONCLUSION

In this chapter some attempt has been made to describe and analyse the traditional and modern roles of the family in the care of the aged in the developing countries and to review future trends. This gargantuan task has been attempted in the firm conviction that there are wide regional and even national variations in the nature of care, problems and needs, and policy approaches. There are indeed considerable differences in the situation of the aging throughout the developing countries, as there are within the same country, depending on the level of development, the degree of modernization, urbanization, and other developmental processes. Nevertheless within the context of tradition and, more specifically, current developmental trends we sense that there are some common grounds for argument, if not in actual individual details. A common development is the increasing number of the aging in these countries who can no longer rely solely on their own or 'family' resources and are therefore in need of some social intervention. Selected countries considered as examples in the discussion from the host of developing countries can best give an idea of what is or what might be.

Notes

1. United Nations World Assembly on Aging, 26 July–6 August 1982, Vienna. National reports of participating countries are on file at the Centre for Social Development and Humanitarian Affairs of the UN Secretariat Vienna. Excerpts and summaries can be found in the UN Publication *The world aging situation: strategies and policies*, (1985). UN, New York.
2. Between 1974 and 1984 I have had the privilege of attending eight international meetings on aging related to the developing countries. Notable among them are the following:
   —— United Nations Inter-Regional Seminar on Aging, 1979, Kiev, USSR;
   —— WHO Preparatory Conference for UN World Assembly on Aging, 8–11 December 1980, Mexico City;
   —— Symposium on 'Aging in the Developing Countries' 1981, Hamburg, Germany;
   —— Group of Experts Meeting, International Centre for Social Gerontology, 4–6 May 1983, Versailles, France.
3. 7–11 July 1981, Hamburg, West Germany. The symposium was attended by representatives of 17 countries from Africa, Asia, and Latin America.
4. Income-generating projects aim to supplement family income through self-help. Examples of such projects include backyard gardening of vegetables, poultry and piggery, cottage industries of simple food processing for local consumption, weaving, dyeing, and other local crafts.

References

1. United Nations (1979). Age–sex composition of population by countries 1960–2000. UN, New York.
2. United Nations (1979). Demographic overview of the aging of populations. UN International seminar on aging, Tables 2, 3, and 4. United Nations Centre for Social Development and Humanitarian Affairs, New York.

3. Lambert, W. W. and Lambert, W. E. (1964). *Social Psychology*. Englewood, New Jersey.
4. Goode, W. J. (1964). *The family*. p. 45. Prentice Hall, New Jersey.
5. Chattergy, V. (1976). View from the Philippines. In Proceedings of the *Hawaii governors bicentennial conference on aging*. State of Hawaii, Hawaii.
6. Adeotkun, L. A. (1983). Demographic determinants of intra family support for the aged in Nigeria. Presented at the Group of Express Meeting of the International Centre for Social Gerontology, Versailles.
7. Guthrie, G. (1966). *Child rearing and personality development in the Philippines*. Pennyslvania State University Press.
8. Goode, W. L. (1970). *World revolution and family patterns* pp. 124–5, 201. The Free Press, New York.
9. Peil, M. and Sada, P. W. (1984). *African urban society*. p. 145. John Wiley, New York.
10. United Nations (1975). *Human settlements and the aging*. Report of the United Nations Centre For Human Settlements, New York.
11. Daghestani, K. (1983). Evolution of the Moslem family in the Middle Eastern countries. *UNESCO International Social Science Bulletin*, **5**, 687.
12. Goode, W. J. (1970). *Ibid* p. 150.
13. Little, K. (1965). *West African Urbanisation*. Cambridge University Press.
14. Caldwell, J. C. (1968). *Population and family change in Africa*. Canberra University Press.
15. Oppong, C. (1974). Family change in Africa-a review. *Institute of African Studies, Legon. Research Review*, **7**, 1–17.
16. Azu, G. (1974). The Ga family and social change. *African studies documents*, Vol. 5. University of Leiden.
17. Birmingham, W. (1967). *A study of contemporary Ghana*. Vol. 2, (ed. Newstadt, J., and Omabos, E. N.) p. 158. Allen and Unwin, London.
18. Rowe, W. (1961). The middle and later years in Indian Society. In *Aging and Leisure* (ed. R. Kleemeir) pp. 104–12. Oxford University Press, New York.
19. Press, I. and Mckoal, M. (1972). Social structure and status of the aged: toward some valid cross-cultural generalizations. *Aging and Human Development*, **3**, 297–306.
20. Arth, M. (1986). Ideals and behaviours: a comment on Ibo respect patterns. *Gerontologist*, **8**, 242–44.
21. Gibson, M. J. S. (1985). *Older women around the world*, p. 13. International Federation on Aging, Washington.
22. Souza, A. de (1982). *The social organization of aging among the urban poor*. Indian Social Institute, New Delhi.
23. Khan, A. (1983). Personal communication.
24. Heisel, M. A. (1989). Women and widows in Turkey: support systems. In *Widows: other places, other times* (ed. Lapata, H. Z.), (Forthcoming).
25. Adeokun, L. A. (1980). Social aging in Yoruba women. Paper presented at the IX International Conference of Social Gerontology, Quebec, Canada, August.
26. United Nations (1982). Demographic indicators of countries: estimates and projections as assessed in 1980. UN publication No. E. 82. XIII.5. UN, New York.

27. United Nations (1985). *The world social situation: strategies and policies.* p. 115. UN, New York.

Further reading

American Association For International Aging (1985). *Aging population in developing countries.* Washington DC.

Apt. N. A. (1972). Urbanization and the aged. In *The family research papers No. 5.* Institute of African Studies, University of Ghana, Legon.

Apt, N. A. (1986). Changing family patterns and the impact on aging in Africa. In *The graying of nations II.* US Government Printing Office, Washington DC.

Symposium report (1981). *Population development and social security aging in developing countries.* Duisberg, Hamburg.

Iliovici, J. (1979). Aging and development humanitarian issues. Working Paper, Interregional Seminar on Aging, Kiev USSR.

International Federation on Aging (1987). *Aging International*, **XIV** (1), 2–3. Washington DC.

Schade, B. and Apt, N. (1983). Aging in developing countries. In *Aging in the eighties and beyond.* (ed. Bergner, M., Lehr, U., Lang, E., and R. Schmits-Sehe) Springer, New York.

23

The role of the family in developed countries

DAISAKU MAEDA

INTRODUCTION

It is impossible to discuss 'the role of the family in developed countries' in the context of social situations in developed countries as a whole, as they greatly differ from each other. This chapter discusses the theme mainly from the standpoint of Japan. Whenever possible, we will try to take into consideration the facts and problems of other developed countries.

THE ELDERLY AND THE FAMILY IN DEVELOPED COUNTRIES

Many people in developing countries tend to think that the elderly in developed countries are abandoned by their offspring and live a solitary and miserable life in general, but this is not true. Elaine Brody, a social gerontologist in the United States, describes the social network of the elderly in her country as follows:

While family structure and composition have no doubt undergone profound changes, the theory of the isolated nuclear family has been discredited. . . . Studies and the observations of practitioners have . . . shown that despite the greatly increased number of old people, personal ties between the generations continue to be strong and viable; families continue to behave responsibly in helping their aged; and when they are unable to do so, a constellation of personal, social and economic forces may be at work. Thus, the collective social and cultural rejection of the aged has not been acted out on the individual or family level.[1]

Barry D. McPherson[2] summarizes aging parent and offspring exchange relationships in developed countries as follows:

Recent demographic changes such as decreased family size, childless marriages, and fewer single adult daughters, combined with an increasing number of middle-aged women in the labour force, have led to a decrease in the availability and opportunity of children to care directly for aging parents. As a result, more social and health care support services are provided by the private and government sectors. Nevertheless, in most societies the family is the first and major resource for the elderly, of whom less than 10 percent are ever institutionalized.

TRADITIONAL FAMILY CARE IS STILL FUNCTIONING IN JAPAN

As McPherson points out, even in the developed countries of the Western world, care for a frail and impaired elderly person is given primarily by a family member, and when the elderly person is widowed then care is most likely given by an adult son or daughter. Unlike in east Asian countries, however, the care is in almost all cases given by one of their offspring living separately from the aging parents because the proportion of the elderly who live with an adult married offspring is very small in Western developed countries compared with east Asian countries.

In east Asian countries, including Japan, where the overwhelming majority of old people live in the same household as their grown children, a far greater proportion of elderly are cared for in their offspring's homes until they die. According to the fundamental survey for the Health and Welfare Administration of 1985, 63.6 per cent of the Japanese elderly aged 65 and over live with their offspring. As shown in Fig. 23.1, this traditional pattern of living arrangement and family care of aged parents is still fairly well preserved, even in the completely industrialized and urbanized metropolitan areas of Japan where the influence of Western culture is felt much more strongly than in other areas. That is, even in such areas, more than 50 per cent of the elderly aged 65 and over live with their offspring. This proportion is significantly higher in less industrialized areas. In rural areas, more than 70 per cent of the elderly aged 65 and over live with their adult offspring.

It should be noted, however, that the proportion of the elderly living thus has been decreasing very rapidly in the last 30 years in parallel with the industrialization and urbanization of Japanese society. As shown in Table 23.1, it has been decreasing at an average annual rate of 0.9 per cent over the last 15 years, but the rate of decrease has accelerated in recent years. However, even if this accelerated rate continues in the future, it will take more than 22 years for the proportion of co-living elderly to decrease to 50 per cent. In other words, even at the beginning of the next century, approximately 55 per cent of elderly persons will be living with their grown offspring in Japan.

The above estimation is made solely by extending the recent numerical trend to the future. Another factor reinforces the prediction. In 1981, the Section on Aging (Roujin Taisaku Shitsu) of the General Executive Office of the National Government carried out a nationwide survey on the opinion of middle-aged persons on life after retirement and the care to be given.[5] According to this survey, as shown in Table 23.2, 58 per cent of married men and women aged between 30–49 think that one of

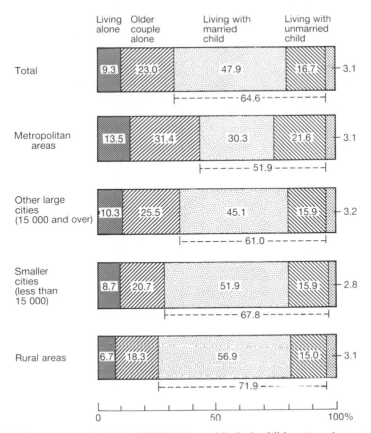

Fig. 23.1 Percentage of elderly (65↑) living with their children in urban and rural areas.[3]

Table 23.1 Decrease in percentage of persons 65 years of age and above living with their children[1]

Year	Living with children	Aged couple Only	Living alone	Others	Total	Decreasing rate of 'living with children' per year
1970	76.9	12.1	5.5	5.5	100.0	
1975	72.5	15.7	6.9	4.9	100.0	0.88
1980	68.7	18.9	8.2	4.3	100.0	0.76 } 0.9
1985	63.4	21.5	9.6	5.5	100.0	1.06

Note: Persons living in institutions were excluded.

Table 23.2 Opinions of middle-aged persons about life after retirement and the care to be given[5]

Conditions of parents	Opinions on living arrangements of aging parents				
	Son's family should live together	Daughter's family should live together	(Subtotal)	Married child should live separately from parents	Don't know/ not available
In general	45.9%	12.3%	(58.2%)	30.4%	11.4%
When one of the aging parents gets frail	62.1%	21.4%	(83.5%)	6.6%	9.9%
When one of the aging parents died	63.2%	20.5%	(83.7%)	5.0%	11.3%

Note: National representative sample (1259) of middle-aged married men and women aged 30–49.

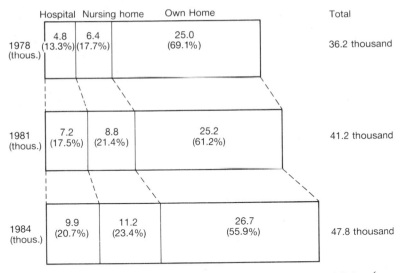

Fig. 23.2 Proportion of bedridden old people by places of living.[6]

their offspring's families should live with aging parents. When they were further asked what they think about the living arrangement of aging parents if one of them gets frail or dies, more than 83 per cent answered that the children's families should live with them.

This result implies that, unless the attitude of the present middle-aged generation changes significantly, which is most unlikely at least in the next 35 years, the living arrangements of Japanese elderly persons will not become similar to that of Western developed countries.

It should also be noted that in Japan most bedridden older persons are cared for in their own homes. A recent nationwide study estimated as 2.7 per cent the proportion of the bedridden who had been in such condition more than 6 months in the population aged 60 and over in 1984.[3] As shown in Fig. 23.2, out of all the bedridden elderly, 56 per cent were cared for by their spouse, offspring, or other relative in their own homes. The proportion of the bedridden elderly institutionalized in nursing homes was only 23 per cent; the remaining 21 per cent were hospitalized.

ATTITUDE OF MIDDLE-AGED JAPANESE PERSONS ON FAMILY CARE OF THE BEDRIDDEN ELDERLY

Some Westerners have attributed the extensive care of bedridden old people in Japan by their families to the limited amount of available nursing home beds. The shortage of beds in institutions, however, seems

Table 23.3 People's plans for the care of their parents when they become bedridden[5] (percentages)

Planned source of care	For husband's parents $n = 1017$		For Wife's parents $n = 1079$	
Parent's spouse	11.1		8.9	
Respondent him/ herself	24.4		10.0	
Respondent's spouse	18.9		6.8	
Brother	13.8	81.7	18.8	83.0
Brother's spouse	16.9		31.4	
Sister	2.0		7.3	
All brothers and sisters	5.8		8.7	
Other family members or relative	0.6		0.7	
Sub-total	93.4		92.6	
Other resources (paid housekeepers, public homehelpers, nursing homes, etc.)	2.9		1.7	
Don't know	3.7		5.7	

to be only a minor reason why the majority of Japanese old people are cared for by their families.

The recent nationwide survey of the opinions of middle-aged married persons cited above[5] also studied people's plans for the care of their parents when they become bedridden. According to the survey, slightly more than 80 per cent answered that the offspring or the latter's spouse would care for them, and approximately 10 per cent answered that the parent's spouse would provide care. Less than 3 per cent answered that they were planning to depend upon resources other than family members (e.g. a paid housekeeper, public home help services, nursing homes, etc.) (Table 23.3). Thus, it is clear that in Japan the overwhelming majority of middle-aged persons still firmly believe that care of bedridden older parents is the responsibility of their offspring.

However, there is a great gap between attitude and fact. As shown in Fig. 23.2, in Japan almost half of bedridden old people are hospitalized or institutionalized. Even if we admit that there are a number of those bedridden old people who do not have offspring, who are too seriously impaired to be cared for by the families, or whose expected caregiver is too old or not healthy enough, this gap between attitude and reality means that many middle-aged persons do not provide the needed care for other reasons—for instance, an expected caregiver might choose to continue his/her career rather than to sacrifice his/her future life, or a bedridden older person might prefer to go to a hospital or nursing home rather than to be cared for by their offspring for fear of being too much of a burden, or the latter might not want to give the needed care because of difficult family relationships.

CHANGE IN THE ROLES PLAYED BY OFFSPRING

Reference was made above to the gap between the attitude and the actual behaviour of middle-aged Japanese persons in relation to the care of bedridden parents. However, the avoidance of a culturally expected role is made possible by the development of formal support and care services. A similar phenomenon can be observed in other aspects of relationships between the elderly and their adult offspring.

Comparing two nationwide studies on the care of older parents in 1974 and in 1983,[7] the proportion of children (married middle-aged male offspring) providing economic support to their aging parents is found to be reduced as follows:

	Percentage	
	1974	1983
Offspring aged 35–39	41	36
Offspring aged 40–44	42	40
Offspring aged 45–49	48	42

In answer to the question of why they do not provide financial support for aging parents (in the 1983 survey), 54 per cent of those who did not answered that their parents were sufficiently well-to-do not to need such support. During these 9 years Japan's economy developed considerably, and the income of these middle-aged men had improved substantially. Therefore, the reduced proportion of economic support to aging parents reflects the greater financial independence of the elderly brought about by the development of public pension programmes.

The importance of the role of adult offspring in health care has also changed greatly recently. As shown in Fig. 23.2, in 1978, 69 per cent of bedridden old people were cared for in their own homes.[3] The same survey done only 6 years later disclosed that this proportion had reduced to 56 per cent.

CAUSES OF DECLINE IN FAMILY ROLE IN THE CARE OF AGING PARENTS

The data above indicate that the pattern of traditional family care of the elderly is still well preserved in Japan, but there has been a significant decline in such family care in the past several decades.

At least four factors should be considered as causes of this decline in the context of social situations in Japan:

(1) change in socio-economic structure of Japanese society as a result of the second industrial revolution;

(2) demographic changes;

(3) the decreased capability of families to care for their aging parents;

(4) development of formal support and care services.

First let us discuss the impact of the second industrial revolution.

Impact of the second industrial revolution

Japan has been experiencing the second industrial revolution since 1955. At that time the proportion of the population who were engaged in agriculture was approximately four-tenths. This proportion reduced to less than one-tenth by 1985.[4] This reduction of the agricultural population had a profound impact on the socio-economic structure of Japanese society. In Japan and also in other east Asian countries when the head of a household is engaged in agriculture all the adult members of the household, including the elderly, also work together in agricultural production to help the work of the household head. In other words, all the household members of east Asian farmers produce collectively and at the same time consume collectively. In a society where this type of household is predominant, it is quite natural and convenient for all family members to live together in the same household.

In industrialized societies, where an older and a younger generation are both engaged in secondary or tertiary industry, the two generations generally have separate incomes. In addition, because of the different lifestyles of the two generations caused by different occupations in many

Table 23.4 Index of increase in number of the older persons (1950–2020)[4,8]

Age	1950	1975	2000	2020
60–69	100	190	360	371
70–79	100	214	499	765
80+	100	323	1193	2398

cases it is more natural, and above all more convenient, for the two generations to live separatively.

Secondly, industrialization has brought about much more frequent geographical mobility of working populations. In industrialized societies, people change their jobs much more frequently than before. Even when they remain in the same firm, most of employees are frequently forced to move to other industrial areas for various reasons. In such cases, aging parents tend to prefer to remain at the original residence rather than move to an unknown place with the offspring's family in order to continue to live together.

Thirdly, in our industrialized areas housing for workers is, generally speaking, not large enough for two generations to live together.

Last, but not the least, the awakening of self among the general public aroused by higher education, higher living standards, and the influence of Western industrialized countries has also played a very important role with regard to the change in living arrangements of the elderly in Japan. That is, these days an increasing number of both older and younger generations prefer to live separately from each other just for the sake for personal independence and freedom.

All in all, Japanese society is now in a conflicting situation with regard to the family care of elderly parents, where the impact of traditional culture and that of industrialization and modernization co-exist side by side.

Impact of demographic changes

One feature of Japan's recent demographic changes is an increase in the number of unmarried and/or childless old people, along with that in the total size of the aged population. Moreover, because of improvements in the general standard of living as well as in the medical sciences, the number of very old persons (aged 80 years or above) has increased significantly, as shown in Table 23.4. The more advanced age of dependent older parents means that the age of their caretaking offspring is also higher. In many cases offspring themselves are already old and their own health is not good enough to provide the needed care.

Decreased capability of families to care for aged parents

Several social factors have contributed to the decreased capability of families to care for aging parents. First, a great migration of the younger generation from rural to urban areas has occurred. On the urban side, the development of industry has brought about a dispersion of industrial areas. Thus, persons who were born and raised in urban locations often find it difficult to get a job in the urban area where their parents live. As a result, in urban as well as rural areas, the proportion of old people living alone or only with their spouse has increased.

Another social factor is the growing number of working women. Many of the married, middle-aged women who were once the most dependable caretakers of dependent older parents are now working outside their homes.

Finally, the number of children born in Japan has decreased rapidly since 1950. As a result, persons with fewer offspring are now gradually entering the aged population. Obviously, when old people have fewer offspring, their chances of depending on them are reduced. This factor will make the need for services for old people, both community and institutional, more acute in the near future.

Development of formal support and care services

Theoretically speaking, formal support and care services were developed to cope with the various problems the elderly and their families are facing in the industrialized society of present-day Japan. However, as economists frequently point out, supply arouses demand. The development of various forms of formal support and care services in recent years has made it possible for people to depend upon them with regard to the care of their aging parents, and thereby has allowed family members to shift at least partially their responsibility. The present situation of our formal support and care services will be discussed later in this paper.

DIFFICULTIES OF FAMILIES CARING FOR IMPAIRED AGING PARENTS

The impact of the demographic and social changes described above has been so strong that the recent development of formal support and care services could not fully meet the expanding needs of the elderly and their families. Thus, impaired elderly are frequently cared for by families whose capability for giving the care needed is not sufficient. In these cases, the quality of care is very poor, and, at the same time, the sacrifice

Table 23.5 Caregivers of bedridden older persons[9]

Caregiver	Bedridden (%)	
	Males	Females
Spouse	61.0	11.4
Offspring (both sexes)	10.8	27.7
Son's wife	21.7	50.4
Grandchildren (including both sexes)	0.8	2.7
Others, unknown	5.7	7.8

of the caring family is very great. Without a doubt, institutional care should be provided in some cases. In other cases support from outside sources can effectively complement the function of the family and, as a result, the level of care will become adequate and the family's burden will become lighter and more bearable.

In order to plan and implement effective social services for the impaired elderly, knowledge of who is actually caring for them and under what conditions is vitally important. Recently a number of such studies have been conducted in Japan. The results of two of these investigations deserve special attention.

The question of who is caring for bedridden older people is answered in Table 23.5, which describes caretakers in relation to the gender of the bedridden elderly. As seen in the table, 61 per cent of bedridden older men are cared for by their aged wives, and 22 per cent are cared for by their son's wives. On the other hand, 50 per cent of bedridden older women are cared for by their son's wives, and 28 per cent are cared for by their own children.

These figures reveal several very serious problems. First, the average age of the caregivers is high. About one-quarter of the people caring for bedridden old people are aged 60 and over; this includes 3 per cent who are aged 80 and over. Second, the majority of caregivers are son's wives or married daughters, who are generally at the prime stage of their lives and are busy with many duties such as work and the care of their own children. Third, in some cases the bedridden elderly are cared for by unmarried sons or daughters who are usually also working full-time. It is often very difficult for such caregivers to have the opportunity to marry, and because of the social pressure dictating that children should take care of their aged parents they seldom place their parents in institutions.

Further evidence of the difficult conditions experienced by Japanese caregivers can be seen in Table 23.6, which is derived from a study conducted in Tokyo by the Sociology Department of the Tokyo Metropolitan Institute of Gerontology in 1981. This table describes the care of physically impaired old people living in the community, in terms of the degree of difficulty experienced by caregiving families.

As can be seen from the bottom row of the table, nearly two-thirds of the impaired elderly are cared for by families whose degree of difficulty in caregiving is very serious. Even among the most seriously impaired older persons who are completely bedridden and/or totally incontinent, more than half are cared for by families whose degree of difficulty is very serious.

From the viewpoint of ascertaining the unmet needs of impaired elderly and their families, the most seriously impaired older persons cared for in a family with the most serious difficulty require special attention. As shown in Table 23.6, these cases account for 6.8 per thousand of the population aged 65 and over living in the community. It is quite clear that such persons should be institutionalized as soon as possible for their own well-being as well as for that of their caregivers. Since this study was done 6 years ago, the proportion now might be a little bit smaller, owing to the development of the institutional services mentioned earlier in this paper. However, as the availability of nursing homes is still seriously inadequate in large metropolitan areas, we are quite sure there are still quite a number of such families waiting for a long time for admission into nursing homes. In many of these families neither the impaired elderly nor their caregivers desire institutionalization because they think that care to the aging parents should be given by their offspring (including the son's wife) in their own homes.

In Table 23.6 the proportion of families whose degree of difficulty in caregiving is very serious accounted for more than 60 per cent of all families caring for the impaired elderly. If one takes into consideration those families for whom caregiving conditions were slightly difficult then four-fifths of the caregiving families reported some difficulty.

Not all of these families need external care services immediately. It is quite likely, however, that most of the families caring for most seriously and seriously impaired older persons will need some form of outside support in the near future. Because community services to support these families are not very well developed, the hardships that they experience are often very serious. The term 'family care' has a beautiful and noble connotation, but in many cases it is accompanied by the painful sacrifice of the caregivers, and the quality of care is frequently poor.

Table 23.6 consists of the results of an objective measurement of the needs of impaired elderly and their families. In the same survey we also

Table 23.6 Prevalence rate of impaired older persons by degree of physical impairment and by degree of difficulty of caring families[10]

393

Degree of impairment	Very difficult	Degree of Difficulty of Caring Families				Totals
		Slightly Difficult	No Difficulty	Unable to care or not caring	Degree of Difficulty not known	
Most seriously impaired	6.8	2.6	—	—	0.2	P1 9.6
Seriously impaired	16.8	2.8	—	1.4	—	P2 21.0
Moderately impaired	20.5	8.1	0.2	7.2	—	P3 35.9
Slightly impaired	5.4	1.2	0.2	6.5	0.2	P4 13.5
Totals	49.5	14.7	0.4	15.1	0.4	80.0

Note: The number in each cell indicates the prevalence rate of the category per 1000 persons aged 65+.

studied the subjective needs in these cases and found that the number of respondents who expressed needs subjectively was much smaller than the number of cases diagnosed objectively as having needs. For example, in our study less than half of the families who were judged as needing a home help service stated that they wanted that service. However, these implicit needs will no doubt become more and more explicit as the number of impaired older persons increases and as our society continues to change. The rising number of married, middle-aged women anticipated to enter the labour force in the future is likely to be especially important in the shift from implicit to explicit needs.

Thus, it is urgently necessary that we develop various types of institutional and community care services for the impaired elderly and their families as well as support and encouragement programmes for those families.

DEVELOPMENT OF PUBLIC SERVICES FOR THE IMPAIRED ELDERLY

In order to cope with the problems of the impaired elderly and their caregiving families, Japan has been developing various kinds of national services ranging from institutional care to tax deduction or tax exemption programmes. The national programmes are all administered by local government with subsidies from the national government. In addition to the programmes subsidized by the national government, a number of local governments have established their own programmes although, generally speaking, their effects are limited compared with those of the nationally supported programmes.

Development of institutional care

Since 1970, the total number of beds in all kinds of institutions for the aged (including those for ambulant but frail elderly) has more than doubled from 75 400 to 205 600 in 1985. The increase in the proportion of institutionalized elderly was less conspicuous, from 1.02 to 1.65 per cent, which is still remarkably small compared with other developed countries.

Development of community services

Japan had no public home care services before 1962, when the National Financial Support Programme for Home Help Services was estabished. Since then, three national programmes have been established: provision of special equipments for bedridden older persons in 1969, short-term stay service in 1978, and day-care service in 1979.

Home help services

In 1970, the number of home helpers throughout Japan was 6100 (full-time). By 1987, the number had increased approximately four times to 25 300. During these 17 years the ratio of the number of home helpers for persons aged 65 and over had increased from one per 1210 to one per 530.

Provision of special equipment for bedridden older persons

The equipment includes special beds and bath-tubs, hot-water heaters, mattresses, special telephones, and so forth.

Short-term stay service

Short-term stay services for the bedridden elderly are fairly well developed in Japan. In 1987, the national government assigned a subsidy for local governments to serve approximately 41 000 bedridden older persons throughout Japan. They can stay a week in a nursing home for any reasons including giving respite to a caregiver. The length of stay can be extended when necessary.

Day care service

In 1986, the national government announced a long-term goal for its development in Comprehensive long-term social security and health and social service programmes for the aging society to establish 3000 day care centres for the frail and impaired elderly throughout Japan in the near future. The programme further says that in the long run approximately 10 000 such centres should be established throughout Japan, including small-scale branch centres. In 1987, approximately 500 such centres have already been established, including those not supported by the national subsidy.

Day care services are expected to provide rehabilitation and reactivation services and thereby enable elderly persons to become independent, or at least less dependent, in their daily living, which will alleviate the suffering of caregivers.

Loans to caregivers who build or remodel their homes

This programme is provided for caregivers who build or remodel a house with an independent room for older parents, or add such a room to an existing home.

Tax deduction or exemption

Income tax credit is given to all taxpayers, regardless of income, who are supporting older persons aged 70 and over whose income is below a certain level. When the old person is the taxpayer's or the spouse's parent and lives in the same household as the taxpayer, the amount of deduction is increased. When the older person is impaired, the caretaker is eligible for additional tax credits, and when the degree of impairment is very serious the deductible amount is further increased. Similar credits are also given for local taxes. The amount that is deductible, however, is rather small compared with the amount actually needed to support an old person in the home. Therefore, this programme should be regarded as a means of encouraging family caregiving rather than as providing a real support.

CONCLUSIONS

The family is, and will continue to be, the most important source of support for the elderly in Japan. In the future, however, the relative importance of the role of family will inevitably decrease because (1) the proportion and real number of frail and impaired older people who are no longer independent in their daily living will greatly increase and (2) the capability of families to care for older parents will decrease owing to demographic changes, industrialization, and urbanization. Therefore, various social services for the frail and impaired elderly and support services for the families who care for them will undoubtedly have to be expanded.

References

1. Brody, E. (1977). Aging. In *Encylopedia of social work* (17th ed), Vol. I. pp. 55–77. National Association of Social Workers Washington D.C.
2. McPherson, B. D. (1983). *Aging as a social process*, p. 136. Butterworths, Toronto.
3. Ministry of Health and Welfare (1985a) *Kousei gyousei kiso chousa houkoku: shouwa 60-nenban.* report of fundamental survey for health and welfare administration (1985 edn). Ministry of Health and Welfare, Tokyo.
4. Statistics Bureau, General Executive Office (1950, 1955, 1970, 1975, 1980, 1985). *Kokusei chousa.* (National Census. General Executive Office, Tokyo.
5. Section of Aging (Roujin Taisakushitsu), General Executive Office (1981). *Rougono seikatsuto kaigoni kansuru chousa*, Survey of opinions about life after retirement and the care to be given. General Executive Office, Tokyo.
6. Ministry of Health and Welfare (1985b). *Kourei hakusho: shouwa 60-nenban.* White paper on health and welfare administration, (1985 edn), p. 45 Ministry of Health and Welfare, Tokyo.
7. Section of Aging (Roujin Taisakushitu), General Executive Office (1974, 1983). *Roushinno fuyouni kansuru chousa.* Survey on the Support and Care of Aged Parents. General Executive Office, Tokyo.

8. Institute of Population Problems, Ministry of Health and Welfare (1986). *Estimated future population of Japan*. Institute of Population Problems, Tokyo.
9. National Council of Social Welfare (1979). *Roujin kaigo chousa houkokusho*. Report of the National Survey on Caretakers of the Elderly. National Council of Social Welfare, Tokyo.
10. Tokyo Metropolitan Institute of Gerontology, Sociology Department (1983). *Zaitaku shougai roujinto sono kazokuno seikatsu jittai, oyobi shakaifukushi need-ni kansuru chousa kenkyuu (3)—toukyouno shitamachino baai*. Study on the Needs of Impaired Old People and their Families (3)—in the case of the older sections of Tokyo. Tokyo Metropolitan Institute of Gerontology, Tokyo.

24

Case management and assessment of the elderly

ROSALIE A. KANE

Over the past two decades, case management has been increasingly recognized in the United States as a way to co-ordinate services on behalf of that subgroup of elderly people with functional impairments and multiple needs.[1-4] Sometimes known by other names such as care coordination or resource coordination, some form of case management has been implemented or considered in Canada,[5] Great Britain,[6,7] Australia,[8] Israel,[9] and many other countries in Europe and even Asia.

Any country with a large percentage (or even large numbers) of elderly people must develop some mechanism for identifying who among the larger group need services to address functional impairment, and for allocating those services fairly. Unless the marketplace is left to determine the amount and type of care the functionally impaired receive, some form of case management or co-ordination is likely to emerge. And the case for case management is strengthened because the marketplace works poorly in distributing care for the functionally impaired, in part due to inequalities in the resources of the disabled, but also to difficulties those with functional impairments are likely to have in identifying and locating an appropriate service.

Although some co-ordinating mechanism is necessary, the form that the case management takes will necessarily vary from country to country, and sometimes from region to region within a country. The particulars of case management and the services that are managed depend on at least two factors: the general system of health and social services that has been established, and culturally determined expectations about appropriate ways of treating persons with functional impairments and their families. The proportion of resources expended on the functionally impaired of all ages, the expectations of how family members will help in providing that care, and the ideal concept for the way in which households should be organized are all decisions that will require each country to analyse its own circumstances in the light of its own collective traditions and values.

Given the diversity in culture, policies, and resources around the world, developing a consensus on the best way to organize for management of care would be presumptuous and undesirable. Instead, this chapter gathers evidence about case management to generate guidelines to be considered by those tailoring a system for use in particular contexts. Without a doubt, however, considerable evidence *does* exist in support of developing some form of case management to improve the quality of care for the functionally impaired (most of whom are elderly) and to rationalize the use of resources on their behalf.[10-12]

CASE MANAGEMENT DEFINED

A 1981 United States statute authorizes public expenditures for case management, or 'management of a specified group of services for a specified group of persons'.[13] This global definition leaves unsettled the boundaries of both the clientele managed and the services managed on their behalf. Indeed, in the United States several configurations for managed care have developed side by side. Thus, case managers may be responsible for managing the care needs of persons enrolled within a prepaid health care system whose care is largely provided or financed by that entity. Or they may be responsible for arranging care for persons in a geographically defined area who perhaps meet some other eligibility characteristics (e.g. income). In this latter situation, the care arranged or purchased may come from a wide variety of providers. Also unsettled by the definition is the scope and duration of the case manager's responsibility—for example, the extent to which acute health care services are managed, or the duties of the case manager to continue the case after a client has entered a nursing home.

Despite the vagueness of the somewhat circular definition presented above, it does capture a duality inherent in case management. On the one hand, the case manager must act as an information source and advocate for the person needing care. On the other hand, the case manager simultaneously attempts to conserve resources in the individual case and use the overall resources well on behalf of an entire group of persons with needs. In some programmes an individual focus predominates; in others it is the obligation to the whole group at risk for care and to the community's resources. In any event, case managers attest that maintaining this dual focus can be stressful. Advocacy and parsimony are difficult ingredients for a case manager to reconcile in a single job description.

More operationally, case management is defined by its component processes. With remarkable consistency, these have been identified as follows: screening and casefinding, comprehensive assessment, care planning, implementation of a care plan, monitoring, and re-assessment (with a repetition of the cycle). We now turn to each of these functions separately before considering general issues about who should be given the responsibility to do case management and how a programme might be organized.

Screening/case finding

The first task of a case management programme is to distinguish those who need a case manager's help and/or special care from the larger group of persons at risk. The case-finding mandate requires that the programme be well publicized and that professionals likely to make referrals (e.g. physicians, social workers, mental health personnel, and hospital personnel) and the elderly themselves are well informed about how to initiate a request. This need for visibility and outreach is coupled with a need for criteria to sort out those initially screened, so that the case manager's detailed assessment and care-planning efforts are devoted to those most likely to be in need.

Screening, which is often accomplished in a telephone call with the applicant or with a referring professional or family member, requires application of a set of indicators to establish both eligibility for the programme and the likelihood that a fuller assessment will find the applicant in need of service. Screening questions usually emphasize functional and cognitive abilities, the nature of the living situation, and the amount and type of help at home currently provided by families.

In the United States (and to a lesser extent in Canada and much of Europe as well), institutional care preceded home care in the historical development of widespread long-term care programmes. Much of the growth of case management in the United States occurring in the last two decades resulted from a general effort to develop home care options as 'alternatives' to nursing homes. These efforts were motivated by a combination of cost consciousness (it was thought that unnecessary and expensive admissions to nursing homes might be avoided) and humanitarianism (most older people prefer to live at home, and for every person in a nursing home several equally impaired persons were known to be struggling in the community, some with insufficient help). By now, at least two decades of community care demonstrations have been conducted in the United States, some with well-designed research to examine the cost-effectiveness of additional home care benefits mediated by case management.[10, 14-17] The aggregated findings from all these studies pinpoint the difficulty in targeting community services to a group that would be likely to enter nursing homes. Even when extremely frail persons are identified, often the use of nursing homes is low in the control group.

Predictions about likely use of nursing homes are surest if the patient has actually been referred to a nursing home by a hospital or physician, if the patient is ready for discharge from an acute hospital and needs substantial care, if he or she has applied to a nursing home, and, of course, if he or she is in a nursing home already. If the case-managed services are meant, even in part, to substitute for nursing home care, the programme must reach these groups. Indeed a very cost-effective community care demonstration in the United States, which was conducted in South Carolina, identified its clientele from a mandatory screening programme that assessed all those entering nursing homes and likely to need public funds soon to pay for the care.[16]

Similar pre-admission screening programmes are developing around the United States; Minnesota, for example, mandates that each applicant for a nursing home, regardless of income, receive a pre-admission screening assessment and further provides case management and payment for community services to all those who would be dependent on public funds within 6 months of admission to a nursing home.[18] Recently, the state established that only those who had made application to a nursing home would be eligible for community care; this policy (which is similar to those in effect elsewhere) was designed to improve the targeting of home care, but renders application to a nursing home meaningless as an indicator of a likely admission.

Comprehensive assessment

Once screening is complete, the next step is a multidimensional assessment that can be used as the basis for a care plan. Such an assessment is usually done according to a systematic protocol that covers a variety of areas and contains within it a number of scales capable of yielding separate scores. Indeed, a wide array of measures have been developed for assessing an elderly population.[19, 20] A comprehensive assessment typically takes 1–2 hours to complete. It is multidisciplinary in the sense that its subject matter and design is the product of more than one profession. It may also literally be administrated by a team (e.g. a nurse, social worker, and physician doing their respective components), but more often a single case manager conducts the assessment.

The assessment generally includes the following areas: general health status, functional abilities, cognitive status, emotional status, social functioning including social resources and social support received from family and friends, and current use of health and social services including care at home. Environmental assessment (including assessment of the safety and adequacy of the clients' home, the safety of the larger surroundings, and the availability of services) is also recommended, but measurement technology is less advanced for tapping this dimension. Increasingly, a comprehensive assessment includes exploring whether the care provided by relatives constitutes a burden to them.

Assessment of functioning tends to follow a well-established path. The case manager determines how well the client can perform basic self-care (such as feeding, grooming and bathing, transferring in and out of bed, and using the toilet). These tasks have come to be known as ADLs (Activities of Daily Living). The assessment of each function usually distinguishes between complete independence, ability to perform the task with the help of others, ability to perform the function with equipment, and complete dependence. More detailed variations examine finer gradations of functioning such as hand dexterity (opening jars), strength (lifting pots of water), and gradations of mobility (climbing stairs, walking several city blocks, using a wheelchair). Other activities related to independence are combined into scales measuring what is known in the jargon as IADLs (Instrumental Activities of Daily Living). These include cooking, house cleaning, laundry, shopping, heavy outdoor work (such as shovelling snow), driving or using public transportation, communicating in writing and by telephone, managing money, and taking medications. ADL and IADL scales are available in a wide variety of lengths and formats and almost invariably are included in a case manager's assessment.

Also almost standard in all assessment protocols is some brief test of cognitive capacity (screening for orientation, recent and remote memory, judgement, and computational ability). These MSQs (Mental Status Questionnaires) play two roles in the assessment; they directly measure cognitive abilities, and they inform the case manager if the older person is unlikely to be able to speak reliably for himself. Typically, the measure of emotional well-being includes items or scales to assess anxiety, depression, and suicidal ideation. Social variables include measures of frequency and type of social contacts (from which one can deduce both degree of isolation and potential for tangible help), and the qualitative aspects of relationships, including presence of a confidante and satisfaction. Sometimes life satisfaction or morale is also measured.

The assessment of physical health done by a case manager does not substitute for a medical assessment. If the case manager first enters the case during or immediately following a client's stay in an acute hospital, the case manager will be likely to have access to current information about health status. Often, however, the case manager sees new clients in the community, where they must form general judgements about the client's physical well-being, any need for referral to a physician or other health care provider, and, if so, the urgency of that need. Protocols for assessing physical status include checklists of symptoms, questions about diagnoses acquired in the past, items on recent utilization of health care and hospitals, recent bed-disability days, and perceptions of health (which have proved to be highly correlated with mortality). Usually the case manager also determines which prescribed and over-the-counter medications the older person is using, including dosage and frequency. A non-physician can readily perform such an assessment and use its results to channel the client to appropriate diagnostic and therapeutic care. Similarly, the review of psychiatric history and psychiatric symptoms, along with standardized tests of depression and cognitive impairment, do not replace a mental health workup and diagnosis but can suggest the need for a referral for complete mental health work-ups.

Care planning

More attention has been given to assessment than to the actual planning of care. Yet the purpose of the comprehensive assessment is to inform the care-planning process. Care planning involves translating the problems and unmet needs identified in the assessment into a service package that is acceptable to the client. If the range of services available in the community are limited, the resulting care plans are also less likely to vary.

Care planning should consider the following:

—— the preferences of the client;

—— the possibility of relying on family members to give service, yet the need to ensure that family members are not unduly burdened or asked to perform tasks beyond their competence;

—— the cost of the plan for both public programmes and the client.

The preferences of the client are expected to enter into the care decisions. Sometimes this participation is formalized by a requirement that case manager and client both sign the care plan. However, even when they have 'signed off', clients may still fail to understand the trade-offs in a plan. For example, one study done in New York City found that, although the clients had agreed to the plans, they had not fully understood the array of options from which their care plans were constructed. Once informed of the 'menu' for services, many stated they would have chosen differently.[21]

Case management programmes are expected to take into account the wishes and needs of family members in formulating plans, and they are also expected to use family help whenever possible. However, guidelines are not available to describe how the wishes and interests of family members and the client should be reconciled, if these indeed differ. One programme developed in a family service organization in Boston is currently testing the concept of training family members to themselves act as case managers for their relatives and, in that capacity, arranging services and monitoring their quality.[22] This is an interesting concept, but one that could jeopardize the autonomy of the clients themselves. The older person may be in substantial disagreement with family about the place of care and the type of services sought.

The need to forecast accurately the cost of care plans may at first be perceived as a difficulty by service-oriented case managers. However, with training, reliable cost projections can be made.[23] Costs may be reduced through use of unconventional services—for example, paying a neighbour rather than a formal agency to look in on the client at intervals. Concerns about liability that may be incurred by the case managers or the quality of the unconventional service may act as a deterrent to cost-conscious flexibility.

Care planning tends to be done on a highly individualized basis. Only recently have critics suggested that guidelines and standards might be developed to suggest appropriate plan in a particular circumstance. Such guidelines might dictate when a full geriatric assessment should be suggested or purchased. They could also provide direction for commonly encountered situations. What, for example, should be the case management response to finding that a client is taking six or more drugs and has not been to a doctor for a year? Under what conditions might the case manager be expected to review a list of medications by telephone with the patient's physician? When might a change of physician be recommended? What should the case manager's response be to a person with moderate dementia living alone? Under what conditions should a case manager seek out legal guardianship for a client? If consensus could be achieved on these and similar questions, auditing the quality of care planning would become feasible.

Implementation

Case managers vary in their direct authority to implement the plans. In some programmes, the case manager is limited to making referrals, assisting the client to acquire services, and providing information to possible caregivers that paves the way for services to begin. Other case managers have some degree of authority over a plan. The power may be derived simply from voluntary agreement of agencies in the community to accept the judgements of the case managers. For example, in many local jurisdictions in the Canadian province of Ontario, hospitals, nursing homes, boarding homes, and other agencies have voluntarily agreed to accept the judgements of a 'placement co-ordination service' that organizes and prioritizes waiting lists. More authority is granted if the case manager is designated by governmental bodies to authorize the client's need for a particular service—for example, a nursing home bed, or a piece of medical equipment. The authority is even more impressive if the case manager can purchase service on behalf of the client; typically such case managers make direct arrangements with vendors, authorizing the actual amounts and types of services that will be reimbursed.

Monitoring

Monitoring takes two forms. The case manager monitors any changes in the condition of the client, and the case manager monitors the reliability and adequacy of the services received. Typically, the client is encouraged to contact the case manager as needed, and a similar invitation is extended to agencies giving care. Some case managers are more pro-active in the monitoring of clients and services, or develop guidelines for when more frequent monitoring is necessary.

Case management programmes differ also in their philosophy of how much personal relationship should develop between case manager and client; in programmes with frequent contact the case manager tends to assumes a counselling function and a therapeutic relationship. The size of the case load also governs the amount of monitoring feasible, since case management involves considerable amounts of paperwork whenever changes are made. One study showed that changes most often were instigated at the request of providers.[24] With a good management information system and a conscientious approach to monitoring, a case management programme has potential to produce detailed information about the quality of care in a community, the gaps in necessary service, the lag times between service orders and receipt of care, the turnover of personnel, and various other information about the service structure that assists in community planning as well as individual care planning.

Re-assessment

Re-assessment should occur at regular intervals—for example every 6 months. Re-assessments are also indicated after a major change in status, such as a hospitalization. Requests by the patient or care providers could also stimulate a re-assessment. In a large ongoing programme, the temptation might be to fall behind with routine reassessments and respond only to requests. In the city of Vancouver in Canada, where case managers have authority to purchase services, large case loads caused a backlog in the 6-month re-assessments. But when all intake was stopped until each client was re-assessed, the resultant re-adjustments included lessened levels of service for some clients as well as increases for others.[25] This seems to reinforce the importance of the periodic re-assessment.

WHO IS CASE MANAGER

The choice of case manager occurs at two levels. First, the question arises about the appropriate professional background and training for case management. Second, a choice must be made about the appropriate organizational auspices for case managers.

Background and training

Most frequently, the case managers are registered nurses or social workers. In some of the early programmes developed in the United States, the case managers were multidisciplinary teams of nurse practitioner and masters-level social workers, but this is an expensive approach and some tension between the disciplines has been reported.[25] Another strategy is to employ a multidisciplinary group of case managers. This permits cross-fertilization of skills, case-by-case consultation, and even specific assignments (for example, nurses for cases with extensive physical complications, and social workers for cases with a complex psychiatric history). Physical therapists, occupational therapists, nutritionists, and health educators could also be part of the staff, carrying their own case loads and serving as resources. No one disciplinary background seems to be required for a case manager, although nursing and social work training both lend themselves to the role. Yet since one study suggests that assessments can differ systematically depending on the profession of the case manager,[26] some effort to standardize the approach and achieve reliability is needed on an ongoing basis.

Schools of social work educate their neophytes to work with the person in the environment, and social work curricula give attention not only to developing skills in psychotherapy and counseling, but also to mobilizing resources. Thus an affinity between social work practice and case management has been noted, leading Austin[27] to question whether case mangement is anything more than 'social work reinvented'. The National Association of Social Workers (a US organization that is more than 100 000 strong) has even promulgated standards for social workers doing case mangement,[28] emphasizing the need to the applicability of ethical principles such as the primacy and self-determation of the client, and confidentiality of information about the client. These standards, however, fail to come to grips with the inherent tension between primacy of the individual client and the gatekeeping roles or the allocation of resources for a population. In their widely used textbook on social work with frail elderly clients, Silverstone and Burack–Weiss[29] developed an 'auxiliary model' for social work with the frail elderly, named for the metaphor of an auxiliary lighting system that is 'triggered to action by failure of a permanent system, fading when power is restored'. An auxiliary function, in this conception, bolsters depleted resources (psychological, physicial, and social). With their emphasis on study, assessment, and plans, and co-ordinating and monitoring of services, the authors recognize that their scheme is consistent with case management. However, they stress that counselling and formation of a therapeutic relationship with the client is integral to the auxiliary model of social work, whereas a personal relationship is sometimes de-emphasized or even precluded from the role of the case manager. Indeed the question of whether case managers should form a close relationship with the client and act as counsellors, in contrast to contracting with or referring to someone else for any necessary counselling, is controversial and unresolved.

Should physicians be designated as case managers? It is sometimes argued that primary care physicians, such as family practitioners and internists, fulfil much of a case manager's function. Not only do they orchestrate referrals to medical specialists, but they also suggest and even arrange a much wider array of health services (e.g. dentistry, eye and hearing services, mental health, home nursing, medical equipment) and even social services (e.g. housekeeping). In some countries, including the United States, the physician is a titular gatekeeper who must endorse the need for post-hospital services such as rehabilitation, nursing home care, and home health care. In the United Kingdom, the geriatric team led by the geriatrician tends to make allocation decisions during a team meeting. In New Zealand, the general practitioner has considerable authority to recommend a range of health and even social services (e.g. housekeeping), which are provided by the hospital boards.

Nevertheless, the physician seems *not* to be the ideal person to perform the kind of case management role that this paper has elaborated, especially in a country which has developed a wide range of differentiated choices. At best, it would be an injudicious use of physician time and, at worst, the client would suffer because of gaps in knowledge and skills in a physician/case manager.

If not case managers, however, physicians must be involved in the continuing assessment and adjustment of care plans for three reasons. First, patients and families, especially of the age group now elderly, tend to turn to their physicians for advice and to regard those suggestions with the force of important instructions. If physicians are not part of the working case-managed system, patients are likely to coalesce their thinking around unnecessarily restrictive plans or, worse, take irrevocable actions without full knowledge of available benefits and services. Second, the physician is logically the one who should determine the need for referrals to other medical specialists and health-related disciplines. Third, if case managers bypass physicians, a grave danger exists that they will conduct an assessment and arrange services to compensate for impairment without first determining whether the functional impairment can be ameliorated through medical diagnosis and treatment, including adjustment of medications.

Experience in the United States to date suggests that detrimental discontinuities can easily arise between a case management system and acute medical care.[10, 15, 30] A demonstration of social health maintenance organizations now under way in four cities which tests the cost-effectiveness of combining health care and some socially oriented long-term care in a single capitation scheme,[31] affords an opportunity to determine how case managers and physicians can work together and establish an appropriate division of responsibility.[32]

Organizational auspices

Related to the question of the disciplinary background of the case manager is the broader question of how the case manager should be positioned in the system of health and social services. Once again the answer cannot be prescriptive and needs to be settled within the context of a particular set of benefits and programmes.

In Canadian provinces, where functionally impaired adults of all ages enjoy universal benefits for both home care and nursing home care, the case managers are housed either in local health departments or in local departments of social service. Their positioning is somewhat similar to that of local social service authorities in Great Britain. Though not usually called case managers, such social workers have discretion over the use of institutional and community resources (homes for the aged, home helps, day care, waiting lists for congregate housing). For convenience, they may be officed in hospitals or physicians' practices or assigned to geriatric teams, but they and their resources are part of the social service establishment.[33]

In the United States, the funding streams for health and social services are fragmented, and the case manager, who attempts to bridge disparate programmes, has been positioned in a variety of agencies. In demonstration projects that aim to test the effects of added entitlements and broader eligibilities, case managers have been housed in senior citizens' programmes, health departments, social service departments, private family agencies, hospitals, and even nursing homes. Sometimes new freestanding entities have been created. Simultaneously, another trend has emerged—namely consolidated care organizations (often with a budget based on a per-person flat fee—that is, capitation) that use case managers to identify who from the larger group of enrollees or patients need additional services, to assess the needs more fully, to authorize services (most of which are either directly provided or purchased by the care entity), and to monitor those services. The social health maintenance organizations already mentioned[31] constitute such a scheme, as do the growing hospital-based community care programmes.[34] In the latter, the hospital organization has expanded its repertoire of services to include much more than acute care (perhaps a nursing home, a home health programme, a day care programme, equipment rental, preventive services, support groups, and even housing), and case managers are used to co-ordinate (and in a way market) the care. At one non-profit hospital in Pasadena, California, where case management programmes are highly developed through the hospitals senior service network, the staff have developed the concept of the hospital as a 'capacity builder' to strengthen the entire community's ability to respond to the chronically ill.[35]

Case management has become such a popular concept in the United States that it is itself in some danger of becoming a fragmenting rather than an organizing force. Some community care schemes have divided the case management functions (e.g. having hospital personnel do the initial assessment for clients who are first refered while in hospital and public health nurses for community-dwelling clients, and perhaps even distributing ongoing case management to agencies on a geographical or other basis). A brisk debate has developed in the United States about whether a 'single-entry' or 'multiple-entry' system of case management should prevail.[36] In the former, all initial requests for care funded by public programmes are channelled through a single authority (which may, of course, be housed in many geographically decentralized locations) authorized to do initial assessments and approve care plans. In the latter, multiple routes would exist towards an assessment, a care plan, and the triggering of benefits. A multiple-entry system is less disruptive of existing patterns of service delivery and perhaps, therefore, more acceptable to organizations, but is less coherent.

In a multiple-entry question, another troublesome issue arises in greater force: that is, should case management be done by organizations that also give concrete services (apart from counselling and advice)? Some argued that if any agency, say a hospital or a home health care organization, delivers the care it authorizes, it is open to charges of conflict of interest. It may direct toward itself more lucrative or desirable clientele. On the other side of the issue, in rural areas in particular, it may be efficient and effective for a public organization that does case management, say a public health nursing department, to recruit, train, hire, and supervise the paraprofessionals who give direct care in the home.

Some other United States trends should be noted. A private practice of case management has emerged, which for the most part markets itself to the worried out-of-town relatives of the elderly.[37] This phenomenon is most prevalent in sun-belt vacation areas such as Florida. Case managers working on a fee-for-service basis have no responsibility for preserving societal resources and thus they can be less conflicted advocates; however, they have interests of their own at stake (most bill on the basis of hours rendered, and some directly sell homemaker services) that influence the client's costs. Finally, proposals for private insurance for long-term care include a concept of case management to determine when the policy holder is eligible for care on the basis of functional impairment and to mediate the benefits; in typical proposals, the insurance plan would contract with case management agencies to act in a combined role of insurance adjustor/case manager, but experience with such plans so far is rather theoretical.

CASE MANAGEMENT AND THE CARE SYSTEM

As important as case management can be in helping the frail elderly make better health care decisions and get better access to service, it is no panacea. Its limitations must be recognized. In particular, case management is an indirect approach to a fragmented service system. Often it might be more appropriate to try to correct the service system at its source. In their review of systems for community care in a number of industrialized countries, Reif and Trager[38] point out that almost everywhere discontinuities between health and social services and fragmented funding streams across either jurisdictional levels or categorical programmes render care systems confusing. Case mangement is one response to such confusion; policy change is another. Countries with less developed health and social service programmes have an opportunity to avoid those problems that negatively affect both quality for the consumer and costs for all concerned—for example, fragmentation between delivery systems and funding lines—and a lack of fiscal responsibility on the part of those who order services.

A potential risk to clients exists as well if case managers are involved, but have a limited service system for referral. Their professional instincts may be to protect the client, at the expense of the client's autonomy. An early, classic study of case management for the frail elderly in Cleveland[39] showed that clients receiving case management were more likely than the randomized control group to enter nursing homes and to have higher mortality rates.

Though case management is, thus, no substitute for a coherent service system, the development of case-managed services can improve overall care and point the way to necessary systematic changes.

Case management and quality control

The more authority wielded by case managers, the more control they can exert over the nature and quality of care. If the case managers purchase services on behalf of the clients, quality guidelines can be developed for eligible vendors. Periodic letting of contracts with home health organizations can be a useful device to clarify expectations and advance standards.

Case management and information

A case-managed system lends itself to the development of management information systems that can be used to improve care and to adjust the flow of resources from one region to another. At the core of this potential is standardized assessment data and a capability (vastly assisted by computerization) to describe the overall population needing care, the services given, the costs, and, importantly, the outcomes. Typically, case management programmes organized within a geopolitical entity each have been allocated a budget from a central authority. Consistent definitions and recording will allow comparisons to be made about needs that could influence the future allocation of funds. Of course, this very prospect is threatening to local communities. Also no good formulas have been developed to determine how to allocate budgets fairly. For example, a debate is currently under way in the United Kingdom to examine whether local social service authorities should be awarded their budgets based on global indicators such as mortality rates or composite indicators of 'needs' in each jurisdiction.[40] Particularly demoralizing for local organizations is the common allocation method that uses historical experience of cost as the basis for future budgets. This seems to reward inefficiency.

A case-managed system generates profiles of care providers as well as regional information. The characteristics of client, the costs, and the outcomes can be aggregated for a particular agency and for agencies of a particular type (for example, nursing homes owned by municipalities versus those owned by philanthropies). Such information capacity can be used to monitor services, improve quality, and set rates.

Rationing and cost constraints

In case-managed services, rationing can occur at two levels: the programme budget and the allocations to individuals. In virtually any jurisdiction, the amount of services that could be supplied will exceed the amount of money to pay for them. Allocating a specific budget to a jurisdiction brings these financial realities to the local level, and ensures that those who generate costs by prescribing services also have fiscal accountability.

Rationing also occurs in the difficult decisions made by case managers at the individual level. Case managers can be encouraged to be generally parsimonious and to calculate the expected costs of their plans.[23] Sometimes the desire to develop a safe plan (and one that frees the organization from legal liabilities) forces reliance on more expensive services from formal agencies rather than those that might be organized more cheaply (for example, rides from a neighbour versus a transportation service). In a well-developed case management programme, for example at On Lok Senior Health Services, which is a case-managed, capitated programme offering a wide range of institutionally based and community-based care, acute and long-term care, health and social services to its members in the inner city 'Chinatown' area, decisions about plans are based on conscious, group discussions about how much service can be fairly allocated to an individual person without depleting the organizations resources. In an anthropological study designed to make the decision rules explicit, Hennessy[41] found, for example that the number of staff needed to move a person from one place to another was highly related to the decision to recommend an institution, because the 'two-person transfer' created a heavy demand on resources.

Case management and the epidemiological outlook

Case management at its best permits an epidemiological perspective on care giving, and is thus highly compatible with a frame of reference derived from established public health principles. At its best, a case management approach considers populations rather than individuals alone. It recognizes that those who present themselves for services may not necessarily represent all those who need care or even those who need care most, and therefore evolves a method of screening and case finding. Then, having assured itself of the ability to find the cases, the programme develops ways to allocate resources available on the basis of greatest need and/or greatest likelihood to be effective.

ISSUES FOR RESOLUTION

After a fact-finding mission to Sweden, Terroir[42] conducted an interesting exercise by calculating the changes in ratio of various services to population that would be needed 'if France were Sweden'. Some services in France actually exceeded the supply of those in Sweden, whereas others were substantially lower. The point seems to be that it would be ill-advised to adopt wholesale the system of another country. With considerable enthusisam, however, for the rationalization of care that some form of case management permits, I conclude this chapter with a short list of features that would seem important for any case-management system, and of unresolved issues that any system must consider.

Desirable features of case management include the following:

—— the case management system is visible and accessible to the users;

—— case managers and their programmes are accountable to the public for the quality and cost of care (including both publicly incurred and privately incurred costs);

—— case managers are able to balance a range of services including both institutionally and community-based services;

—— case managers base their judgements on a comprehensive assessment that is predicated on the importance of assessing functional abilities;

—— medical care is incorporated into the case-managed system in such a way that efforts are made to improve functioning before care is introduced to compensate for functional impairments;

—— preferences of those receiving care and their family be incorporated into the programme.

Issues for resolution include the following;

—— Should eligibility for the case-managed system of services and benefits include an age criterion as well as a functional one, or should an integrated case management system also serve younger populations with functional impairments, such as the chronically mentally ill, the physically handicapped (e.g. spinal chord injuries, multiple sclerosis, brain-injured younger adults), the developmentally disabled, and terminally ill of all ages (including persons with AIDS)? The elderly will be the largest group served in any event—is their interest better served by an age-specific or an age-blind programme?

—— What responsibility should be expected of family members to provide part of the care authorized under a plan?

—— What risks should the persons whose care is managed be permitted to assume? Supposing they were unlikely to harm others, when should their preferences to continue in a situation that professionals deem unsafe be honoured?

—— Should those who provide case mangement also deliver services?

—— Is a single-entry or multiple-entry case management system preferable?

—— How much flexibility should case managers be permitted in arranging unconventional plans? When, if at all, would it be desirable to give money directly to the older person to hire someone to provide the care?

—— What will be the duration and intensity of the case managers involvement? Once receiving a referral does the case manager continue to monitor the client regardless of whether any services are needed? Once the client enters a nursing home as a permanent arrangement, should the case manager have a continued involvement? And to what extent does the case manager maintain a personal relationship with the client?

The case management effort should, of course, be evaluated. Yet it is extremely difficult to evaluate the effectiveness of case management apart from looking at the effectiveness of the services available for the case managers to suggest, broker, authorize, monitor, and adjust. It will be possible to develop process and outcome criteria to determine whether case managers are doing their technical job well (e.g. the reliability of their assessments, the efficiency of their plans, the satisfaction the consumers express with their performance). However, to examine the effectiveness of a case-managed system of care in general, one must return to the value-laden questions raised at the beginning of the chapter. First, it must be determined what outcomes are being sought for older people and their families, and then a method can be developed to see if the case-managed system of care is achieving those outcomes.

Note

Prepared for the WHO Conference on Care of the Elderly, Geneva, October 1987.

References

1. Steinberg, R. M. and Carter, G. W. (1982). *Case management and the elderly*. D. C. Heath, Lexington, MA.
2. Weil, M. Karls, J. *et al*. (1985). *Case management in human service practice*. Jossey–Bass, San Francisco.
3. Austin, C. D., Low, J., Roberts, E. A. and O'Connor, K. (1985). *Case management: a critical review*. Pacific Northwest Long-Term Care Gerontology Center, University of Washington, Seattle.
4. Austin, C. D. and O'Connor, K. (1989). Case management: components and program contexts. In *Health care of the elderly: an information source book*, (ed. Petersen M. D. and D. White D) pp. 167–205. Safe, Newburg Park, CA.
5. Kane, R. L. and Kane, R. A. (1985). *A will and a way: what the United States can learn from Canada. About caring for the elderly* Columbia University Press, New York.
6. Davies, B. and Challis, D. (1987). *Matching resources to needs in community care: an evaluated demonstration of a long-term care model*. Gower Publishing Company, Aldershot, Hants, UK.
7. Boldy, D. and Canvin, R. (1984/1985). Community care of the elderly in Britain: value for money. *Home Health Care Services Quarterly*, **5**, 109–22.

8. Coombs, E. M. (1984/1985). Home support services in Australia: a confusion of intergovernmental responsibilities and provision. *Home Health Care Services Quarterly*, **5**, 175–206.
9. Hirschfeld, M. J. (1984/1985). Toward a social policy on caring for the aged in Israel, *Home Health Care Services Quarterly*, **5**, 269–82.
10. Kane, R. A., and Kane, R. L. (1987). *Long-term care: principles, programs, and policies*. Springer Publishing Company, New York.
11. Pelham, A. O. and Clark, W. F. (ed.) (1986). *Managing home care for the elderly: lessons from community-based agencies*. Springer Publishing Company, New York.
12. Zawadski, R. T. (ed.) (1983). *Community-based systems of long-term care*. Haworth Press, New York.
13. United States Senate Special Committee on Aging (1985). *Developments in aging: 1984*. Government Printing Office, Washington.
14. Capitman, J. A., Haskins, B., Bernstein, J. (1986). Case management approaches in community-oriented long-term care demonstrations. *The Gerontologist*, **26**, 289–97.
15. Carcagno, G., Applebaum, R., Christianson, J., Phillips, B., Thornton, C., and Will, J. (1986). *The evaluation of the national channeling demonstration: planning and operational experience of the channeling projects*. Vols, I and II. Mathematica Policy Research Inc, Princeton, NJ.
16. Kemper, P., Applebaum, R., and Harrigan, M. (1987). *A systematic comparison of community care demonstrations*. University of Wisconsin Center for the Study of Poverty, Madison, WI.
17. Weissert, W. G., Cready, C. L., and Pawelak, J. E. (1989). Home and community care: two decades of findings. In *Health care of the elderly: an information source book*, (ed. Peterson, M. and D. White), pp. 39–126 Sage Publications, Newbury Park, CA.
18. Moscovice, I., Davidson, G., and MacCaffree, D. (1987). *Evaluation of Minnesota's preadmission screening and alternative care grant program*. Center for Health Services Research, University of Minnesota, Minneapolis.
19. Kane, R. A. and Kane, R. L. (1981). *Assessing the elderly: a practical guide to measurement*. D. C. Heath, Lexington, MA.
20. Israel, L., Kozarevic D., and Sartorius N. (1984). *Source book of geriatric assessment*. Vol. I & II (English Ed). Karger, Basel/New York.
21. Frankfather, D. L., Smith M. J., and Caro, F. G. (1981). Family care of the elderly: public initiatives and private obligations. D. C. Heath, Lexington, MA.
22. Seltzer, M. M., Simmons K., Ivry, J., and Litchfield, L. (1984). Family–agency partnerships: case management of services for the elderly. *Journal of Gerontological Social Work*, **7**, 57–71.
23. Rickards, S. (1985). Cost projections in the channeling care planning process. In *Case management: a critical review* (ed. Austin, C. D., J. Low, E. A. Roberts, and K. O'Connor) pp. 154–68, Pacific Northwest Long-Term Care Gerontology Center, University of Washington, Seattle.
24. Schneider, M. J., Hirsch, C., Galper, M. K., Rickards, S. W., and Sterthous, L. M., (1984). *A year in the lives of clients and case managers*. Temple University Institute on Aging, Philadelphia.
25. Amerman, E. (1985). The nurse/social worker dyad in community-based long-term care. In *Case management: a critical review* (ed. Austin, C. D., J.

Low, E. A. Roberts, and K. O'Conner) pp. 188–93 Pacific Northwest Long-Term Care Gerontology Center, University of Washington, Seattle.

26. Hennessy, C. H. and Shen, J. (1986). Sources of 'unreliability' in multidisciplinary team assessment of the elderly. *Evaluation Review*, **10**, 178–92.

27. Austin, C. D. (1987). Case management: reinventing social work? Paper delivered at the Annual Meeting of the National Association of Social Workers, New Orleans, LA, September 9.

28. NASW (1984). *Standards and guideline for social work case management for the functionally impaired*. Professional Standards, No. 12. National Association of Social Workers, Silver Springs, MD.

29. Silverstone, B. and Burack-Weiss, A. (1983). *Social work practice with the frail elderly and their families: the auxiliary function model*. Charles C. Thomas, Springfield, IL.

30. Peters. B. (1986). The ten commandments of case management during hospitalization. In *Managing home care for the elderly: lessons from community-based agencies* (ed. Pelham, A. O. and W. F. Clark) pp. 67–76 Springer Publishing Company, New York.

31. Leutz, W. N., Greenberg, J. N., Abrahams, R., Prottas, J., Diamond, I. M., and Gruenberg, L. (1985). *Changing health care for an aging society*. D. C. Heath, Lexington, MA.

32. Leutz, W. N., Abrahams, R., Greenlick, M., Kane, R. A., and Prottas, J. (1988). Targetting expanding care to the aged. Early SHMO experiences. *The Gerontologist*, **28**, 4–17.

33. Goldberg, E. M. (1971). *Helping the aged*. Allen & Unwin, London, UK.

34. Brody, S. J. and Persily, N. (1984). *Hospitals and the aged: the new old market*. Aspen, Rockville, MD.

35. White, M. and Simmons, J. (1989). Case management in hospitals. *Generations*, **12**, 34–8.

36. Pitkialis, D. S. and Callahan, J. (1986). Organization of long-term care: should there be a single or multiple focal points for long-term care coordination. In *The impact of technology on long-term care* (ed. Grana, J. M. and D. B. McCallum) pp. 147–72. Project HOPE Center for Health Affairs, Millwood, VA.

37. Secord, L. (1987). *Private case management for older persons and their families: practice, policy, potential*. InterStudy, Excelsior, MN.

38. Reif, L. and Trager, B. (ed.) (1984/1985). International perspectives on long-term care. *Home Health Care Services Quarterly*, **5**, 1–341.

39. Blenkner, M., Bloom, M., and Nielson, M. (1971). A research demonstration of protective services. *Social Casework*, **52**, 483–99.

40. Mays, N. (1987). Measuring need in the National Health Service resource allocation formula: standardized mortality ratios or social deprivation? *Public Administration*, **65**, 45–60.

41. Hennessy, C. H. (1987). Risks and resources: Service allocation decisions in a consolidated model of long-term care. *Journal of Applied Gerontology*, **6**, 139–55.

42. Terroir, P. (1984/1985). Report of a mission from France to review care provided to the aged in Sweden. *Home Health Care Services Quarterly*, **5**, 207–28.

25

The efficacy of geriatric assessment programmes

LAURENCE Z. RUBENSTEIN

Geriatric assessment can be defined as a multidimensional—usually interdisciplinary—diagnostic process designed to quantify an elderly individual's medical, psychosocial, and functional capabilities and problems with the intention of arriving at a comprehensive plan for therapy and long-term follow-up. Assessment has assumed a pivotal role in geriatric care because of the complexity of the frail elderly patient, the vast number of unmet needs facing the rapidly growing older population, and the fact that assessment has been increasingly associated with improvements in care outcomes. This chapter will provide an overview of geriatric assessment and a summary of its proved and probable benefits.

ORIGINS OF GERIATRIC ASSESSMENT

The concept of geriatric assessment traces its origins to the British geriatric pioneers of the 1930s such as Marjory Warren, Lionel Cosin, and Sir Ferguson Anderson. These physicians noted a disturbingly high rate of long-term institutionalization among disabled elderly patients, most of whom had never been carefully evaluated from a medical or psychosocial standpoint nor given a trial of rehabilitation. These early geriatricians uncovered a very high prevalence of readily identifiable remediable problems among both institutionalized and non-institutionalized patients. They also found that most of these patients could show improvement, often dramatic, when provided with appropriate therapy and rehabilitation. From this work of these pioneers, two basic principles of geriatrics emerged: first, many elderly patients need a special diagnostic and therapeutic approach to their care—one that is more interdisciplinary and geared to the complex problems common among aged individuals; second, no patient should be admitted to a long-term care facility without a careful medical and psychosocial assessment and, for most patients, a trial of rehabilitation.[1-2]

When the British National Health Service was founded in 1948, geriatric medicine was accorded full specialty status, largely based upon the successful experiences of the earlier pioneers. In the British system, geriatric specialists are in charge of geriatric services that include acute hospital care for the elderly as well as an assortment of co-ordinated special care programmes such as day hospitals, geriatric rehabilitation units, and home visit services. Under the British system of 'progressive geriatric care', elderly patients requiring admission to hospital, except those requiring intensive medical care, are usually first admitted to an acute-care geriatric assessment/evaluation unit. There each patient receives a comprehensive assessment of medical, functional, and psychosocial problems during an approximately 2- to 3-week length of stay. Care plans are established on the unit, usually by an interdisciplinary team, and the next level of care and placement is decided on—whether discharge to home, to a rehabilitation or chronic-care ward, or to a long-term care facility. The geriatric assessment units also accept patients in need of assessment from other institutions, often for periodic re-assessment. Several other countries (including Sweden, Australia, Norway, Israel, and the Netherlands) have built, or are building, geriatric care systems with many similarities to the British system, most with centrally located geriatric assessment units as focal points for entry into the care system.[1, 3–4] Less intensive assessments are provided to elderly patients through other programmes such as consultation clinics, home visit systems, and day hospitals.

In the United States, growing awareness of the unmet health care needs facing the elderly and realization of how Britain and other countries have met similar needs are promoting the concept of American geriatric assessment programmes. An enlarging body of evidence is indicating that the most striking of the unmet needs—inappropriate institutionalization, incomplete medical diagnosis, lack of co-ordination of community support services, overprescription of medications, and under-utilization of rehabilitation[5–6]—can be ameliorated through the use of geriatric assessment services. Though the United States lacks a national health service, which in other countries has facilitated development of comprehensive geriatric care systems, many components of such a geriatric care system are already present. Medicare, the government-sponsored medical insurance plan for those past retirement, pays for most acute hospital care and outpatient visits for persons 65 and older. Another government insurance programme, Medicaid, covers the cost of long-term and acute care for the indigent. In addition many local and regional programmes exist for providing other vital services such as case management, day care, hospice care, meals-on-wheels, supplemental income, and visiting nurse care. Unfortunately, the separate funding sources of these programmes often interfere with optimal provision and co-ordination. While a large-scale American system for geriatric assessment and case management has not been developed, many local programmes have been created—most in the past decade. Geared to specific local needs and conditions, these programmes vary in many of their structural and functional components as well as in their stated purposes.

The major types of geriatric assessment programmes, both in the United States and abroad, are as follows:

—— acute hospital inpatient units:
     Geriatric assessment/evaluation units;
     Geropsychiatric assessment units;
     Geriatric rehabilitation units;
—— chronic hospital inpatient assessment units;
—— inpatient geriatric consultation services;
—— hospital outpatient departments;
—— home visit assessment teams;
—— office settings or free-standing units.

Some are located within inpatient hospital wards, while others are outpatient or home visit programmes. Some are carefully targeted to the most frail elderly populations while others are open to virtually anyone over a certain age of eligibility. Nevertheless, they share many common characteristics. A listing of the primary purposes for geriatric assessment programmes is as follows:

—— multidimensional diagnostic assessment;
—— planning therapy;
—— providing limited or more extensive treatment;
—— arranging for rehabilitation;
—— determining optimal placement;
—— facilitating primary care and case management;
—— optimizing use of health care resources;
—— geriatric education and research.

Most existing programmes incorporate at least three or four of these purposes, and a few attempt to accomplish them all. Virtually all provide multidimensional assessment, using one or more sets of measurement instruments to quantify functional, psychological, and social parameters. Most use interdisciplinary teams to pool expertise and enthusiasm in working toward common goals. Many programmes, both outpatient and inpatient, provide at least limited treatment and are sites for geriatric education and research. To a large extent, their structures influence their purposes; for example, as a rule only inpatient units are able to provide extensive treatment and rehabilitation while, on the other hand, outpatient programmes are better able to provide longitudinal primary care and case management. Costs are greater for inpatient programmes, but so are the variety of services able to be offered.

PROCESS OF GERIATRIC ASSESSMENT

The process of geriatric assessment varies considerably between programmes. Most are organized around an interdisclipinary core team of providers including a physician, a physician assistant or nurse practitioner, a nurse, and a social worker. To this core is added a variety of other specialists, who either participate in the basic assessment or are called in as consultants (e.g. psychologist or psychiatrist, occupational therapist, physical therapist, audiologist, dentist, optometrist or ophthalmologist, dietician, public health nurse). The size of the team is influenced by several factors, including programme goals, setting, patient load, and funding levels. While large teams offer certain advantages, the bulk of the assessment process can be performed by the core team alone.

Most programmes include a multidimensional assessment including the areas of physical health, functional ability, psychological status, and social support structure. Table 25.1 lists the most important of the measurable dimensions of geriatric assessment. Some programmes use a comprehensive test battery or a multidimensional instrument to perform assessment; others use several of the existing unidimensional instruments suited to their particular programmes; still others rely primarily on judgements and use no particular instrument. While in some programmes individual team members may complete separate assessment forms or specific parts of the multidimensional instrument corresponding to their own areas of expertise, other programmes may appoint a single person to complete the entire multidimensional instrument. Many make special efforts to ensure reliability and validity of their instruments in their own settings, while others simply use instruments validated in other places and assume reliability and validity. Some programmes use instruments from which data are easily computerized, while others are not concerned with tabulation of data.

Although geriatric assessment *per se* does not absolutely require specific instruments and scales, the use of easy-to-administer, well-validated assessment instruments encompassing the major domains of geriatric assessment makes the process of assessment more reliable and considerably easier to perform and to teach. In addition, these instruments facili-

Table 25.1 Measurable dimensions in geriatric assessment

Physical health:
Traditional problem list
Disease severity indicators
Self-ratings of health or disability
Quantification of medical services used
Disease-specific rating scales (e.g. gait dysfunction, parkinsonism, dementia)

Overall functional ability:
ADL scales
Instrumental ADL scales

Psychological health:
Cognitive function (mental status) tests
Affective function (depression) tests

Social–environmental parameters:
Social interactions network
Social support needs and resources
Environmental adequacy and safety

tate transmission of understandable clinical information between health care providers, permitting smooth teamwork to occur, meaningful and valid data to be tabulated, and the therapeutic progress to be measured over time.

Several recent publications provide analysis of the existing geriatric assessment instruments and describe in detail which ones are best for each particular setting and patient population.[7-9] In the author's experience, the instruments most useful in supplementing the standard medical history and physical examination have been in the areas of psychological functioning (a cognitive function screen[10-12] and a screen for depression[13-15]) and overall functional status (a scale for measuring basic and advanced activities of daily living[9, 14, 16]).

Following the assessment itself, which can take between a few hours and a few days to accomplish depending on the patient's level of need and the complexity of data to be collected, planning for treatment occurs. This is usually accomplished during a team conference, or at least via interdisciplinary discussions. Subsequent therapeutic measures (medical treatment, rehabilitation, psychosocial interventions) can take place in the same location (either inpatient or outpatient setting depending on the therapy involved) or elsewhere via referral. Arranging for long-term follow-up and case management is an important aspect of the overall programme.

EFFECTIVENESS OF GERIATRIC ASSESSMENT

In 1982, the author and co-workers published an analytical review of the then available reports on geriatric assessment programmes in the North American literature that summarized data on their impacts.[17] Since then, several controlled studies and many other descriptive reports have appeared. This article considerably expands the previous review on outcome studies of geriatric assessment programmes by adding reports of more recent studies and including studies from outside North America. It is an attempt, through several literature searches, to include all published papers that include outcome data on geriatric assessment programmes.

Table 25.2 lists the several beneficial outcomes that various studies have shown to be derived from geriatric assessment programmes with the types of study evidence available (experimental, quasi-experimental, or descriptive) and the specific study references. Some kinds of benefits can be identified readily by descriptive studies. These are primarily process of care benefits such as improved diagnosis and reduced prescribed medications. Other benefits, including the most important outcomes (e.g. improved use of services and survival) require more sophisticated studies to document, involving equivalent control group designs with longitudinal follow-up.

Table 25.3 summarizes each of the published studies on impacts of geriatric assessment programmes. As can be seen, most of the earlier studies have been descriptive or quasi-experimental. Not surprisingly, considering that most of the papers were written by geriatric practitioners, they abound with glowing reports of programme benefits (e.g. many new diagnoses, improved placement over what had been anticipated, improvement in functional status). Policy makers' often appropriate scepticism of reports stemming from uncontrolled trials makes the more recent reports of controlled trials especially important. Fortunately, most of the controlled trials show even more striking benefits than do the previous non-controlled studies.

Though admittedly the table cannot do justice to the individual papers in what is now a sizeable literature, one can appreciate the growing body of data supporting the idea that the frail elderly population can derive great benefit from assessment programmes. Of the 33 studies included, only 13 employed control groups,[25, 30–1, 35–7, 40, 44, 45–7, 50–1] and 9 of these used random allocation.[25, 30–1, 37, 40, 44, 45, 47, 51] All 20 of the papers describing non-controlled studies report positive results. Of the 13 studies employing control groups, all but 2 report at least some major positive benefits of the programme compared with the controls. Neither of the 2 studies that did not demonstrate major programme impacts[44, 50] employed true randomization and, perhaps more importantly, neither targeted their

Table 25.2 Improvements in patient outcomes derived from geriatric assessment programmes

Outcome	Program type	Study type and references
Improved diagnostic accuracy	GAU/GARU	D[18-21], RCT[22]
	ICS	D[23,24], RCT[25,51]
	OAS	D[27-9], RCT[30-1]
	HVT	D[32-3]
Improved placement location	GAU/GARU	D[20-1,26,34], MC[35-6], RCT[37]
	ICS	D[24,38]
	OAS	D[27-8,39]
	HVT	RCT[40]
Improved functional status	GAU/GARU	D[18,20-1,41-2], MC[35], RCT[37]
	OAS	D[29], RCT[30]
	HVT	D[32]
Improved affect or cognition	GAU/GARU	D[18,20,41-2], RCT[37,44]
	ICS	RCT[51]
	OAS	D[29]
	HVT	RCT[45]
Reduced prescribed medications	GAU/GARU	D[18,21], MC[36]
	ICS	RCT[25,51]

Table 25.2 (*cont.*)

Outcome	Program type	Study type and references
Decreased nursing home use	GAU/GARU	D[20-1, 26, 34], MC[35-6], RCT[37]
	ICS	D[24]
	OAS	D[39]
	HVT	RCT[40]
Increased use of home health services	GAU/GARU	MC[36]
	ICS	MC[46], RCT[51]
	OAS	RCT[31]
	HVT	RCT[40, 45]
Reduced use of acute hospitals	GAU/GARU	D[26], MC[36], RCT[47, 7]
	ICS	D[38, 48]
	OAS	RCT[30-1]
	HVT	RCT[40]
Reduced medical care costs	GAU/GARU	RCT[37, 47]
	OAS	RCT[31]
	HVT	RCT[40]
Prolonged survival	GAU/GARU	RCT[37, 47]
	ICS	RCT[51]
	HVT	RCT[40, 45]

GAU = Inpatient geriatric or geropsychiatric assessment unit; GARU = Inpatient geriatric assessment and rehabilitation unit; ICS = Inpatient consultation service; D = Descriptive (before-after study; MC = Matched control study; OAS = Outpatient assessment service; HVT = Home visit team; RCT = Randomized controlled trial.

Table 25.3 Geriatric assessment programmes: summary of published studies designed to measure impacts

Reference	Programme studied	Study population	Outcome measures	Study design	Major impacts reported
Williamson et al.[33] Scotland	Home assessment team	Pts >65 in practices of three GPs (n = 200)	Diagnoses and disabilities, known and unknown	Descriptive	Mean of 3.2 problems found per male pt, 1.9 unknown to GP (3.4 and 2.0 per female)
Lowther et al.[32] Scotland	Home assessment service	Pts >65 living at home deemed 'high risk' (n = 300)	Diagnoses detected, improvement at $1\frac{1}{2}$–$2\frac{1}{2}$-year f/u	Descriptive, with f/u	Mean of 2.3 problems detected; 65% had 'major' problem detected; 23% showed improvement at f/u
Williams et al.[39] New York	Outpt assessment programme	Ger outpts referred for NH placement (n = 322)	Placement location and appropriateness (expert judgement)	Descriptive, with pre-intervention comparison group	Only 38% needed NHs. 23% able to remain at home, 39% to board & care homes; 84% appropriately placed, vs. 50–60% before intervention
Bayne and Caygill[27] Ontario	Outpt assessment and placement service	Outpts referred for NH placement (n = 2005)	Placement; diagnoses of medical and psychiatric problems	Descriptive	60% to long-term care facilities, 40% to homes or board & care; 2.8 diagnoses per referral documented

Table 25.3 (cont.)

Reference	Programme studied	Study population	Outcome measures	Study design	Major impacts reported
Poliquin and Straker[20] California	Inpt psycho-ger eval and rehab unit (20 beds)	Pts >60 referred for psychiatric problems ($n = 47$)	Placement: diagnoses of psychiatric and medical disorders: response to treatment	Descriptive, with before–after measures	79% discharged to board & care facilities rather than NHs; 66% had treatable psychiatric disorders, 72% had associated medical problems uncovered; 74% achieved some remission
Brocklehurst et al.[28] England	Outpt assessment clinic	Frail elderly awaiting admission to a residential care facility ($n = 100$)	New findings. placement improvement	Descriptive	80% had new finding or needed treatment change; placement improved for 32%
Schuman et al.[26] Ontario	Assessment and rehab programme in a chronic-care facility	Ger pts referred for continuing care and rehab	Placement; length of stay	Descriptive, with before–after and parallel group comparisons	33% reduction in LOS; increase discharge home (from 28 to 40%)
Burley et al.[38] Scotland	Inpt ger consult service	Pts ≥65 admitted to acute medical services (n:before = 856; after = 866)	LOS, placement	Time series comparison (year before vs. year after services)	LOS shorter (females only), discharges to home increased

Cheah and Beard[19] Arkansas	Psychiatric eval on a ger unit (10 beds)	Pts on and inpt ger eval unit (n=241)	Diagnosis of psychiatric problems	Descriptive	75% had new psychiatric diagnoses made
Chekryn and Roos[49] Manitoba	Inpt rehab unit (160 beds)	Ger pts needing rehab	Functional status, mental status, and life satisfaction scores	Descriptive	No significant correlation between recorded care processes and outcomes
Tulloch and Moore[30] England	Outpt assessment and f/u clinic	Pts ≥70 of a general practice (n:cases = 145, controls = 150)	New diagnoses, resolution of problems, functional status, use of services	Randomized controlled trial, 2-year f/u	Mean of 0.9 new problems detected, 33% of these resolved at follow-up; cases had fewer hosp days and maintained independence longer
Balaban[44] New Jersey	Hosp assessment and rehab unit	Chronically ill pts > 55, treated on unit (n = 85) vs. elsewhere in hosp (N = 110)	Placement; re-hospitalization rates; functional status and well-being; use and costs of services	Partially randomized controlled trial with serial assessments	Beneficial effects on emotional status and well-being*; no significant effects on rehospitalization, functional status, or costs

Table 25.3 (*cont.*)

Reference	Programme studied	Study population	Outcome measures	Study design	Major impacts reported
Reifler and Eisdorfer[29] Washington	Outpt psychoger assessment unit	Geriatric outpts referred to NH placement (*n* = 82)	Mental and physical functioning; f/u questionnaire	Descriptive, with before–after comparisons	32%—reversible cognitive impairment; physical health improved—38% and mental functioning—24%; 71%—satisfied
Sloane[34] Florida	Special ward for eval & rehab (30 beds)	Geriatric pts referred for NH placement (*n* = 74)	Placement; functional and mental status scores at discharge	Descriptive, with before–after measures	28%—improved placement; small improvement in function
Spar *et al.*[43] California	Geropsychiatric assessment ward (20 beds)	Geriatric pts referred for psychiatric assessment and therapy (*n* = 122)	Psychiatric profile (IPSCE scale)	Descriptive, with before–after measures	Consistent improvement in IPSCE scores from admission to discharge
Rubenstein *et al.*[21] California	Inpt ger assessment and rehab unit (15 beds)	Inpts veterans over 65 from acute medical and surgical wards (*n* = 74)	Placement; functional status; analyses of medications and diagnoses	Descriptive, with before–after measures	48%—improved placement; 67%—improved functional status; (mean) 4 new treatable diagnoses; mean prescribed drugs reduced by 32%.

Study	Setting	Sample	Measures	Design	Results
Applegate et al.[18] Tennessee	Inpt ger assessment & rehab unit in acute hosp (10 beds)	Frail elderly pts needing rehab and at risk of NH placement (n = 100)	New diagnoses, functional status, affect, motivations & medication changes	Descriptive, with before–after comparisons	Many new treatable diagnoses, ADLs improved*, drug reductions*, depression & motivation improved*
Berkman et al.[46] Massachusetts	Inpt ger consult service	Pts ≥75 admitted to acute general medicine services judged in need of discharge planning (n:cases = 35; controls = 17)	New diagnoses, LOS, re-admission rates, use of social work services	Matched control group with 10-month follow-up	Longer LOS than controls*, used more services*, and had fewer rehospizations*
Lefton et al.[35] Ohio	Ger unit in a rehab hosp (14 beds)	Pts ≥70 admitted to rehab hosp (n = 14 beds)	Placement, functional status, LOS, 3–6 month f/u	Matched control group with before–after measures	Entered NHs less often*, functioned better at discharge*, were more likely to live at home at f/u*
Popplewell and Henschke[36] Australia	Inpt ger assessment unit (14 beds)	Pts ≥75 admitted to acute-care hosp (n:cases = 50, controls = 50)	Placement, drugs used, LOS, use of services	Matched control group with before–after measures	Less likely to enter NH*, took fewer drugs at discharge*, had a shorter LOS, but used more services* than controls

Table 25.3 (cont.)

Reference	Programme studied	Study population	Outcome measures	Study design	Major impacts reported
Teasdale et al.[50] Texas	Inpt ger assessment unit in acute hosp	Any pt ≥75 requiring acute hosp care (n:cases = 62, controls = 62)	Placement, mortality, LOS	Matched control group	Longer LOS. No difference in placement or survival.
Hendriksen et al.[40] Denmark	Home assessment & referral team	Pts ≥75 living at home (n:cases = 285, controls = 287)	Mortality, NH placement, home services, hosp admission, costs	Randomized controlled trial, 3-year f/u	Lower mortality*, fewer hospizations or emergency visits*, used more home services*, and had lower costs*
Lichtenstein and Winograd[24] California	Inpt ger consult service	Frail elderly inpts referred for consults (n = 35)	New diagnoses, placement of pts slated for NH (n = 35)	Descriptive	Many new diagnoses (0.7 per pt); 51% slated for NH had 'improved' placement
Rubenstein et al.[37] California	Inpt ger assessment & rehab unit (15 bed)	Frail pts ≥65 randomized from acute hosp services (n:caes = 63; controls = 60)	Placement; 1 year mortality; functional status, affect, mental status changes; use of services & costs	Randomized controlled trial, 1-year f/u	50% lower mortality*, lower NH use*, lower rehospitalization rates*, higher improvement rates in functional status & morale*, lower 1-year costs

Study	Intervention	Population	Outcomes	Study design	Results
Vetter et al.[45] Wales	Homes assessments by heath visitors	Pts ≥70 of several urban & rural GPs (n:cases = 279,289; controls = 270,291)	Survival, functional status, affect, use of home services	Randomized controlled study, before–after measures	Urban study pts had lower mortality*, higher affect*, and used more home services* than controls; rural pt effects NS
Barker et al.[48] New York	Inpt ger consult service	Inpts ≥70 judged at high risk for long stays at 6 acute hosp (n = 366)	Monthly census and LOS of pts in hosp not needing acute care	Time series comparison (before and after project)	Monthly census and LOS not needing acute care decreased
Collard et al.[47] Massachusetts	Special ger nursing units in 2 private hosps (10 beds each)	Pts ≥65 admitted to acute hosp (n:cases=218. controls=477)	Placement, use of restraints, complications, LOS, hosp charges	Randomized controlled trial, before–after measures	In one hosp, unit pts had a lower mortality*, fewer restraints, shorter LOS*, and lower charges*; in other hosp, effects NS
Gross[41] Australia	Inpt ger assessment unit in acute hosp	Pts ≥65 admitted to unit from home or hosp (n = 399)	Changes in drugs prescribed, functional status and mental status changes	Descriptive, with before–after comparisons	70%—drug changes (31%—decreased, 38%—increased), 50%—improved in ADLs, 30%—improved in mental status

Table 25.3 (*cont.*)

Reference	Programme studied	Study population	Outcome measures	Study design	Major impacts reported
Katz et al.[23] New York	Ger inpt consult service	Pts ≥64 referred from acute inpt services for consultation (n = 51)	Identification of new diagnoses, drug problems, and MD compliance with recommendations	Descriptive	51%—new problems detected, 75%—treatment changes indicated; MD compliance was disappointing (15–35%)
Liem et al.[42] Arkansas	Inpt ger rehab unit (28 beds)	Disabled elderly pts needing inpt rehab (n = 190)	Functional status, speech, mental status, changes	Descriptive, with before–after measures	Major improvements in function, mental status, and speech*
Allen et al.[25] North Carolina	Inpt ger consult service	All consenting inpts ≥ 75 admitted to acute VA hosp (n:cases = 92, controls = 93)	New diagnoses, need for treatment changes, MD compliance with recs for study pts	Randomized controlled study	Recs made (mean = 6.1 recs/pt), 72% of recs carried out on study pts vs. 27% of controls; no major outcome differences
Williams[31] New York	Outpt ger consult service	Frail home-living elderly (n:cases = 58, controls = 59)	Survival, new diagnoses, hospitalizations, use of services, costs	Randomized controlled study, before–after measures	Fewer hosp days, many new diagnoses, lower costs: no change in survival or NH use

| Hogan et al.[51] Nova Scotia | Inpt ger consult service | All inpts ≥75 meeting targeting criteria (n:cases = 57, controls = 56) | Survival, LOS, mental status, use of services, drugs | Randomized controlled study | Lower mortality*, greater improvement in mental status*, more drug reductions*, unchanged LOS |

f/u = follow-up; NH = nursing home; GP = general practitioner; outpt = outpatients; hosp = hospital; pt(s) = patient (s); inpt = inpatient; recs = recommendations; LOS = length of stay; rehab = rehabilitation; * = p < 0.05; NS = non-significant; consult = consultation; MD = physician; VA = Veterans Administration; ger = geriatric; eval = evaluation.

study patient populations to those particularly likely to benefit. (Thus these two 'negative' studies provide a great service by highlighting the need to target geriatric assessment programmes to patients particularly likely to benefit.)

A consistent area of demonstrated impact from these assessment programmes has been improvement in diagnostic accuracy, usually indicated by the diagnosis of new, treatable problems. Many found substantial numbers of previously undiagnosed problems among patients undergoing geriatric assessment. Depending on each study's criteria for considering newly documented problems as new diagnoses (some included all new diagnostic labels while others only counted major problems which were treatable), new diagnoses were found in frequencies varying from just under one per patient to over four per patient. Discovery of these new diagnoses stemmed from several factors, including the geriatric assessment process itself (which includes a careful search for treatable problems), a longer period of time to evaluate the patient, and a probable lack of diagnostic throroughness in the referring services.[18–22, 23–5, 27–33, 51] Though it is virtually impossible to prove cause and effect, it is likely that this improved diagnostic accuracy helped to produce many of the other reported benefits.

The first report that an assessment programme could improve placement location and decrease the use of nursing homes was published in 1973 on data from T. Franklin Williams' pioneering outpatient assessment programme in Monroe County, New York.[39] This assessed all patients referred for nursing home placement in the county and found that only 38 per cent of these actually needed such skilled nursing care, whereas 23 per cent were able to return to their homes and 39 per cent were able to go to board and care facilities or retirement homes following careful assessment and recommendations for specific therapy. Expert judgements made by an independent team of observers indicated that major improvements in placement decisions were being made by the programme. Several subsequent reports, including two from controlled studies,[37, 40] have shown similar assessment-related improvements in placement locations.[20–1, 24, 26–8, 34–8, 40]

Several reports have examined patient functional status before and after treatment on geriatric units, particularly on units providing rehabilitation. These reports have usually used a validated measure of functional status to document change over time. They show that the majority of patients improve during their stays in the units. The absence of control groups in most of the reports prevents the differentiation of the effect of time from that arising from the geriatric programme itself. However, two controlled studies clearly showed that patients in geriatric programmes were more likely than controls to improve and to retain their improvement.[30, 37]

Impacts on psychological parameters, such as cognitive status and affect, have also been examined. Both cognitive function and affect have been consistently shown to improve over time in non-controlled studies.[18, 20, 29, 41–3] Controlled trials have primarily shown positive impacts on affect,[37, 44–5] though one showed a positive impact on cognition.[51]

Improvement in quality of treatment is difficult to quantify. One measurable parameter—use of prescription drugs—has been reported. In these reports, drug prescribing was made generally more appropriate, usually resulting in a decreased quantity of prescribed drugs, despite concurrent increases in the number of treatable diagnoses identified.[18, 21–2, 25, 36, 51]

Use of hospital services has been examined in several studies, involving inpatient units, inpatient consultant services, and outpatient assessment services. All studies that included long-term follow-up of at least a year report reduced use of acute hospital services and reduced total health care costs over time.[22, 30, 37, 40] When only the initial hospitalization period is compared, the results are mixed—some show a prolonged length of stay (LOS) associated with the assessment.[21, 37, 46] while others show a shorter LOS.[26, 36, 38, 47–8] Whether the initial LOS is shortened or prolonged is a function of, among other things, the intensity of the intervention as well as the speed and thoroughness of the hospital services used by control patients. The reduction in acute hospital use and total health care costs over time from assessment services primarily reflects a reduction in rehospitalization rates, which stems both from the initial assessment itself and from the often improved quality of follow up services.

The only reliable way for measuring programme impact on survival is to use a control group, preferably one assigned randomly, and to follow subjects for a substantial period of time. The Sepulveda randomized controlled trial showed a 50 per cent reduction in 1-year mortality compared with the control group.[37] The Danish randomized trial showed a 25 per cent reduction in 3-year mortality from a group of home-living elderly receiving periodic in-home assessments.[40] Similar positive impacts on survival were reported in the Welsh trial of home assessment and the Canadian trial of intensive inpatient consultation.[45, 51] On the other hand, Mark Williams' study of an outpatient assessment programme failed to show impact on survival, although, as the author discusses, the control group received additional diagnostic care from well-trained internists.[31]

As mentioned above in connection with the two studies failing to show a substantial programme effect, targeting programmes to the most appropriate patients is a key issue. Although geriatric assessment programmes can clearly be effective, it is important to identify accurately which subgroups of patients can be expected to benefit most in order to make maximal use of scarce resources. Although it might be argued that the majority of elderly probably could benefit from careful assessment, the bulk of older people are generally healthy, and the relative yield of assessment tends to be lower for healthy than for the frail or ill elderly. In general, individuals most likely to benefit from assessment are those who are on the verge of needing institutionalization, who are in the lower socio-economic groups, who have inadequate primary medical care, and who have poor social support networks. On the other hand, patients in the end stages of a terminal illness or irreversible dementia would be less likely to derive much benefit. The proportion of at-risk elderly who can derive especially great benefits from assessment programmes appear to constitute between 5 and 10 per cent of the hospitalized elderly and a currently undetermined proportion (perhaps 2 to 5 per cent) of the non-hospitalized elderly. In systems of care where the average level of health of the elderly population is lower, the proportions who would benefit would probably be much higher.

CONCLUSIONS

The data reviewed in this chapter and tables suggest that geriatric assessment programmes are effective, practical, and vitally important. They can lead to better diagnosis, treatment outcomes, functional status, and living location, and lower use of long-term institutional care services. Perhaps the greatest remaining dilemma in starting a geriatric assessment programme in today's world climate of fiscal restraint is how to establish and maintain adequate funding sources. Despite evidence cited earlier that geriatric assessment programmes can lead to long-term financial savings in the care of frail elderly patients by reducing days in acute hospitals and nursing homes, mechanisms for establishing and paying for them do not yet exist in many health care systems. At present, these programmes are most readily established within large prepaid systems, such as in national health services or, in the United States (which lacks a national health service) in the Veterans Administration or in the larger health maintenance organizations. In places without such systems, smaller-scale programmes using three-person teams of geriatrically skilled professionals can be important first steps. In all cases, careful effort to target frail elderly persons most in need of assessment services is vital to assure maximum cost-effectiveness. It is hoped that funding for geriatric assessment programmes throughout the world will become more readily available when efficacy and cost-effectiveness studies, reviewed in this chapter, are fully considered by policy makers.

References

1. Brocklehurst, J. C. (ed.) (1975). *Geriatrics care in advanced societies*. University Park Press, Baltimore, Maryland.
2. Matthews, D. A. (1984). Dr Marjory Warren and the origin of British geriatrics. *Journal of the American Geriatrics Society*, **32**, 253–8.
3. Kane, R. L. and Kane, R. A. (1976). *Long-term care in six countries: implications for the United States*. Fogarty International Center Proceedings No. 33. United States Government Printing Office, Washington DC.
4. Schouten, J. (1979). Modern ideas about organization of services for elderly patients in the Netherlands. *Journal of the American Geriatrics Society*, **27**, 258–62.
5. Butler, R. (1975). *Why survive? Being old in America*. Harper & Row, New York.
6. Kane, R. L. and Kane, R. A. (1978). Care of the aged: Old problems in need of new solutions. *Science*, **200**, 913.
7. Kane, R. L. and Kane, R. A. (1981). *Assessing the elderly: a practical guide to measurement*. DC Heath, Lexington, MA.
8. NIA Technology Assessment Conference (1983). Evaluating the elderly patient: the case for assessment technology. *Journal of the American Geriatrics Society*, **31**, 636–64, 721–65.
9. Rubenstein, L. Z., Schairer, C., Wieland, G. D. *et al.* (1984). Systematic biases in functional status assessment of elderly adults: effects of different data sources. *Journal of Gerontology*, **39**, 686–91.
10. Folstein, M. F., Folstein, S. E., and McHugh, P. R. (1975). Mini-mental state: a practical method for grading the cognitive state of patients for the clinician. *Journal of Psychiatric Research*, **12**, 189–98.
11. Kahn, R. L., Goldfarb, A. L., Pollack, M. *et al.* (1960). Brief objective measures for the determination of mental status in the aged. *American Journal of Psychiatry*, **117**, 326–8.
12. Pfeiffer, E. (1975). A short portable mental status questionnaire for the assessment of organic brain deficit in elderly patients. *Journal of the American Geriatrics Society*, **23**, 433–41.
13. Beck, A. J. (1973). *The diagnosis and management of depression*. University of Pennsylvania Press, Philadelphia.
14. Lawton, M. P. (1975). The Philadelphia Geriatric Center morale scale-a revision. *Journal of Gerontology*, **15**, 851–89.
15. Zung, W. W. K. (1965). A self-rating depression scale. *Archives of General Psychiatry*, **12**, 63–70.
16. Katz, S., Downs, T. D., Cash, H. R. *et al.* (1970). Progress in the development of the index of ADL. *Gerontologist*, **10**, 20–30.
17. Rubenstein, L. Z., Rhee, L. and Kane, R. L. (1982). The role of geriatric assessment units in caring for the elderly: an analytic review. *Journal of Gerontology*, **37**, 513–21.
18. Applegate, W. B., Akins, D., Vanderzwaag, R. *et al.* (1983). A geriatric rehabilitation and assessment unit in a community hospital. *Journal of the American Geriatrics Society*, **31**, 206–10.
19. Cheah, K. C. and Beard, O. W. (1980). Psychiatric findings in the population

of a geriatric evaluation unit: implications. *Journal of the American Geriatrics Society*, **28**, 153–6.

20. Poliquin, N. and Straker, M. (1977). A clinical psychogeriatric unit: Organization and function. *Journal of the American Geriatrics Society*, **25**, 132–7.

21. Rubenstein, L. Z., Abrass, I. B. and Kane, R. L. (1981). Improved care for patients on a new geriatric unit. *Journal of the American Geriatrics Society*, **29**, 531–6.

22. Rubenstein, L. Z., Josephson, K. R., Wieland, G. D., Pietruszka, F., Tretton, C. *et al.* (1987). Geriatric assessment on a subacute hospital ward. *Clinics in Geriatric Medicine*, **3** (1), 131–44.

23. Katz, P. R., Dube, D. H., and Calkins, E. (1985). Use of a structured functional assessment format in a geriatric consultative service. *Journal of the American Geriatrics Society*, **33**, 681–6.

24. Lichtenstein, H. and Winograd, C. H. (1985). Geriatric Consultation: a functional approach. *Journal of the American Geriatric Society*, **33**, 422–8.

25. Allen, C. M., Becher, P. M., McVey, L. J., Saltz, C., Feussner, J. R., and Cohen, H. J. (1986). A randomized controlled clinical trial of a geriatric consultation team: compliance with recommendations. *Journal of the American Medical Association*, **255**, 2617–21.

26. Schuman, J. E., Beattie, E. J., Steed, D. A. *et al.* (1978). The impact of a new geriatric program in a hospital for the chronically ill. *Canadian Medical Association Journal*, **118**, 639–45.

27. Bayne, J. R. and Caygill, J. (1977). Identifying needs and services for the aged. *Journal of the American Geriatrics Society*, **25**, 264–8.

28. Brocklehurst, J. C., Carty, M. H., Leeming, J. T. *et al.* (1978). Medical screening of old people accepted for residential care. *Lancet*, **2**, 141.

29. Reifler, B. V. and Eisdorfer, C. (1980). A clinic for impaired elderly and their families. *American Journal of Psychiatry*, 1399–403.

30. Tulloch, A. H. and Moore, V. (1979). A randomized controlled trial of geriatric screening and surveillance in general practice. *Journal of the Royal College of General Practitioners*, **29**, 733–42.

31. Williams, M. E. (1987). Outpatient geriatric evaluation. *Clinics in Geriatric Medicine*, **3** (1), 175–84.

32. Lowther, C. P., MacLeod, R. D. M., and Williamson, J. (1970). Evaluation of early diagnostic services for the elderly. *British Medical Journal*, **3**, 275–7.

33. Williamson, J., Stokoe, I. H., Gray, S. *et al.* (1964). Old people at home: their unreported needs. *Lancet*, **1**, 1117–20.

34. Sloane, P. (1980). Nursing home candidates: hospital inpatient trial to identify those appropriately assignable to less intensive care. *Journal of the American Geriatrics Society*, **28**, 511–14.

35. Lefton, E., Bonstelle, S., and Frengley, J. D. (1983). Success with an inpatient geriatric unit: a controlled study. *Journal of the American Geriatrics Society*, **31**, 149–55.

36. Popplewell, P. Y. and Henschke, P. J. (1983). What is the value of a geriatirc assessment unit in a teaching hospital?: a comparative study. *Australian Health Review*, **6** (2), 23–5.

37. Rubenstein, L. Z., Josephson, K. R., Wieland, G. D. *et al.* (1984). Effectiveness of a geriatric evaluation unit: a randomized clinical trial. *New England Journal of Medicine*, **311**, 1664–70.

38. Burley, L. E., Currie, C. T., Smith, R. G., and Williamson, J. (1979). Contribution from geriatric medicine within acute medical wards. *British Medical Journal*, **263** (2), 90.
39. Williams, T. F., Hill, J. G., Fairbank, M. E. *et al.* (1973). Appropriate placement of the chronically ill and aged: a successful approach by evaluation. *Journal of the American Medical Association*, **226**, 1332–5.
40. Hendriksen, C., Lund, E., and Stromgard, E. (1984). Consequences of assessment and intervention among elderly people: three year randomized controlled trial. *British Medical Journal*, **289**, 1522–4.
41. Gross, P. F. (1985). *Evaluation of a geriatric assessment unit in an acute general hospital in a rural region of Australia.* Long Term Care Project, Working Paper No. 3, Institute of Health Economics and Technology Assessment, Sydney, Australia.
42. Liem, P. H., Chernoff, R., and Carter, W. J. (1986). Geriatric rehabilitation unit: A 3-year outcome evaluation. *Journal of Gerontology*, **41**, 44–50.
43. Spar, J. E., Ford, C. V., and Liston, E. H. (1980). Hospital treatment of the elderly neuropsychiatric patients II. *Journal of the American Geriatrics Society*, **28**, 539–43.
44. Balaban, D. J. (1980). *Chronic care study: a randomized longitudinal study of patients with chronic diseases treated on a special care unit.* Final Report. Leonard Davis School of Health Economics, Philadelphia.
45. Vetter, N. J., Jones, D. A., and Victor, C. R. (1984). Effects of health visitors working with elderly patients in general practice: a randomized controlled trial. *British Medical Journal*, **288**, 369–72.
46. Berkman, B., Campion, E., Swagerty, E., and Goldman, M. (1983). Geriatric consultation team: Alternate approach to social work discharge planning. *Journal of Gerontological Social Work*, **5** (3), 77–88.
47. Collard, A. F., Bachman, S. S., and Beatrice, D. F. (1985). Acute care delivery for the geriatirc patient: An innovative approach. *Quality Review Bulletin*, 180–5.
48. Barker, W. H., Williams, T. F., Zimmer, J. G. *et al.* (1985). Geriatric consultation teams in acute hospitals: impact on back up of elderly patients. *Journal of the American Geriatric Society*, **33**, 422–8.
49. Checkryn, J. and Roos, L. (1979). Auditing the process of care in a new geriatric evaluation unit. *Journal of the American Geriatrics Society*, **27**, 107–11.
50. Teasdale, T. A., Schuman, L., Snow, E. *et al.* (1983). A comparison of outcomes of geriatric cohorts receiving care in a geriatric assessment unit and on general medicine floors. *Journal of the American Geriatrics Society*, **31**, 529–34.
51. Hogan, D. B., Fox, R. A., Badley, B. W., and Mann, O. E. (1987). Effect of a geriatric consultation service on management of patients in an acute-care hospital. *Canadian Medical Association Journal*, **136**, 713–17.

26

The role of geriatric medicine

R. A. BARKER

INTRODUCTION

The British Geriatrics Society has defined Geriatrics as 'that branch of general medicine concerned with the clinical, preventive, remedial and social aspects of illness in the elderly'. There have been a number of modifications of this definition and some would disagree that geriatrics should be a specialty. Whatever one's view, this remains the most generally useful definition as it covers the various aspects of activity which are required in providing services and facilities for the elderly.

The modern approach to the care of the elderly was initiated by Marjory Warren[1] in London, England. She made the fundamental observation that direct admission to any chronic care facility was unsatisfactory and inevitably led to the risk of misplacement of old people. Comprehensive geriatric services developed first in the United Kingdom. Some services have developed in most developed countries. Some, such as Canada, Australia, and New Zealand, have adopted similar systems to the UK but with some modifications.

Geriatrics was born in the chronic disease hospitals. At the end of the 1950s, I worked in such a chronic disease hospital typical of its kind at that time. It was an old army hospital built as a temporary structure during the Second World War. The patients were cared for in long open wards with no provision for privacy. Even in the toilets two elderly ladies sat looking at two other old ladies on opposite sides of a small room. Blankets, linen, and ward equipment were sent from the acute hospitals when they were too old for use in the 'more important hospitals'. The elderly patients, stripped of every vestige of dignity, lived and died *sans* hope, *sans* everything.

There was a deep conviction among the public and among many members of the health professions that nothing could be done for the elderly. And if nothing could be done it was perfectly logical to argue that not much was needed to do it with and not many people were needed to do it. Such hospitals in many parts of the world were housed in shocking accommodation and grossly understaffed. On this unlikely basis, many of us built geriatric services.

I provide this fragment of history so that readers may recognize the origins of some of my prejudices, but also I think it is important for the young to appreciate what the past has contributed, what the present holds, and to base on that their aspirations for the future. Or, to put it more simply, you don't know where you are going unless you know where you have come from.

THE NEEDS OF THE ELDERLY

The aging are not a race apart. The common diseases from which the aging suffer are found also in younger people but not with the same frequency. If the aging have health problems they are due to disease not to age. The elderly are not a homogeneous group and in grouping their needs one must take care to preserve their individuality. Neither are the elderly of today the same as the elderly of tomorrow. Each cohort will have lived through different times and seasons.

However, in some important respects, the characteristics of the aged sick are different from those of other aged groups and these differences have an important bearing on the best ways in which to meet their needs.

Acute disease in the elderly can easily become chronic unless it is promptly and effectively treated. There must be nothing second rate about such treatment. On the contrary, because there is as a rule only one chance, it must be of a particularly high order at all levels of staffing and facilities and provide for skilled diagnosis and treatment. In many cases, acute disease appears on a background of chronic disease.

Chronic disease also has certain aspects that must receive attention in planning care. Disease processes are seldom single. Old age affects the whole body and often the mind as well and a programme that concentrates on a single disability will often be frustrated if others, often unassociated, are neglected. This does not mean that one should set off on a relentless pursuit of total pathology by undertaking a multitude of tests at great expense and often at considerable discomfort to the patient. Asymptomatic problems in the elderly seldom impair the patient's function or alter the quality of life.

Besides the physical and emotional aspects of chronic disease, the whole social background has to be considered. Are there relatives able and willing to support the patient? What is the physical environment in which the patient lives and what changes can be made which would reduce handicap? What supporting services are available to the patient in the home?

Recoverability of the aged patient has in the past been greatly underestimated by both the health professions and the public. It is important to ensure that the elderly are not confined to institutions unless all the potentialities for their recovery have been explored. No person should be admitted to long-term care except after thorough assessment and rehabilitation. Rehabilitation, if it is to be effective, must begin early in the course of an illness and be continued until maximum function has been attained, bearing in mind that recovery is often very slow in the aged and that potentialities for recovery may show themselves even after hope of it has been given up.

Physical illness is often intimately related to mental health problems. It is important to treat the underlying causes of these problems as in such cases the mental health problems are often reversible. Preventive and curative mental health services should therefore form an integral part of an organized geriatric service.

Movements of the elderly from one place to another, such as admission to hospital, can sometimes cause confusion and deterioration in the patient's physical condition. Such movements should therefore be avoided if possible. However, if admission to hospital will provide the appropriate care, the patient should not be deprived of this benefit purely for the sake of keeping him in one place. If the main reason for admission of the patient is the strain on the family, a prolonged delay in admission will result in the family being strained to the utmost and admission comes as a relief from an intolerable situation which the next of kin are determined not to allow to occur again. Prompt admission would avoid this and make discharge correspondingly easier.

Multiple pathology, insidious onset, and atypical presentation of symptoms make diagnosis difficult in the elderly. Management of the patient must also pay due regard to certain attributes such as differing responses to therapy and to the sensation of pain, the ability to maintain posture, the perception of ambient temperature and the impairment of the response to water deprivation by thirst.[2]

SERVICES AND FACILITIES

Kay *et al.*[3] describe the main component of a modern geriatric service orientated towards preventive care as follows:

(1) an organization and administrative structure which facilitates integration on a practical level of the various services provided by the local authority, the family doctor and the hospitals and it might be added, as far as possible, the voluntary bodies;

(2) a scheme of ascertainment of those aged most likely to need help such as the infirm, the isolated, the widowed and bereaved, the very old, those with defective sight and hearing, and those suffering from economic hardship;

(3) a number of lines of defence within the community designed to serve old people with differing needs such as domiciliary services of various kinds, club and day centres, outpatient clinics, and day hospitals;

(4) hospital inpatient services that can be used not as a last resort but at appropriate stages and often for short periods only within the total programme of care.

Primary health care

Contrary to popular belief, the majority of the elderly are not disabled or dependent[4] and they live in their own homes or in the homes of their relatives.[5] The major area of activity in the health of the elderly will therefore be in primary health care, a subject which is covered by Dr Gary Andrews (Chapter 21). It is appropriate to say here that any geriatric service, if it is to be effective, must have close co-operation with the primary health services and be prepared to assist with services in the home and with short- or longer-term assistance in hospital.

Institutions and institutional services

The early geriatric units grew out of the old chronic disease hospitals and many were divorced from the activities of the general hospital. Most people would now accept that a geriatric service is an essential part of the function of any general hospital. The elderly acutely ill patient should have ready access to all the services and facilities available for younger patients and the assessment and rehabilitation unit should also be part of the general hospital.

In the siting of long-stay units, attention should be paid to the needs of elderly relatives and younger relatives with children who would be better served by having the unit not too far distant from their home. The care of these patients, however, should remain the responsibility of the geriatric service. No patient should be admitted to a long-stay unit unless they have first been evaluated in an assessment and rehabilitation unit. There is considerable variation in the provision of long-stay units. In the Netherlands they are operated by non-profit organizations and funded by the sick funds. In Australia they are run by private profit-making organizations but funded by government. In Denmark they have abolished the distinction between residential homes for the frail aged and hospital units for the severely disabled. All levels of disability are cared for in the same unit and admission follows assessment by the geriatric service.

Provision should be made in the hospital for short-term admissions to give relatives a rest from continuing care, for outpatient attendance, and also for day care for patients who do not require admission or for those recently discharged from inpatient beds.

Assistance in the home should be provided by a full range of support services which may include home help, meals-on-wheels, laundry service, district nursing service, physiotherapy and occupational therapy services, and equipment loan service. Such home services are sometimes based in the hospital and sometimes on private or voluntary agencies. Such services avoid admission of some patients and expedite the discharge of some inpatients, but make their greatest contribution by improving the quality of care of severely disabled patients who are being nursed by their relatives and are not applicants for admission to hospital.

RELATIONSHIP OF GERIATRIC SERVICES TO ACUTE SERVICES

There has been debate about the relationship of the geriatric service to the remainder of the acute medical services and a number of patterns of organization have emerged.

In the early 1960s Gibson[6] in Newcastle, New South Wales, Australia would consult automatically on all patients in acute medical wards who had been in hospital for twice the average number of days stay. Barker *et al.*[7] have described the shortening of average number of days stay and reduction of blocking of beds following the introduction of a geriatric team to an acute medical service. Burley *et al.*[8] also described the introduction of a geriatric consultant team to acute wards and reported a reduction of average number of days stay, an increase in the number sent home, and an increase in the number staying in hospital for less than 2 weeks. Evans *et al.*[9] point out that three-quarters of the 65–74 age group go to the acute medical wards and claim that the geriatric service should be organized on an age-related basis, taking all medical patients 75 and over. Other age-related services have been described by O'Brien *et al.*[10] and Bagnall *et al.*[11] Evans[12] described the integration of geriatric services with general medicine in Newcastle. Among other benefits he cited the co-ordination of the acute service with the rehabilitation service, a single referral point for general practitioners seeking emergency admission of elderly patients, a more efficient use of general hospital beds, ready access of elderly patients to a full range of hospital facilities, and better training of junior medical and nursing staff.

The view in the USA is that 'geriatric medicine should not be a separate speciality but that gerontology and geriatrics be recognized as academic disciplines within the relevant medical specialties.'[33]

In Sweden there is no geriatric speciality as such, but specialists in rehabilitation medicine care for disability in both the young and the old.

Williamson[14] argues that geriatrics is at the cross-roads, with three options open to it: to abandon the specialty, to make it an age-related specialty like paediatrics, or to foster integration with the rest of medicine while preserving what has been achieved. He favours the last.

A Working Party of the Royal College of Physicians of London[15] has recommended that all acute medical and geriatric facilities in the district general hospital should evolve into one integrated operational unit but believes that different patterns of care may evolve in each area.

All of these patterns of care are no doubt successful in their time and place. My own belief is that the development of geriatric medicine will evolve in the general direction of the integration of general medical and geriatric services along the pattern of the Newcastle service, but I think this will be a slow evolution and not a rapid change. How rapidly integration occurs will depend on a multitude of factors such as the effectiveness of undergraduate and postgraduate training, the attitude of general physicians, changes in public and professional attitudes to the elderly, the acceptance by medical staff of more flexible use of hospital beds and services, and the type of health delivery system operating in any particular country. The inertia inherent in any health delivery system is such that major changes will be possible only over long periods of time. In the immediate future there will continue to be wide variation in the delivery of health services to the elderly but this should not be looked at askance. The principles on which the care of the elderly should be based are well delineated. Various methods of delivery can therefore be measured against these principles.

The requirement of close association with other services is not confined to the medical wards. All the other services with the exception of paediatrics and obstetrics will have elderly patients and should be able to seek consultation about them from the geriatric service. Orthopaedics and psychiatry, however, need a much closer and more formal relationship. Devas and Irvine[16-17] have described a geriatric orthopaedic unit where there is close working together of the orthopaedic surgeon and the geriatric physician in the care of the elderly orthopaedic patients, particularly those with femoral neck fractures. This type of management has been followed in many units with considerable success.

Mental health problems are often associated with physical problems, and a close association between the psychiatric and geriatric services is essential. Because of the considerable overlap, joint services as described by Robinson[18] in Edinburgh have proved very successful. There is a wide variation in what has been accomplished in this area—at the one extreme good jointly administered services and at the other a virtual abdication of their responsibilities by psychiatrists leaving the geriatric physician to manage mental disorder in the elderly as best he can. The conflict and collaboration between medicine and psychiatry in the aged has been reviewed by Godber.[19]

Williamson[20] has described the development of geriatric services in the

UK and most of us have emerged from the time when a great deal of effort was spent in an endeavour to establish a service in an impossible environment in a rejected specialty in the face of unbelieving physicians. There are good prospects of building on what has already been accomplished in those countries which have accepted the UK model or modifications of it. For those, like the USA who are taking another path, it is imperative that they measure what the results of a non-specialty approach to geriatrics will be. One thing is certain: with the demographic changes that are occurring there is no way of avoiding the task that faces us and, whatever the fears of the cost of providing an adequate geriatric service, the economic and social cost of failure will be much greater than that of success.

EVALUATION OF GERIATRIC UNITS

Most of the earlier accounts of geriatric units were descriptive. The function of these units, most of which were modelled on the UK system, have several goals which include increasing the level of the patient's functioning, improving diagnosis and treatment, achieving more appropriate placement, reducing the use of institutional services, and generally increasing the quality of care delivered to elderly patients. In the early days we concentrated on providing an improved environment for patients in hospital and applying the basic requirements for diagnosis and treatment. With this type of activity it was not difficult to double the turnover in the geriatric unit within a short time.[21] In more recent years there has been a call for controlled trials of the effectiveness of geriatric units[22]— always a difficult problem when what is being tested has long been accepted as an effective system.

Over the years many methods of measuring function in the elderly have been developed and have become an essential tool for the geriatric physician. Measures of physical, mental, and social function, and multi-function measures have been reviewed by Kane and Kane;[23] they conclude that further improvements in methods are still required.

In a series of four papers, Rubenstein *et al.*[24-7] provide an analytical review of geriatric assessment units in caring for the elderly across America, a description of the establishment and 1-year outcome of a new geriatric evaluation unit, a 4-year outcome study of the same unit, and a randomized clinical trial of the effectiveness of the geriatric evaluation unit. In this latter study, it was shown that at 1 year patients assigned to the unit had lower mortality than the controls, and were less likely to have initially been discharged to a nursing home, or to have spent time in a nursing home in the follow up-period. The control group had substantially more acute-care hospital days, nursing home days, and acute-care hospital re-admissions. Patients in the geriatric unit were more likely to have improvement in functional status and morale than controls. Direct costs for institutional care were lower for the experimental group, especially after adjustment for survival.

In a controlled trial Teasdale *et al.*[28] found their unit patients were better on discharge but there was no significant difference 6 months from discharge. Sainsbury[29] in New Zealand compared the provision of assessment and rehabilitation beds and long-stay beds and waiting lists in eight hospital districts and showed that areas with an active geriatric evaluation unit had fewer long-stay beds and a short or no waiting time for admission. There is increasing evidence to confirm the original observation of Marjorie Warren that direct admission of the elderly to a chronic disease facility can commonly lead to misplacement.

EDUCATION

Battersby[30] studied the attitudes of children aged 7–10 to the elderly and found negative and unfavourable stereotypes were already well established and reinforced by schoolbooks, parents, teachers, and the media, particularly television. Rachel aged 10 wrote: 'I know I won't like being old. I will be cut off from the world and be put away like in jail. I'm afraid of being lonely and having no one near when I need them. I'm going to be useless I know but I don't want to have no one there and only the occasional visitor.' If in 7 years Rachel is a nursing or medical student there will be great difficulty in reversing these stereotypes.

In view of the major demographic changes occurring in all countries, it is essential that education of the health professions includes health of the elderly throughout the course. Svanborg and Williamson[31] have made suggestions with regard to training health professionals in the care of the elderly, namely that:

—— students learn the biology and physiology of aging as part of the teaching in biology and physiology;

—— age-related changes in mental and social function be taught in behavioural sciences classes;

—— students be able to recognize the clinical differences between normal aging and changes due to disease, as well as the susceptibility of elders to overtreatment;

—— community health teaching emphasize the importance in old age of preventive care and healthy lifestyles;

—— students have an opportunity to observe old people in their own homes to see how they cope with illness and disability and to become familiar with the varying ways in which the community and families rally to them.

Most people would agree with this in broad terms.

There are reviews of training in Asia and Oceania[32] and medical education for care of the elderly in the USA by the Institute of Medicine[13] among others. It is apparent that, although there has been commendable progress in undergraduate education in some areas, in others there has been only token acceptance of the important place aging has in a modern curriculum.

Postgraduate medical education in aging has been advanced also. In countries which have adopted geriatric medicine as a speciality, provision is made for special training for postgraduate qualifications. In New Zealand the basic programme is in general medicine, and advanced training can include varying periods of time in geriatrics or in general medicine. A general physician can therefore include some time in geriatric medicine and a geriatric physician can vary his length of experience in general medicine. General physicians wishing to transfer to geriatric medicine at a later date find this arrangement flexible enough to meet their needs. If physicians are to follow the Newcastle pattern of organization of services[12] such a flexible postgraduate education is necessary.

The importance in both basic and post-basic nursing programmes in the health needs of the elderly is at least as great as in medicine. Adequate nursing education is difficult where the concept of nursing as a hospital-based service persists. New Zealand, along with some other countries, has moved from a hospital-based to an education-based training with nurses obtaining a much more community-orientated training than previously. Such a move is essential if nurses are going to be able to serve the needs of the elderly and to practice modern views of rehabilitation and promotion of independence.

CONCLUSION

The twentieth century has witnessed in many regions of the world the control of perinatal and infant mortality, a decline in birth rates, improvements in nutrition and basic health care, and the control of many infectious diseases. This combination of factors has resulted in an increasing number and proportion of persons surviving into the advanced stages of life.

In 1950 there were approximately 200 million people over 60 years of age throughout the world. By the year 2000 it is estimated this number will have reached 590 million. Whereas in 1975 52 per cent of all persons over 60 lived in developing countries, by the year 2000 60 per cent will do so.[33] The problems of the aging are therefore becoming urgent for developing as well as for developed countries.

The extension of the average expectation of life at birth and the changing spectrum of disease with which this has been associated has meant, as Fries[34] has pointed out, that the practical focus on health improvement over the next decades must be on chronic instead of acute disease, on morbidity not mortality, on the quality of life rather than its duration, and on postponement rather than cure. Health delivery systems must therefore be designed to deal with these new problems.

A variety of patterns of care have developed in a number of countries and some of these have been mentioned in this paper. There is no agreement on the 'best' way to deliver care to the elderly and this is not even to be expected as each country must find its own solution which will best suit its own social and cultural pattern. Many developing countries may have to develop an entirely new structure to meet the needs of this emerging elderly population. In this they may be fortunate in not having to battle with old entrenched views and old facilities.

With a new service the emphasis should be on primary health care and the delivery of services in the home. Outpatient and day-care services can follow and thus limit institutional care to a minimum.

It may well be that the key to successful care may be as much in changing public attitudes to the aging as to the development of appropriate services and facilities with well-trained staff. When I was 40 I wrote 'when I am old I will expect no more from society than I do when I am young but equally I will expect no less'; 25 years on I see no reason to change this opinion. Society must recognize and provide for the particular needs of the aging as it does for any other age group. But while grouping our needs it must preserve our individuality.

The health care of the elderly has emerged from a position of neglect to being accepted as an important and complex area of health care. The broad range of problems affecting the elderly demand a multi-disciplinary approach of professionals with special training and skills in the care of the elderly.

These are not skills which can be picked up in passing because there are 'plenty of old people in the acute wards'. The proper care of the elderly is not a matter of charity but of social justice.

There can be no international pattern of the delivery of services. The differing social and cultural structure of each country makes it important for each to develop a delivery pattern peculiar to its own needs. But we can learn from each other and borrow other peoples ideas to fit our own needs and—in the words of the Maori proverb: '*Tau rau rau takü rau, ka ora te manuhiri*' ('With your basket of fruit and my basket of fruit, we will feed the multitude').

References

1. Warren, M. W. (1946). Care of the chronic aged sick. *Lancet*, **1**, 841–3.
2. Anderson, W. F. (1976). *Age and Ageing*. **5**, 194–7.
3. Kay, D. W., Roth, M., and Hall, M. R. (1966). Special Problems of the aged and the organisation of hospital services. *British Medical Journal*, **2**, 967–72.
4. Jack, A. (1981). *Physical disability*. Special Report Series No. 59. New Zealand Department of Health, Auckland.
5. Salmond, G. (1976). *Accommodation and service needs of the elderly*. Special Report Series No. 46. New Zealand Department of Health, Auckland.
6. Gibson R. M. Personal communication.
7. Barker, W. H., Williams, T. F., Zimmer, J. G., Van Buren, C., Vincent, S. J., and Pickrel, S. G. (1985). Geriatric consultation teams in acute hospitals: impact on backup of elderly patients. *Journal of the American Geriatrics Society*, **3** (6), 422–8.
8. Burley, W. E., Currie, C. T., Smith, R. G., and Williamson, J. (1979). Contribution from geriatric medicine in acute medical wards. *British Medical Journal*, **2**, 90–2.
9. Evans, G. J., Hodkinson, H. M., and Mezey, A. G. (1971). The elderly sick: who looks after them. *Lancet*, **ii**, 539.
10. O'Brien, T. D., Joshi, D. M., and Warren, E. D. (1973). No apology for geriatrics. *British Medical Journal*, **ii**, 3; 277.
11. Bagnall, W. E., Datta, S. R., Knox, J., and Horrocks, P. (1977). Geriatric medicine in Hull: a comprehensive service. *British Medical Journal*, **ii**, 102.
12. Evans, J. G. (1983). Integration of geriatric with general medical services in Newcastle. *Lancet*, **i**, 1430–3.
13. Institute of Medicine (1978). *Aging and medical education: report of a study*. National Academy of Sciences (Pub. 10M-78-04), Washington DC.
14. Williamson, J. (1979). Notes on the historical development of geriatric medicine as a medical speciality. *Age and Ageing*, **8**, 144.
15. Royal College of Physicians of London (1977). Medical care of the elderly: report of a working party. *Lancet*, **21**, 1092.
16. Devas, M. B. and Irvine, R. E. (1969). The geriatric orthopaedic unit: a method of achieving a return to independence in the elderly patient. *Journal of the Royal College of General Practitioners*, **6**, 19–25.
17. Irvine, R. E. (1985). Rehabilitation in geriatric orthopaedics *International Rehabilitation Medicine*, **7** (3), 115–19.
18. Robinson, R. (1965). A psychiatric geriatric unit. Psychiatric disorders in the aged. *WPA Symposium*, pp. 186–205. Geigy.
19. Godber, C. (1978). Conflict and collaboration between medicine and psychiatry. In *Recent Advances in Geriatric Medicine*. (ed. Isaacs, B) Churchill Livingstone, London.
20. Williamson, J. (1979). Geriatric medicine: whose speciality? *Annals of Internal Medicine*, **91**, 774–7.

21. Barker, R. A. (1972). Submission to Royal Commission on Hospitals and Related Services, New Zealand.
22. Petersen, O. L. (Editorial) (1978). *Annals of Internal Medicine*, **89**, 279.
23. Kane, R. A. and Kane, R. L. (1981). *Assessing the elderly: a practical guide to measurement*. DC Heath, Lexington, Mass.
24. Rubenstein, L. Z., Rhees, L., and Kane, R. L. (1982). The role of geriatric assessment units in caring for the elderly. *Journal of Gerontology*, **37**, 513–21.
25. Rubenstein, L. Z., Abrass, I. B., and Kane, R. L. (1981). Improved care for patients on a new geriatric evaluation unit. *Journal of the American Geriatrics Society*, **29**, 531–6.
26. Rubenstein, L. Z., Wieland, D., English, P., Josephsen, K., Sayre, J., and Abrass, I. B. (1984). The Sepulveda V. A. geriatric evaluation unit data on 4 year outcomes. *Journal of the American Geriatrics Society*, **32**, 503–12.
27. Rubenstein, L. Z., Josephson, K., Wieland, G. D., English, P., Sayre, J. A., and Kane, R. L. (1984). Effectiveness of a geriatric evaluation unit: a randomised clinical trial. *New England Journal of Medicine*, **311**, 1644–70.
28. Teasdale, T. A., Shuman, L., Snow, E., and Luchi, R. J. (1983). A comparison of placement outcomes of geriatric cohorts receiving care in a geriatric assessment unit and on general medical floors. *Journal of the American Geriatrics Society*, **31**, 529–34.
29. Sainsbury, R. (1984). Address to Christchurch Conference on Health of the Elderly.
30. Battersby, D. (1986). Address to Seminar of NZ Social Sciences Research Fund Committee.
31. Svanborg, A. and Williamson, J. (1980). *Health care for the elderly: implications for education and training of physicians and other health professionals*. WHO Regional Office for Europe, Copenhagen.
32. WHO/International Organization of Gerontology (1983). *A review of training programmes in Asia and Oceania*. Report of an international workshop.
33. United Nations (1982). *Report of the world assembly on aging*. UN, New York.
34. Fries, J. F. (1980). Aging, natural death and the compression of morbidity. *New England Journal of Medicine*, **303**, 130–6.

27

Home care and day care for the elderly
BETTY HAVENS

INTRODUCTION

Home care is usually viewed as the in-home or community-based option for providing long-term care to elderly persons. While the majority of this chapter will address precisely this option, two points should be noted: home care may also be provided to persons of all ages, not just the elderly, and some persons require home care only as a short-term (usually defined as less than 60 days) care solution.

The most essential element in long-term care is assessing the individual's type and level of care. Only then, as a last step in the assessment process, should the most appropriate location for that care be considered. The assessed need and level-of-care decision are totally different from the location or site of care decision. If the location decision—that is, whether or not the individual is eligible for nursing home care—is made first, that decision will come to drive the whole system. When this occurs, long-term health care costs will necessarily escalate as it becomes necessary to build, staff, and operate additional nursing homes in lieu of using the more cost-effective solution of providing care in the elderly person's home.

Home care rests on several principles: it must be consistent with a cultural tradition which hallows home and family, it must help individuals and their families or other informal network members to cope with illness and disability, it must link to both health and social services, it must acknowledge the centrality of the community in the lives of individuals, it must promote the use of appropriate services, it must enhance the continuity of care, and it must guarantee universal access regardless of ability to pay or age, or type and duration of disability.

The most typical non-community alternative to home care is care in a nursing home; however, in some instances the alternative may be care in an acute, rehabilitation, chronic, or extended treatment hospital. Where appropriate this chapter will make reference to institutional care to include all the residential options, and in other cases specific reference to nursing homes will be made. The chapter makes three assumptions: knowledge of the aging process, knowledge of pertinent disease processes, and knowledge of population aging, all based on content contained elsewhere in this volume.

Throughout this chapter most of the specific examples will be drawn from the Manitoba Continuing Care Program with suggestions for application to programmes in developing and developed countries. Because no programme operates in a vacuum, the first part of the chapter provides a brief overview of the Manitoba programme and the context within which it operates. This is followed by a section on the principles of evaluating the efficacy of home care programmes, a section on the evidence of benefits from home care, and a section on the linkages of home care with other service components, including existing informal care.

THE MANITOBA CONTINUING CARE PROGRAMME AND ITS CONTEXT

It is important to an understanding of the Manitoba model to know that, while health services are publicly insured in Canada, each of the 10 provinces retains autonomy in the delivery of health care and in developing health programmes. Therefore, while the government of Canada establishes certain minimum standards of health service provision as the basis for the federal share in funding health programmes, each province may develop its own programme and may supplement the requisite core standards as is appropriate to its jurisdiction. As a result the Manitoba system can be and is very different from programmes in other provinces. For example, in Manitoba there are no premiums as the insured services are publicly funded from taxes, but some provinces do levy premiums. Many provinces insure some aspects of long-term care but the components vary across the provinces.

The population of Manitoba is slightly over 1 000 000, with over 600 000 living in the capital city of Winnipeg. The population of seniors (65+) represents approximately 12 per cent of the total population. The oldest-old (80+) constitute over 20 per cent of seniors.[1] Manitoba is an extremely large province: 240 000 square miles. With so much of the population in Winnipeg, the remaining 400 000 persons are scattered in much smaller widely dispersed communities.

Within this setting Manitoba has developed a community-based social care programme, which fits it in an historical and national context.[2-6] Until the 1970s, community care consisted mainly of: (1) fee-for-service payments to physicians; (2) a number of fragmented home care programmes to encourage early discharge from hospital; and (3) some provincial social allowance home support programmes (cost-shareable with the federal government from 1966), providing some long-term care to indigent elderly.

By the 1970s, universally insured hospital and medical services had provided all Canadians with access to these services when sick, and

eliminated pauperization consequent to illness. However, these developments and their timing produced three unfortunate legacies.

First, provincial priorities began to be shaped to a large extent by
cost-sharing programmes. Rather than designing a model best suited to
meeting needs, most provinces allocated monies for short-term home care
to hospital budgets to benefit from cost sharing. This fostered a medically
oriented, short-term home care model which was very limited in its
potential to serve the needs of most elderly persons.

Secondly, any service model which becomes entrenched, regardless of
its merits, becomes perceived by professionals and institutions as their
exclusive territory. The development of a new model, even if superior,
which involves relinquishing or sharing control inevitably encounters resistance.

Finally, not including long-term community care within the insured
services meant no cost sharing was offered for the services needed by the
majority of elderly persons. Further, little disincentive was created as it
was cheaper to stay in hospital than to go home if resources beyond the
family were required.

In the early 1970s, the organization and delivery of health care were
re-appraised. The most serious problems were fragmentation, waste, and
inefficiency. One result of this re-appraisal was a series of provincial
initiatives in the field of community care. As a consequence, between
1974 and 1982 almost every province developed some community-based
home care services.

The Manitoba Continuing Care Program[2-5, 7-11] is a province-wide,
universal, no-cost-to-consumer programme which was initiated by the
provincial government in 1974 and gradually expanded throughout the
province in 1975. The programme staff assess persons requiring care,
whether for placement in nursing homes or for home care. The programme delivers services to those who remain at home. It is a co-ordinated
service programme which provides a broad range of services to meet the
needs of persons who require assistance or support to remain at home, or
whose functioning without home care is likely to deteriorate, making it
impossible for them to stay at home in the community. Upon identification of needs, services are organized to avoid deterioration and to maintain and enhance health. This is accomplished within established policy
guidelines, through the existing departmental health the community services network, and in conjunction with relevant voluntary agencies.

The service delivery framework is based upon professionally co-ordinated
and conducted assessments of need, care planning, and supervision of
service delivery. Ongoing services in the home are delivered both by paid,
professionally and paraprofessionally skilled persons and by volunteers.

For those of any age who are referred from any source (i.e. self, family, friend, neighbour, doctor, nurse, or hospital) determination of need for services is based upon a clinical, a health-functioning, and a social-functioning assessment. Assessment is focused to identify those who, without services, would be at risk of not being able to remain at home but who, with home-delivered services, could have their care needs managed appropriately.

Programme guidelines call for each person to be assessed fully using a comprehensive multidimensional assessment instrument, including identification of those activities which the person can perform, those which family members, friends, or neighbours can realistically perform, and those which require placement of services. A care plan is developed to provide for needed services which exist within the programme. When needed services are not available within it every effort is made to secure such services from other community sources as part of the care plan. Services provided by the programme are to be the minimum required to meet need and to foster independence. Delivery is to be organized so that services are provided by the person with the minimum skill required to perform the task.

Establishment of an assessment process which can be used within the programme itself and with components of both the health and social systems is an essential ingredient for success. The case of Mr S illustrates this principle. A common assessment for care at home or in a nursing home allowed the case co-ordinator to determine that placement in a nursing home was neither the most suitable solution nor necessary if Mr S's home could be modernized. Much more effort, time, and professional staff involvement would have been required if a common assessment procedure had not been in operation within the programme and across system components.

Mr S

Mr S is 88 years old and lives alone on a small farm at the edge of a small village. He has lived on this farm all his life, he has never married, and his siblings have predeceased him. His only relatives, nieces and nephews, live many miles away and seldom visit except occasionally during the summer. Mr S had been coping relatively well on his farm until he suffered pneumonia 8 months ago. Since that time, he has been unable to haul water from the well and chop the necessary firewood for cooking. He also had not built up his stock of wood which he uses for heating in the winter. The grocer has taken to delivering supplies as Mr S was finding it increasingly difficult to drive to town (about 12 miles each way) to do his banking and shopping.

A niece referred him for placement in a nursing home. The assessment for care indicated that he did need care but none of the staff in the neighbouring nursing home spoke Ukrainian and Mr S spoke very little English. In any case, he did not want to leave his farm. The assessment team had grave concerns about providing home care to him without water or reliable heat in the house. Mr S was not opposed to having water and plumbing in the house, he had just not needed them. He had had electricity for years but had not used it for heat, although he had begun doing much of his cooking on a hot plate and an electric frying pan after his pneumonia related hospital stay.

The case co-ordinator, a Ukrainian speaking social worker, began to negotiate with the local municipality for assistance with bringing water into the house under a special senior citizen's assistance programme. This took several months and many phone calls, visits, and forms to complete.

In the mean time, the case co-ordinator found a neighbouring teenager who agreed to haul water from the well on a daily basis. The case co-ordinator also helped Mr S to arrange with the electrical utility company to install electric heating and a hot-water tank in the house with provision for the cost of the installation to be added to his monthly electrical bill. The grocer agreed to continue delivering his supplies on a regular basis and the public health nurse added him to her case load to monitor his continued recovery and general health status.

Finally, late in the fall, water was brought into the house and with the help of the case co-ordinator Mr S contracted with a local plumber to install a kitchen sink ordered from the Sears catalogue and to attach the hot-water tank. A toilet with an external septic holding tank was installed in a hallway between the kitchen and the bedroom, which also served as the clothes closet. Had Mr S required financial assistance for this latter contract, it would have meant more time and potential frustration in negotiating with another government agency to accomplish the task. Fortunately, Mr S had sold some property and farm equipment just before his stay in hospital and was able to pay the plumber and suppliers.

His neighbour continues to visit Mr S a couple of times a week helping a bit around the place even though the water no longer needs to be hauled. After all this work was completed, the case co-ordinator closed the case as Mr S is able to continue living at home on his own without home care services and is no longer a candidate for an unwanted placement in a nursing home. Mr S and his relatives know they can contact the case co-ordinator if the situation changes. They explain that this has given them a greater sense of security. In this example, the case co-ordinator acted much as a surrogate for a caring family member.

Maintaining the balance between supporting independence without incurring dependence is critical and seldom easy to accomplish. If the case co-ordinator had not been committed to maintaining and supporting independence, Mr S would probably have been placed in a nursing home at the request of his niece. The creativeness of the case co-ordinator in assisting Mr S in modernizing his house not ony allowed him to remain at home but, in fact, even made it unnecessary for home care services to be provided in his home. This solution enabled him to maintain his home, his health, and his independence.

Assessments for care typically concentrate on client weaknesses and functional deficits. However, by operating in the community from a premise of maintaining independence, assessments are more appropriately focused on the strengths of the client and his/her informal support network. The assessment of Mrs B demonstrates this focus on strengths.

Mrs B

Mrs B has been referred for an assessment for care by the local public health nurse who has been visiting the family household as part of her case load for many years. Mrs B has lived with her son and daughter-in-law since she was widowed 30 years ago. The son and daughter-in-law have worked all their adult lives and Mrs B looked after their five children as they grew up. The youngest grandchild has finished university and is about to move to another city. One of the grandchildren is married and living two blocks away with his wife and two small preschoolers. The granddaughter-in-law works three half days a week and leaves the great-grandchildren with Mrs B while she works. She has noticed that Mrs B no longer picks up the children when they are fussing in the bed or playing on the floor. She has commented that she is not as limber as she used to be and has fallen several times just doing her usual tidying around the house.

During the assessment interview the nurse and social worker determined that Mrs B is mentally alert. She is able to get about the house, prepare meals, and generally tidy up her room, the kitchen, and help with other cleaning. Her daughter-in-law does all the shopping for her now, as she no longer trusts herself to walk the few blocks to and from the store alone, even to buy milk or bread. Occasionally the grandaughter-in-law brings bread or milk when she picks up her two children after work.

The assessment team was impressed with the strengths of Mrs B at 86 years of age and the mutual supportiveness of her family. However, they were also concerned about her reference to falls and her hesitation to walk out of doors or to pick up her great-grandchildren. They know that the family can respond to all the identified needs of Mrs B; however, they recommended that she attend the nearby day hospital programme for a full geriatric clinical assessment to be undertaken to determine the cause of her falls. Following a consultation from the assessment nurse, Mrs B's physician agreed to make a referral to the geriatrician at the day hospital for the days when she does not baby-sit with her great-grandchildren. Pending the outcome of that geriatric clinical assessment the home care assessment team made no further care plans. They forwarded their assessment findings to the day hospital, where the common assessment process enables better communication across portions of the system.

The referral of Mrs B to the geriatric day hospital programme for a comprehensive clinical assessment provides an example of innovative use of the full care system. The home care nurse assessor consulted with the family physician to arrange the referral to the geriatrician at the day hospital. The clinical assessment findings will be provided to the family physician and to the home care team should follow-up services be required. In the mean time, Mrs B will remain at home and will continue to baby-sit for her great-grandchildren while she is being assessed at the day hospital. Consequently, she will be retaining her independence and will continue to contribute to her own and her family's well-being.

The examples highlight the strengths of both clients and the informal support networks. However, each example also identifies some weakness within the client or the informal network, either temporarily or relatively permanently. The ability of an assessment to identify the strengths initially, and then to proceed to identifying weaknesses which inhibit independence, allows the assessment team to assign a case co-ordinator and develop a care plan which will provide only those services which fill gaps in supporting a client's independence and in maintaining his/her informal support network.

Seldom does a client need just a single service to remain in their own home in the community, so co-ordination of services becomes a major concern of both a providing agency and the client. If the community-based long-term care programme does not include service co-ordination in its functions, clients or their family are left with the time- and energy-consuming task of trying to co-ordinate a variety of service deliverers at the very time when they need to conserve their diminished energies and restricted time. All of these providers are employed by and responsible to a variety of organizations. For the community-based programme to co-ordinate health and social services from a variety of public, private, and voluntary agencies with those tasks performed by the client and his/her family, friends, and neighbours, a comprehensive multidimensional assessment is essential.

The range of programmes that may be classified as day care is very broad and varies considerably from one jurisdiction to another. As a general rule, day-care programmes can be distinguished from home care in that they are congregate programmes which occur in various commu-

nity facilities outside the individuals' homes. In Manitoba, these programmes include support services projects such as congregate meals
(often with additional capacity to provide heat and serve meals and meals-
on-wheels), transport (with escorts for shopping or medical appointments
when required), information dissemination (with referral if appropriate),
and handy person services. Adult day care programmes are usually located
in nursing homes but are also found in senior citizens' housing units,
health centres, senior centres, and local churches. In these programmes
the participants have the opportunity to socialize, share a nutritious meal,
have their health care monitored, and have their medication supervised.
Respite care programmes are usually located in a nursing home but may
occur in a hospital or in the client's home and provide complete care for
the client for a few hours as scheduled within the care plan up to a few
weeks to provide often much-needed holiday relief. Finally, day hospital
programmes provide multidisciplinary clinical assessments, medical supervision, and therapeutic treatments (occupational therapy, physiotherapy,
speech therapy, and psychotherapy) in addition to the elements of adult
day care. These programmes may be used alone or in combination, depending on the assessed need and based on the care plan, which incorporates the care required to maintain the informal support system—typically
family caregivers.

There is a certain satisfaction for a professional in successfully resolving
a problem with an individual client and his/her support network. This is
true when a solution is relatively straightforward and all components of
the solution are readily available and internal to the programme. However, it is even more challenging and satisfying when the components of
the solution are external to it. One of the components which can help
many families continue to maintain care with minimal formal service supports is respite care. This allows the primary caregiver(s) to do both
essential things such as banking or shopping, and other things that they
wish to do such as attending club meetings, joining friends for lunch, or
taking a necessary vacation. It may be provided in the client's home, in a
nearby nursing home, or in a hospital. In many instances adult day care
attendance by a client can fulfil most of these same goals. The changes
made in the case of Mrs L reflect a balanced interdependence.

Mrs L

Mrs L is a home care client who is severely disabled with arthritis and
mildly disoriented. She lives with her husband and their 62-year-old
widowed daughter, who works at a nearby computer centre. The case co-
ordinator has reviewed Mrs L's care plan on a quarterly basis for the past
4 years, during which time episodes of disorientation have become more

frequent. An occupational therapist monitors Mrs L's progress in maintaining her physical functioning and a homemaker assists with household maintenance 3 hours a week.

As Mrs L has become more disoriented, Mr L has had to stay with his wife unless their daughter or the homemaker is at home. As a result, Mr L and his daughter have found it increasingly difficult to do the household shopping, their own shopping, the shopping for Mrs L, the laundry, and yardwork. Mr L has also had difficulty getting to the bank. Both Mr L and his daughter have ceased to attend social activities and seldom have contacts with friends except when they drop in to see Mrs L or, in the daughter's case, at work. Mr L has become less agile physically, less outgoing, and more apathetic.

As a result of these changes the daughter contacted the case co-ordinator with a request for more homemaking time. She felt that her father was becoming less able to cope with preparing meals for her mother. The case co-ordinator reviewed the case and, in discussion with Mr and Mrs L, decided that respite care for Mrs L would vastly improve the situation. A revised care plan maintained the 3 hours of homemaking and provided 4 hours a week of home attendant care for Mrs L. This allowed Mr L to do more outside the home. In addition, arrangements were made for Mrs L to spend 1 out of every 6 weeks in a nearby nursing home. This provided respite for both Mr L and his daughter, which enabled them to maintain more of their social contacts and to do the major tasks in their home and yard.

This solution enabled the family to continue to care for Mrs L for 46 weeks of the year with only 7 hours a week of formal services. All components of this solution are within the services of the home care programme, but the use of a nursing home for respite care had to be arranged with the facility administrator and approved by the provincial funding authorities. This solution was successful in meeting Mr and Mrs L's needs. Without going outside the programme, the case co-ordinator probably would have eventually had to oversee the permanent placement of Mrs L in a nursing home.

The example of Mrs L highlights the importance of the case co-ordinator being able to keep on top of his/her case load. While it is essential to maintain the independent functioning of the client and the support network, clearly without essential gap-filling services which respond to and compensate for weaknesses in a given situation the whole situation can fall apart. When cases fall apart, no matter how small or simple the missing service is, the typical response is to seek placement in a nursing home. In most instances, the client and his or her support network can cope with an occasional gap in services or slowness in placing or replacing in-home services. But repeated occurrences generally discourage the client, frustrate their support network, put undue burden on other formal caregivers or service deliverers and case co-ordinators, and may ultimately become an incentive to either unnecessary service increases or premature nursing home placement.

When a common assessment process is used across all sectors of long-term care and the assessment itself is designed to establish types and amount of care required, the last step in the process is to determine the most appropriate location for that care. If the location decision is made first, it begins inappropriately to drive the whole system. What one needs to know is not whether or not the individual is eligible for nursing home care but whether or not the individual needs a level of care equivalent to nursing home care, regardless of its source. Then one can look at the potential sites at which this care can be provided and make the location decisions. These are very different kinds of decisions; that is, the assessed need and level-of-care decision is different from the location or site-of-care decision.

The importance of this order of events is most clearly demonstrated in the case of Mr S, who was referred to the assessment team by a niece who believed that he should be placed in a nursing home. If the team had assessed his situation on the basis of eligibility for placement in a nursing home rather than on the basis of his strengths, care needs, and desire to remain at home, he most certainly would have been placed in a neighbouring nursing home. However, the assessment revealed that, while Mr S required assistance and while his own home left much to be desired as a location within which to deliver services, it was possible to modify his home sufficiently to enable him to care for himself.

In a milieu of fiscal responsibility and economic constraint, responsiveness to changing client needs will have to be accomplished through redirection of existing resources. As such, it will become even more essential to assure adequate programme staffing and to maintain sufficient direct service staffing flexibility. If the Manitoba Continuing Care Program has learned one thing through painful experience, it is that there are no savings to be made from curtailing programme staffing. Unrealistically large case loads inhibit prompt assessment, slow down case reviews, mitigate against appropriate and timely reassessments, and preclude innovative solutions. They incur either client dependence through delays in withdrawing unneeded services or increased costs by employing easy solutions. This often means providing more costly services that are integral to the programme even if personnel are overskilled for requisite tasks. Programme-staffing patterns must be adequate to this impending challenge or the institutionally easy and more costly decisions will prevail.

In order to provide a brief overview of the present (1986/1987) statistics for users of continuing care, Table 27.1[12] shows the relationship of in-

Table 27.1 Relationship of in-home and in-nursing-home users and those waiting placement as a percentage of the total population aged 65 and over

Description	Number	Percentage
Home care only	10 325	7.7
Home care pending placement	494	0.4
Hospital pending placement	595	0.4
Personal care home	7 645	5.7
Other elderly	114 169	85.7

Table 27.2 Home care case loads

	1982–1983	1983–1984	1984–1985	1985–1986	1986–1987
March 31	10 631	10 933	11 848	13 193	13 608
Percentage change		2.8	8.4	11.4	3.1
Yearly admissions	9 696	9 761	10 438	11 479	11 827
Yearly discharges	9 202	9 479	9 549	10 183	11 409
Total receiving	19 716	20 392	21 371	23 327	25 020

home and in-nursing-home users and those waiting placement as a portion of the total population aged 65 and over. This is further detailed in Tables 27.2 and 3,[12] which deal with the home care case loads and admissions to personal care homes (nursing homes) from 1982/1983 to 1986/1987.

Most people also want to know about the costs of these programmes; therefore Table 27.4[12] presents a summary of *per diem* rates and home care costs during the same period. The costs per person served by home care have been calculated in two ways. A cost per person per month figure was calculated using the average of the maximum number served in the month for 1986/1987. The cost per person for the year was calculated using the number at the beginning of the year plus admissions. The costs for last year do not include some of the direct service costs, which are related to term positions and the cost of medical supplies from the Medical Supplies and Home Care Equipment Branch. Costs for hospital co-ordination and homemaker co-ordination are included. Table 27.4 and the related calculations continue to support the findings of the *Manitoba/Canada Home Care Study*[13] that home care is a less costly alternative than institutional placement in those cases where non-institutional locations for care are appropriate.

Table 27.3 Manitoba personal care home first admissions

	From community	From hospital	From other	Total
1984/1985:				
Outside Winnipeg	392	365	4	761
Winnipeg	498	455	12	965
Manitoba total	890	820	16	1726
1985/1986:				
Outside Winnipeg	355	375	14	744
Winnipeg	519	456	13	988
Manitoba total	874	831	27	1732
1986/1987:				
Outside Winnipeg	345	406	11	762
Winnipeg	438	481	19	938
Manitoba total	783	887	30	1700

Table 27.4 A summary of the highest *per diem* rates[a] experienced in each region (in $)

	Level 1[b]	Level 2	Level 3/4
1984/1985 fiscal year:			
Non-proprietary personal care homes	44.70	57.00	73.85
Proprietary personal care homes	46.05	46.05	63.70
1985/1986 fiscal year:			
Non-proprietary personal care homes	44.05	74.75	85.80
Proprietary personal care homes	47.70	47.70	66.05
1986/1987 fiscal year:			
Non-proprietary personal care homes	45.20	98.20	98.65
Proprietary personal care homes	49.10	49.10	68.00

[a] The gross *per diem* rates listed include the residential charge of: $14.80 *per diem* payable by the resident in 1984/1985; $16.60 *per diem* payable by the resident in 1985/1986; and $18.40 *per diem* payable by the resident in 1986/1987.

[b] Proprietary personal care homes are required to staff for any Level 1 residents in their facility as though they were assessed as a Level 2.

Home care costs 1984/1985:
$142.43 average cost per client per month = $4.75 average *per diem*.
$992.53 average cost per client per year = $2.72 average *per diem*.
Home care costs 1985/1986:
$153.51 average cost per client per month = 5.05 average *per diem*.
$1069.85 average cost per client per year = $2.93 average *per diem*.
Home care costs 1986/1987:
$198.12 average cost per client per month = $6.60 average *per diem*.
$1287.37 average cost per client per year = $3.58 average *per diem*.

There may be concern about whether or not families will 'dump' their older family members into a home care programme or into an insured nursing home. In other words, the position of those persons who are opposed to publicly insuring or subsidizing integrated, community-based continuing care is fear that families will neglect their familial or financial responsibility for their older members. Manitoba has found home care to be an enabling programme to ensure that families can and will continue to care for older family members, and universality of home care and insured nursing home care is a further guarantee of support by families, not a deterrent. In Manitoba, 80 per cent of the care provided to persons over age 65 is still provided by the family and/or other members of the informal support system. This rate was 80 per cent before home care was introduced, it was 80 per cent before the insured nursing home program was introduced, and it is still 80 per cent.

Furthermore, the rate is 80 per cent in at least three additional Canadian provinces. The 80 per cent rate is a fairly constant level. Virtually all of the literature in the United States and Europe and at least two studies in developing countries also indicate that 80 per cent of the care is provided informally. This is not a new piece of information, but it is an issue which is constantly raised as something that it is feared will change when alterations are made to insure nursing homes or home care. This has not been Manitoba's experience at all.

As a matter of fact, there are many elders whom it is hard to believe are able to be maintained in the community. Two of the most widely used programme components for this purpose are the adult day care programme and the respite programme. With these programmes, families continue to cope with their elderly relative, as do neighbours and friends. Nursing home and hospital staff are often amazed by the ability of families and neighbours in the community to cope with such heavy care. There has been ample opportunity to observe that this formal care has supported the informal care system, not detracted from it.

Finally, before moving on to the section on evaluation, it seems appropriate to make a final comment on the chronology of health and social system events which, as noted at the beginning of this section, have had a lasting impact on the Manitoba programme. Having been faced with the medically oriented and higher-cost services being insured and accessible prior to establishing policy relative to both institutional and community long-term care, and having had the institutional policy implemented first, this sector continues to influence the programme. If one could start in a rational manner to create a system, one would want to start with health promotion and to support informal assistance in a community-based and locally 'owned' manner, add community-based care, then nursing home care, then chronic or extended treatment, then rehabilitative hospital care, and only then would one add acute or general hospitals and the insuring of physician services.

It is doubtful that any jurisdiction, today, could start with a totally clean slate to design a rational system. However, at whatever stage the system is, one should plan to incorporate first of all those elements which foster independence and wellness and support the informal system. This is one area in which most of the developing nations could learn from historical mistakes and move to implement a system which is, from very nearly the beginning, more rational and really would be built from the informal caring networks in the community to more elaborate, costly, and medically oriented institutional forms of care.

The epitome of a lack of system rationality in Manitoba was the addition of projects for support services to seniors in 1984, a full decade after home care and over two decades after hospital and medical insurance. Support services to seniors[14] are local community projects which support frail elderly persons in the community. These projects provide services which: support independence, assist with the ordinary, basic but essential, daily living activities, are locally planned and managed, involve essentially voluntary efforts by community members including the participants, and involve very minimal governmental funding (average government project cost in 1986/1987 was $12262, and most projects provide almost daily services to at least 60 different people in a year) to preclude the necessity for care. In other words, why would one have to have a homemaker prepare meals or receive meals-on-wheels if one can cook but cannot shop? Support services in this case might: involve the individual in a congregate meals programme; arrange transport including an escort, if one were required, to enable the person to shop; or arrange for the shopping to be done and delivered by a volunteer on either a short-term or relatively lengthy basis. These projects have enabled home care to be used more appropriately and have contributed to a reduction in waiting lists for nursing home placement in those communities with support services to seniors projects.

Manitoba administrators would have preferred to have a fully developed health promotion and support service programme in place prior to the universal home care programme and to any of the institutional elements. As history could not be rewritten or altered, certain systems savings were at best delayed and at worst lost in the top-down development of the Manitoba system. In spite of these unfortunate facts, Manitoba has reduced its total number of hospital beds and has not increased its supply of nursing home beds at a rate even near the rate of growth in the elderly population.

PRINCIPLES OF EVALUATING EFFICACY

Many of the principles of evaluating home care efficacy are those appropriate to evaluation of any social or health programme. Because the aim of most home care programmes is to provide care and to preclude or curtail use of some other system component (eg. nursing home or hospital), evaluation of home care is fraught with all the problems of evaluating any preventive programme. That is, the most important effects are usually unable to be measured for many years and involve many more components than the programme in question—in this case home care. Further, the measuring capability is limited and the available instruments are crude.

An additional problem in determining the efficacy of home care is the degree to which it is bound by the system of which it is a part and by the sociocultural context within which that system exists.[5, 10, 15-20] Consequently, comparative or even multiple-site studies are virtually impossible to mount. Because home care programmes are implemented to meet the needs of already vulnerable persons, even demonstration projects are seldom able to pursue evaluations wherein the designs are suitable to determining efficacy. For example, outcome studies based on the initial randomized assignment of persons to home care, to any alternative care, or to no care conditions is sufficiently repugnant to most caregivers, program administrators, policy makers, funders, and society at large to necessitate the use of inadequate designs.[13, 21-3]

Setting aside these methodological concerns, other than to note that multiple methodologies and longitudinal designs should be encouraged, it is possible to identify many elements to be included in any sound evaluation of home care. While these elements will not be described in this chapter, it seemed useful to list them. The following listing is not in any priority order, nor is it to be considered exhaustive but simply as a guide to those seriously designing home care evaluations, planning and implementing home care programmes, and developing relevant policies. In addition to the references cited with the individual elements, evaluators would be well advised to study those evaluation reports[7, 11, 13, 15, 22-3] which deal with the majority of these items.

The elements in evaluating home care efficacy include:

(1) costs, costing, cost-effectiveness, and cost savings;[17, 18, 24, 26-30]

(2) precluding or inhibiting impoverishment, pauperization, or 'spending down';[5, 18, 27-31]

(3) accessibility to care regardless of ability to pay, age, or type of disability;[5, 13, 17, 27-31]

(4) degree of universality;[5, 27, 28, 30]

(5) client (or patient) health outcomes and inclusion of chronic illness or disability;[5, 18, 23, 28]

(6) improvement in quality of life or life satisfaction;[18, 26-8]

(7) degree of support to social networks or informal care, including considerations of living arrangements, caregivers' health, and quality of life;[5, 17, 18, 25-9]

(8) evidence of communication with clients and informal supporters;[17]

(9) evidence of multidimensional assessments based on functional capacity;[6, 17, 28]

(10) mechanisms for and degree of service or case co-ordination;[5, 25, 29]

(11) analysis of the sociocultural context and value structure;[6, 15, 19, 20]

(12) degree of 'local' fit or community 'ownership';[5, 7, 28, 29]

(13) breadth of the continuum of health and social services, including community and institutional care;[5, 17, 24-6, 29, 31]

(14) encompassing of all relevant programmes and policies;[17, 19, 26]

(15) degree to which service components are available singly, as opposed to a 'total package', and whether the least-trained person appropriate to the care actually provides it;[1, 5, 17, 25, 29]

(16) whether new, high-technology aids are included; i.e. is technology seen as a viable alternative to some forms and amounts of 'hands on' caregiving?;[17]

(17) the degree to which home care is seen as social care versus the medical model;[5, 27 8, 30]

(18) evidence of the political will to implement or change home care programmes.[5, 15, 17, 19, 27]

THE EVIDENCE OF BENEFITS

While it would have been desirable to go through the list above and cite the evidence of benefits element by element, based on methodologically sound evaluations of home care efficacy, given the primitive state of this field of knowledge this goal cannot be accomplished. Therefore, based on the various studies already cited in this paper and with particular attention to the case examples derived from the Manitoba Continuing Care Program, several benefits of home care will be identified in this section.

While the jury is still out on the cost-effectiveness and cost savings of home care programmes,[15–16, 18, 24–5, 28, 30] there is evidence that, when taken as a programme in its own right or where savings are viewed as deriving from a broad systems perspective, home care is cost-effective.[4, 10, 12–13, 16, 32] Similarly, several reports exist on successes in inhibiting pauperization in the face of long-term care[4–5, 9, 10, 15–16, 28] without bankrupting the systems or the societies of which they are a part.

Accessibility to care and universality are hallmarks of the Manitoba model, as evidenced particularly by the case examples cited earlier in this chapter and elsewhere.[4–11, 13, 15] The unique solutions mounted for Mr S and the modifications to the care plan for Mrs L to allow Mr L and their daughter to continue to care for her are striking examples of the benefits accruing from this principle. While less is known about health outcomes, some studies[5–6, 18, 23] have addressed this issue.

Many studies have looked at quality of life but few have used adequate measurements.[5–6, 11, 18, 23, 28] The degree of support to the social networks of clients and documentation of the caregiver's health status and quality of life is also scant but some does exist.[4–6, 17, 18, 26–8] Communication with the client and their informal support system and the use of high technology as a substitution for 'hands on' caregiving are virtually non-existent topics other than in Kane and Kane's[17] recent work. Multidisciplinary assessments are also seldom studied,[6–8, 11, 17, 23, 28] although nearly every source acknowledges multidimensional assessment as a principle important to home-care programmes. This is certainly apparent in the cases of Mrs S and Mrs B. In the area of supporting caregivers, it should be noted that the 'thinning' of the adult offspring generation, which is typically the source of much caregiving,[10, 18–20, 26] will become even more marked in the developing nations[34] and will make such supports less possible than has been the case among the developed nations. This may produce strengths, as suggested in the earlier discussion of support services,[14] or may create a virtual stampede to institutional models[7, 10, 18–20] of care. These discussions[7, 10, 14, 18–20, 34] also highlight the importance of 'local fit' for home care programmes—as was particularly obvious in the case of Mr S.

The benefits of a full continuum of services, of adequate case co-ordination, of respect for the sociocultural context of services, of the ability to use single programme components and the use of the least-trained personnel resources are all critical components of the solutions arrived at for all three of the case examples in this paper. These topics have been documented[5–7, 15, 17, 19–20, 24–6, 29, 31] to a greater extent than some of the other elements.

Finally, the case of Mr S reveals the importance of maintaining home care as social care without overmedicalization[4, 5, 7, 15, 27–8, 31–3] of either the care or the system. Those jurisdictions which do not have home care in place, especially if little institutional care exists relative to the size of the aging population (e.g. in many developing nations[18-20]), have the potential of learning from the more developed programmes and of creating much more appropriate models and solutions. However, none of these strategies can be implemented without the 'political will'[15] to bring them about. In this context, political will has a much broader definition than simply politicians, it must be seen to include all the health professions, administrations, funders, consumers, and society at large[5,15,19,27] if the benefits of home care are to be realized.

LINKAGES WITH OTHER SERVICE COMPONENTS, INCLUDING INFORMAL CARE

It may have become obvious to the reader that home care is largely a conceptual extension of the informal care and support provided to the elderly in every society historically and in the present. Women have been still are the primary providers and consumers of this care. As many studies have pointed out, approximately 80 per cent of all care provided to the elderly population is provided by the informal support networks of these elderly persons. The care provided by the formal care system builds on that informal care, supports it, and enables it to carry on in the face of extremely difficult situations.

The full continuum of health and social services includes not only informal care, support services (as described earlier in this chapter), home care (including adult day care and respite care), nursing home care, extended and rehabilitative institutional care, day hospitals, acute care, and care from physicians and other health professionals, but also the broad spectrum of social services, including pensions (or other income security measures), affordable housing, special interest groups, senior centres, older adult centres, senior educational programmes, and all the age-integrated social programmes. The most effective home care programmes will have easy access to any and all of these components, enabling solutions (such as those described in the case examples) to be developed *with* the client and his or her support system and to be changed or modified as required.

The forging of these linkages requires each component to negotiate across its boundaries and to be open to such boundary crossings, creating a type of functional reciprocity throughout the system. This process of linking components will be much more successful and easier if a common multidimensional assessment for service/care is available to and used by all the components, and if service/care is co-ordinated on behalf of the client and his/her informal support system by one player in the overall system. That co-ordinator may change from time to time and will surely vary from person to person but the assessment and co-ordination roles must be performed if home care is to be viable as care in its own right or as an alternative to any other care component.

Note

Second Expert Committee Report on the Health of the Elderly, WHO, Geneva, November 1987.

References

1. Manitoba Health Services Commission (1987). *Population of Manitoba health region*, Vol. 5. *Regional summaries by age and sex*. Manitoba Health Service Commission, Winnipeg, MB.
2. Havens, B. (1986). *Manitoba model of continuing care*. Paper presented at National Conference of State Legislatures Annual Meeting, New Orleans, LA.
3. Havens, B. (1985). *The Manitoba model*. Paper presented at the Ontario Hospital Association Annual Meeting, December. Toronto, ON.
4. Chappell, N. L. (1988). Long-term care in Canada. In *North American elders: United States and Canadian perspectives*, (ed. Rathbone-McCuan, E. and B. Havens) Greenwood, Westport CT.
5. Berdes, C. (1987). *Warmer in winter*. Report to World Health Organization Fellow Program. Northwestern University, Chicago, IL.
6. Shapiro, E. (1987). *Multidisciplinary health assessments of the elderly in Manitoba Canada*. Paper presented at International Work Group Meeting on Multidisciplinary Health Assessment of the Elderly, Göteborg.
7. Havens, B. (1986). Boundary crossing: an organizational challenge for community-based long-term service agencies. In *Managing home care for the elderly: lessons from community-based agencies*. (ed. Pelham, A. O. and W. F. Clarke), pp.77–98. Springer Publishing Co., New York.
8. Havens, B. (1987). Assessment for care: the Manitoba Model. *Provider*, **13**, 26–9.
9. Havens, B. (1985). Statement of Betty Havens, provincial gerontologist, Manitoba, Canada. In *Select Committee on Aging, House of Representatives. Continuing care: international prototypes for America's aged*. pp. 17–22, 81–188. (Comm. Pub. No. 99–523). US Government Printing Office, Washington DC.
10. Havens, B. (1985). A long-term care system: a Canadian perspective. In *The feasibility of a long-term care system: lessons from Canada*, (ed. Kane, R. L.) pp. 19–27. University of South Florida, Tampa, FL.
11. Shapiro, E. (1986). Patterns and predictors of home care use by the elderly when need is the sole basis for admission. *Home Health Care Services Quarterly*, **7**, 29–44.
12. Office of Continuing Care (1983–1987). *Annual statistical reports*. Manitoba Health, Winnipeg, MB.

13. Policy Planning and Information Branch Department of National Health and Welfare (1982). *The Manitoba/Canada home care study, an overview of findings.* Health and Welfare Canada, Ottawa, ON.

14. Interagency Committee on Support Services to Seniors (1983, revised 1985). *Policy paper on support services to seniors.* Manitoba Health, Winnipeg, MB.

15. Kane, R. L. and Kane, R. A. (1985). *A will and a way: what the United States can learn from Canada about care of the elderly.* Columbia University Press, New York NY.

16. Kane, R. L. (1985). *The feasibility of a long-term care system: lessons from Canada.* University of South Florida, Tampa, FL.

17. Kane, R. A. and Kane, R. L. (1986). *Health care for the elderly in the year 2000: a profile of service needs in the year 2000.* Paper presented at Health Care for the Elderly in the Year 2000 Symposium, Victoria, BC.

18. Health Care Financing Administration (1986). *Long-term care for the elderly provided within the framework of health care schemes.* International Social Security Association, Geneva.

19. Havens B. (1987). Intra and inter national proposals. In *Economic Council of Canada. Aging with limited resources.* pp. 18–22. Minister of Supply and Services Canada, Ottawa, ON.

20. Lopez, A. D. and Cliquet, R. L. (ed.) (1984). *Demographic trends in the European region: health and social implications.* WHO Regional Publications, European Series No. 17. World Health Organization, Copenhagen.

21. Mathematica Policy Research, Inc. (1982). *National long-term care channeling demonstration: initial research design of the national long-term care demonstration.* NTIS No. PB86–234366/AS. US Department of Health and Human Services, Washington, DC.

22. Mathematica Policy Research, Inc. (1986). *National long-term care channeling demonstration: the evaluation of the national long-term care demonstration: survey data, collection design and procedures.* NTIS No. PB86-235330/AS. US Department of Health and Human Services, Washington, DC.

23. Wan, T. T. H. (1986). Evaluation research in long-term care: scope and methodolgy. *Research on Aging,* **8**, 559–85.

24. Hughes, S. L., Manheim, L. M., Edelman, P. L., and Conrad, K. J. (1987). Impact of long-term home care on hospital and nursing home use and cost. *Health Services Research,* **22**, 19–47.

25. Brody, J. J. (1987). Strategic planning: the catastrophic approach. *The Gerontologist,* **17**, 131–8.

26. Brody, E. M. (1986). Institutional versus community health care of the elderly: the delicate balance of social policy, position paper. *Home Health Services Quarterly,* **7**, 113–29.

27. Estes, C. L. (1986). Institutional versus community health care of the elderly: the delicate balance of social policy, a national perspective. *Home Health Services Quarterly,* **7**, 135–41.

28. Mathematica Policy Research, Inc. (1986). *National long-term care channeling demonstration: analysis of the benefits and costs of channeling.* NTIS No. TR-86B-12. US Department of Health and Human Services, Washington, DC.

29. Mathematica Policy Research, Inc. (1987). *National long-term care channeling demonstration: channeling effects on formal community-based services and*

housing. NTIS No. TR-86B-10. US Department of Health and Human Services, Washington DC.

30. Kane, R. L. (1986). Overview: who should pay for long-term care and how? In *National debate on health care, proceedings*. pp. 75–81. Texas Department of Human Services, Dallas TX.

31. Rice, D. P. and Estes, C. L. (1984). Health of the elderly: policy issues and challenges. *Health Affairs*, **3**, 25–49.

32. Levin, P. J. (1985). A comparison, from a hospital administrator's viewpoint, between three Canadian provinces long-term care programs and the US non-system. In *The feasibility of a long-term care system: lessons from Canada*, (ed. Kane, R. L.) pp. 28–36. University of South Florida, Tampa, FL.

33. Chappell, N. L., Strain, L. A., and Blandford, A. A. (1985). *Aging and health care: a social perspective*. Holt, Rinehart and Winston of Canada Ltd., Toronto, ON.

34. Nusberg, C. (1987). Policy-makers urged to act now on economic consequences of aging populations. *Aging International*, **14**, 9–13.

28

Nursing home care for the elderly

MIRIAM J. HIRSCHFELD and RACHEL FLEISHMAN

INTRODUCTION

The purpose of this chapter is to ask a few basic questions about nursing homes and to shed some light on the issues involved. Hopefully, these arguments and data will prove helpful to a thoughtful consideration of social policy issues regarding long-term care in both developed and developing countries. It is not the purpose of this chapter to review the vast literature on nursing homes, which covers topics such as quality of care, over-and undersupply of beds, regulations, descriptions of life in nursing homes and personal and literary descriptions of residents' experiences, the effect upon nursing home residents of a wide variety of nursing home characteristics as numerous accounts on the misuse of nursing homes, and other related topics.[1-11]

The following questions are crucial issues of relevance to all countries, despite the vast regional differences.

1. Which needs should nursing homes fulfil for the individual old person, which for the family, and which for society?
2. What are the demographic and epidemiological trends influencing the need for nursing home beds?
3. What are the origins of the nursing home, its utilization, and the needed supply rates?
4. What are the intrinsic effects of the nursing home upon the old person's well-being and what are they related to?
5. How is nursing home utilization related to other services?
6. How do quality of care and 'dependency' affect quality of life in nursing homes?
7. What are the social policy implications for developed and developing countries in regard to nursing homes?

THE ROLE OF THE NURSING HOME

For the individual elderly person, the nursing home is above all an answer to one major need—the need for tending, whenever there is a deficit in self-care ability. Tending is the work performed in looking after those who cannot do so for themselves: feeding, washing, lifting, toileting, protecting. Often the nursing home is the answer to two additional basic needs—the need for shelter and the need for human comfort. These needs are so basic to human existence that whenever they are unmet an old person is likely to experience what Rabinowitz and Nielsen[12] describe in their classic study as the desperate trinity of fear, despair, and persuasion, bringing her or him into the nursing home. Catastrophic illness, frailty, or a major loss in the social support system, more likely with each advancing year, are often the background leading to nursing home admission. For the family the nursing home is meant to fulfil the surrogate position of both usages of the term 'care':[13] first the idea of caring about, of concern and moral involvement, and second the direct work of tending. This does not mean to say that families abandon their elderly. To the contrary, research and clinical experience from many countries demostrate the vital role that families have in the care of the elderly.[14-18] But when a family, for whatever reason, feels or becomes unable to care for an elderly person and decides upon institutionalization, the nursing home is expected at least to share family caring and tending functions, if not to be solely responsible for these functions.

Much of the evidence presented in the literature reinforces the notion that for society the major purpose of the nursing home is that of a human 'warehouse' for its physically, mentally, socially, or financially dependent members. With that, major changes are now occurring in the social awareness regarding quality of life for the dependent aged. A vast literature on quality of care in nursing homes, on regulations, and quality assurance is shedding new light on society's means of developing nursing homes as places for 'full living'. The role of the nursing home for society is influenced by social forces, family commitment, and the values discussed below. It is also influenced by the balance allotted to the various components of the long-term care system as socio-economic provisions, community care, and institutional care which are interdependent parts of the wider picture.

As Townsend[1] stated in his classical study, the role of the nursing home for society is still manifold and in need of careful consideration: It is a permanent refuge for infirm persons who cannot care for themselves in their own home and who cannot be supported in their homes by any practicable system of domiciliary services. It is a temporary refuge for frail persons recovering from illness or malnutrition or seeking to give relatives or workers in the domiciliary services a hard-earned rest or perhaps a chance of improving the facilities available at home. And in addition it may simply be a rescue device for the present generation of elderly whose differing needs cannot be met because good housing, adequate pensions, and comprehensive local domiciliary services are not yet provided.

The tendency in developed countries today seems to point in the direction of providing more social and health services in the community and reserving the role of the nursing home for the very impaired elderly, needing intensive nursing and medical care.[11,19] In summary, the role of the nursing home for the individual elderly person, for the family, and for society must be taken into account when considering a sensible long-term care policy providing optimal quality of life in appropriate settings.

DEMOGRAPHIC AND EPIDEMIOLOGICAL TRENDS INFLUENCING THE NEED FOR NURSING HOME BEDS—FOR INSTITUTIONALIZATION

Reductions in fertility, infant mortality, and death from infectious disease, and increased life expectancy for those with chronic disease, have resulted in the aging of populations. Starting in richer and industrialized countries and spreading at various rates, there has been a continuous rise in both the numbers and the proportion of elderly. Not only have populations grown older, but there are now increased proportions of the very old and frail within the elderly population itself.[20]

While the majority of elderly live autonomous lives, frailty and dependency increase more rapidly after 75 years of age than before it. Over the last decade, life expectancy at the age of 85 has increased from about 6 months to 4.6 years for men and 5.6 years for women. In many countries the 80+ group is the fastest growing one and is expected to double in size by the end of the century.[21] In industrialized countries old age is associated with widowhood, one-person families, reduced income, a greater risk of poverty, survival of one's children, and institutionalization. While the demographic forecasts (size and composition of aged population) for the WHO region of the Eastern Mediterranean region, for instance, are less impressive than those from Europe or the United States, the social, economic and political developments may have severe repercussions upon the aged population world-wide: an Egyptian report[22] and the country reports of Pakistan and Kuwait to the United Nations World Assembly on Aging, 1983[23,24] mention such factors as urbanization and modernization, migration of the young to the cities and abroad, and a trend towards nuclear families. All these trends are known to have negative effects upon the situation of the elderly. One example from Egypt is the establishment of small housing units in new urban housing projects which do not permit the accommodation of elder family members. This latter reality was one factor which greatly encouraged institutionalization of the aged in Israel, a development which is today bitterly regretted.[25]

Increasing survival brings increasing frailty and morbidity from chronic disease. The ill elderly live longer and, because of this, in developed countries diseases are managed rather than cured.[26, 27] Mental and functional impairment reduce self-care ability and more people become dependent upon long-term care services. The examples of Kuwait and Fiji may highlight future trends in developing countries. In Kuwait, rapid economic development and a very high standard of living have brought about an increase in obesity, diabetes, hypertension, cardiovascular diseases, and cancer. In a very different part of the world, the Western Pacific, the mortality and morbidity pattern is also changing from that of communicable diseases to chronic diseases with accompanying disability. Cardiovascular disease, cancer, and diabetes are the leading causes of death among both main ethnic groups in Fiji: the Indians and the Fijians.[28] The proportion of aged is rising and the absolute numbers of old people are expected to double by the year 2000.

What these demographic forecasts and epidemiological developments tell us is that the problems associated with an aging population are problems not only for the developed world, but are at the doorstep of developing countries as well.

All these changes affect the need for long-term care services and, in particular, that for nursing homes.

ORIGINS OF THE NURSING HOME; ITS UTILIZATION AND SUPPLY

Nursing homes have developed out of different custodial types of facilities, most of which were originally designed to serve the poor. Institutional care was thus the solution to poverty and social problems such as mental illness, or for the chronically ill of all ages over many generations.[1, 4] In the last century the contemporary nursing home has come to serve not only the poor and disabled, but also individuals formerly treated or housed in acute care hospitals, mental institutions, and other types of institutional settings. Today institutional care for the aged spans a wide gamut. In much of the literature 'the nursing home' is the *pars pro toto* of all such care.

If one lives to advanced old age, the odds of being institutionalized in a nursing home are at least one in five in the United States. For most this residence is likely to be a permanent one. The percentage of institutionalized persons rises from 1.2 per cent in the 65–74 age group to 23.7 per cent in the over-85 group.[4] The comparative figures in Israel, a country 'midway' on the development continuum, are 0.6 per cent among ages 65–9, 1.5 per cent among ages 75–9, 10 per cent among ages 80–4, and

20.1 per cent among those aged 85+.[29] The lower rates of institutionalization in Israel compared with the United States can be explained in at least two different ways. The first argument would emphasize the lower rate of socio-economic development and the lack of nursing homes in Israel.[30] The other argument would emphasize the cultural component; an international comparison of patterns of informal social support of the elderly showed rates of about 25 per cent of elderly receiving instrumental informal help in Europe and the United States and about 40 per cent receiving effective support, while Jewish populations in Israel and other countries showed a stronger family-oriented pattern with 40 per cent receiving instrumental help and 85 per cent receiving effective support.[15]

A strong family-oriented informal social support system for the elderly may serve as an alternative to institutionalization. In many European countries the quantitative emphasis in terms of costs and numbers of people cared for is in the institutional domain. The Netherlands tops the list with 13.7 per cent of the elderly living in institutions (10 per cent in residential homes), but the trend is to reduce this to 7 per cent. Denmark reports 6.2 per cent of the over-65s living in institutions, most of them in nursing homes. In Austria nearly 4 per cent of the over-60 population live in institutional households and the supply rate is 34.5 per 1000 population aged 65 and over.[19] But the under- or oversupply of nursing home beds is a controversial issue influenced by a wide variety of ideological, economic, legal, and other issues. In the United States, there is a considerable variance in the supply of nursing home beds across States, from 212 beds per 1000 elderly in Arizona to 89 beds in Wisconsin.[31] Federal funding and the de-institutionalization of aged patients from state mental hospitals in the 1960s and 1970s led to a rapid growth of the nursing home industry. Nursing home utilization is negatively related to the percentage of the aged population in mental hospitals.[31-4] There seems to be little agreement upon the rate of nursing homes for appropriate utilization.

THE EFFECTS OF INSTITUTIONALIZATION UPON ELDERLY PERSONS' WELL-BEING

Elderly persons who enter long-term care institutions do so to assure survival and to improve their quality of life. Their goals would seem congruent with an institutional setting that has the provision of health care within a structured social environment as its purpose. Yet these same institutions have been charged with having most detrimental effects on the elderly. These are assumed to result from two major factors. The first suggests that institutionalization in itself has a negative impact upon 'the inmate',[6,35] while the second factor is related to low quality of care, lack of regulations, the profit motive, etc.[2-4,7,36] The institution is perceived as a coercive environment often causing more incapacity than it cures in terms of de-individuation, aculturation, isolation, stimulus deprivation, and even premature death.[1-2,4,37]

In a methodologically thorough and sophisticated study of 175 nursing homes and some 7000 residents in Wales, Booth[6] set out to answer his questions on the relationship between environment and behaviour in homes for the elderly. He concluded that the difference between homes must be seen as a veneer covering the massive uniformity of institutional life. Underneath lies the same crushing control over the lives and doings of residents. His main conclusion was that we must face up to the fact that the only sure way of limiting the harmful effects of residential care is to stop admitting people who, given the chance, could manage with other kinds of support. In his study a sizeable proportion of residents in all homes were quite independent and could have managed in the community.

In an Israeli study on the quality of institutional care,[38] national supervisors assessed institutions as either 'good' or 'poor'. While this distinction made some difference in the psychosocial indicators, even residents of the 'good' institutions reported loneliness (46 per cent) and lack of autonomy; individuality and environmental control were severely restricted.

While these arguments reinforce the notion that institutionalization *per se* is potentially harmful, a large literature attests to the wide array of means which can make a decisive difference in the quality of nursing homes. This literature also emphasizes the point that quality of nursing homes is directly related to the quality of life of the old residents.[39]

THE NURSING HOME IN RELATION TO OTHER SERVICES

The major issue is the question of comparative balance in resource allocation. In an Israeli study on elderly awaiting institutionalization,[40] the rate of elderly whose institutionalization could be prevented in the opinions of the professional caregivers in charge of each case and of the elderly and their families was: 75–94 per cent of the semi-independent elderly, 53–90 per cent of the frail elderly, and 21–68 per cent of the nursing elderly. An independent review of the cases by an expert multi-disciplinary team corroborated the finding that many elderly (about 30 per cent) in Israel's three major cities are capable of remaining in the community with the help of additional services. The services demanded by the families and the elderly did not usually exceed those recommended by professionals. Families, in fact, indicated their willingness to continue to provide a large part of the total care, even when offered unlimited care. According to this study the cost of required community services was below institutional costs for about two-thirds of the elderly capable of remaining in the community. This was true for all three cities and all functional levels.

When all is said about institutional care and nursing homes, there remains no doubt that they are an essential, vital part of the long-term care system. There will always be a proportion of the elderly in need of nursing home care, whether for their multiple needs, which make home care untenable from a cost of feasibility perspective, or whether from preference of the old person her/himself for a guarded secure environment.

The question which remains is the centrality of institutional care and the proportion of the budget and of manpower invested into institutional versus community care. In Israel, for every shekel spent for community care 5 shekel are spent for nursing home care. The comparative ratio of manpower allocation is even more strikingly in favour of institutional care. Also in other countries the proportional investment in nursing home care is tremendously high. This remains so, despite the declarations of the urgent need to develop comprehensive community services. In Amann's study on open care for the elderly in seven European countries,[19] the motto of geriatric care is 'encourage the elderly to remain in their own homes for as long as possible'. If this is to be more than a motto the appropriate balance between institutional and community services must be addressed. It is then necessary to develop a wide range of services, a topic which is dealt with elsewhere.

QUALITY OF CARE AND ACCEPTANCE OF DEPENDENCY

Despite all the criticism of nursing homes and the often pernicious effect of institutional care, it remains a vital service for many old people. How can we ensure that this service becomes a blessing rather than a curse for those in need of it? It seems that the answers lie in two main areas that we have to deal with. The first is quality of care and the second lies on an emotional, perhaps ideological level—the acceptance of dependency needs. We shall first discuss the broad area of quality of care.

Quality of care

Two broad aspects of the concept of quality of care will be addressed in this chapter: What are the factors influencing quality of institutional care? And what is quality assurance?

Quality of care is a very broad concept, especially in regard to that in long-term care institutions. All areas of an elderly person's life within the institution should be considered as being within the care domain. Nursing home care is both a treatment and a living situation. It encompasses both the health care and social support services provided to individuals with chronic conditions or disabilities and the environments in which they live. For many residents the nursing home is their home, not merely a temporary abode in which they are being treated for a medical problem.[39, 41]

Factors influencing quality of care

At the individual's level, changes in the quality of care are a function of: (a) the success of technical care in increasing benefits and limiting risks (this area includes the level of skill and safety in actual nursing care provision as well as the availability of technical aids—e.g. lifting devices, medical equipment, pads), (b) the professional norms and values of the caregivers, and (c) the expectations and aspirations of the clients.[42] The latter two issues are decisively influenced by a culture's and a society's acceptance of dependency. But first let us look at the more measurable structural and institutional factors: the quality of the institutional care given to the elderly resident is also influenced by these (Fig. 28.1).[36, 43]

The structural factors described in the model (government supervision, reimbursement policies, staff education and training policies, and referral policies) in turn influence the institutional factors (management, recording, manpower ratio and training, physical institutional conditions, family involvement, and inadequate placement) and the performances in the process of caregiving. In turn, institutional factors influence the direct performances in the care-giving process. The interweaving of all these factors determines, to a large extent, the quality of the care given to the elderly resident.[36, 43–4]

Government supervision.   Among the important causes of shortcomings in care are a number of areas that are related to government supervision of institutions—for example, lack of clarity as to the institution's areas of responsibility, partial enforcement of existing rules or regulations, and the existence of institutions operating without license. Supervisory methods in many countries are generally neither uniform nor methodical, there is a lack of reliable and comprehensive supervision instruments, and supervisors generally have little access to various enforcement measures.[45] An example of excellent development of methods and instruments for government supervision constitutes the new surveillance process applied in New York State.[46]

Although good supervision does not ensure good quality of care, a supervisory system may play an important role in improving the quality of care provided. It can upgrade the quality of care by enforcing the rules

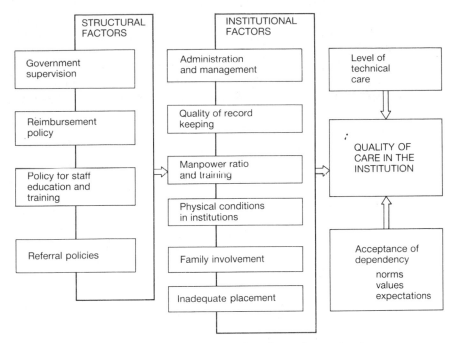

Fig. 28.1 Factors influencing quality of care in nursing homes.

and raising the requirements. An additional function is performed by regulatory systems as in Israel. Supervisors advise institutional staff in the process of corrections of deficiencies.

Reimbursement policies. Such policies may constitute a rewarding structure associated with different levels of performance. Nursing homes for the elderly and old age homes tend to follow different reimbursement models. The majority of old age homes receive payments directly from residents or their families, not from a third party. Nursing homes operate within a more constrained reimbursement environment. For most nursing homes, the major source of income is third-party payments, especially governmental. Homes therefore operate in accordance with regulations that qualify them to receive these reimbursements. Most countries have adopted 'facility-related' reimbursement plans, in which state payments are based on the costs incurred by the home. Another type of reimbursement is the case-mix reimbursement for nursing home services, in which payment is directly related to residents' needs and functional disabilities and/or to services deemed necessary to meet these needs. A few states have complex reimbursement formulas, which depend on the quality of the nursing home, and a very few use the 'flat-rate' reimbursement in which the payment is identical for all patients in a category in every nursing home in the state.

The different reimbursement schemes provide inducements for particular sorts of dysfunctional adaptations. In the facility-related reimbursement, on each activity covered by the government the home spends enough to ensure home accreditations for the activity but no more, since actual costs do not enter into the reimbursement formula. In the case-mix reimbursement, there is little incentive for encouraging patient improvement since this would reduce income. Flat-rate reimbursement is even more pernicious since each expenditure on a patient comes out of the home's potential profit. Schemes related to quality designate, by omission, the features of homes and the array of potential services that will not enter into the reimbursement calculations. Facilities respond to the inducements of regulations, thus often the physical needs of patients are adequately cared for, but in an environment that is sterile socially, intellectually, and emotionally.[47]

Staff education and training.   One other factor that affects the quality of care is the level of training among institutional staff. Some institutions have no registered nurse, and some have no trained social workers. Most workers undergo no special training for working with elderly people. Suitable training programmes could alleviate some of the administrative problems, as well as improve the level of recording and encourage family involvement. Training is needed mainly to ensure a concept of rehabilitative and supportive care of the residents, instead of the 'maintenance' concept that views the elderly person as someone nearing the end and in need only of a roof over his head in his remaining year. Statements of national or regional policies seem necessary to address this issue.

Referral policies.   These may influence quality of care when high concentrations of functionally impaired patients or cognitively impaired are referred to nursing homes which do not have the adequate structure to care for those patients. Referral and admission policies should seek a uniform distribution of patients according to the need of patients and capacities of the homes to cover these needs. Periodical assessments of residents are very necessary to keep the balance between capacity of the home to give care and the specific needs of residents.[48]

Administration and management.   Institutions have administrative problems such as: a lack of job descriptions and clear division of responsibilities, lack of written work procedures, little internal supervision, and lack of ongoing in-service training for staff. In addition, there are no special incentives for attracting and motivating workers to work in nursing homes. Nursing patients are more likely to exhibit problematic behaviours and tend to suffer from physical disabilities and cognitive impairment, and presumably staff are less likely to care for persons who are more problematic.

Record keeping. A good record-keeping system is the basis for good quality of care. Without recording, the formulation and follow-up of both care plans and further development of residents' conditions are very difficult. Shortcomings in follow-up and recording in medical and nursing as well as in social records are frequently found. Internal supervision, government supervision, and education of staff are the main factors which could influence the quality of record keeping.

Staffing. In many institutions, the staffing rates and skill levels are below the required standard. There is a serious shortage of nursing staff at all levels (nurses, aides) and of staff for psychosocial care (social workers and recreational workers).

Physical and structural conditions. The physical conditions of some institutions detract from the quality of life and the quality of care provided to the residents. For example, a lack of hot water around the clock, a shortage of toilets, and overly crowded rooms may have an adverse effect on the residents' health, nursing, and psychosocial condition.

Lack of family and community involvement. Families and prior communities of residents are not sufficiently involved in supervising the institutions. In many countries there are no organizations representing the families of institutionalized elderly, and communities seem unconcerned. There are no established procedures for registering complaints. Ombudsman organizations are also in a developing stage.

Quality assurance

Quality assurance is the mechanism or process for promoting a high quality in the performance of care. But in most of the government regulatory systems the concept of high quality has been replaced by the concept of 'adequacy', which in turn has been interpreted as the 'minimum' acceptable standard. There are two standards of accreditation of nursing homes: (a) a governmental one which provides a licence to operate a nursing home at a minimum level under governmental regulation (e.g. ref. 49) and (b) a private one which certifies a higher level of quality given in the nursing home, this being an optional alternative under the facility's responsibility. (e.g. refs. 50, 51)

Thus, quality assurance may be achieved by combining these four systems of supervision: the governmental supervisory system, the private certification committee, the internal supervisory system of the facility, and the ombudsman system.

Acceptance of dependency

The need for others, dependency, is a basic human need that is independent of functional capacity. In geriatric care, and in particular when considering institutionalization, dependency needs are linked to functional performance. Actual need for help often overrides the choice on how physical dependency needs, which now merge with emotional and social dependency needs, become met.

But does this have to be so? It is argued below that a different approach in caring professions has the potential to respect a changing mix of physical, emotional, and social dependency and independency needs. This approach to self-care is argued to have the power to minimize the negative effects of the institution upon the aged resident.[52, 53] In the community and more so in the institution, for instance, the nurse–patient relationship includes many dependency situations. Few are as complete as the dependency relationship with the physically impaired old person who needs help with toileting, feeding, and bathing.

A dependency situation can either lead to a human interaction where people are not embarrassed to need one another, or to a situation where one person's vulnerability is the occasion for another's mastery and dominance. In the latter, helplessness leads to humiliation, passivity, and withdrawal, but in a relationship where embarrassment and fear of manipulation are absent, the encounter becomes marked by warmth, openness, and spontaneity. But too often the old and mentally impaired person 'provokes' frustration and anger in his caregivers. Competence as well as learning to accept one's limited capacity to help someone in need are asked for. The crucial condition for such a functional relationship is the full recognition of all involved that the other is a human being—no more and no less. Thus the dependency relationship becomes interdependent with the power of giving comfort to all involved in the harsh reality.[54–5]

The issues raised above touch upon professional competencies as well as value issues. The values of dependency and interdependency are in no way universally accepted. While Jewish and Japanese tradition consider them positively,[55–7] Western tradition considers independence to be a basic human value and goal.[7] There is little agreement about the level of preparation required of staff in nursing homes. While family caregivers do provide the bulk of tending in the home, there is a profound difference between family members giving care to a single relative (and also this is not without problems[58]) and formal caregivers. In fact, the consistently documented negative effects of nursing homes might be explained by the large percentage of 'hands-on' caregivers who are minimally trained. Creating relationships where unavoidable dependency is not embarrassing or humiliating, and enabling an impaired person maximum autonomy despite severe functional dependency, seems to ask for skills usually only attainable in years of study, equivalent to a professional degree.

If our society would value caring as it values curing, commensurate to its social importance, it might not seem so ironic to ask for well-prepared nurses. Shamans and other 'volunteers' fulfil curing functions in traditional societies. Does this mean that their education is the desirable standard for medical education? The skill of promoting self-care ability and encouraging autonomy despite changing physical and mental capacity is the nursing skill commensurate with the skill needed for medical diagnosis and treatment; it is the skill needed to work with this population.

In summary, the factors influencing the quality of care in nursing homes discussed above are manifold. They are the key to creating nursing homes as true human environments.

SOCIAL POLICY ISSUES

The questions which must be addressed lie on several planes. There are those questions related to who becomes admitted to nursing homes and whether the alternative of home care is feasible. Then there is an entirely different plane of questions on the quality of care within institutions—an issue addressed above. A third plane is that of the nature of the nursing home as part of a wider community. How open and responsive is it to the needs of elderly in the neighborhood and how much are the residents still integrated into the wider social setting? The crucial issue seems to be how 'untotal' can an insitution be? And how can it become an integral part of community services by offering, for example, meals, physiotherapy, entertainment, respite services, etc. to the elderly in the neighbourhood? Today's trend in those countries which have a high rate of institutionalization and many even excellent nursing homes as The Netherlands, Denmark[19], and Canada[59] is towards de-institutionalization and policies that would reduce the proportion of elderly in institutions by a massive extension of community resources.

For those countries where services have not been developed yet, the question is one of 'primary prevention', of creating conditions where the need for nursing homes in the future will be kept to the unavoidable minimum. This is determined by the sometimes unavoidable triad of severe impairment, lacking social support, and fears as the concomitants of advanced old age. In much of the developing world, the need for long-term care is still small, but this need is about to grow drastically. In Israel it took less than 20 years for the major challenge of communicable diseases and malnutrition to turn into a major challenge of managing the multiple needs requiring long-term care. Nursing homes are still isolated phenomena in developing countries such as Fiji, the Philippines, or Kuwait. It is difficult to convince even very enlightened health care professionals, and even more so politicians, that nursing homes and institutionalization are not only the result of Western mores and the waning commitment of families to their elderly in the industrialized world. The very typical response when asked about the care of old people in developing countries is: 'With us it is different, in our culture we respect the elderly; our families take care of their aged members and are proud to do so'. Residents of the few existing nursing homes are assumed to belong either to another ethnic group or to be social outcasts. Fijians would say, 'Well, you will see, those homes are for Indians or Whites' and Indians would assert 'You know, of course, Fijians and Whites are in those nursing homes'.[60] It is hard to accept that, no matter how strong cultural and family values might be, other forces will have their impact. Changing demography and morbidity, as well as social developments accompanying industrialization as urbanization, migration, and changes in family structure, will create a reality where prolonged dependency will have to be dealt with on a scale unprecedented in human history. Industrial societies have found the major solution in institutional care. A vast literature attests to the fact that this solution is not only expensive, but also costly both in human terms for those institutionalized and in human and moral terms for families and society at large. But long-term care, and in particular institutional care, is part of a much wider picture. Dependency is in part socially constructed. It is not the inevitable outcome of demographic changes and the process of aging, but influenced by societal forces as poverty and forced retirement. Industrial societies under capitalist and state socialist regimes alike have created realities where legal, economic, and political institutions socially structure conditions of dependency for the aged. The low status in which old people are then held publicly is often in sharp contrast to the important roles they play within the families.[61-4]

This argument is not meant to minimize the problem of physical or mental dependency, nor to negate the necessity for nursing homes. It is meant to raise the crucial question of where the nursing home fits in long-term care, social, and health policy. The issues must be understood and argued from an ideological basis in developed and developing countries alike. In developed countries the toll of inequity, agism, poverty, and partially avoidable institutionalization is already enormous. The hope that cultural values and traditional family ties in the developing world will prevent these trends in those countries is bleak. The realities of demographics, morbidity, and disability, as well as of social, political, and economic developments, are forces that would have to be dealt with pre-actively. Adequate income maintenance for the aged is a major factor to be planned for, taking the effects of migration and urbanization into account. Laws and social mores will have to deal consciously with providing opportunity for continued participation of elderly in social and work life. Since developments are so rapid, the challenge of social planning for the developing world is urgent. This is a challenge most difficult to meet, since resources are usually scarce and it is most difficult to advocate needs of the future over the pressures of those of the present. Todays demands for economic investments, for education development, and often for military spending are very real. All these demands compete for limited resources. Nevertheless, if the near-future dependency needs are ignored in the developing world as they were in most of the industrially developed countries then institutionalization and nursing homes will become 'the solution' by default. This blanket solution for biological and socially constructed dependency has a high toll for individuals, families, and societies alike.

But when nursing homes are needed, both developed and developing countries alike will have to consider the factors influencing quality of care and quality assurance. Nursing homes will then truly promote quality of life for very dependent elderly.

References

1. Townsend, P. (1964). *The last refuge. A survey of residential institutions and homes for the aged in England and Wales.* Routledge and Kegan Paul, London.
2. Tobin, S. S. and Lieberman, W. A. (1976). *Last home for the aged.* Jossey-Bass, San Francisco.
3. Vladeck, B. C. (1980). *Unloving care. The nursing home tragedy.* Basic Books, New York.
4. Johnson, C. and Grant, L. A. (1985). *The nursing home in American society.* Johns Hopkins University Press, Baltimore.
5. Barton-Smith, D. (1981). *Long-term care in transition. The regulation of nursing homes.* AUPHA Press, Washington.
6. Booth, T. (1985). *Home truths. Old people's homes and the outcome of care.* Aldershot. Hants. Gower,
7. Kane, R. L. and Kane, R. A. (1982). *Values and long term care.* Lexington Books, Lexington, MA.
8. Jansson, T. (1977). *Sun city.* Avon Books, New York.
9. Sarton, M. (1973). *As we are now.* W. W. Norton, New York.

10. Hazan, H. (1986). 'Existential boundaries in an institutional setting. the care of the aged: In *People in institutions: the Israeli scene* (ed. Kashti J. and M. Arieli), pp. 239–56, Freuna Publishing House, London.
11. Committee on Nursing Home Regulation, Institute of Medicine (1986). *Improving the quality of care in nursing homes*. National Academy Press, Washington DC.
12. Rabinowitz, D. and Nielsen, Y. (1971). *Home life. A story of old age*. Macmillan, New York.
13. Parker, R. A. (1980). *The state of care*. The Richard M. Titmuss Memorial Lecture. Joint (JDC) Brookdale Institute of Gerontology and Adult Human Development, S-3-80, Jerusalem.
14. Shanas, E. and Sussman, M. E. (ed.) (1977). *Family, bureacracy and the elderly*. Duke University Press, Durham, NC.
15. Fleishman, R. and Shmueli, A. (1986). Patterns of informal support of the elderly: an international comparison. *The Gerontologist*, **24**, 303–72.
16. Brody, E. (1981). 'Women in the middle' and family help to other people. *The Gerontologist*, **21**, 471–480.
17. Krulik, T. and Hirschfeld, M. J. (1985). The continuation of home care to severely impaired children and aged in Israel: family attitutdes. In *International perspectives in long-term care*, (ed. Reif, L.) pp. 283–313. Hayworth Press, New York.
18. Goodman, C. (1986). Research on the informal carer: a selected literature review. *Journal of Advanced Nursing*, **11**, 705–12.
19. Amann, A. (ed.) (1980). *Open care for the elderly in seven European countries. A pilot study in the possibilities and limits of care*. Pergamon Press, Oxford.
20. Davies, A. M. (1984). *The epidemiology of aging*. International Forum. IF-2-84. Brookdale Institute of Gerontology, Jerusalem.
21. Siegel, J. and Hoover, S. (1982). Demographic aspects of the health of the elderly to the year 2000 and beyond. *World Health Statistical Quarterly*, **35**, 133–202.
22. Ali, F. A. (1982). *Aging in the Arab republic of Egypt*. Unit on Aging. UN Office, International Center, Vienna.
23. Firoza, A. (1982). *Aging in Pakistan: problems and plans*. Social Welfare and Development, Ministry of Health and Social Welfare, Islamabad.
24. Kuwait National Committee of International Year on Aging—1982 (1982). *Kuwait report on the care of the aging in the state of Kuwait*, July.
25. Hirschfeld, M. J. (1987). The World Health Organization's regions of the eastern Mediterranean and Europe: aging of the population and nursing care. *Journal of Advanced Nursing*, **12**, 151–8.
26. Gruneberg, E. (1977). The failure of success. *Milbank Memorial Fund Quarterly*, **55**, 3–24.
27. Brody, J. (1982). Life expectancy and the health of older persons. *Journal of the American Geriatrics Society*, **30** 681-3.
28. Bavadra, T., Olakowski, T., and Rausavanua, E. (1982). *Population and health problems in Fiji during past 100 years*. Ministry of Health, Fiji.
29. Bergman, S., Factor, H., and Kaplan, I. (1986). *Census of long-term care institutions in Israel, 1983. Population, functional level and financing*. S–26–86. Brookdale Institute of Gerontology and Adult Human Development, Jerusalem (Hebrew with English Abstract).

30. Habib, J., Factor, H., and Beer, S. (1987). Evaluating the needs for long-term services and their cost. *Social Security*, **30**, 103–19, (Hebrew with English abstract).
31. Swan, J. H. and Harringon, C. (1986). Estimating under-supply of nursing home beds in States. *Health Services Research*, **21**, 57–83.
32. Dunlop, B. D. (1976). Determinants of long term care facility utilization by the elderly; an empirical analysis. Working Paper. Urban Institute, Washington DC.
33. Gruenberg, E.M. and Archer, J. (1979). Abandonment of responsibility for the seriously mentally ill. *Milbank Memorial Fund Quarterly*, **57**, 485–506.
34. Rose, S. M. (1979). Decipering deinstitutionalization: complexities in policy and program analysis. *Milbank Memorial Fund Quarterly*, **57**, 429–60.
35. Goffman, E. (1961). *Asylums: essays on the social situation of mental patients and other inmates*. Doubleday, Garden City.
36. Fleishman, R. and Tomer, A. (1986). *Evaluation of quality of care in long-term care institutions in Israel: the tracer approach*. Discussion paper 125–86. The Brookdale Institute of Gerontology, Jerusalem.
37. Lieberman, H. and Tobin, S. (1983). *The experience of old age: stress, coping and survival*. Basic Books, New York.
38. Tomer, A, Fleishman, R., and Schwartz, R. (1986). *The quality of institutional care: psycho-social aspects*. D-137–86. Brookdale Institute of Gerontology, Jerusalem.
39. Fleishman, R. and Ronen, R. (1986). *Quality of care and maltreatment in the institutions for the elderly*. Paper prepared for the International Workshop on Stress, Conflict and Abuse in the Aging Family, August 25–7, Jerusalem.
40. Habib, J., Factor, H., Naon, D., Brodsky, J., and Dolev, T. (1986). *Adequacy of care for elderly receiving community services and for elderly awaiting institutionalization*. D-133–86. Brookdale Institute of Gerontology, Jerusalem.
41. Committee on Nursing Home Regulation, Institute of Medicine (1986). *Improving the quality of care in nursing homes*. National Academy Press, Washington DC.
42. Donabedian, A. (1982). *Exploration in quality assessment and monitoring*. Health Administration Press, Michigan.
43. Fleishman, R., Bar-Giora, M., Mandelson, J., Tomer, A., Schwartz, R., and Ronen, R. (1987). Institutional care for the elderly in Israel: study and application. *Social Security*, No. 30, pp. 120–7. (Hebrew with English Abstract).
44. Penchansky, R. and Taubenhaus, L. (1965). Institutional factors affecting the quality of care in nursing homes. *Geriatrics*, **20**, 591–8.
45. Day, P. and Klein, R. (1987). Quality of institutional care and the elderly: policy issues and options. *British Medical Journal*, **294**, 384–7.
46. Axelrod, D. and Sweeney, R. (1984). *Report to the governor and the legislature on the new surveillance process for New York State residential health care facilities*. Office of Health Systems Management, New York.
47. Spilerman, S. and Litwak (1983). Rewards structure and the organizational design of institutions for the elderly. In *Evaluating the welfare state: social and political perspectives* (ed. Spiro S. and E. Yutzchman-Yaar) pp. 233–52. Academic Press, New York.
48. Fleishman, R., Rosin, A., Tomer, A., and Schwartz, R. (1987). Cognitive

impairment and the quality of care in long-term care institutions. *Comprehensive Gerontology B*, **1**, 18-23.

49. Government of Ontario (1980). *Nursing homes act*. Toronto
50. Canadian Council on Hospital Accreditation (1985). *Standards for accreditation of Canadian long-term care centres*. Ottawa.
51. Joint Commission on Accreditation of Hospitals (1985). *Principles of quality assurance for long-term care professionals*. Chicago.
52. Underwood, P. (1980). Facilitating self-care. *Psychiatric nursing. A basic text*, (ed. Pothier, P.) Little, Brown and Company. Boston.
53. Underwood, P. (undated) *Tools for implementation of self-care deficit theory*. University of California, San Francisco.
54. Hirschfeld, M. J. (1985). Ethics and care for the elderly. *International Journal of Nursing Studies*, **22**, 319–28.
55. Hartman, D. (1979). Moral uncertainties in the practice of medicine: the dynamics of interdependency from a Halakhic perspective. *Journal of Medicine and Philosophy*, **4**, 98–112.
56. Doi, T. (1973). *The anatomy of dependence*. Kodansha International, San Francisco.
57. Minami, H. (1982). *The construction and validation of a measure of amae network*. Unpublished doctoral dissertation. University of California, San Francisco.
58. Krulik, T. and Hirschfeld, M. J. (1986). Hard labor: workers in family caregiving, *Israel Social Science Research*, **4**, 84–98.
59. Canadian Medical Association (1984). *Health: a need for redirection*. Report of a task force on the allocation of health care resources. Ottawa.
60. Hirschfeld, M. J. (1983). *Health care of the elderly in Fiji*. Assignment Report ICP ADR 003. World Health Organization, Suva.
61. Estes, C. L. (1980). Constructions of reality. *Journal of Social Issues*, **36**, 2.
62. Walker, A. (1980). The social creation of poverty and dependency in old age. *Journal of Social Policy*, **9**, 45–75.
63. Phillipson, C. and Walker, A. (1986). *Aging and social policy a critical assesment*. Gower, England.
64. Townsend, P. (1986). Ageism and social policy. In *Aging and social policy* (ed. Phillipson, C. and A. Walker,), pp. 15–44. Gower, London, England.

29

Hospice care for the elderly

DAVID S. GREER

INTRODUCTION

As countries develop, the terminal phase of life is delayed and prolonged; people die older and from chronic rather than acute illnesses. Coincidentally health care systems become more sophisticated, technological, and intensive. The natural tendency is to apply the increasingly sophisticated technology to the terminal period in an attempt to prolong life. Unfortunately that effort is often fruitless, painful, and expensive.

In some developed nations, notably Great Britain and the United States, this technology-biased trend has matured to the point where a reaction has set in. Among the major manifestations of that reaction has been a philosophy and a service system called 'hospice' by its originator, Dame Cicely Saunders, dedicated to palliation (pain and symptom relief), social and spiritual support, and dignity for the dying and their families. Hospice is 'low-tech–high-touch' caring, an alternative to the aggressive technological imperative which characterizes developed health care systems.

Hospices vary widely in size and structure, particularly in the United States, which has no national health system to encourage uniformity. After the introduction of the concept to the USA in 1974 by Dame Cicely, the hospice movement grew rapidly; in about a decade it was estimated that there were over a thousand hospices in the country. Sponsorship varied from churches and charitable organizations with no experience in health care to established hospitals and home care agencies. Congress came under pressure to acknowledge and provide support for this new approach to care. It responded by ordering the National Hospice Study (1980–1983), which is the basis for the report in this chapter.

To place the study in context, it is important to note that hospice is a program, a system of care, rather than a specific type of institution or facility. It consists of an integrated collaboration of health professionals (physicians, nurses, social workers, psychologists, etc.) organized to address the needs of terminally ill patients and their families. The professionals need not be based in a single site, nor (in the USA) need they be employed by a single agency; contractual and professional relationships may suffice to co-ordinate services (in contradistinction to hospices in countries with a national health system like Great Britain where they tend to be more uniform and based in institutions, often hospitals).

Hospices have focused their efforts on patients with cancer, although they do not generally exclude patients dying of other diseases. They apply primarily low-technology, non-invasive methods designed to support and comfort both the patients and their families. The patient–family is the unit of care. Although no attempt is made to hasten death, prolongation of life is not an objective; rather, death in comfort and dignity is the goal. Hospice care is therefore appropriate only when cure is not attainable.

Hospices, particularly in America, shift some of the burden of care from the 'formal' to the 'informal' caregivers, from professionals to family members, friends, and volunteers. Frequently, an individual (usually a family member) is designated as the primary liaison between the professionals and the patient; that individual is designated as the primary care person. Utilization of primary care persons reduces costs and enhances the intimacy of care but frequently places substantial burdens on families.

Hospice is not long-term care. The median length of stay in the National Hospice Study was 35 days.[1] The burden on families is therefore not usually prolonged and is generally predictable.

METHODS

Forty hospices distributed throughout the United States were the basis of the study. Twenty-six were chosen by government authorities to receive funding sufficient for them to provide optimal hospice care; 14 were studied in their 'natural' state, without additional funding. Half of the hospices had units with inpatient beds ('hospital based') and half did not ('home care based'). The hospices were compared with 14 conventional cancer care programmes (i.e. normative care in the US health care system). Quality of life of patients and families and costs were the principal outcomes examined, although much additional data were obtained and have been reported.[1–14]

Data were obtained on 13 374 hospice and 670 conventional care patients. A subsample of 1457 patients/families was more intensively studied; these had weekly or bi-weekly interviews by research personnel. Data collection occurred over a period of approximately 2 years. A third source of data for this report was a substudy of the NHS conducted in Rhode Island to examine health care costs of cancer decedents using death certificate and insurance payment (Blue Cross–Blue Shield) records.

OVERVIEW OF NATIONAL HOSPICE STUDY RESULTS

To place the current report in perspective, a review of the major findings of the National Hospice Study is helpful.[4,5] Using a quasi-experimental design to compare the costs and outcomes experienced by terminal cancer patients served in hospice and conventional oncological care settings, few differences in the quality of patients' lives were observed. Patients served in hospital-based hospices did appear to manifest less pain and fewer symptoms than did non-hospice patients, and their family members reported being somewhat more satisfied with the care the patient received. In most other respects, the findings with respect to emotional, physical, nd overall quality of life were similar. Surviving primary care persons (generally family members) of patients in hospice were no more likely than conventional care survivors to experience increased hospitalizations, physician visits, or other indicators of secondary morbidity. Surviving primary care persons of hospital-based hospice patients did somewhat better than home care survivors, manifesting less grief reaction and symptoms of depression in the postmortem period.[4]

While there were few differences in the outcomes experienced by patients and their primary care persons, there were substantial differences in the pattern of care received. Hospice patients were significantly less likely to receive 'intensive' medical interventions (e.g. surgery, thoracentesis), diagnostic tests, and blood transfusions than were cancer patients being conventionally treated. On the other hand, after adjusting for differences in the mix of patients, hospice and conventional care did not differ in their use of supportive care procedures such as oxygen administration, although hospice patients were more often at home and remote from such care.[15]

Comparisons of the health care costs incurred by hospice and non-hospice patients revealed that patients served in home care hospices had substantially lower costs than either hospital-based hospice or conventional care patients. While hospital-based hospice patients had lower costs than conventional care patients in the last weeks and months of life, higher costs in hospice earlier in the terminal period largely offset any savings associated with the hospital-based hospices. Home care hospice patients had lower costs because they used hospitals less than did either hospital-based hospice or conventional care patients; hospital-based hospice patients spent almost as much time in hospital as conventional care

Table 29.1 Characteristics of the population of hospice patients by age ($n \approx$ 10 212)

	Age				
	21–24 (*n* = 635)	45–54 (*n* = 891)	55–64 (*n* = 2053)	65–74 (*n* = 3364)	75+ (*n* = 2804)
Female (%)	56.8	57.1	53.2	51.6	50.7
Married (%)	53.5	67.8	67.2	60.6	47.5
Patient lives alone (%)	5.7	9.1	11.3	16.9	18.9
Non-white (%)	15.9	12.8	8.8	5.9	4.8
Family income under $10 000 (%)	46.0	42.0	45.6	52.6	61.7
Primary care person (%)					
spouse	48.7	64.3	63.3	56.2	41.4
child	8.9	17.1	21.2	26.4	38.6
female	62.1	60.9	65.2	70.0	77.6
Patient requires (%)					
catheter	18.9	16.3	15.0	19.0	22.5
oxygen	15.0	17.4	18.7	21.4	17.6
Cancer (%)					
colorectal	8.4	10.2	12.2	14.8	17.7
lung	18.4	27.2	27.7	26.0	18.1
breast	17.9	17.6	13.2	10.0	8.0
prostate	1.0	1.5	3.8	6.8	11.3
brain tumour	10.4	5.2	4.6	2.7	2.0
Average length of disease (yrs)	2.6	2.8	2.9	2.6	2.6

patients but they used fewer high-cost ancillary services (laboratory, X-ray) when hospitalized.[2, 4, 8]

A description of the elderly in the National Hospice Study

Table 29.1 presents the characteristics of hospice admissions for whom complete demographic and medical data were available, organized by age groups. In view of the very large sample sizes, most differences of a few percentage points between groups reach statistical significance. Since differences that small may not be meaningful, no statistical interpretation of this table is presented.

Table 29.2 Characteristics of hospice patients' discharge disposition by age

	Age				
	21–44	45–54	55–64	65–74	75+
Length of stay (d)	53.8	50.2	51.2	51.9	53.0
Location of death (%) for those discharged dead (total 92%)					
home	42.0	36.9	40.9	39.2	39.6
inpatient hospice	21.1	28.6	27.6	27.1	30.1
acute hospital	34.3	31.8	29.3	30.6	26.8
other inpatient	2.6	2.7	2.3	3.1	3.5

Approximately 65 per cent of all hospice admissions were 65 years of age or older; 27.4 per cent were 75 or older. Hospice obviously attracts and serves an elderly population. However, as can be seen from the characteristics presented in Table 29.1, the hospice population of elders was not typical of the traditional aged long-term care population. Only half were female and, except for the oldest age group, a majority were married. The older the patient, the more likely it was that he/she lived alone at the time of hospice admission and the lower the household income. As could be anticipated, the older the patient, the less likely the spouse was to be the caregiver, and the more likely it was that the role was assumed by a child. In view of the increasing prevalence of female caregivers with increasing age of the patient, it is obvious that daughters were predominantly assuming the caregiving responsibility.

Older patients were not more functionally impaired on admission; however, the older groups were somewhat more likely to be catheterized (incontinent). Differences in cancer-type distribution mirror the age-related prevalence of these diseases.[16] Disease duration was comparable across all age groups and was highly variable since the major determinant of survival is cancer type.

Table 29.2 presents data summarizing the length of stay and discharge disposition of the hospice patient population by age. Age was not related to how long a patient was served in hospice. Since in the vast majority of cases (92 per cent) discharge was due to death, length of hospice stay is essentially an indicator of survival. Thus, in this terminal cancer population, age was unrelated to survival. This finding is borne out by more detailed studies of the predictors of survival already reported.[17] Aged patients were no more and no less likely than younger patients to die at home, although they were somewhat less likely to have died in hospital. The principal determinant of where hospice patients died in this study was whether they were served in a hospital-based or home-based hospice; the latter were more likely to die at home.[7] Since dying at home requires substantial support from the family as well as the help of hospice staff, the lack of an age differential suggests that the support systems of aged and younger hospice patients are similarly resilient, even though they have different relationships to the patients (younger patients have spouses; older patients have daughters).

Outcomes experienced by aged hospice patients

The range of outcomes examined in the National Hospice Study was limited by the amount and type of data that could reasonably be gathered from terminally ill patients.[18] Of patients who gave signed consent to participate in the study, as many as 40 per cent were unable to respond to interviews that occurred within the last week or two of life. The implication of this attrition, which did not differ by age, is that most patient outcome data were obtained from the patients' primary care persons, who were in the best position to comment upon the patients' condition.[4] Patient mood state and satisfaction data were examined only in those patients able to respond to interviews. No significant differences between hospice and non-hospice patients were observed, and no significant relationship was observed between patient age and self-reported mood state and satisfaction.

Table 29.3 summarizes two symptom measures which were age correlated. Older patients were less likely to report moderate to severe pain in the last weeks of life.[12] Similarly, older patients reported experiencing fewer symptoms (e.g. nausea, dyspnoea, trouble with swallowing) than did younger patients.[13] On the other hand, many of the functionally based indicators of quality of life such as the Karnofsky Performance Status index reveal no relationship to age; physical function declines progressively independently of age. Measures of patient awareness and social interaction also revealed no difference with respect to age.

Outcomes of aged primary care persons

A major goal of the hospice movement is to reduce postmortem morbidity (physical and psychological) by helping family members to cope with the stress of their caregiving responsibility by giving assistance and education while the patient is alive, and by providing bereavement counselling after the patient's death. Since the stress of caregiving might have a greater impact on older caregivers, we conducted a series of analyses to explore the bereavement outcomes experienced by older and younger primary care persons. The outcomes we specifically examined were con-

Table 29.3 Hospice patients' outcomes in last weeks of life by age

	21–44	45–54	Age 55–64	65–74	75+
Percentage of patients in pain based on primary care person report in:					
last week of life	0.717	0.725	0.655	0.608	0.548
3rd to last week	0.652	0.700	0.629	0.553	0.463
Average number of 10 symptoms reported in:					
last week of life	4.9	5.4	5.1	5.0	4.7
3rd to last week	5.2	5.0	4.8	4.6	4.2
Interviewer judgement, Karnofsky Performance Status[a] in:					
last week of life	20.9	24.4	22.8	22.9	22.3
3rd to last week	28.9	30.9	29.2	29.5	27.0

[a] Range – 100 (fully independent) to 0 (dead).

crete indicators of secondary morbidity such as hospitalization, physician visits, and tranquillizer or alcohol use. As expected, older primary care persons had higher rates of physician and hospital use, but once prior illness and their relationship with the deceased was statistically controlled, there was no relationship between any of these outcomes and the primary care person's age.[10] The most important factor was the person's prior health and whether he/she was the spouse of the patient. Regardless of age, loss of a spouse was a major predictor of increased secondary morbidity.

Pattern of services

As noted above, hospice patients were significantly less likely than conventional care patients to receive intensive medical and diagnostic interventions. Home care patients may have achieved this result by staying out of the hospital (they had fewer inpatient days), but hospital-based hospice patients spent almost as many days in the hospital as did conventional care patients. The philosophy of care apparently determined the hospice treatment plan even in hospitalized patients. Older patients were as likely as younger patients to receive some aggressive treatments in conventional care. Comparing hospital and home care hospices, in the latter younger patients were more likely to continue to receive some aggressive treatment (e.g. chemotherapy).[1, 14, 15]

Other indicators of treatment differences may be related to the earlier data contrasting patients' symptoms. Older hospice patients were less likely to have analgesics prescribed (they complained of less pain).[19] Older hospice patients also complained of fewer symptoms (specifically nausea and vomiting) and were therefore less likely than younger patients to be consuming anti-emetics.[3, 13]

Cost and utilization experiences of aged hospice patients

We examined patient costs in hospice from a variety of different perspectives.[1, 2, 4, 8] Costs during patients' stay in hospice were primarily determined by the length of stay and the amount of time spent in an inpatient setting. The latter factor was largely attributable to the type of hospice serving the patient (hospital versus home care) and was unrelated to age. Age was therefore found to be unrelated to costs in hospice.

A measure of the intensity of hospice care was developed based upon costs incurred per hospice day. There was no difference in service intensity attributable to age in either type of hospice. On the other hand, age was negatively related to cost in inpatient stays, in either an acute hospital or an inpatient hospice unit[20] (i.e. older patients incurred lower hospital costs per stay).

Analyses of the hospitalizations that hospice patients experienced well before they were admitted to hospice revealed that the cost per inpatient day, our measure of intensity, was significantly related to age, with older patients having substantially lower costs. This was true for hospitalizations that occurred at the time of cancer diagnosis as well as for hospitalizations occurring between diagnosis and hospice entry. This suggests a potential age bias in the treatment of cancer. Various authors have discussed this possibility, and a series of National Cancer Institute sponsored investigations are currently examining the proposition that chronological age influences the treatment of cancer patients.[21]

DISCUSSION

Hospice is not long term or chronic care but rather an alternative to aggressive acute care for the terminally ill. Evidence from the United States National Hospice Study supports the notion that hospice care is a viable alternative, with outcomes comparable to or better than conventional care, and that hospice is as effective for elderly persons as it is for the younger age group. Hospice costs no more than conventional terminal care and can be less costly under certain conditions (i.e. if home care is substituted for institutional or hospital care.)

Kane *et al.*, in the only other large scale study of hospice care in the United States, reported findings similar to those of the NHS.[22] In their Veterans Administration hospital population, patient and long term family outcomes were comparable in hospice and conventional care.[23, 24] They noted shorter-term improvement of family anxiety and greater satisfaction of both patients and families with hospice care.[25] A number of smaller studies, most frequently from England and Canada, have yielded results more favourable to hospice.

There is evidence from recent American studies[26] of a bias against aggressive curative therapy for elderly patients with cancer. It is important, therefore, that health care providers be especially vigilant in assuring appropriate application of hospice care for elderly patients to avoid premature abandonment of curative care in favour of palliation. Cure and prolongation of useful life remain preferable despite the efficacy of hospice care for the elderly.

Hospices emerge from the finest ideals and objectives of health care professionals: relief of suffering, human support, love, and spiritual considerations. These ideals evoke sympathetic responses from lay populations and are capable of recruiting widespread support in societies receptive to the message. For its success, therefore, hospice requires certain cultural and social conditions, but it can also exert a salutary influence on society by dramatizing humanitarian values in a highly visible manner and in an emotionally laden environment.

As societies develop and modernize, health care systems tend to evolve in the direction of specialization, sophistication, and increasing reliance on technology. Humanitarian care tends to be shunted aside by aggressive, scientifically based, cure-oriented treatment, often to no avail. Low-technology care, often ministered by less-sophisticated professionals or lay persons, is devalued. Costs escalate in proportion to the application of technology.

Developing nations can learn much from the hospice experience in the developed nations. Rather than accommodate to the specialized, high-technology imperative until a reaction such as hospice occurs, they might temper the apparently inevitable enthusiasm of most medical professionals for progressively more complex and technical medical modalities by insisting on balanced health care development: care as well as cure, appropriate development and utilization of low-technology as well as sophisticated personnel and methods, and science balanced by liberal doses of humanism. In even the most sophisticated health care system the need for personal attention, family and community support, and spiritual nourishment remains. In a world of limited resources and incessant pressure for 'modernization', these traditional values need protection. The hospice experience demonstrates the public desire for and the efficacy of traditional methods for the care of the incurably ill.

In the developed nations, the last year of life is often the most expensive for the health care system, largely owing to inappropriate and frequently futile in-hospital aggressive therapy. Funds spent on the dying, usually elderly, are diverted from the needs of the younger population. Hospice care can reduce the costs of the terminal period of life, but it does not do so inevitably. The key to economy is emphasis on out-of-hospital care and appropriate utilization of lower-level professionals, family, and friends. The proper time to switch from the pursuit of cure or prolongation of life to the provision of solace and comfort is often debatable, but further research should provide us with better information on which to base rational decisions.

References

1. Mor, V. (1987). *Hospice care systems: structure, process, costs, and outcome.* Springer Publishing Company, New York.
2. Birnbaum, H. and Kidder, D. (1984). What does hospice cost? *American Journal of Public Health*, **74**, 689–97.
3. Goldberg, R. J. and Mor, V. (1985). A survey of psychotropic use in terminal cancer patients. *Psychosomatics*, **26**, 745–51.
4. Greer, D. S., Mor, V., Morris, J. N. *et al.* (1986). An alternative in terminal care: results of the National Hospice Study. *Journal of Chronic Diseases*, **39**, 9–26.
5. Greer, D. S., Mor, V., Sherwood, S. *et al.* (1983). National Hospice Study analysis plan. *Journal of Chronic Diseases*, **36**, 737–80.
6. Laliberte, L. and Mor, V. (1985). An examination of the effect of reimbursement and organizational structure to the use of hospice volunteers. *Hospice Journal*, **1**, 21–44.
7. Mor, V. and Hiris, J. (1983). Determinants of site of death among hospice cancer patients. *Journal of Health and Social Behavior*, **24**, 375–85.
8. Mor, V. and Kidder, D. (1985). Cost savings in hospice: final results of the National Hospice Study. *Health Services Research*, **20**, 407–22.
9. Mor, V. and Laliberte, L. (1984). Burnout among hospice staff. *Health and Social Work*, **9**, 274–83.
10. Mor, V., McHorney, C. and Sherwood, S. (1986). Secondary morbidity among the recently bereaved. *American Journal of Psychiatry*, **143**, 158–63.
11. Mor, V., Schwartz, R., Laliberte, L. *et al.* (1985). An examination of the effect of reimbursement and organizational structure on the allocation of hospice staff time. *Home Health Care Services Quarterly*, **6**, 101–18.
12. Morris, J. N., Mor, V., Goldberg, R. J. *et al.* (1986). The effect of treatment setting and patient characteristics on pain in terminal cancer patients: a report from the National Hospice Study. *Journal of Chronic Diseases*, **39**, 27–35.
13. Reuben, D. B. and Mor, V. (1986). Dyspnea in terminal cancer patients. *Chest*, **89**, 234–6.

14. Wachtel, T. J. and Mor, V. (1989). Utilization of health resources by physicians for terminal cancer patients: clinical setting versus physician specialty. *Southern Medical Journal*, (in press).
15. Mor, V., Greer, D. S. and Kastenbaum, R. (1988). *The hospice experiment: is it working?* John Hopkins University Press, Baltimore.
16. American Cancer Society (1985). *Cancer facts and figures: 1984*. American Cancer Society, New York.
17. Mor, V., Laliberte, L., Morris, J. N. *et al.* (1986). The Karnofsky performance status scale: an examination of its reliability and validity in a research setting. *Cancer*, **53**, 2002–7.
18. Mor, V. (1986). Assessing patient outcomes in hospice: what to measure? *Hospice Journal*, **2**, 17–35.
19. Goldberg, R. J., Mor, V., Wiemann, M. *et al.* (1986). Analgesic use in terminal cancer patients: report from the National Hospice Study. *Journal of Chronic Diseases*, **39**, 37–45.
20. Mor, V., Wachtel, T. J., and Kidder, D. (1985). Patient predictors of hospice choice: hospital versus home care programs. *Medical Care*, **23**, 1115–19.
21. Yancik, R. (1983). *Aging, Vol. 24: Perspectives on prevention and treatment of cancer in the elderly*. Raven Press, New York.
22. Kane, R. L., Wales, J., Bernstein, L. *et al.* (1984). A randomized controlled trial of hospice care. *Lancet*, **1**, 890–4.
23. Kane, R. L., Bernstein, L., Wales, J. *et al.* (1985). Hospice effectiveness in controlling pain. *Journal of the American Medical Association*, **253**, 2683–6.
24. Kane, R. L., Klein, S. J., Bernstein, L. *et al.* (1986). The role of hospice in reducing the impact of bereavement. *Journal of Chronic Diseases*, **39**, 735–42.
25. Kane, R. L., Klein, S. J., Bernstein, L. *et al.* (1985). Hospice role in alleviating the emotional stress of terminal patients and their families. *Medical Care*, **23**, 189–97.
26. Samet, J., Hunt, W. C., Key, C. *et al.* (1986). Choice of cancer therapy varies with age of patient. *Cancer Therapy*, **255**, 3385–90.

30

Housing for older people: the North American approach

NORMAN BLACKIE

Since the Second World War, the governments of Canada and the United States have intervened directly in the housing market to assist persons with special needs. Federal governments in Canada and the United States have employed three major forms of housing assistance: public housing, subsidized newly constructed units (built by the public and private non-profit sector), and assistance to households living in existing units in the private market. The recipients of this assistance have been low- and moderate-income households. Elderly persons have qualified for housing assistance not on the basis of age but because of low income.

A HISTORICAL OVERVIEW

Throughout history there have been various forms of housing for those in need. Traditionally, the first recourse has been family. Children provided for aged parents, and younger siblings provided for older brothers and sisters. The disabled and mentally impaired were cared for in a similar way; however, when circumstances did not permit it, institutions stepped in to provide accommodation.

Even in ancient Greece, housing the aged was primarily a responsibility of children, on whom societal scorn and possible loss of citizenship would fall if the latter defaulted. However, if an elderly person was without children of his own, or was too ill for the children to provide care, the '*Asclepieion*' or health resort was the place of refuge. The *Asclepieion* was organized aesthetically and with therapeutic value—it had proper ventilation and heliotherapy and hydrotherapy—to prolong and extend life.

During the third and fourth centuries, the Christian Church set up institutions to care for those in need; '*gerontochia*' for the elderly, '*nosochomia*' for the sick, and '*ptochia*' for the poor. Monastic orders established similar institutions. For example, an analysis of the plan of the twelfth century Monastery of St Fall shows an elaborate health facility for aged and infirm monks. The monastery at Cluny, France provided a supportive environment for a large population of retired monks, paying pensioners, and even nobles. The retired were expected to participate to the degree they were able in the physical, mental, social, and the spiritual life of the community.

When the monasteries disappeared in England and Wales in the six-teenth century, responsibility for the poor was taken on by the parish churches. Parish 'poor houses' sheltered young and old, sick, disabled, mentally impaired, and destitute. These facilities were also known as workhouses. In an 1893 report, it was estimated that nearly a half of the occupants of a typical workhouse were 'aged and impotent' persons.[1]

The practice of housing all of the destitute of society in one institution continued in the nineteenth century. Larger and larger institutions were built, serving larger geographical areas. Thomson[2] reported that, by the middle of the nineteenth century, the aged formed a majority of most workhouse populations, but it was not until the last years of the century that official documents made reference to the elderly and their special needs.

European practices were carried over to North America. For example, in Lower Canada during British rule, care for the sick, insane, and foundling was undertaken by private philanthropy and by the Roman Catholic Church. In Upper Canada, municipal councils provided relief for the destitute. However, welfare from municipal governments was difficult to obtain. The assumption that destitution was the result of an idle life was as prevalent in North America as in Victorian England.

In the Canadian province of Ontario, during the period 1840 to 1900, many charitable organizations were incorporated. Most of these estab-lished houses of refuge for poor and infirm elderly people. Provincial legislation was introduced, following a severe depression in 1867, requir-ing that houses of refuge be built. Opposition was so strong that the mandatory part of the legislation was dropped. However, in 1890, legisla-tion was approved to provided grants to counties for the purchase of land and the construction of houses of refuge. Even in Colonial America, to be old and poor was to be despised. Ships unloading in New England ports were searched for 'old persons' as well as 'maimed, lunatic or vagrant persons'.[3]

By 1900, housing for elderly people in Canada and the United States was still the responsibility of their children, but this was changing. Elderly people were becoming known as a 'societal problem' and society was to become their caretakers. Even though efforts to assure family responsibil-ity for elderly members was still widespread, the United States govern-ment created in 1937 a public housing programme. Canada followed in 1938 with a similar programme called Low Rental Housing.[4]

CHARACTERISTICS OF HOUSING FOR THE ELDERLY

It is important to recognize that the housing situation of elderly people is very different from that of their younger counterparts. Several distinguishing characteristics set it apart. The dwelling unit and the surrounding neighbourhood are of greater importance to older people than to the young because of the greater proportion of time they spend in and around home. Another distinguishing characteristic is the pattern of necessary housing services. These depend on factors such as income level, household composition, and health status. The loss of a spouse or change in functional ability will affect the pattern of housing services required. A third characteristic is that older people do not like to make major housing adjustments. They are less ready than younger people to change their housing situation when confronted with a major change in their life situation. A final characteristic is that the definition of housing for older people must be much broader than that typically used. For example, the the definition encompasses the concept that the older occupant can use the dwelling independently without special equipment or personal assistance.

HOUSING NEEDS

On the basis of available data there are four major areas of housing need: (1) affordability, (2) assistance in making timely housing adjustments, (3) adequate housing quality, and (4) promotion of independence. Housing affordability is the most widely discussed issue with respect to housing needs generally, including those for elderly people.

Certain groups of households headed by an elderly person have particularly severe affordability problems. Assistance in making major housing adjustments to such changes as reduced income due to retirement, the death of a spouse, or children leaving home has only recently begun to be recognized as an important characteristic of the housing needs of elderly people. The physical conditions of the dwelling unit have traditionally been used as an indicator of housing need. The health status of elderly people is directly related to such needs. At issue is the extent to which the dwelling unit can promote independence. Institutionalization may be required when functional ability is severely diminished, but current efforts are directed at assisting people to remain in the community for as long as possible. This trend has given rise to the housing concept of 'aging in place'.[5]

Affordability

Many would argue that the single most important housing problem is affordability. The Report of the President's Commission on Housing in 1982 concluded:[6]

While the public sector has provided housing for lower income persons through new construction and substantial rehabilitation, forces at work in the private sector have produced steady and dramatic improvements in both the quality and quantity of available housing. In fact the ability to pay for decent housing has become the predominant housing problem faced by the poor.

Similarly in Canada, The Canada Mortgage and Housing Corporation's Consultation Paper on Housing (1985) points out:[4]

Canadians still have unmet housing needs. Sizeable numbers of people remain unable to afford decent shelter whether rented or owner-occupied.

Those particularly hardest hit in the United States are renters: 38 per cent of renters spend over 35 per cent of their annual incomes on housing, compared with only 10 per cent of homeowners without mortgage debit.[7] According to Brotman[8] almost 20 per cent of households headed by older persons pay a disproportionate part of their annual income on housing. Households headed by women living alone are particularly hard hit. They are very likely to be paying more than 30 per cent of income on shelter.

Individuals who purchased a home earlier in life are better able to retain that home after retirement and have lower shelter costs than those who remain renters. In 1980 Stryk and Soldo[9] found that the average household headed by an elderly person in a dwelling without a mortgage devoted only 23 per cent of its income to housing, versus 20 per cent in other households. The difference was negligible. Furthermore, elderly persons, especially couples who owned their homes, appeared to be more financially secure than those who were renting.

People in the United States with very low incomes have excessive housing cost burdens. About half of elderly people living below the poverty line devote more than 45 per cent of their income to housing. Being in poverty overlaps with living alone.

In Canada in 1971, 45 per cent of women aged 75 years and over and living alone paid 50 per cent or more of their income for shelter in rented dwellings. However by 1981, this proportion had been reduced to 20 per cent.[10] The same is true for men, but to a lesser degree. The very significant improvements in the ratio of housing costs to income can be largely attributed to improvements in income.

The impact of living alone is shown by comparison with those living as couples. Less than 10 per cent of couples aged 55–65 in Canada pay more than 30 per cent of their income for housing. Furthermore the proportion steadily declines with age.

Golant[11] claims that both older American homeowners and renters live in housing inappropriate for their declining personal resources and distinctive lifestyles. This problem is more severe for suburban dwellers.

Housing adjustments

Struyk[12] has argued that a major problem for older Americans is the difficulty they face in making timely housing adjustments in response to major changes in their life situation. Reductions in income, the death of a spouse, a son or daughter moving out or returning, or the onset of physical limitations are factors which affect older persons' ability to pay for and maintain their current dwelling unit, or to search for and locate alternative situations in the community.

The most dramatic housing adjustment is a move to another location. A commonly held belief is that older people who move within their community do so to reduce the size of their dwelling unit and the associated expenses. The available data suggest that there is very little consistency in the moves; substantial numbers move into larger units as well as smaller ones. Some patterns do, however, emerge. For example, the loss of a spouse usually triggers a move into a smaller living unit. Husband and wife relocations appear to increase housing expenses, while single-person household relocations reduce them. A shift from home ownership to renting is evident when physical limitations increase for the head of the household. For example, 61 per cent remain homeowners when they relocate, while 39 per cent shift to becoming renters. Conversely, only 15 per cent of those that rent shift to being homeowners on moving.[13]

Moving is the least-preferred way of adjusting to major life events, however. This is borne out by the evidence that in US Metropolitan areas only 4 per cent of elderly homeowners will move in any 12-month period. The rate is higher in renters of whom 11 per cent will move.[14]

Mobility patterns are very similar in Canada. Moves by older people between 1976 and 1981 were mainly over short distances within the same municipality. Only 15 per cent of those aged 65 and over moved within the same municipality, and only 3 per cent elderly people changed their province or territory.[10]

Housing quality

What evidence do we have to suggest that elderly people live in inadequate housing, and are more likely to do so than younger people?

Discussions of housing quality have traditionally focused on the three areas of incomplete plumbing, overcrowding, and the condition of the structure. In the United States, when data were first collected on housing condition by the Census Bureau in 1950, there was a high prevalence of deficiencies in all three areas. Today, most observers would agree that the prevalence of such deficiencies has declined considerably over the last three decades. Housing experts have also agreed that the definition of housing condition has been too narrow. The old three-factor definition has been broadened to include the 'flow of services' coming from the structure and its component systems. For example, it is not only important to have complete plumbing; it is equally important that it works in a dependable manner. It is not only the number of rooms and their size that matter, but also the condition of the walls, ceilings, and floors.

On the broader indicators, old people in the US have higher rates of plumbing and kitchen inadequacies than do younger people. For other indicators, any differences are generally small. Other interesting patterns do, however, emerge. Renters' units have deficiencies at about twice the rate of those of homeowners. Lack of a complete kitchen, heating break-downs, and poor maintenance are especially difficult problems for renters compared with homeowners.

Husband–wife households have the lowest prevalence of deficiencies. The rate of deficiencies of plumbing and kitchens of elderly-person house-holds living in rural areas is several times the rate of those living in urban areas.

Households of elderly blacks in the United States have a high preva-lence of housing deficiencies. Older people whose income is at or below the poverty line are several times more likely to live with housing de-ficiencies than are people whose income is higher. The prevalence of housing deficiencies decreases as income rises.

Another important aspect of housing quality is the extent to which dwellings have been modified to accommodate people with disabilities. Modifications can include specially equipped kitchens, bathrooms mod-ified for wheelchairs, and any type of special feature like grab bars, ramps, and specially equipped telephones. The 1978 US Annual Housing Survey reported about 1.7 million households equipped with some form of special feature. The survey pointed out that homeowners were more likely than renters to live in dwelling units with special features.

It is important to note that temporary inadequacies do not necessarily mean that the housing unit is deficient. When major physical deficiencies persist over time, the is a more reliable indicator of deficiency. For example, survey date over time in the United States shows that elderly renters, especially in rural areas, are more likely to occupy units that have some major physical deficiencies that persist over time than are younger renters or homeowners of both age groups.

The situation in Canada with regard to housing quality is different from that in the United States. The age of the housing stock in Canada is much younger than in the United States. Fifty per cent of the housing stock in Canada was built in the last 20 years and only 21 per cent of the housing stock prior to 1940. According to the 1982 Household Facilities and Equipment Survey, as reported in the Fact Book on Aging in Canada,[10] 72 per cent of Canadian households reported that their housing only needed regular maintenance, 15 per cent needed only minor repairs, and just 13 per cent needed major repair work. Little differences were reported between older and younger households in the proportion of their housing needing repair.

Promotion of independence

A central concern of those involved in housing for the elderly is the relationship between health and housing needs. The housing situation of older people is influenced by health limitations. At issue is the extent to which housing policies and programmes directed at older people promote independent living in the community and prevent premature or unnecessary institutionalization. There is recognition of the fact that older persons have widely varying health and housing needs requiring a wide range of housing options and choices. The options range from completely independent living arrangements to institutional facilities.

Data show that roughly 45 per cent of the non-institutionalized American population aged 65 and older had a health limitation that restricted activity.[15] This is a particular problem for those over 75 years of age; more than half in this group reported that health problems limited the type of activity they could perform.[16] This presents particular problems for homeowners who live alone. Physical limitations may affect not only personal care, but also the maintenance and repair of the dwelling unit, and even its day-to-day upkeep.

Another concern is how to compensate for limitations in functional ability. Formal and informal services, some provided by the family, can assist older people to remain independent. Another approach is to modify the dwelling unit to make it more usable by older people with functional limitations. Studies like the US Annual Housing Survey indicate a low overall incidence of special features being added to dwelling units. Where modifications are made, they are primarily to bathrooms to facilitate wheelchair use.

The older population as a whole in Canada is remarkably healthy and remains functionally well until advanced age.[17] Approximately 80 per cent of persons over the age of 65 in Canada are capable of living independently.[17] This is in spite of the fact that 75 per cent of older people suffer from at least one chronic health problem.[17]

GOVERNMENT RESPONSE

How have the governments of Canada and the United States responded
to the special housing problems of their older citizens? The response in
both countries has been through the creation of many different forms of
assistance.

The US government's response

For more than four decades, the government of the United States has
responded actively to the needs of various groups, including elderly
people. The centrepiece of federal housing policy has been the provision
in the tax code which permits homeowners to deduct property taxes and
interest paid on their mortgages. Other programmes have included housing subsidies and the construction of public housing. Federal, state, and
local governments all play a similar role in the housing sector.

Federal government housing policies have relied on direct financial
outlays to suppliers (supply-side programmes) and to households themselves (demand-side programmes). Supply-side programmes attempt to
increase the supply of housing through the construction of new housing
units. Demand-side programmes, on the other hand, augment the effective demand for housing through mechanisms such as rent subsidies or tax
credits for home purchasers.

The government's assistance can also be distinguished by tenure—
assistance to renters versus assistance to homeowners. The federal government has directed its assistance programmes primarily towards renters
through various renter assistance programmes. The assistance towards
homeowners had been mortgage interest and property tax deduction
provisions in the tax code. Elderly homeowners have, with a few exceptions, received relatively fewer benefits from these provisions, as most
elderly homeowners own their homes outright.

The system of housing programmes prior to 1981 grew tremendously in
terms of budgetary commitments and the number of households served.
By the end of 1980, over one-third of those assisted by renter programmes were elderly persons. However, January 1981 marked a turning point
in American housing policy as a fundamental redirection of housing
assistance programmes took place when the Reagan administration came
into office. The goal of that administration was to cutback drastically on
the overall level of assistance. The new assistance policy essentially proposed that there be no further increase in the number of households
receiving housing subsidies.

Instead the objective was to move in the direction of greater reliance
on the private market for the provision of housing. The federal govern-

ment decided to rely heavily on the existing housing stock for its housing policy, and thereby shift from a supply-side policy to a demand-side policy.

Renter Programmes in the USA

Elderly renters have been assisted through a variety of programmes since the Second World War. At the end of 1980, approximately 40 per cent of all rental-assisted units were occupied by the elderly.[7]

Public housing.   Launched in 1937, the Public Housing Program is the oldest and largest federally supported housing programme. Public housing is low-rent housing and it was begun with objectives which included generating jobs and eliminating slums. Its present objective is to assist poor households to live in adequate housing. Some public housing projects are especially designed for elderly persons.

Public housing units are owned and operated by local housing authorities. The federal government pays for constructing the units and also pays a portion of the operating expenses. The local housing authority must meet the remainder of the operating costs from rents and utility charges. The property management responsibilities rest with the local housing authority.

By 1980, there were 1.2 million federally supported units of public housing of which 37 per cent of the units were occupied by households headed by elderly people.[7]

'Section 8'.   As the supply-side programmes began to expand in the 1960s and early 1970s, the US Congress enacted the 1974 Housing and Community Development Act, which created the 'Section 8 Program'. The purpose of the Act was to give local governments more flexibility to provide housing assistance consistent with local conditions. By the end of 1980, the Section 8 Program was larger than the public housing programme with 1.1 million units occupied and several hundred thousand units under development.

The Section 8 Program consisted of four subprogrammes: existing, moderate rehabilitation, substandard rehabilitation, and new construction. Approximately 70 per cent of the occupied units were accounted for by the 'existing' segment of the programme. This segment helps households to rent units from the existing rental housing stock which meet prescribed physical standards. The programme pays the landlord the difference between the actual market rent, capped at a level called the 'fair market rent' and the household's share of the rent calculated at 30 per cent of adjusted gross income. The Section 8 Program has been successful in offering households freedom in choosing their own units.

The household has the freedom to remain in their current unit, or to find another one, provided the unit meets set standards and is within rent limitations. Zais *et al*,[7] pointed out that approximately 65 per cent of elderly participants stayed in their preprogramme dwellings.

The 'new construction' segment of the Section 8 Program provides a guaranteed rental income to developers who build or rehabilitate units under the programme. The federal government pays the difference between the tenant's contribution and the actual rent. Mortgage financing is obtained privately or from the Department of Housing and Urban Development (HUD) through the Government National Mortgage Association or from a State or local housing agency.

'Section 202'. The Housing Act of 1959 created the 'Section 202 Program', which subsidizes new construction. It is restricted to serving the elderly, handicapped, and disabled, and relies exclusively on non-profit sponsors to develop and operate projects. Projects are financed by a direct loan to the sponsor. This programme has been adjusted several times to include more low-income households, to revise applicable interest rates, and to allow for a Section 8 subsidy to be applied to individual units. The Section 202 Program accounts for only a small fraction of the subsidized units in the government stock. However, the proportion of elderly participants is estimated at about 80 per cent, the highest of any HUD renter assistance programme.

Homeowner programmes

For older homeowners, assistance has been in the form of loans and grants for housing maintenance, rehabilitation, and weatherproofing. Property tax relief and income tax subsidies were programmes introduced in the early 1970s that attempt to deal directly with the property tax burden on older homeowners.

Rehabilitation and repair loans and grants. The introduction of rehabilitation loans and grants in the mid 1970s was in keeping with the federal governments intent to save money, since subsidies for new construction were considerably higher than relying on the existing housing stock.

Section 312 Rehabilitation Loan Program. This programme provides below-market interest rate loans to property owners to finance the cost of rehabilitation. Loans from this programme are available for rental properties; however, the largest majority of loans to date have gone to homeowners. Two conditions applied to this programme: first, the homes had to be located in neighbourhoods designated for other general assistance and, second, the owner had to be unable to obtain a comparable loan from other sources. Low- and moderate-income owners who intended to occupy the property once the rehabilitation work is completed were given priority.

Community Development Block Grant (CDBG) Program.   The purpose of the CDBG Program has been to provide cities and urban counties with greater flexibility in dealing with problems of urban decay. While low- and moderate-income households are to be the recipients of the block grant funds, the funds need not be restricted to deteriorating areas.

CDBG funds have been used to fund repair and rehabilitation approaches. Some plans have offered financing for work through grants, loans, loan guarantees, and interest rate subsidies. Other approaches have been to provide the repair and rehabilitation work directly through local home maintenance and repair programmes. Between 1975 and 1981 more than $23.3 billion was provided to help local governments deal with community needs. More than one-quarter of these funds was aimed at activities related to housing rehabilitation. The largest proportion of dollars, 70 per cent, went to the rehabilitation of private single-family houses. Roughly one-third of the assistance went to elderly renters and about 43 per cent to older homeowners.[16]

The Section 502 and 504 Rural Housing Loan Program.   This programme was administered by the Farmers Home Administration, Department of Agriculture. It provided loans to homeowners at reduced interest rates for the purpose of constructing or repairing a dwelling unit or site. The objective of the programme was to increase housing purchases.

Section 504 took up where Section 502 stopped. Households that are too poor to meet the 'sufficient income' requirements of Section 502 were elibible for Section 504 grants or loans.

Taxation relief

Property tax relief programs.   The most common approach to property tax relief is through programmes in which States underwrite some proportion of the property tax levy on the homes of elderly homeowners. Eligibility is based on income below some defined level. The higher the tax burden or the lower the income, the greater is the tax relief. The benefit usually takes the form of a credit on State income tax returns. Some States provide direct payments from their general revenues.

Another tax relief programme is the homestead exemption and credit. Homestead exemptions are a dollar amount or a percentage share of the property valuation that is exempted from property taxes. Homestead credits are a dollar or percentage reduction in taxes on property.

Federal income tax subsidies to homeowners.   Three provisions of the Internal Revenue Code: the absence of a requirement to declare imputed income from ownership, the deductibility or property taxes, and the deductibility of mortgage interest payments, account for the most significant and sizeable class of subsidies to homeowners regardless of age. Elderly homeowners benefit as much as their younger counterparts from these programmes.

One other provision in the Internal Revenue Code that benefits older homeowners is the one-time exclusion of a capital gain realized on the sale of a principal residence.

Weatherization assistance.   Weatherization Programmes existed for many years with a primary purpose of improving the weather proofing of dwellings. The intent was to lower utility costs and improve comfort levels.

The Weatherization Assistance Programme, administered by the Department of Energy, provided assistance for the installation of insulation, storm windows and doors, and caulking. Homeowners as well as renters were eligible for this type of assistance. Nearly 200 000 dwellings of both elderly and non-elderly persons were weatherized prior to 1980.[18]

Weatherization assistance was provided through a credit on federal income tax returns. The homeowner was responsible for having the work done. The tax credit was a 15 per cent subsidy on the first $2000 of material and labour.

The Canadian government's response

Passed into law in 1944, Canada's National Housing Act was the legislation that brought the Canadian federal government into the housing field. The Canada Housing and Mortgage Corporation (CMHC) was created by the legislation to be the vehicle through which the federal government would participate in the housing sector.

Housing supply in Canada is the responsibility of the provinces. Consequently, the Canadian government is limited in its direct influence. However, the federal government exercises considerable influence throught budgetary outlays. From 1944 to 1954, CMHC worked at encouraging the banking community to make more funds available for housing. In 1954, the National Housing Act was amended to permit the corporation to insure loans made by lenders approved by the corporation as long as certain terms and conditions were met. These terms included the use of standard mortgage documents, conforming construction standards, and acceptable interest rates. The result of this early intervention was the introduction of the Canadian National Building Code for Residential Buildings.

Little was done to promote housing for elderly Canadians between 1944 and 1954. By 1949, there was a recognized need to provide shelter for poor people. The resulting action was the creation of a public housing programme. While not specifically directed at elderly people, this did provide accommodation for those elderly persons who qualified on the basis of low income.

In 1954, in addition to being empowered as an insurer of loans, CMHC was given the authority to act as a direct lender. The purpose of this change was to ensure a flow of money into the housing industry when private lenders were not making funds available. CMHC continues to play this role today, but the number of loans it makes is very small.

Throughout the federal housing programmes, older persons have not been singled out for special treatment. Rather, the policy has been to develop programmes which take into account the needs that are commonly associated with older persons. For example, housing was built for occupants where the monthly rent would not exceed 25 per cent of gross income and a considerable number of elderly people qualified for this. Income rather than age was therefore the criterion to end in a project of this type.

Over the past 25 years, CMHC has provided assistance to older Canadians directly or indirectly through a variety of programmes. These include:

—— Rent Supplement Program: Section 44 (1) (b) and 44.1 (a);

—— Assisted Rental Program;

—— Non-Profit and Co-Operative Housing Program: Section 56.1;

—— Home Improvement Loans Program;

—— Residential Rehabilitation Assistance Program: Section 34.1;

—— Federal/Provincial Public Housing Program: Section 40;

In 25 years approximately 146 000 dwelling units and 47 000 hostel beds have been provided for elderly people through programmes directly funded by CMHC. Another 40 000 units, occupied largely by elderly people, have received a rental subsidy through CMHC.

In 1979, the federal government amended the national Housing Act to disentangle itself from costly and ever-mounting capital and operating subsidies, and in effect passed the responsibility for supplying housing to provincial governments. This shift in policy to reduce budgetary outlays was very similar to that which took place in 1980 in the United States.

Currently, the overall objective of the Corporation is to promote the construction of new houses, the repair and modernization of existing homes, and to improve housing and community living conditions. CMHC's major thrust with respect to older Canadians is through loan repayment assistance to: lower-income homeowners, tenants living in substandard units, and non-profit groups. Under the current programme, CMHC will ensure a loan granted by an approved lender (banks, insurance companies, trust companies) of up to 100 per cent of the loan and will write down the interest costs to as low as an effective 2 per cent interest rate. The amount of the write-down in non-profit projects is dependent on the income mix of the occupants. The underlying rationale is to encourage non-profit groups to have an income mix in their projects for both social and economic reasons. In 1985–1986 $161 million was committed to loan forgiveness, agent fees, and administration.[4]

In 1987 the Residential Rehabilitation Assistance Program (RRAP) made loans of up to $10 000 per unit, of which up to $5000 could be forgiven. A large proportion of those loans went to seniors. The average age of a borrower was 55 years.

Other CMHC programmes include insuring loans made to the purchaser for the acquisition of a home owned by an elderly person, and encouraging rental housing to be developed so that older people can sell their homes and have a wider range of rental accommodation to choose from.

The provinces

Provincial housing programmes, like federal programmes are heavily oriented toward social objectives. All provinces participate in the public non-profit, public housing, and rent supplement programmes. This participation occurs mainly under federal/provincial programmes. The provinces, in general, are particularly active in providing assistance to elderly households, both rental and owner-occupied, and in the area of renovation.

Several provinces operate shelter allowance programmes directed at older people. Provincial renovation programmes are directed to assisting lower-income households and to upgrading core areas, as well as to promoting general improvements to the housing stock.

In Newfoundland, Prince Edward Island, and Saskatchewan, CMHC owns and manages housing projects for older people, in partnership with the provinces, under Section 40 of the National Housing Act. Under this section, the federal government provides 75 per cent of the investment capital for the project and subsidizes 75 per cent of the operating losses that occurs with tenants paying rent geared to income. In Ontario the cost-sharing arrangement is 50–50.

In the province of Manitoba, shelter allowances are a general programme of cash grants to a broad range of qualified tenant households, defined primarily by the proportion of income spent on rent but subject to a maximum limit. The grant amount is calculated as a proportion of the amount by which the householder's rent exceeds a specified proportion of his or her income. The programme is not subject to minimum housing standards for unit quality. The underlying philosophy of a shelter allowance is one of subsidizing 'the person' as opposed to 'the place'. Affordability is the primary housing need being met. The Manitoba shelter allowance programme is called SAFER—'Shelter Allowances For Elderly Renters'. It is defined as a catalyst to assist older persons to 'freely choose' his or her own accommodation in the marketplace.

Shelter allowance programme are widespread across Canada. However, they are currently affecting only some 40 000 households. This is very small when compared with public housing, which affects some 350 000 to 400 000 units.

The province of Ontario has the most extensive array of provincial housing assistance programmes for older persons of any of the provinces. The Ontario programmes are broadly based and recognize the consumer's need for flexibility and choice. The assistance programmes include:

—— The Ontario Home Renewal Program;

—— The Rehabilitation Program for Low-Rise Apartments;

—— The Home Renewal Program for Disabled Persons;

—— The Convert-to-Rent Program;

—— Homesharing;

—— Portable Living Units for Seniors (PLUS Units);

—— Senior Co-Ownership Project;

—— Retirement Community Planning;

—— Multi Level Housing;

—— Peer Counselling for Seniors;

—— Housing Registries.

Home Renewal Program. The Home Renewal Program provides low-income homeowners, many of whom are elderly, with special assistance to make home repairs. Since 1974, $158 million in grants have been made in amounts up to $7500 per unit. To qualify, an applicant must have an annually adjusted household income of $20 000 or less. Depending on the applicant's income, up to $4000 can be forgiven. Sixty per cent of the loans have been made to persons over 55 years of age whose average income was $9500.

Rehabilitation Program for Low-Rise Apartments. The objective of this programme is to retain low-rise apartments in the housing stock so that they may continue to provide affordable rental housing for low- and moderate-income tenants. There are some 52 000 units in the province of Ontario, of which 18 per cent are occupied by persons over 65 years of age. The programme offers landlords forgivable loans of up to $5000 per unit. A building, in order to qualify, must be less than five storeys, contain two or more rental apartments, and have been built before 1960. The funds are to be used to improve the physical condition of low-rise buildings, while retaining their marketability for low- and moderate-income tenants. The rehabilitation work must also prevent physical deterioration and extend the building's life by at least 15 years. Three thousand units have been rehabilitated under this programme.

The Ontario Home Renewal Program for Disabled Persons.   In 1987, $3.15 million was directed to this newly created programme. It assists disabled homeowners or homeowners with disabled dependent family members to undertake necessary modifications to their homes. This loan programme is capped at $15 000 per home. The loan is interest-free regardless of income.

The Convert-to-Rent Program.   Buildings such as warehouses, vacant factories, and schools can be converted under this programme into housing units. Interest-free loans of up to $7000 per unit are provided to persons who want to convert non-residential property into moderately priced self-contained apartments, where zoning laws permit. Shared accommodation suitable for single persons including old people can be created under this programme. Since 1985, over 6000 units have been created and the expectation is that over 10 000 units will eventually be created.

Homesharing.   Two-year grants to municipalities or municipality-sponsored agencies who are interested in operating home-sharing services are available in Ontario. The grants are up to $20 000 per year to set up matching services. This is a cost-sharing programme where the grant covers 50 per cent of the operating costs. Eleven matching services have been started as a result of this programme.

Portable Living Units for Seniors (PLUS).   This programme is the well-known 'granny flat' housing option. To date, 12 PLUS units have been installed and occupied for 1 year in three participating municipalities in Ontario. The Ontario Ministry of Housing is taking the initial financial risk in developing this innovative form of housing. During the demonstration period the units are owned and maintained by the province, and the occupants rent the premises. Two types of units are part of the demonstration: a one-person model and a two-person model. They measure 530 to

670 square feet (49 to 62 m^2) respectively and are completely self-contained. The exteriors are attractive and unobtrusive. The double occupancy units are wheelchair accessible. Zoning by-laws remain a major obstacle to this innovative housing solution.

The Senior Co-ownership Project. Co-ownership tenure provides residents with the privacy of individual housing units and the companionship of sharing common social and recreational facilities. Older people sell their homes and use the equity from the sale to purchase shares in an equity co-operative, condominium, or a life lease. The Ontario project provides incentive grants to sponsoring groups who wish to convert non-residential buildings into multiple-unit projects that will be sold as co-ownership residences. Funding is available in amounts of $13 000 for start-up assistance. Conversion projects are eligible for an additional $5000 per unit created up to a maximum of $30 000.

Retirement Community Planning incentive grants. Incentive grants are being offered to muncipalities to accelerate and streamline their approval procedures for setting up retirement communities. The Ontario Senior Retirement Community Project will give selected municipalities $2000 for each unit sold or leased in a planned retirement community. The grants are intended to help muncipalities defray a number of costs that new retirement communities introduce, such as new sewer and water services, fire protection services, and extended transit systems.

THE PRIVATE SECTOR'S RESPONSE

Changing domestic priorities in the early 1980s redirected social housing policies in Canada and the United States. Greater reliance on the private sector and, in particular, on use of existing housing stock became important goals of the new social housing policy. An abrupt freeze on financing for construction of new units created a gap that the private sector has only slowly begun to fill.

The non-profit private sector

In the early 1980s in the United States the non-profit private sector picked up the challenge than had been laid down by the federal goverment. National advocacy organizations, professional associations, and public interest groups convened conferences and task forces to consider new and innovative housing and living arrangements that would be consistent with the new domestic priority of economic restraint. New housing concepts as well as old ones surfaced, including shared housing, accessory apartments, granny flats, home equity conversion instruments, co-operative housing, and life-lease rental agreements.

Advocates for each of the options emerged by the mid 1980s. Non-profit private organizations became sponsors and developers of specific housing options. As demonstration projects were created, evaluations were launched to measure the willingness of older persons to accept these new options, and to determine how satisfied they were with these arrangements. Shared housing, accessory apartments, granny flats, and home equity conversion instruments received the most attention and scrutiny because these options utilized existing housing stock and required no government funding.

Shared housing. Shared housing is not a new idea; people have been 'doubling up' for years for a variety of reasons. Shared housing in the 1980s, however, has come to be defined as a living arrangement where at least two or more persons, usually unrelated, share a household. Each member of the household has a private room but shares common areas such as the kitchen, living room, and dining room. Family qualities are an important part of the definition and emphasis is placed on shared decision making, and having primary responsibilities for the management of the household.

Two types of shared housing programme have emerged as a result of the renewed interest in this old idea. The first type is housing oriented and is referred to as 'naturally occurring' households. The second type is service oriented and is called 'agency-sponsored' shared housing. The naturally occurring shared households are the most common and the least visible. Most naturally occurring shared households are small in size, accommodating between three and four people. The benefits of this type of living arrangement include affordability, companionship, greater safety and security, and mutual assistance. Single family detached homes are the most common type of dwelling unit used for this type of shared housing.

The agency-sponsored shared housing programme are considerably larger in size, usually accommodating eight to ten people. A paid staff member provides basic housekeeping and meals, and assists the residents as required. The presence of staff around-the-clock distinguishes this type of sharing from the former type and aligns it more closely with the formal social service delivery system. Another distinguishing feature is that the residents of agency-sponsored programme tend to be older, more frail, and more in need of assistance.[19] The benefits to the residents are about the same, although for some frail older persons agency-sponsored shared housing is an alternative to institutionalization.

Intergenerational shared households are another variation on this model. Mutual assistance, a family environment, and affordability are some of the benefits of intergenerational shared households.

Home sharing is not for everyone. Jaffe and Howe[20] suggest that home-sharing programmes are more likely to emerge in some kinds of community than in others, and that community characteristics such as age structure, housing stock, and housing price will influence whether the programme is housing or service oriented. Current estimates in Canada and the United States suggest that only 7–10 per cent of older persons would consider home sharing as an option. However, it has great potential for elderly people who have a variety of housing and service support needs. Through sharing, people obtain shelter, companionship, security, and home support all in one package, and at very little cost to the public.

Accessory apartments.　In the United States there are more than seven million home-owning households in which one member is 65 years or greater, the household consists of two persons or less, and the home has five rooms or more, not counting the basement or garage.[21] Individuals and organizations have advocated the conversion of this underused space into housing for older persons. This approach is known as accessory apartments.

The accessory apartment model has several benefits. The elderly homeowner making the conversion receives added income and security. Additional units are added to the national housing stock and there is little or no government assistance involved. Conventional bank financing is used for the conversion that can range up to $15 000 a unit.

Government assistance is available in Canada for accessory apartment conversion. In the Canadian province of Ontario, the Ministry of Housing has established a programme called Convert-To-Rent. Under the programme, interest-free loans of $7000 per unit are available to create a self-contained rental unit in a single family dwelling.

The granny flat.　Self-contained, detached, temporary dwellings that can be placed on the property of an adult child to be occupied by the elderly parent is another option that has been developed and promoted by the non-profit private sector. The concept known as the 'granny flat' or 'echo housing' has been gaining momentum since its development in Australia over a decade ago. Some 4500 units have been created in Australia.

The units are usually created for either one- or two-person households. They measure from about 500 to 700 square feet (49 to 62 square metres) respectively. The units are completely self-contained, with a living room, kitchen, bedroom, and bathroom.

The exteriors are attractive and unobtrusive. They are portable and constructed to high standards of energy efficiency. Sewage, water, and electrical utilities are generally linked to the services of the existing home.

In the United States and Canada, municipal zoning by-laws have made it difficult to install the granny flat. Neighbourhood protests against granny flats being located in existing neighbourhoods centre on the potential devaluation of surrounding property, parking problems, and increased loads on sanitary sewers. Evidence would suggest that none of these situations are likely to happen.

As described above, in the Canadian province of Ontario, the Ontario Ministry of Housing has played a leading role in promoting interest in granny flats through a demonstration project in three participating municipalities. Twelve units have been occupied for over a year. The ministry has started a formal evaluation of the project to determine the social acceptability of the units and the market demand associated with the concept.

Home equity conversion instruments. At the same time as the various dwelling unit and living arrangement options were being developed and promoted, attention was also being directed to the development of innovative financing instruments, generally referred to as home equity instruments. These instruments are designed to allow homeowners to borrow against their accumulated home equity without relinquishing their occupancy. Repayment of the loan may be delayed until the sale of the home, or the death of the homeowner. The instruments that permit deferral of payments are known as home equity conversion instruments.

This option has intuitive appeal but the willingness of homeowners to realize their home equity appears limited. A US National Consumer Finance Survey in 1983 showed that only 11 per cent of homeowners were users of home equity[22]. Nelson[23] reviewed the socio-economic characteristics associated with the preference for home equity. He found those most in need of realizing it—widows over the age of 75 with low incomes—were the least interested.

Home equity is a major source of wealth for the older homeowner. Willingness to access it, though, remains very much dependent on the circumstances surrounding the loan.

Co-operatives and life-leases. Co-operative housing and rental housing involving a life-lease have been put forward as options where government involvement is substantially reduced. Both options require a sizeable down-payment on the cost of the unit. Under the co-operative arrangement, the person purchases the unit. The difference between the down-payment and the purchase price is financed by a government programme or through the financial resources of the co-operative. The owner is free to sell the unit at a pre-arranged price that takes into account the original purchase price plus the cost of any improvements that have been made. Any increase in the value of the unit due to appreciation or inflation is not reflected in the sale price. This approach keeps home ownership within the range of those with modest incomes or limited equity from a previous home.

The life-lease option in rental accommodation requires a tenant to contribute between 35 and 100 per cent of the unit cost. This initial payment substantially lowers the monthly rent. It also reduces the amount of financing needed by the sponsor. Rents can be increased as operating and management costs go up. However, any increase in rent will be considerably lower than it would be in private market housing. The equity contribution is returned when the tenant vacates the property, minus a small administration fee. Numerous non-profit private sponsors in Canada are developing this type of housing arrangement for older persons.

The profit sector

The involvement of the for-profit sector in elderly persons housing goes back many decades, and is not just a result of the recent policy shift in social housing programmes. In the post-World War II period, private builders in Florida and in other parts of the United States became aware of the growing market for retirement housing in locations offering a mild climate with recreational and scenic attractions. As a result they began to build what they called retirement housing.

The retirement village was the model most often constructed. The village consisted of low-density, age-restricted developments, constructed with private capital and offering extensive recreational services. The individual units were for purchase and at relatively low cost. The retirement villages and other planned age-segregated communities came to be known as 'retirement communities'. Today retirement communities have come to be defined as aggregates of living units, intentionally planned for at least 100 residents, who for the most part are over 50 years of age, healthy, and retired.[25]

Early studies[24] found that residents preferred to live in a community where everyone is retired, rather than in one in which some people are working. The highly supportive environment created in retirement communities was cited as very important to the residents' perception of well-being. More recent studies[25] suggest that retirement communities are successful in their ability to support the needs of their elderly residents.

The 'life-care' concept, after a disastrous start in the 1960s, is undergoing a major resurgence. Under this concept, the individual pays a large 'founder's fee', sometimes as high as $20 000 or more, and high monthly

costs for shelter and care. In return the person is guaranteed housekeeping services, personal assistance, meals, and medical care when needed
until he/she dies. The attractiveness of this option is that it provides a
sense of security. This type of arrangement serves a very small proportion
of older persons, but represents a significant investment of capital for the
private market.

HOUSING AND SERVICES

The discussion to this point has focused exclusively on housing-oriented
programmes and the respective roles played by government and the private sector. What follows touches on the last issue to be dealt with in this
chapter, namely the issue of the integration of housing and services.

In early times, elderly men and women continued to live in the community as long as they were able to be independent. If illness or disability
interfered with their independence, the family provided services and
meals, usually in the home. When the family was not able or was unavailable to provide assistance, the only solution was institutional care—a
move which often involved a complete separation from the community.
This situation has changed in some ways with the expansion of support
services. These services range from assistance with dressing, bathing, and
preparing meals, to help with shopping and housework.

The distribution of these services in the United States varies considerably, and access is often based on individuals' ability to pay. In other
countries, like Canada and the United Kingdom, they are universal, and
virtually free to consumers. The premise behind such services is that they
may act to prevent or delay institutionalization.

In spite of the proliferation of housing-oriented programmes and support services, the housing and service sectors have seldom been integrated
in the United States and Canada. In Norway, Sweden, and the Netherlands shelter and services are integrated and viewed as part of a 'living
continuum'. In the United States and Canada the two sectors are perceived as separate entities. Social services are part of the welfare system
that exists to maintain a national minimum level of health and welfare,
and a minimum standard of living. Housing, though regarded as a basic
need, has rarely been accorded the same status. The fact that housing
policy has not fallen within the social welfare context has kept the two
sectors apart. Conversely, the welfare definition in a social welfare state
like the United Kingdom brings social services, housing, health care, and
labour into an all-encompassing concept.

Several approaches to a more comprehensive co-ordination of shelter
and services have been attempted. Congregate housing (a shelter and

support service combination) and facilities with multiple services and levels of care (life-care communities) have been introduced in the United States. The US Department of Housing and Urban Development, US Department of Agriculture—Farmer's Home Administration, and the Administration on Aging jointly sponsored a congregate demonstration project in the early 1970s. Extensive research was done in the 1970s on Highland Heights, a health-service oriented congregate housing project in Fall River, Massachusetts.

Another major problem which has limited the expansion of congregate housing in the United States is the issue of assured funding for the services in the housing. Market forces in the United States have been presumed to provide the services where needed, as long as the recipient is able to pay. A limited 'safety net' of welfare programme exists for those poorer persons unable to pay for the services at cost. The expansion of this model has been further limited by a lack of information on alternative funding models which sponsors can use such as traditional realizing of other resources, sliding rent systems, sliding fee scales, legislative revisions to Medicaid for full community-based care, and incentives for family care.

Health care in Canada is a provincial responsibility, with each province administering its own health care progrmmes. Apart from meeting certain general conditions in regard to universality and the portability of programmes across provinces (in order to qualify for federal government cost-sharing monies), the provinces make their own decisions about the nature of benefits and how services are organized. It is also needs to be pointed out that as part of Canadian health care policy there are five levels of institutional care: (1) residential, (2) extended care, (3) chronic, (4) rehabilitation, and (5) acute.

Non-profit sponsors in Canada have developed housing initiatives which provide residential care. The definition of residential care or Level 1 care varies somewhat from province to province. In Manitoba[26] Level 1 indicates minimal dependence on nursing time. The individual requires weekly supervision and/or assistance with personal care and/or some encouragement or reminders to wash, dress, and attend meals and/or activities. He/she may need both administration of medication on a regular basis and to use mechanical aids.

Another variation on the integration of housing and services is where health treatment and supportive services are provided in the home under an insured programme like home care. Such programmes provide a variety of health, treatment, and support services to people in their own homes including nursing care, physiotherapy, occupational, respiratory and speech therapy, medical supplies, and drugs. Home making, handiman services, meals-on-wheels, and the support of a social worker may also be provided. These services are delivered to older people in their own homes, as well as in public housing. For example, the province of Manitoba's home care (continuing care) programme is to provide community supportive services within the client's home, unless the cost of the services would exceed the cost of similar care in an institutional setting.[27]

Eligibility for home care and homemaker programme, as well as their components, vary from Canadian province to province.[27] One other variation of the integration of housing and support services is agency-sponsored home sharing. Agency-sponsored home sharing is a community-based arrangement that meets the housing and service needs of older adults. This option responds to a wide range and changing set of needs within a private residence.

CONCLUSION

Following on the previous discussion about the housing needs of older persons in the United States and Canada, and how the respective governments and the private sector have addressed these issues, one can rightly ask what is an appropriate role for a central government in the housing sector?

The motivation for governments to be involved in the housing sector is the issue of equal access to housing of a standard quality. The recipients most often targeted to receive the benefits of government housing policies are those in greatest economic need. However, housing policy plays a much broader role than just to guarantee equal access to quality housing. Housing policies play a pivotal role in the achievement of a country's national objectives. For example, the housing/construction sector plays a vital role in the economic growth of a country. It creates jobs as well as goods and services. Consequently, national housing policies are created to achieve a blend of economic and social objectives. Government involvement in other sectors, such as labour and finance, also affect housing market activity.

A high degree of government involvement in the housing field produces a regulated market and can result in lower housing costs for all households, or governments can limit their involvement to benefit a selected few, such as those unable to obtain decent housing in the private market. The challenge for governments is to develop housing policies within the broader economic and political framework that ensures the availability of proved shelter solutions and guarantees access to those opportunities for those in greatest need. The elderly are one such group.

References

1. Townsend, P. (1962). *The last refuge. A survey of residential institutions and homes for the aged in England and Wales.* Routledge and Kegan Paul, London.
2. Thomson, D. (1983). Workhouse to nursing home: residential care of elderly people in England since 1840. *Ageing and Society,* **3,** 43–69.
3. Forbes, W. F., Jackson, J. A., and Kraus, A. S. (1987). *Institutionalization of the elderly in Canada (perspectives on individual and population aging series).* Butterworths, Toronto, Ontario.
4. Canada Mortgage and Housing Corporation (1985). *Consultation paper on housing.* Canada Mortgage and Housing Corporation, Ottawa, Ontario.
5. Blackie, N. K. (1986). Aging in place. In *Aging in place: housing adaptations and options for remaining in the community* (ed. Gutman, G. M. and N. K. Blackie), The Gerontology Research Centre, Simon Fraser University, Burnaby, BC.
6. *The report of the President's Commission on housing.* (1982). US Government Printing Office, Washington, DC.
7. Zais, J. P., Struyk, R. J., and Thibodeau, T. (1982). *Housing assistance for older Americans the Reagan Prescription.* The Urban Institute Press, Washington DC.
8. Brotman, H. B. (1982). *Every ninth American: 1982 edition. An analysis for the Chairman of the Select Committee on Aging.* House 97th Congress, 2nd Session. US Government Printing Office, Washington, DC.
9. Struyk, R. and Soldo, B. (1980). *Improving the elderly's housing.* Ballinger Publishing Company, Cambridge, Mass.
10. Fact Book on Aging in Canada, (1983). Minister of Supply and Services, Ottawa, Ontario.
11. Golant, S. M. (1984). Factors influencing the nightime activity of old persons in their community. *Journal of Gerontology,* **39** (4), 485–91.
12. Struyk, R. J. (1977). The housing situation of older Americans. *The Gerontologist,* **17,** 130–9.
13. US Department of Housing and Urban Development (1979). *Annual housing survey: 1973. Housing characteristics of older Americans in the United States.* US Government Printing Office, Washington, DC.
14. US Bureau of the Census (1981). *Annual housing survey. 1979 Part C, Financial characteristics of the housing inventory.* US Government Printing Office, Washington, DC.
15. US Public Health Service (1981). *The 1980 national health interview survey.* US Government Printing Office, Washington, DC.
16. Newman, S. J., Zais, J. and Struyk, R. (1984). Housing older America. In *Elderly people and the environment,* (ed. Altman, I., M. P. Lawton, and Wohlwill J. F.) Plenum Press, New York.
17. Health and Welfare Canada and Statistics Canada (1982). *Canada health survey.* Minister of Supply and Services, Ottawa, Ontario.
18. US Department of Energy (1980). Residential energy consumption survey: conservation. US Government Printing office, Washington, DC.
19. Streib, G., Folts, E. and Hilker M. A., (1984). *Old homes—new families: shared housing for the elderly.* Columbia University Press New York.

20. Jaffe, D. and Howe E., (1988). Agency-assisted shared housing: the nature of programs and matches. *The Gerontologist*, **28**, 318–24.
21. Hare, P. (1988). Peter Pan housing and the remodelling industry. *Canadian Housing*, **5** (1).
22. Sullivan, H. and Jensen, H. H. (1985). Recent evidence on the elderly's use of home equity. *The proceedings of the 31st annual conference on the American Council on Consumer Interest*, March 28–30.
23. Nelson, D. (1980). A profile of elderly homeowners. In *Unlocking home equity for the elderly*, (ed. Scholen, K. and Yung-Ping Chen) Ballinger Publishing Company, Cambridge, Mass.
24. Hoyt, G. C. (1954). The life of the retired in a trailer park. *American Journal of Sociology*, **59**, 361–70.
25. Marans, R. W., Hunt, M. E., and Vakalo, K. L. (1984). Retirement communities. In *Elderly people and the environment*, (ed. Altman, I., M. P. Lawton, and Wohlwill J. F.) Plenum Press, New York.
26. Kane, R. L. and Kane, R. A. (1985). *A will and way. What the United States can learn from Canada about caring for the elderly*. Columbia University Press, New York.
27. Lang, C. and Shelton, C. (1982). *The directory: programs for senior citizens across Canada*. Canadian Pensioners, Conceed Inc. Ontario Division, Toronto, Ontario.

31

Technology development and use for elderly people

KATIE MASLOW

Technology for older people encompasses an enormous range of devices, procedures, and systems for biomedical research, health and long-term care, housing, employment, information, communication, transportation, and environmental design. In this century, technological advances in public hygiene, sanitation, treatment of infectious diseases, and general health care have led to increased life expectancy and rapid growth in the size of the older population, and these trends will continue for the foreseeable future. Technology has the further potential to maintain the functional ability of elderly people and enhance the quality of their lives. Yet many factors combine to limit the development and appropriate use of technology by and for elderly people.

The Office of Technology Assessment (OTA) is a government research agency that provides the United States Congress with analysis of public policy issues related to scientific and technological developments and change. Since 1983, it has conducted several studies in the area of technology and aging, including an overview of the technologies that affect elderly people,[1] a study of life-sustaining technologies and the elderly,[2] and one of technologies for biomedical research and clinical and long-term care of persons with Alzheimer's disease and other diseases that cause dementia.[3]

OTA's assessments of technologies for older people always begin with a focus on specific devices, procedures, or services and the question: 'Do they work for this population?' This question inevitably leads to other questions: How often are the technologies used for elderly people? Are they used appropriately? Are they adapted to the needs of the elderly? Are elderly people, their families, and others who routinely interact with the elderly aware of the technologies? Are there individuals who are trained to assess the needs of elderly people relative to specific technologies and to help them identify potentially beneficial technologies, obtain them, and learn to use them? Can elderly people, their families, and others find these 'experts'? Lastly, are the technologies affordable, or, is there a source of public or private third-party funding for them?

The answers to all of these questions affect the extent to which technologies are used and, in turn, the demand for them. In the United

States, research on and development of technology are generally responsive to demand. When elderly people, their families, and others are not aware of available technologies, cannot locate someone to help them assess need and identify potentially beneficial technologies, or lack a means to pay for them, the technologies are not used. In such circumstances, there may be little demand for existing technologies and little incentive for research and development of new technologies, or for further adaptation of existing technologies to meet the needs of elderly people. To a greater or lesser degree, this scenario describes the current situation with regard to many technologies.

In the circular interaction of technology use, demand, development, and adaptation, the attitudes of elderly people, their families, and society as a whole are extremely important. Negative stereotypes about elderly people, their futures, and their capacity for sustained independent functioning discourage attempts to develop, adapt, and use various technologies. In some cases, these negative stereotypes are the main obstacle to the development and use of technologies.

Another obstacle to the development and adaptation of technologies for elderly people is the current lack of knowledge about important physical, mental, emotional, behavioural, and social aspects of aging. It is usually necessary to understand a problem in some detail before selecting or designing a technology to solve it. Many problems of elderly people are not yet well enough understood for this purpose.

More information is needed about common physiological processes of aging and shared characteristics, experiences, and problems of elderly people. In many respects, however, elderly people are more different from each other than they are the same. The heterogeneity of people over age 60 or 65 is remarkable—across nations, in one country, and even within a single socio-economic or cultural group or a single family. This heterogeneity greatly complicates the processes of development and diffusion of technology. It means that no one device, procedure, or service can be appropriate for all or even most of this population. For an elderly individual, it means that a thorough understanding of that person's physical, mental, emotional, behavioural, and social characteristics is needed before appropriate technologies can be identified.

On a societal level, the heterogeneity of elderly people raises important questions about the validity of age-based programmes and initiatives. The complex conceptual issues involved in focusing on age vs. need in addressing the problems of elderly people are beyond the scope of this chapter. Suffice it to say that, in the United States, political and social realities and the way in which public programmes have developed historically create a strong tendency toward age-based approaches to solving these problems. This age-based focus causes difficulties in technology development and diffusion, however, and complicates many aspects of the process of matching people with technologies that will benefit them.

A final general consideration in the development and adaptation of technology for elderly people is the impact of cognitive impairment on a person's ability to use or benefit from a particular device, procedure, or service. In the United States, assistive medical devices, environmental and housing technologies, and information, communication, and transportation technologies are widely cited as ways to maintain and support the independent functioning of elderly people, and thus, to limit the public cost of institutional care for them. Clearly, these technologies have the potential of supporting independent functioning for many elderly people. However, even though only a small proportion of those over age 65 are cognitively impaired, there is evidence that this includes many of those elderly people who require institutional care or extensive personal care at home. It is not obvious that cognitively impaired people can use the recommended technologies effectively and thereby avoid the need for institutional care or costly personal care services at home. Assessment of technologies for elderly people should include an analysis of the impact of cognitive status on a person's ability to benefit from the technology. Likewise, this factor should be taken into account in projections about the likely effect on public long-term care costs of introducing or promoting the use of a given technology.

The remainder of this chapter discusses the preceding considerations and questions with regard to assistive devices, life-sustaining medical technologies, and medical and long-term care for persons with Alzheimer's disease and other diseases that cause dementia.

ASSISTIVE DEVICES AND ELDERLY PEOPLE

As average lifespan has increased in this century, individuals who might previously have died at a young age of infectious diseases or other acute conditions now live long enough to develop functional impairments related to chronic diseases. Chronic diseases with especially high prevalence in the elderly include heart disease, hypertension, arteriosclerosis, osteoarthritis, diabetes, and urinary system diseases. In some individuals, these diseases result in an inability to perform basic self-care activities (e.g. bathing, dressing, toileting, and eating) and instrumental activities of daily living (e.g. shopping, cleaning, preparing meals, using a telephone, and managing money). Diseases that cause visual and hearing loss are also common in the elderly and can interfere with a person's ability to care for himself or herself independently.[3]

Medical diagnosis is not a good predictor of functional impairment, however, and individuals with the same diagnosis vary greatly in their functional status. For example, some individuals with heart disease, chronic respiratory disease, or degenerative osteoarthritis require 24-hour care, whereas others manage well on their own.

The prevalence of functional impairment increases greatly with age. According to a 1979 survey in the United States, 7 per cent of persons aged 65 to 74, 16 per cent of those aged 75 to 84, and 44 per cent of those over the age of 85 need the help of another person in one or more self-care or instrumental activities of daily living.[4]

Elderly people often measure their own health in terms of functional ability. They may say that they are in good health when they are able to function independently in spite of underlying chronic diseases. Likewise, they may fear the frailty and dependency associated with functional impairment more than the effect of specific diseases.[5-6]

In some cases, medical technologies can cure or substantially alleviate chronic diseases that cause functional impairment, but cures are not available for most of the chronic conditions that affect elderly people. Technologies that do not cure disease can, nevertheless, improve an individual's functional status. Thus, assistive devices that compensate for functional impairments can help an individual to remain independent despite underlying disease conditions. Devices that allow a person to bathe, dress, and feed himself or herself independently, for example, can lessen functional impairment although the disease that caused the functional impairment is not affected.

Even relatively small improvements in functioning can make an important difference in people's lives. For example, an individual with severe tremor due to Parkinson's disease can continue to feed himself using devices such as splints and special eating utensils, thus avoiding the need to be fed and associated feelings of dependence and loss of control.

Assistive devices range from such simple devices as a long-handled soaper that allows an individual with limited arm motion to bathe himself to such highly sophisticated devices as voice-controlled robots for bedridden patients. Some examples of assistive devices to compensate for common functional impairments of elderly people are shown in Table 31.1.

Despite the availability of thousands of assistive devices, several problems limit their use by elderly people. First, some elderly people suffer from multiple chronic diseases with resulting functional impairments. This affects the kinds of assistive devices they can use effectively because assistive devices are often designed to compensate for functional impairment by substituting one ability for another. Such substitution is difficult when a person has multiple impairments.[7] For example, an elderly individual who cannot walk because of an amputation, hip fracture, or

Table 31.1 Examples of assistive devices for the functionally impaired elderly[a]

Impairment	Simple devices	Complex devices
Vision	Lighted magnifying glass Large-print books	Electronic reading machine that converts printed material to speech
Hearing	Hand-held speaking tube or horn	Infrared hearing system that transfers an audio signal via infrared light beam to a receiver worn by the listener, thus suppressing background noise that is a problem for hearing aid users
Speech	Manual communication board; the individual points to a symbol of what he wants to say	Electronic communication board with memory and print-out capability. The individual uses a switch to activate a cursor on the board to indicate words or messages. Portable speech synthesizer
Memory	Pad to keep notes for reminders	Clock radio system that verbalizes reminders and automatically controls some appliances
Mobility	Braces and splints	Computerized electrical impulse device to stimulate muscles and allow paralysed persons to walk
	Canes, walkers, and wheelchairs	Voice-controlled, electric wheelchair that can open doors and manipulate switches
	Ramps	Electric chairlift for stairs
Upper extremity weakness	Reachers and grippers Levers to facilitate turning door knobs and faucet handles	Prosthetic control system using electronic sensors and mechanical transducers to operate a prosthetic arm

Bathing	Shower or bathtub chair Long-handled soaper	Hydraulic bath lift Horizontal shower
Dressing	Velcro fasteners Clothing that opens in front	No complex devices known
Eating	Utensils with built-up handles	Automatic feeding machine
Toileting	Bedside commode	Commode with automatic toilet flusher, warm water bidet and hot air drying in a push-button unit
Shopping	Shopping cart for a wheelchair user Prepackaged, freeze-dried meals	Shopping by computer
Cooking	Suction gripper to hold a jar to be opened	Robot that can prepare meals
Environmental control	Switches and controls on extension cords that can be reached by the patient	Computerized remote environmental control system to allow a bed- or chair-bound patient to adjust lights, radios, TVs, thermostats, and other electrically controlled appliances

[a] These devices were selected to illustrate the kinds of assistive devices that are available. Thousands of other devices are also available.

osteoarthritis may not have the stamina to use crutches or a walker because he or she also has cardiac or respiratory disease.

Careful assessment of a person's functional impairments and residual strengths is a prerequisite for matching the individual and appropriate devices. Locating devices for a person with multiple impairments also requires a wide knowledge of the devices that are available. For a family member, friend, or health care provider with good intentions but no specific knowledge of available devices, this can be a frustrating process. It is likely that many assistive devices purchased for elderly individuals with multiple impairments are never used because the individual lacks the residual abilities needed to use them.

Physiological changes that occur with normal aging can also affect an elderly person's ability to use some assistive devices. These changes include decreases in visual acuity, hearing, touch sensitivity, fine motor control, and grip strength. Although these changes may not limit the functioning of a healthy elderly person, they can lessen that person's capacity to compensate for impairments resulting from acute or chronic disease.[8] For example, decreased grip strength may not interfere with the functioning of the healthy elderly person but can hamper the ability of a mobility-impaired individual to use a cane or grab-bars effectively. Awareness of the physiological effects of normal aging is essential for the design of assistive devices and the selection of appropriate devices for elderly people.

The impact of cognitive impairment on the ability of elderly people to use assistive devices has received little research attention, although anecdotal evidence indicates that it is an important factor. Persons who are confused as a result of Alzheimer's or other diseases that cause dementia may not be able to learn to use assistive devices such as walkers, hearing aids, or simple devices for dressing, bathing, or eating. Sometimes it is even difficult for them to remember what the device is for. Failure of caregivers to assess an older person's cognitive ability in addition to his or her other functional abilities may result in the purchase of inappropriate devices.

Negative beliefs about the inevitable mental and physical deterioration of elderly people are widespread, and the sense of hopelessness that often results from these beliefs is a significant barrier to the use of assistive devices. On the one hand, because of these negative stereotypes, some elderly persons resist thinking of themselves as old and deny impairments that they think make them seem old. They may refuse to use assistive devices such as canes, walkers, and hearing aids that call attention to impairments, even though use of these devices might help them to function independently. Other elderly people, especially those who are suffering from debilitating acute or chronic illnesses, accept the negative stereotypes, regard themselves as old, and lose hope about eventual recovery or rehabilitation.[7] In this state of mind, they are not receptive to suggestions about devices that could improve their functioning and quality of life.

Family and friends of disabled elderly persons can be an important source of motivation and concrete assistance in obtaining assistive devices and helping the elderly person to learn to use them. Family and friends who accept the stereotyped view that mental and physical deterioration is inevitable in aging are unlikely to offer encouragement and assistance in obtaining such devices, however.

Some health care professionals and others who work with elderly people share society's negative stereotypes about the elderly. As a result, they may not recommend assistive devices that could benefit the older person.

Ongoing difficulties in the production, marketing, funding, and repair of assistive devices also restrict access to and use of these technologies by elderly people. Some potentially useful devices are invented but never produced or marketed because companies are reluctant to invest in manufacturing a device without an identifiable market for it. In some cases, the number of people who could benefit from a certain device is relatively low, and potential users are difficult to identify. Small companies that are frequently the source of innovative products may lack the financial or staff resources to launch the kind of marketing campaign needed to reach potential users.[9]

Lack of information about assistive devices is an ongoing problem. Computerized data systems and catalogues of devices have been developed to solve the problem, but the information gap persists. Researchers complain that this results in frequent instances of 're-inventing the wheel'. Elderly people, their families, and service providers continue to have difficulty finding out about appropriate technologies. Meanwhile, companies with innovative products struggle to find ways to make people aware of them.

Lack of funding also restricts access to potentially beneficial assistive devices. Although some devices are inexpensive, many are expensive, sometimes because of the cost of designing and marketing products for a relatively small number of potential users or because of the cost of adapting a device to meet the needs of a given individual.

In the United States, the public programmes that pay for medical care for elderly people do not cover many kinds of assistive devices. Furthermore, public and private programmes that do pay for assistive devices have uncoordinated and inconsistent definitions of who is eligible and what devices will be paid for. Decisions about whether a device is covered under a certain programme may vary from one part of the country to another and are sometimes made retro-actively, so that neither the individual nor the provider knows in advance whether the device will be paid for.[10]

Lastly, difficulties in obtaining repair services for devices such as hearing aids and wheelchairs limit their usefulness. Repairs sometimes take weeks or even months and are often costly. Replacement parts are hard to find. For someone who is dependent on the device for an important functional disability, the time spent waiting for repair of the device can be very difficult.[11]

The many problems in development, adaptation, diffusion, and access to assistive devices for elderly people suggest a need for government initiatives in several areas: basic research on normal aging and diseases that cause functional impairment; applied research on assistive devices to compensate for functional impairment; public education about such devices; manpower and training programmes to increase the availability of persons qualified to assess functional impairment, identify appropriate devices, and help elderly people obtain and learn to use them; and increased public funding for the devices. In the United States, both government and non-government agencies and groups are involved in testing assistive devices and evaluating their safety, quality, and effectiveness. These important functions require greater co-ordination and the commitment of more public and private resources.

LIFE-SUSTAINING TECHNOLOGIES AND THE ELDERLY

In the past few decades, the discovery and development of life-sustaining medical technologies have been followed by rapid expansion in their availability and use. As equipment and procedures have been refined and experience accumulated, the clinical criteria guiding use have been broadened. The types of patients who become candidates for life-sustaining technologies have changed, and their numbers have increased sharply.

OTA's study *Life-sustaining technologies and the elderly*[2] focuses on five technologies: cardiopulmonary resuscitation (CPR), mechanical ventilation, dialysis, tube and intravenous feeding, and antibiotic therapy. It discusses the outcomes of the treatments for elderly people, modifications that might improve outcome, and manpower and funding issues. As use of the technologies has increased, so has concern about inappropriate use for patients who may not want the technologies or do not benefit from them and for whom suffering may be prolonged. Thus, OTA's study also addresses questions about how decisions are made on the use of the

Table 31.2 Utilization of life-sustaining technologies for patients of all ages, and for elderly patients, in all settings combined, United States 1985[a2]

	Total number of patients (all ages)	Patients over age 65	
		Number	% of total
Dialysis[b]	90 621	27 641	31
Resuscitation (CPR)[c]	370 000 to 750 000	204 000 to 413 000	55 (est.)
Mechanical ventilation	3 755[d] to 6 575[e]	1 250[d] to 2 200[e,f]	34
Nutritional support[a]	1 404 500	680 000	48 (est.)
enteral (tube)	848 100	450 000	53 (est.)
parenteral (intravenous)	556 400	230 000	40 (est.)

[a] 1984 industry data and contractor estimates.
[b] 1985 HCFA data for ESRD Program.
[c] Contractor estimates, hospitalized patients only.
[d] 1985 data for 37 States, patients dependent on ventilator 14 days or longer.
[e] National estimates extrapolated from survey in Massachusetts.
[f] Elderly defined as over 70.

technologies and whether patients are sufficiently involved in the decision-making process.[2]

In the United States, elderly people constitute a large proportion of all people who receive these technologies. As indicated in Table 31.2, more than half of all patients who receive CPR and tube feeding, and about one-third of patients who receive mechanical ventilation, dialysis, and TPN (an intravenous feeding procedure), are over the age of 65.

It is often assumed that elderly people will not do well on these technologies. In fact, mortality is high for people of all ages who receive life-sustaining technologies, but outcome is difficult to predict in individual cases. As a group, elderly people are more likely than younger adults to die or to develop serious complications of treatment, but age by itself is not a good predictor of outcome. The best predictor is a patient's physiological status—particularly whether he or she suffers from multiple acute or chronic diseases. Elderly people vary greatly in their physiological status, as stated earlier, and many elderly people who receive life-sustaining technologies do as well or better than younger patients. Thus, age is a poor basis for treatment decisions.

Modification of equipment and procedures to reflect physiological changes that occur with normal aging might improve the outcome of life-sustaining technologies for some elderly people, but OTA found little evidence that such modifications are made. Age-related changes in drug metabolism are now well recognized, for example, but antibiotic doses and dose intervals are generally standard regardless of a patient's age. Similarly, although it is well established that nutritional requirements change with age, these changes are not well understood, and most tube-fed patients, especially in nursing homes, receive standard, prepackaged formulas that are not adjusted to reflect individual needs. For CPR, mechanical ventilation, and dialysis, the possibility that clinical outcomes for elderly patients might be improved if modifications were made either in the equipment or in procedures has received relatively little attention.

In many instances, appropriate modifications would require greater understanding than is now available about physiological aspects of aging and the mechanisms of acute and chronic diseases in the elderly. Modifications to the technologies for elderly patients would also require more physicians, nurses, and allied health professionals who are trained in both geriatrics and in the use of the technologies, or greater use of treatment teams in the care of elderly patients.

One of the most important developments in life-sustaining technologies in the last 10 years is the increased feasibility of providing them outside hospital intensive care units. All the technologies OTA studied can now be safely provided for some patients in general hospital units, nursing homes, or their own home. Care outside a hospital requires, however, that support services are available and that the physical environment is suitable. Moreover, equipment for home use must be easy to operate, reliable, self-monitoring, and generally smaller and lighter than hospital equipment. Recent advances in computerization, communication systems, and miniaturization have allowed the development of equipment appropriate for home use.

Life-sustaining technologies are expensive. In 1985, in the United States, the cost of mechanical ventilation for a hospitalized patient (including the cost of hospitalization) averaged about $850 a day, and TPN averaged $196 (not including the cost of hospitalization). For patients at home the technologies can cost $12 000 to $200 000 a year. Moreover, the cost of the technologies is sometimes only a small part of the cost of caring for severely debilitated patients whose lives they have extended.

Some people believe that expensive life-sustaining technologies are wasted on elderly patients. Yet rationing these technologies on the basis of age would clearly result in the deaths of many people who could survive with a quality of life that is acceptable to them. Research on factors that affect treatment outcome is needed to provide information to assist patients, families, physicians, and others in making treatment decisions.

Decisions about the use of life-sustaining technologies for some patients—notably those who are terminally ill, severely debilitated, or in persistent vegetative state—raise difficult legal and ethical dilemmas. In hospitals and nursing homes, many people are involved in caring for a patient. These individuals have different values, beliefs, and experiences that can lead to intense disagreement about treatment decisions. Currently in the United States, decisions about tube or intravenous feeding engender the most controversy.

Some hospital and nursing homes have institutional ethics committees to assist with difficult treatment decisions. Others have formal policies that define required and/or recommended decision-making procedures for the facility. At present, most such policies address only decisions about CPR. Institutional policies for decisions about other life-sustaining technologies are also needed.

Government initiatives to support appropriate use of life-sustaining technologies and improve quality of care include: basic research on aspects of normal aging and acute and chronic diseases that affect the use of the technologies, applied research on modifications of the technologies to meet the needs of elderly patients and to adapt technologies for home use, manpower and training programmes to familiarize health care professionals and others with the special needs of elderly patients who receive the technologies, and regulation of the safety and reliability of the equipment, particularly if it is intended for use in the home. The potential role of government in encouraging hospitals and nursing homes to develop formal institutional policies for decision-making is the subject of another OTA report published in the summer of 1988.

TECHNOLOGIES FOR MEDICAL AND LONG-TERM CARE OF PERSONS WITH DEMENTIA

In the United States, an estimated 1.5 million people suffer from severe dementia—that is, they are so incapacitated that others must care for them continually. An additional 1–5 million have mild or moderate dementia. Prevalence increases with age, from about 1 per cent of those aged 65–74 to 7 per cent of those aged 75–84, and 25 per cent of those over the age of 85. Ten times as many people are affected now as were at the turn of the century, and the number is expected to increase by 60 per cent by the year 2000 (see Fig. 31.1).

More than 70 diseases and conditions can cause dementia. A few of them can be reversed with treatment, but truly reversible dementia occurs only in a small proportion of cases. Most diseases that cause dementia are not reversible with available treatments. Alzheimer's disease, which

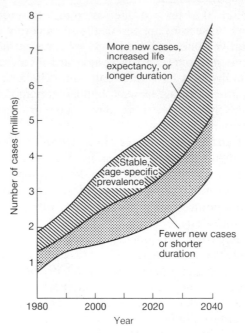

Fig. 31.1 Current and projected cases of severe dementia in the United States, 1980–2040.[12]

accounts for more than 60 per cent of all cases, is the prime example.

The ultimate solution for the problem of dementia is a 'technical fix'—a fully effective way to prevent all dementing diseases, or a drug or surgical procedure to reverse their symptoms. There is no assurance that such a solution is possible at all, and it is certainly not likely in the next several years. In the mean time, methods must be developed to care for those who now have dementia or will develop it before there are technical means to prevent it or reverse its symptoms.[3]

Although most diseases that cause dementia are not reversible, the condition is treatable. A system of care for dementia includes several components: patients must be medically evaluated; any coexisting illnesses must be identified and treated; the severity of the dementia, associated functional impairments, and residual strengths of patients must be assessed; care needs must be identified; and services to maintain patients' functioning and support family caregivers must be located, arranged, and paid for.

Medical management of persons with dementia begins with an accurate diagnosis. A consensus statement developed at a 1987 conference sponsored by the US National Institutes of Health[13] describes accepted procedures for differential diagnosis of dementing diseases. Accurate diagnosis is important both to rule out reversible causes of dementia and to give families and other caregivers a basis for understanding the patient's condition and planning for his or her future care needs.

Medical management also includes treatment for any coexisting physical or emotional conditions that may exacerbate a patient's cognitive deficit and further impair his or her functioning. Dementia is most prevalent among the very old, who are also at greatest risk of multiple acute and chronic diseases that can cause excess disability and complicate their care. Younger patients are also at risk, however. All persons with dementia need ongoing medical supervision.

Comprehensive assessment of a patient's cognitive deficits, self-care abilities, and behaviour provides information about the severity of the patient's condition and is essential in determining care needs. A variety of assessment technologies have been developed specifically for dementia patients. Many include measures of caregiver burden and evaluation of the patient's physical environment and social support system.

All persons with dementia eventually require supervision and personal care. Families and friends provide such care informally for most patients, and some patients never use any paid services. Other patients have no family or friends who are able and willing to provide care, and many patients require paid services in addition to the care that family and friends can give.

Support for families and other informal caregivers is an important component of treatment of many dementia patients. Although lip service has been paid to the concept of paid services to support family caregivers, only in the past 5 years has that concept been realized to any extent in the care of elderly people in the United States. One form of family support is respite care, including any services that provide supervision and personal care for the patient so that the primary caregiver is temporarily relieved of caregiving responsibilities. A second example is family support groups, which give informal caregivers an opportunity to discuss problems, share feelings, and learn about health and long-term care agencies and services in their communities.

In the United States, respite care programmes and family support groups have been initiated primarily by voluntary groups, notably chapters of the Alzheimer's Disease and Related Disorders Association. Public and private agencies are now beginning to experiment with provision of these innovative services.

An increasing number of nursing homes, adult day care centres, board and care facilities, and even hospitals are developing specialized services for persons with Alzheimer's disease and other diseases that cause dementia. These specialized services generally consist of a staff that is trained to care for dementia patients, adaptations to the physical care setting, and activities designed for cognitively impaired people.

Specialized services for dementia patients are not yet widely available in the United States. In 1987, for example, only about 2 per cent of nursing home residents with dementia were in special care units. There is still no consensus about appropriate structural or organizational principles for specialized services, and philosophies and methods for administering them differ markedly. The ferment caused by the development of specialized services is resulting in innovative care techniques, however, and may eventually raise the standard of care generally by focusing attention on the needs of these patients.

Provision of high-quality medical and long-term care for persons with dementia presumes the availability of trained staff. Yet, the sudden increase in awareness of dementia and the care needs of dementia patients means that most of those who care for persons with dementia have no specialized training.

Another obstacle to high-quality treatment for these patients in the USA is the lack of adequate public and private funding for comprehensive assessment, family support services, and many specialized long-term care services. A third obstacle is lack of an effective information and referral system whereby patients, families, and others could be referred to knowledgeable professionals and appropriate services.

A final obstacle to the development of high-quality systems for treating dementia patients is a sense of futility among some health care professionals, government officials, and others about the process of caring for people with irreversible, progressive dementia, many of whom are very old. Fortunately for these patients, many of their families refuse to give up. The political pressure created by these families in the past decade has resulted in greatly increased government spending for biomedical and health services research and increased, although still inadequate, funding for necessary services. The next step is the development of an effective service delivery system and technologies for assuring quality of care.

References

1. US Congress, Office of Technology Assessment (1985). *Technology and aging in America*. US Government Printing Office, Washington, DC.
2. US Congress, Office of Technology Assessment (1987). *Life-sustaining technologies and the elderly*. US Government Printing Office, Washington, DC.
3. US Congress, Office of Technology Assessment (1987). *Losing a million minds: confronting the tragedy of Alzheimer's disease and other dementias*. US Government Printing Office, Washington, DC.
4. US Department of Health and Human Services (1983). Americans needing help to function at home, National Center for Health Statistics, *Advancedata*, no. 92.

5. Kutza, E. A. (1983). Overview. Unpublished report prepared for the Office of Technology Assessment, November 1983.
6. Mezey, M., (1983). Letter to the Office of Technology Assessment.
7. Bruer, J. M. (1982). *A handbook of assistive devices for the handicapped elderly*. Haworth Press, New York.
8. Baker, G. T. and Krauser, C. K. (1982). *A catalogue of products and services to enhance the independence of the elderly*. Drexel University, Philadelphia, PA.
9. LaRocca, J. and Turen, J. (1978). *The application of technological developments to physically disabled people*. The Urban Institute, Washington, DC.
10. Mittlemann, M. and Settele, J. (1982). Insurance reimbursement mechanisms for rehabilitation equipment and environmental modifications. *Archives of Physical Medicine and Rehabilitation*, **63**, 279–83.
11. Corcoran, P. J. (1982). Independent living in Berkeley and the Bay Area of California. In *Technology for independent living* (ed. Stern, V. W. and M. R. Redden) pp. 41–5. American Association for the Advancement of Science, Washington, DC.
12. Cross, P. S. and Gurland, B. J. (1986). *The epidemiology of dementing disorders*. Contract report prepared for the Office of Technology Assessment.
13. National Institutes of Health (1987). Differential diagnosis of dementing diseases, *Consensus Development Conference Statement*, **6** (3).

32

Assessing the impact of introducing new technologies and interventions for the elderly

HENK A. BECKER

INTRODUCTION

In most developed and developing countries the 'greying of society' has become recognized by now as one of the major problems for years to come. Demographical data have been extrapolated and the costs for the cure and care of the elderly have been estimated. Some countries will experience this rise in costs relatively early and heavily, while others still have some time to get accustomed to this development, or will undergo the 'greying' to a relatively light degree only. Table 32.1 summarizes the prospects for a number of countries.

An overview as given in Fig. 32.1 does not take an important aspect into account, however: the elderly of the future will differ markedly from the elderly of our times. Let us look at some examples. People born in the 1930s have been in their formative years during or shortly after World War II. Each new cohort in the West born in the 1930s enters the category of the elderly (at 55) with more formal education than its predecessors. The new elderly belong to the generation that has profited substantially from the golden years of economic prosperity (1955–1965). Members of this generation on the average have had speedy careers, they have been able to become owners of a house while relatively young, and their old-age pensions are relatively favourable. We are speaking about a generation that has practised physical exercise in a considerable way, and therefore enjoys a relatively favourable mental and physical condition. Religious affiliations are less pronounced than in former generations. Many individuals born between 1930 and 1940 know how to handle products of modern technology like the personal computer. In short: the elderly of the near future will differ from the elderly we are used to. There are social science publications for those who want to study this in more detail.[2]

The characteristics of birth cohorts have a direct relationship with the main theme of this paper: assessing the impact of introducing new technologies and interventions for the elderly. How will the elderly in the cohorts concerned react to new technological opportunities? Which new technologies are on their way? Some examples are:

Table 32.1 Ranking of countries by size of population 65 years of age and over, 1980 and 2000 (thousands)[1]

Ranking	1980		2000	
1	China	53 924	China	85 747
2	USSR	26 659	India	38 332
3	USA	24 928	USSR	37 471
4	India	20 729	USA	31 822
5	Japan	10 275	Japan	18 037
6	Federal Republic of Germany	8 842	Italy	9 978
7	United Kingdom	7 817	Indonesia	9 521
8	France	7 102	Brazil	9 461
9	Italy	6 782	Federal Republic of Germany	9 216
10	Brazil	4 395	United Kingdom	8 465
11	Indonesia	3 761	France	8 111
12	Spain	3 571	Spain	6 188
13	Poland	3 245	Poland	4 975
14	German Democratic Republic	2 737	Mexico	4 535
15	Mexico	2 470	Bangladesh	4 365
16	Argentina	2 321	Pakistan	4 240
17	Canada	2 174	Nigeria	3 978
18	Bangladesh	2 097	Turkey	3 898
19	Pakistan	2 071	Argentina	3 441
20	Romania	2 039	Viet Nam	3 383
21	Nigeria	1 891	Yugoslavia	3 319
22	Yugoslavia	1 837	Romania	3 303
23	Turkey	1 810	Canada	3 200
24	Czechoslovakia	1 792	Republic of Korea	3 015
25	Viet Nam	1 642	Thailand	2 991
26	Phillipines	1 591	Egypt	2 986
27	Egypt	1 488	Phillipines	2 929
28	Netherlands	1 473	German Democratic Republic	2 479
29	Belgium	1 362	Burma	2 422
30	Hungary	1 332	South Africa	2 234
31	Republic of Korea	1 252	Czechoslovakia	2 152
32	Sweden	1 239	Netherlands	2 010
33	Thailand	1 238	Iran	1 948
34	Australia	1 183	Australia	1 937
35	Burma	1 133	Greece	1 687
36	Austria	1 126	Colombia	1 666
37	Greece	1 108	Hungary	1 641
38	Iran	1 084	Zaire	1 555
39	Bulgaria	952	Belgium	1 546
40	Portugal	930	Bulgaria	1 509

	Context A (a future society with prosperity developing according to recent trends)	Context B (a future society with substantially more prosperity)	Context C (a future society with substantially less prosperity)
1. Characteristics of the context in more detail			
2. Characteristics of the 'focal system' (the elderly in society for instance)			
3. Characteristics of the innovation proposed (home monitoring for the elderly for instance)	Modest version of the innovation	Bold attempt at leap ahead	Very limited version would be possible only
4. Implementation of the innovation (how will the diffusion be attempted?)	Modest activities to introduce	Large-scale introduction possible	Only volunteers available for the introduction
5. Consequences of contexts on focal system (effects and side-effects)			
6. Consequences of innovation on focal system (effects and side-effects)			
7. Conclusions (is innovation to be introduced at all? which priorities? which adaptations? which safeguards?			

Comments: the reader is invited to elaborate the exercise by filling up each cell. A considerable number of rounds of filling up and correcting is necessary, maybe five to ten. Try alternatives: for instance, what would be the consequences of a bold strategy under the conditions of Context C?

Fig. 32.1 Format for assessing the impacts of innovations by using instant scenario analysis.

—— home care technology;[3, 4]

—— intelligent protheses, more or less self-regulating;[5]

—— communication technology enabling the elderly to live on their own for a longer period of time than is possible now.[5]

Each of these examples shows some aspect of 'physical' technology, but on the other hand none of these innovations would have an impact if the elderly concerned would refuse to take advantage of them. We also need 'social' technology to facilitate the diffusion of the innovations.

Each time an innovation is considered we have to explore the effects and side-effects to be expected first. A problem analysis is required, in order to get a preliminary insight into the innovative process that we want to initiate. This problem analysis has to tell us also whether a 'high' or a 'low' impact is to be expected. An assumption about the kind of impact is necessary in order to decide in a systematic way which kind of assessment and diffusion of the innovation we need. Small-scale, medium-scale, and large-scale approaches to the preparation of innovations are available. Ultimately we have to consider which perspectives we face with regard to these kinds of future research related to the care for the elderly.

The questions to be answered in this chapter are: (1) how do we accomplish a problem analysis prior to the introduction of new technologies and inventions for the elderly? (section 2); (2) how do we handle a small-scale, medium-scale, or large-scale assessment and diffusion process related to the introduction of new technologies and inventions for the elderly? (sections 3 and 4); (3) how could we improve our capabilities to innovate for the benefit of the elderly? (section 5).

PROBLEM ANALYSIS

Proposals, actors, and interests

The first thing we have to do is take a careful look at the innovation that is proposed. Is it just one proposal or are we confronted with a whole complex of innovations? In this way a number of questions have to be asked.[6] Next we have to look at the actors involved, and their interests. How do those interests affect the consequences of the innovation that is proposed? In order to focus the discussion in this and the following paragraphs I shall take one specific example as a starting point: home monitoring. As Banta[3] pointed out home monitoring could become common especially for the elderly. Imagine an elderly person of 75, still living on his or her own but going to need 'a watching eye'. Nowadays an elderly person in this situation would have to go to a home for the aged.

Home monitoring would give him a chance to stay in his own appartment for some more years. This involves electronic surveyance equipment, cameras, and a monitoring team able to arrange for help as soon as it is needed by the monitored persons. Not only the elderly themselves but other actors would be interested also. For instance, government will be interested in the question, to which extent home monitoring would lower the costs of caring for the elderly. But experts warn that home care technology in general, if adequately introduced and managed, might be not less expensive than care in a hospital or a nursing home. Neighbours, members of the family of the elderly person, and his or her friends are involved also. With a little help from them, perhaps the monitoring would become a success.

Predictability of the processes involved

Of course the best basis for taking decisions in situations like these are prognoses. A prognosis is a statement about future events given in numerical terms, based upon regularities found in the past and related to an explanatory model. Only a few statements about future processes meet these requirements, however. Processes in social life as a rule show 'disorder' (also called 'chaos' or 'systems noise') to such an extent that prognoses often are not feasible. Recent analyses of social developments provide arguments for this pessimistic view.[7] If a relatively large amount of disorder reigns, futures research has to adopt other approaches than prognoses. Present research starts by formulating assumptions, as plausible as possible, and next studies future processes by performing 'simulations' on a model of the social system whose future interests us. Nowadays exploration of the future along these lines is often done by applying scenario projects. The methodology of scenario projects will be introduced in the next paragraph.

Expected impact of the processes involved

If developments have a low impact only, and their probability is low, nobody will bother to assess impacts. In social life, developments as a rule belong to one of the following categories, however: 'high probability, high impact' or 'low probability, high impact'. A new branch of policy-oriented social research has been developed—impact assessment—to provide early warnings to policy makers and other actors involved.[8, 9] With regards to home technology this new field of research will have to accomplish a 'technology assessment', in a restricted or an elaborate way, as we shall see later.

Is innovation as planned change feasible?

Of course installing home monitoring would be useless if the elderly refused to take advantage of it. As soon as the intrusion upon their privacy irritated them, they could just hang a towel on the camera and restore their privacy. To what extent can social scientists predict the effects of planned social change? Rogers has evaluated more than three thousand cases of 'diffusion of innovation' and has elaborated general conclusions and guidelines.[10] We have enough experience now to estimate the chance of success whenever we consider embarking upon a new attempt to innovate.

Type of assessment and diffusion

Policy-oriented social research to prepare and introduce an innovation (like home monitoring for the elderly) consists of assessment (estimating effects and side-effects) and diffusion (assisting in the implementation of the innovation). Policy-oriented research like this can be done by *instant projects* (taking less than one man-week to accomplish), *mini projects* (up to 1 man-year), *medium-scale projects* (1 to 5 man-years), and *large-scale projects* (more than 5 man-years). If little impact is expected, instant or mini projects are appropriate. If research has to be done under pressure of time, for instance during negotiations, instant or mini projects might do also. If the innovation has to be elaborated first, considerable impacts are foreseen, and diffusion of the innovation may prove difficult, medium- or large-scale projects are required. Of course small-scale projects (for instance a mini project) can be used to prepare the ground for a larger project. Under extreme conditions, for instance in developing countries with little financial resources and no specialized manpower, a small-scale project may be the only feasible approach, even in a situation that in fact requires a large-scale assessment and diffusion of a specific innovation.

SMALL- AND MEDIUM-SCALE ASSESSMENT AND DIFFUSION

Instant assessment projects

Let us suppose that a policy maker has not more than 1 week to prepare an opinion on a proposal for the introduction of home monitoring, and that not more than one scientist is available to do this assessment. In this case a quick survey of the literature available, a small number (perhaps three) of group discussions with experts, and an analysis 'with pencil and paper' is about all that could be accomplished. An outline of a format for an assessment along these lines is given in Fig. 32.1. The scheme contains the basic elements for a scenario project.

The steps we take in a small scenario project can be summarized as follows. We start with a short problem analysis. Next a number of contextual scenarios are elaborated (as a rule, three contexts are sufficient). The focal system is described (in our example the elderly in society). The innovation proposed is described, often elaborating alternative versions fitting the contexts. The implementation of the innovation is made explicit. Next the consequences of the contexts on the focal system and the innovation on it are elaborated, taking effects and side-effects (both positive and negative) into account. Then the innovation and its implementation are analysed with regard to their relevance and feasibility, as a rule adapting the original version of the innovation and its implementation until they fit each of the contextual scenarios. Ultimately the policy maker makes up his or her mind and takes a decision. In instant assessment projects, public participation is not feasible. Neither is assisting in the diffusion process.

Mini assessment projects

In the next type of assessment a bit more time and resources are available. If one expert works for 1 year, or three experts co-operate for 4 months, for instance, a project can be launched that provides a survey of expert opinion on a broader basis than in the instant project. Now, for instance, a small Delphi project is feasible. The Delphi method was developed in the 1950s in order to replace 'brainstorming' with a more sophisticated approach. A Delphi project implies that the respondents are interviewed (as a rule by mail questionnaire) separately. Let us look at such a project using three rounds of questioning. In the first round, the respondents reply to open questions, providing an exploration of the subject matter to be studied. The answers are analysed and each participant is given an overview of the answers, but without the names of participants. In the second round, questions are asked that are more focused. For instance, in which year is an innovation expected? Again all participants get an overview of all the answers, but in an anonymous way. The participants are invited to revise their answers. The third round of the Delphi project brings questions that are still more focused. As a rule the ultimate results show a high degree not only of sophistication but also of consensus between the participants.

What use could be made of a mini assessment in preparing an innovation regarding the health of the elderly? If the elderly need help, younger people have less and less time available. Intergenerational solidarity is waning, and might even disappear altogether. On the other hand a lot of elderly persons are capable of helping other people of their own age, and a sizeable number of the elderly are willing to do so. Such intragenerational solidarity among the elderly might be stimulated, and perhaps in the future elderly people helping each other will develop into a substantial resource. If an elderly person still living on his own and relying on home monitoring could be assured that as soon as help is needed a person living nearby will come to his rescue, the willingness to stay in one's apartment would be high. Exploring the ins and outs of a home monitoring system in some detail could be accomplished in a Delphi project demanding up to 1 man-year and relying on the knowledge of a large number of experts (perhaps including insiders from the group of the elderly themselves). In a project like this, assisting in the process of diffusion of the innovation will not be possible because of lack of manpower.

Medium-scale assessments

Banta assessed the '*Potentials for home care technology*'[4] in a medium-sized subproject of his larger study. As we have already mentioned, he expects that these technologies will become common especially for the elderly. In the field of diagnosis the major change that he envisions in the future is more diagnosis in the home using kits, either by a health care provider or by the patient him- or herself. A number of kits will be marketed directly to the public. This move promotes autonomy, but it also has dangers. Lay people are not taught to perform tests, nor to interpret their results. With regard to clinical monitoring, self-monitoring by the patient might include diabetes and hypertension (high blood-pressure). The monitoring of hypertension is relatively simple: it takes about 20 minutes for a nurse to explain the principles and train the patient. In the field of treatment, Banta assesses home parenteral nutrition, drug delivery systems, cancer chemotherapy, management of respiratory failure, and renal and peritoneal dialyses.

   Technologies may be addressed to improving functioning also. In this field, prosthetics are analysed. Also telecommunications and computers in home care receive attention. Banta concludes that, in general, special attention needs to be paid to the relations between people and devices used in the home (the 'man–machine interface'). Equipment used in the home needs to be specially designed for easy use and it needs to be particularly reliable. Little is known about the effects of equipment use in the home, especially medical equipment such as dialysis machines and respirators. The selection of patients and the human support for effective use need much attention. Devices have to be designed that avoid errors in use and do not need much strength to handle. Special attention has to be paid to maintenance and the availability of spare parts. If the report by Banta were to be discussed in workshops and explained to the public at large, especially the elderly, assessment and diffusion would go hand in hand. A medium-scale project can indeed combine both aspects of the innovation process.

LARGE-SCALE ASSESSMENT AND DIFFUSION

An example in detail

The most relevant example comes from the field of mental health research and development. Fairweather and his colleagues[11] have undertaken studies during a period of more than 20 years in an attempt to discover what could be done about the problem of increasing chronic hospitalization that has constantly plagued the mental hospitals in the United States and in other countries. In an initial survey they found that 39 per cent of the patients stayed in hospital for more than 90 days, with a high likelihood of rather permanent residence. A second project was a quasi-experiment comparing patients who stayed less than 90 days with those who remained for a longer period. Persons who tended to remain in the hospital were more often single, diagnosed as psychotic, judged to be severly incapacitated upon entry, considered legally incompetent, and did not indulge in the use of alcoholic beverages. These five characteristics were used to predict length of stay with considerable accuracy.

The third project was an experiment comparing four treatment methods: (1) individual psychotherapy, (2) group therapy, (3) group living, and (4) a work-only programme. In the process of selecting participants, matching and randomization have been applied. The results of this study showed very clearly that the current treatment programmes available in the hospital setting yielded few if any more beneficial results than simply assigning an individual to preferred in-hospital work. Persons who were considered 'chronic patients' failed completely, regardless of the type of treatment they had had in hospital, so that 74 per cent had returned to a hospital setting by the end of 18 months.

From this study it seemed clear that a new type of programme needed to be innovated which would lead to a more adaptive community adjustment for long-term hospitalized patients. The fourth project consisted of small groups in treatment programmes. The idea had taken shape among the researchers that if small cohesive groups of mental patients could be developed in the hospital they might function to maintain each other in the community and thus lead to a reduction in recidivism and an improved adjustment in the community. The results of this study showed that the small-group social model enhanced all aspects of within-hospital adjustment contrasted with the traditional programme. However, these comparative differences disappeared when the patients lost their groups by returning to the community individually. The evidence further suggested that, unless new and supportive community conditions were created, the high return rate to the hospital would continue.

The fifth project was again an experiment. One social model linked the within-hospital small-group programme with traditional community health agencies. A second social model linked the within-hospital small-group programme with a newly created small society run by ex-patients (the Community Lodge), so that the hospital training would permit the continuation of cohesive small-group membership in the community. Even though the small group had been well trained in the hospital to care for its members and made reasonable and adequate decisions, the immediate move to the community was chaotic. The group decision process and organizational structure broke down, partly because it had been so closely linked to the hospital structure itself.

This led to the sixth project. New training procedures were introduced and the lodge society developed its own rules, its own work situation (gardening and janitor service), and gradually progressed through periods of staff-structured activities to the development of a cohesive, totally autonomous small society. The sixth project became a success. Following this project two replicates were established. Both replicates yielded positive results similar to those found for the original model.

Project seven brought a national dissemination experiment. An experimental design was created to compare the effectiveness of alternative approaches to inducing hospitals to adopt the lodge programme. To accomplish this, 255 mental hospitals were randomly assigned to different conditions of persuasion and supportive assistance. The experiment in which the hospitals were involved compared written brochures, face-to-face workshops, and social change agents in order to assess their effectiveness in persuasion. From this experiment, several principles of approaching, persuading, and activating social models were discovered and used as feedback to create another experiment (project eight) with those hospitals that did not accept that lodge model during the course of the seventh project.

Technological innovation for the elderly on a large scale

Major innovations like the introduction of various types of home care technology for the elderly[3, 4] demand large-scale projects for the preparation, assessment, and diffusion of the new hardware and software. The most important steps in such a major operation are: (1) further designing and testing, *inter alia* adaptation of devices for use by the elderly in a specific country, region, and social class; (2) diffusion on a small scale, using the methodology of experimental innovation, adapting the innovation until it is adequate; and (3) dissemination on a large scale, monitoring of the use of the new technology by the elderly, repeating information processes, and inducing the social network of the elderly to become involved. Major innovations in the medical field; for instance, basic research to find out more about the causes of epilepsy and to find pharmaceutical and surgical solutions to treatment problems regarding epilepsy demand series of projects lasting for 10 to 20 years. Major innovations in the field of developing, testing, and introducing new technology for home care of the elderly is an enterprise of about the same magnitude. The example described in the previous section illustrates the ups and downs to be expected.

Designing, testing, re-designing, and testing again...easy solutions do not last long as a rule. If we want reliable and precise knowledge about the needs of the elderly and their reaction to new technology, social experiments including control groups are necessary. The individuals participating in experiments have to be randomized and matched. Experiments like these abstract from the everyday institutionalized social setting of the elderly. Utilization of new technology ultimately will have to take place in everyday settings. This implies that abstract experiments have to be followed by try-outs in replicates, following the example of Fairweather and Tornatzky. Next, nationwide diffusion has to be taken care of. This huge task demands attention toward social and cultural differences among the elderly. As I pointed out in the beginning of this chapter, differences between birth cohorts (and generations as 'clusterings' of birth cohorts) have to be taken into consideration. We have to find the situations that evoke resistance to change. We have to find out also to what extent this resistance to change is a healthy reaction towards an innovation not yet adapted enough to specific situations. We have to enlist help from both individuals (members of the family, friends, neighbours) and organizations.

Special attention has to be paid to the category of the elderly with regard to try outs of new technologies, treatment, etc. on samples of the population in general. In these try-outs the elderly are often excluded for reasons of convenience; the research team responsible for the try-outs eliminates everybody older than 55 or 65 in order not to confound the analysis with complicated preconditions of participants. As a result of these eliminations, new technologies and therapies may be denied to the elderly because no research results are available with regard to side-effects on older individuals. Such biases produce a paradoxical situation in which older persons may be excluded from benefits for a technology or therapy because there is no evidence that the treatment or technology works for them, but there is no proof because they were eliminated from the tests.

Developing countries will find it hard to meet requirements like these. This implies that the developed countries will have to co-operate, for instance by taking responsibility for pilot projects. In the WHO strategy 'Health for all by the year 2000', examples can be found of co-operation between countries, some of them contributing pilot studies.[5]

PERSPECTIVES

A lot of knowledge and know-how necessary to assess and diffuse new technology for the elderly is available already. The diffusion of innovations[10] has been analysed in depth and new projects can profit from the experiences gained. Of course knowledge and know-how have not reached a final state, and never will reach. But nevertheless medical, technological, and social scientists do not face the challenges completely unprepared.

The expertise available is restricted to a small number of researchers and public servants, however. Only a few teams of experts are available. This shortage of manpower and institutes hampers the introduction of new technology for the elderly in developed and developing countries alike. If the present shortage of money and other resources continues, most of the prospects will have to be left unused. Unless international co-operation induces national governments to allocate the resources needed, no progress with regard to technological assistance of the elderly will be accomplished.

References

1. United Nations (1980). *Selected demographic indicators by country, 1950–2000; demographic estimates and projections as assessed in 1978.* Medium variant projections. UN Department or International Economic and Social Affairs.
2. Becker, H. A. (1987). *Generations and social inquality.* Van Arkel, Utrecht.
3. Banta, D. (ed.) (1987). *Anticipating and assessing health care technology*, Vols. I and II, p. 114. Martinus Nijhoff Publishers, Dordrecht.
4. Banta, D. (ed.) (1987). *Potentials for home care technology.* Martinus Nijhoff Publishers, Dordrecht.
5. Hollander, C. F. and Becker, H. A. (ed.) (1987). *Growing old in the future.* Martinus Nijhoff Publishers, Dordrecht.
6. Porter, A. L., Rossini, F. A. *et al.* (ed.) (1980). *A guidebook for technology assessment and impact analysis.* North Holland, New York.

7. Boudon, R. (1984). *La place du désordre*. Presses Universitaires de France, Paris.
8. Becker, H. A. and Porter, A. L. (eds.) (1986). *Methods and experiences in impact assessment*. Reidel, Dordrecht.
9. Becker, H. A. and Porter, A. L. (ed.) *Impact assessment today*, Vols. I and II. Van Arkel, Utrecht.
10. Rogers, E. M. (1983). *Diffusion of innovations*, (3rd edn). The Free Press, New York.
11. Fairweather, G. W. and Tornatzky, L. G. (1977). *Experimental methods for social policy research*. Pergamon, Oxford.

Further Reading

Dunning, A. J. and Wils, W. I. M. (ed.) 1987. *The heart of the future*, Vols. I and II. Martinus Nijhoff Publishers, Dordrecht.
Finsterbusch, K. and Motz, A. B., (1980). *Social research for policy decisions*. Wadsworth, Belmont.
Russell, L. B. (1979). *Technology in hospitals*. Brookings, Washington.

Part IV

Education and personnel needs

33
Introduction

D. MACFADYEN

SELF CARE

Health professionals are responsible for only a small proportion of the care given to elderly people. This applies to the whole range of care, from prevention to acute care, long-term care, and terminal care. The role of the professional carer is therefore 'enabling', that is to say fortifying of family and friends in their caring roles so that they may perform their supporting tasks with knowledge, confidence, and skill. The knowledge which families have as a basis for providing care comes from a growing literature of self-health care materials produced largely by volunteer organizations or by specific family support groups. In developing countries, family and lay care are the predominant forms of care. Despite this, few simply written texts are available for use in a developing country situation.

Day care is an important adjuvant to family care, especially in situations where women family members are in the formal work-force. It is exceptional to find that the aides who staff day care centres are trained, advised, or supported by health or social service professionals.

VALUES AND ATTITUDES

The values and attitudes of the society are reflected in the readiness of staff to elect to work with elderly people as a career of first choice. Where elderly people are valued, there is little difficulty in attracting able young persons to train and work in this area.

THE CARE SETTING

Very little training for elderly care is conducted in a multidisciplinary setting, despite the consensus that the care of elderly people demands the co-ordinated attention of many disciplines. While there is agreement on the desirability of expanding training sites, too few educational programmes offer training in non-institutional settings, especially those in which the trainee comes into contact with healthy and vigorous elderly people.

PEDAGOGY

Formulation of explicit educational objectives for professional training is most commonly encountered in nursing. Appraisals of the achievement of attitudinal and performance objectives are rarely used in assessing student competence.

RESEARCH

Manpower planning can ease the adjustments which the new aging countries are having to make in order to provide effective care to the increasing number of elderly citizens. Estimates of future manpower needs are aided by research on health and social status such as that being conducted in a number of countries with support from the World Health Organization.

GERIATRIC SPECIALISTS AND ACADEMIC LEADERSHIP

All health personnel in primary care and all specialists, save those in child health or paediatrics, should learn how to meet the health needs of elderly people. Where it is affordable, specialist geriatric expertise is an important resource for elderly people when this is focused on maintaining their autonomy, providing support to their primary care attendants, and giving expert consultation and guidance in the management of very complex cases. A small number of specialists should be trained to provide leadership in teaching and research.

34

Educating lay persons about the care of the elderly

ESTHER CONTRERAS DE LEHR

DEFINITION OF THE CONCEPT OF LAY CARE

The organization of formal health and social services is frequently complex and subject to bureaucratic rules and professional procedures. Moreover, in developing countries, health services are available to only a small minority of the aging population owing to financial constraints.[1] However, a solution must be found for the growing number of the aged who require appropriate care for their needs. Such a solution is already being sought through the informal health care system, which is made up of lay persons. These groups, however, require better preparation and greater awareness of everything involved in the aging process so that they can provide care for the elderly on a sounder basis.

Ambiguous and interchangeable usage of the terms 'lay' and 'self' care is often made in literature, and an attempt to define these is therefore necessary.

The informal lay care system should be understood as a non-professional system made up of persons who participate and contribute to prevention, maintenance, and recovery of their own health and that of the community.[2] The characteristics of such a system are:

1. The people who provide this support are not experts in the field.
2. As a rule they are not paid for their services, but offer them altruistically.
3. Aid is directed to third parties.

Lay care is a generic term that implies that individuals share responsibility for their own health and that of others across the entire spectrum of health; that is, from prevention, maintenance, acute care and care of chronic conditions, to terminal care.[3]

Care provided by lay persons involves a strategy of:

1. *Rationality*—on the one hand, as the cost of professionals and institutions is reduced the need for lay care is reduced; lay care may offer on the other hand increased effectiveness, since the bureaucracy of the

formal health care system often prevents the services from being rendered when they are needed.

2. *Co-operation*—because relations and bonds are initiated or strengthened, through the intervention of various groups, like family, friends, and neighbours, and these in turn give rise to new support networks for the elderly.

3. *Economy*—since public spending can be substantially decreased when lay persons are active, the organization of such a system could be politically significant for the official health establishment.

It can be assumed that the lay care system is extremely widespread among the general population, particularly in the care of the aged, and is largely underestimated. Probably two-thirds to three-quarters of the care during episodes of illness of the aged is provided by lay persons without resorting to professional services.

Although the elderly still have a great deal of support from family, neighbours, and friends in many countries and, especially in the Third World, this is now decreasing markedly because of the changes in social structures caused by modernization[4] (migration, urbanization, family disintegration, etc.). Nevertheless, there is very little information on which to base an objective assessment of the present state of lay care for the elderly.

SCOPE OF ACTION OF LAY PERSONS

Lay persons are moved by internal motivation, and they set their own objectives. Their sphere of action covers the entire continuum of health care itemized earlier, including the phases of:

(1) health prevention;

(2) health maintenance;

(3) acute care;

(4) care for chronic conditions;

(5) terminal care;

Lay care groups are particularly significant as regards disease prevention, but in the curative and rehabilitation stages their support is indispensable from the psychosocial viewpoint, since they provide company for the elderly and are involved throughout the illness and associated crises.

The lay persons involved as health providers in this continuum are the individual concerned, the family, and the community (neighbours, friends, volunteers).

Self-care

The concept of self-care is not new. Ever since humanity began its struggle for survival, people have taken health-related actions to remain in good health for as long as possible and to overcome disease and infirmity. For centuries people had no medical care other than what they provided for themselves, and there are still places in the world, and especially in developing countries, where this is the only form of health care.

For a very long time the efforts of the elderly to maintain and improve their own health were underestimated or viewed as inadequate. Their competence and skill in caring for their own health were insufficiently recognized, while the role played by health professionals was stressed and little importance was given to what they could do for themselves.

However, the World Health Organization is promoting both lay and self-care as one of the strategies to attain health for all in the year 2000. In 1977 Dr Mahler, Director General of WHO, made the following statement: 'If health doesn't start with the individual, the home, the family, the working place and the schools, then we shall never get to the goal of health for all...Any significant improvement in physical, mental and social well-being to a large extent will depend on the individual's and the community's will to fend for themselves.'[5]

In recent years, both in Europe and in the United States, a host of self-care programmes for the elderly have sprung up, some of them documented by health professionals, and others implemented by the aged themselves with counselling from professionals.[6] However, there is no doubt that, for the successful implementation of such a quantity and variety of programmes, information and awareness of the elderly population about the responsibility they can exercise in regard to their own health is indispensable, as is an appropriate attitude on the part of health professionals towards the involvement of the individuals concerned in the health–disease process.

Self-care is a form of lay care consisting of all the actions and decisions of an individual to prevent ill health and to maintain and improve their own good health.[3] In the particular case of the aged, defeatist attitudes should be avoided, and elderly persons should be encouraged, counselled and made aware of their own competence to maintain and improve their health. This information should be clear, simple, specific, and easily understandable, and should take into account the level of education of the aged persons, especially in developing countries where the majority of the elderly in rural areas are illiterate. The cultural patterns and traditions of the region should also be considered.

Health education addressed to the elderly should include information and actions aimed at:

—— Doing away with the negative bias that health is a product that can be bought, or that it is predetermined by fate, God, or luck, and that it is the doctor's responsibility. The aged should understand that health is a way of living and behaving, and therefore it is their own responsibility.

—— Developing self-care skills based on an elementary knowledge of the body's functions, organs, and systems, and of the changes that take place with aging, with all its biological, psychological, and social repercussions. Armed with such knowledge and their own experience, they will be able to distinguish normal from abnormal conditions, and to solve some minor health problems, identify alarm signals and recognize diseases that require professional health care.

—— Preventing self-medication and the use of unknown treatments of questionable reputation. The widespread presence of quacks and a variety of ancestral customs and prejudices in all developing countries distorts and weakens a good health care system.

—— Teaching people to keep their own clinical record by keeping their lab test reports, monitoring their own functions through simple physical observations, learning the normal levels of vital signs (blood-pressure, temperature, pulse, etc.).

—— Participating actively and responsibly in the control of chronic or disabling conditions, so that they can be properly managed (diabetes, hypertension, myocardial infarctions, etc.). In such diseases in particular, a clear and detailed explanation is very important so that the elderly person can understand why they should do certain things and so that they learn to recognize the body's alarm signals.

For these and other actions health professionals, and especially doctors, need to change their attitude. A common stereotype among physicians, as a result of the image of old age as a handicap, is that old age is seen as a synonym of illness, and the diseases most frequently found at this time of life are considered to be the result of age. Older people frequently hear from the doctor: 'We can do nothing for you, because this is due to your age. I will just give you something to get along meanwhile'.

Nor is it uncommon for health professionals to think that it is not worth while to invest resources and efforts in aged people. When the latter are treated in this way they feel rejected and put down, they give up, and then their condition truly becomes hopeless.

The arrogance of doctors and their lack of communication with patients make the latter passive, dependent subjects, poorly informed about their own health. The tradition that only the physician knows and can make decisions about the health of another person should be challenged. The commonly held attitude that old people are not strong or clever enough to take care of themselves, or intelligent enough to make decisions about their own health should also be changed.

The sensitive, respectful, encouraging, and informative participation of professionals in the health care of the elderly is fundamental. Professionals should be chief educators of the community, the family, and the elderly persons themselves. The responsible and active behaviour of the aged person in their own health care depends on the relationship established by the doctors.

Family care

Another highly important provider of health care for the elderly is the family. In developing countries the family is the main natural resource for care. However, the growing trends towards urbanization, modernization, and migration are giving rise to significant changes in family structure. The traditional family, where two or more generations share the same home, is in the process of transition.

Migration of young people from the countryside to urban centres and the increasing number of women who enter the labour market are changing family dynamics. The entry of women to economically productive activities affects their traditional role as protectors and custodians of the aged.[7]

In spite of the general belief that in developed countries families participate less in the care of their old people, it has been proved that the majority of the aged, even though they may live by themselves, are in frequent touch with their children and other relatives.[8]

In any event, both in industrialized societies and in developing countries, the family is the most consistent and reliable source of emotional and material support for the aged. However, in most cases it is not sufficiently well informed to deal appropriately with the biological and psychological changes that take place during that time of life, and this may give rise to erroneous expectations about the behaviour of old people, and consequently tension in family relations.[9]

It is therefore indispensable for health professionals to provide information and counselling to the family, giving them practical guidelines about the aging process, preferably as to prevention, while the old person is still self-sufficient, in order to:

—— avoid the unnecessary loss of the elderly person's functional capacity;

—— prevent and cope with health problems that adversely affect the quality of life of the elderly person;

—— adapt the physical facilities where the elderly person is housed, if necessary, in order to optimize their surroundings so that they can preserve the greatest possible degree of self-sufficiency and mobility, in keeping with their capacity and skill, and to prevent accidents;

—— avoid dependency and overprotection from the family.

Chronic diseases like dementia or stroke disease can cause anxiety and guilt feelings in the family, but they can be alleviated if the doctor, in addition to providing extensive information about the disease and its prognosis in a way that can be understood, also establishes a relationship of understanding and empathy with the family so that they feel they are not alone with their problem.

Almind *et al.*[10] refer to three forms of interaction between the family and the elderly person in critical circumstances. First, when the person's functions have steadily deteriorated, and therefore a considerable need for increased care by the family, there is a sudden weakening of family support. Second, acute disease episodes can also cause a loss of family support and, eventually, an acute breakdown.

A third problem of interaction between the family and the aged person may occur when the person's functional condition remains stable but a family problem arises because of the death of a spouse, divorce, change of job, etc., and then family support fades and leaves the elderly person in the midst of an acute crisis.

In order to prevent the loss of family support when it is most needed by the elderly person, health professionals need to bring into play additional resources, such as temporary relief services (day care centre, social clubs, vacation centres for the aged, etc.) so that the family can recover from the stressful situation. In developed countries there are a variety of such services but in developing nations their lack may bring about a grave burden for the family, and therefore the intervention of friends and neighbours as a support resource plays a major role in the care and well-being of the aged person.

In this context is should also be borne in mind that in addition to the family's role as a direct care provider, it also performs the function of mediator between the elderly person and medical and welfare services. This is fundamental for the aged, because in times of trouble the encouragement and love that can be given only by the family and the communication bridge they establish with health professionals and institutions are more effective than the alternative of choosing institutionalization.[11]

In order for the family to play their role of mediators properly and feel supported, it is essential for health professionals to reassure them and give them information and advice about the services that can be made available to the elderly person involved, and about the way in which the care they give can be joined to that of others.

When there is no family support because the family is absent or it has broken up (poor relationships, or unmanageable distances), health professionals should see this as a risk factor and should investigate the elderly person's social network so as to provide support and the services required in good time.

Community care (neighbours, friends, volunteers)

Community implies something more than just a physical area: it means a group of persons joined by close bonds and common interests, and it is a medium in which social participation and collective action take place.[12] Above all, the community, as an extension of the family, provides a social network that is fundamental for the well-being of the elderly in many developing countries. The lack of organized services for the elderly that is to be found in developed countries are partly made up for in the Third World by the participation of the neighbourhood, friends, and in some cases groups of volunteers. Such traditional support networks, of course, are also found in industrialized nations, and especially in rural or stable areas of residence.

The elderly may find in their neighbours, friends, and volunteers different forms of support and personal care: (1) emotional support (affection, trust, esteem, respect, interest, etc.), (2) instrumental support (help at work, in shopping, in housekeeping, etc.), (3) informational support (advice about available community services, suggestions, updating of information, etc.), and (4) appraisal support (social acceptance and comparison).[13] An important alternative communication for an elderly person, next to family and friends, is the relationship with neighbours who, because of their proximity and their mobility, can serve as a significant care resource.

For the actions and programmes of health professionals in the community to be effective and have the desired impact on the health care of the elderly the following goals should be set:

—— to strengthen the existing relationships of the aged person, which are characterized by being emotionally supportive and reciprocal;

—— to detect the needs of the aged persons, their access to the various community services, and their support resources;

—— to strengthen the active participation of the elderly in on-going interventions and facilitate self-determination;

—— to develop and train the care-giving skills of friends and neighbours.

One way of developing new support networks for the elderly in the community is to identify people with similar needs or diseases and to involve them in mutual aid activities in which they can all be both recipients and providers of support and services.[14] By building these groups it is possible to share common problems and experience that will give emotional, material, and informational support, as well as access to new contacts. Moreover, the resources and skills of each member can be identified, and thus an exchange of services can be established.

In various places, and especially in the Third World, there is some experience in organizing such groups.[15] Health professionals should serve as resource persons in the process of creating and maintaining effective and autonomous groups. They should also counsel and advise the latter, providing the appropriate information about the aging process, the functions of the body's organs and systems, the use of medication, etc.

The organization of volunteer services and agencies is fairly well developed in industrialized countries, and these are highly flexible and respond rapidly to perceived needs. In such countries, volunteers provide a significant support for the elderly—as is the case in Europe where they provide daily telephone contacts with the housebound elderly, home health care, delivery of newsletters, warm meals for the ill and dependents who live in their homes, etc.

The volunteer organizations made up of the elderly themselves are one of the great breakthroughs of industrialized societies, as through this vehicle the aged have focused on their own situations and have proposed important services for their own benefit. Their actions are given serious consideration by governments.

In developing countries the type of support given by volunteers in institutions or in the community is not as highly organized, and therefore, may require more advice and counselling. In any event, both in industrialized nations and in the Third World, there is a great need to train and educate volunteers about aging.

To the extent that these groups of lay persons become more knowledgeable and skilled in basic gerontology they will be able to provide more effective care. Good will is important but it is not always enough to care for the needs of a sick elderly person.

HEALTH EDUCATION ABOUT AGING FOR LAY PERSONS

There is agreement in literature that health education about aging, both for the aged themselves and for other groups, is influenced by two primary aspects:

1. *The image society has of the aged.*   In industrialized nations this image is characterized above all by certain negative stereotypes of loneliness, passivity, dependence, and the loss of capacity and skill. The image may be transmitted by the mass media, books, and even by health professionals, and it not only influences the attitude of friends, family, neighbours, and volunteers, etc., but also shapes the self-image of the elderly person and imposes limits on behavioural patterns.[16]

2. *The beliefs and attitudes of the aged and their community in regard to health.*   The cultural factors in various societies, and their customs and traditions in regard to disease and treatment, interfere and hamper the health education measures undertaken by health professionals. Both the aged person and the community in some societies attribute magic powers to disease, and resort to ancestral customs to expel the evil spirits that have seized the body of the patient; or they may believe that illness is determined by fate or by God, and therefore passively accept whatever happens.

In principle, health professionals should be made aware of the falseness of their stereotyped and negative image of old age by means of good gerontology training which stresses the normal aging process, teaching techniques with a community approach so that health professionals may be better prepared to fulfil their function as educators.

As to the health education about aging for the elderly, health professionals should first of all give due consideration to the beliefs, customs, and needs of the aged. The latter are:[17]

(1) coping needs (adjustment to stressful life events, economic self-sufficiency, use of leisure, physical health);
(2) expressive needs (teaching the person to express and accept his or her emotional needs, engaging in activities for their own sake);
(3) contributive needs (to be useful and wanted in society);
(4) influence needs (agents of social change).

With knowledge of these needs and of the aged person's social support network, health professionals will be better equipped to design educational programmes and materials. There are no teaching techniques specifically designed for the aged; educators must be flexible enough to choose, adapt, and apply methods in keeping with the characteristics of the population to whom the information is addressed (education, literate or illiterate, occupation, interests, etc.),

However, it has been shown that one of the most effective teaching techniques for the elderly, if they have any difficulties learning, is that of learning from models—that is, by showing them someone who does the thing that they are supposed to learn.[18] I believe this is not only one of the best techniques for the elderly, but also for the lay persons in general, since health subjects such as body organ and system functions, measurement and monitoring of vital signs, and so forth must be taught with sufficient illustration to achieve adequate comprehension, especially if dealing with an illiterate population (as is often the case in developing countries).

The direct instruction method, in which the subject is told how to perform a task, has been less useful with the aged because their abstractive capability, or fluid intelligence, may deteriorate with age. The method is not very successful with persons who have not already developed this capacity.

Moreover, it is important for instructions to be brief, precise, and spaced. Feedback techniques help to correct or re-affirm learning. Efforts should be made to allay anxiety, especially in the elderly persons, by first allowing them to become familiar with new learning elements and giving them continuous encouragement.

Health professionals have the responsibility of transmitting basic knowledge about normal and pathological aging to the group of lay persons (the aged, family, friends, neighbours, volunteers) and also that of continously counselling and encouraging them. Health education programmes directed to this group could include some elementary facts about:[19]

—— what aging is;

—— psychological changes and developmental tasks of old age;

—— social changes: retirement, loss of spouse, friends, etc.;

—— notions of normal adult anatomy and physiology and biological changes with age;

—— normal function of body systems and organs;

—— clinical case history and check-up;

—— what the vital signs and symptoms are;

—— making out the person's own case history;

—— how to do a medical examination at home;

—— what the diagnostic methods are;

—— what the clinical tests are;

—— administration of medication;

—— first aid;

—— what to expect from the doctor;

—— how to exercise correctly;

—— what good nutrition is;

—— smoking, drinking, and overweight as enemies of good health;

—— most frequent heart diseases of the elderly: prevention and care;

—— stroke: prevention and care;

—— most frequent mental disease of the elderly: management of senile dementia;

—— kinds of tumours and their care;

—— diseases of bones and joints: prevention and care;

—— endocrine diseases: diabetes mellitus, its care;

—— diseases of the kidney and urinary tract: prevention and care;

—— orodental problems: prevention and care.

This is obviously just an outline of the subjects that could be discussed by health professionals. They must consider for each case according to the problems that are more significant in the community what should be discussed with the elderly person, the family, and the community.

HEALTH EDUCATION FOR THE ELDERLY AND THEIR COMMUNITY: THE CASE IN MEXICO

Significant progress has been made in Mexico in the twentieth century in the control of infant and perinatal mortality, reducing the birth rate, the control of infectious diseases, and the improvement of basic health care. The result is that there is an increasing number and proportion of people who live to old age.

In 1975 there were only some 3 million persons over 60 years of age, but according to UN projections this sector of the population will grow to 7 million in the year 2000, and to 12 million in 2025. There are now more than 4 million people who are 60 years of age or older, or nearly 6 per cent of the total population.

With the purpose of assisting toward the optimal development of the elderly persons' potential, the DIF (or National System for Total Family Development), a government national institution in charge of all the government welfare programmes, has tried to preserve the integration of the aged persons within their community and family by organizing self-managed groups called *councils of elders*.

The essence of these councils is awareness as a group, a sense of belonging, and of autonomy to meet the members' own requirements. By free communication of problems, concerns, and mutual wishes, proposed solutions are generated within the groups.

The councils of elders try to foster the development and maintenance of physical and mental skills by having the people take part in productive activities that serve to stimulate all their functions, but also to avoid marginalization and a loss of the sense of being useful.

Individuals are given information about the aging process and all the associated biological, psychological, and social aspects by means of teaching sessions. They are also given counselling to help them remain productive and not a burden for the family.

Sports, recreational, and cultural activities are also organized to help develop and improve the overall potential of the elderly persons. Physical fitness training, basic and recreative exercises, bodily expression, and directed organized games and meant to help develop the psychomotor and sensitive capacities, body handling, and recognition and to develop skill, balance, endurance, and strength.

The DIF system conducts self-care programmes in the community and in the homes for the elderly designed to prevent disease and physical deterioration and to keep the elderly persons autonomous. In order for elderly persons to use self-care techniques it has been necessary to hold health education sessions that cover basic explanations about the function of the body's organs and systems, the aging process, and diseases such as diabetes mellitus and heart, infectious, and urinary diseases and their risk factors, sight and vision deficiencies, and dental problems and their consequences.

The participation of the family and community in activities to foster the health of the elderly has also been stressed. The family is a fundamental part for implementation of self-care techniques, as the family members too must be familiar with preventive measures to support the health of the aged person.

In order to implement self-care techniques and primary health care, a self-care record (a card) is given to every aged person in the programme, so that they keep a record of the basic information about their health. It bears the title 'I care for my own health'.[20] This record comprises:

—— identification of the council of elders and of the person in particular;

—— data to assess social risk factors;

—— monthly record of vital signs and of location of disease processes;

—— charts of blood sugar, blood-pressure, and weight;

—— general recommendations on nutrition, hygiene, and exercise.

One copy of this record is always kept by the elderly person and another by some health professional (health promoter, social workers, nurse, physician, etc.).

It was decided to use a colour code to identify organs as healthy or impaired: green represents good health, yellow the remission of some disease, and red a disease or an alarm signal. The reason for colour

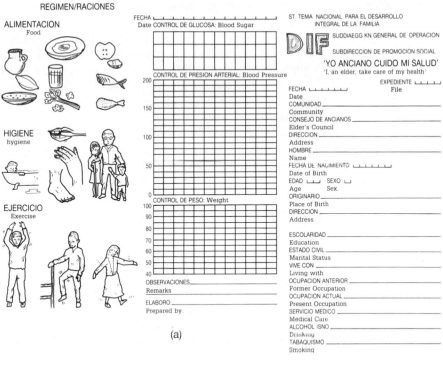

(a)

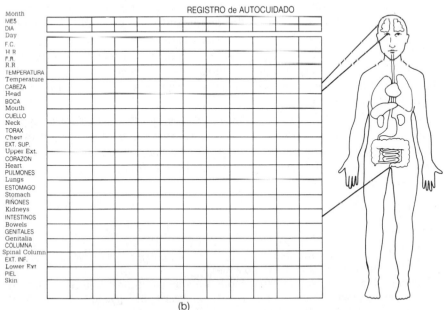

(b)

Fig. 34.1.

coding was a high rate of illiteracy among the elderly population in Mexico.

Fig. 34.1 shows the two sides of a simple chart to record the health condition of the elderly person, who can personally (or the family can do it) fill in the chart about alarm signs that require attendance at a health centre, or on the control of disease during treatment. The chart is easily understood by anyone, even those who cannot read.

Since the record cards have been in use for a very short time no assessment has been made of their impact on the health of the elderly. However, it has been observed that elderly persons are becoming less passive about their health and more aware and concerned about what is happening within their body; also they are demanding more attention from health professionals. They carry these records with them with great pride and care for them as their most important documents.

SUMMARY

The organization of formal health and social services is frequently complex and subject to bureaucratic rules and professional procedures. Besides this, in developing countries health services are available to only a small minority of the aging population due to financial constraints in these countries.

The lay care system is extremely widespread among the general population, particularly in the care of the aged, and is largely underestimated. Probably two-thirds to three-quarters of the care during periods of illness of the aged is provided by lay persons without resort to professional services. Therefore, these groups require better preparation and greater awareness of the aging process so that they can provide care for the elderly on a sounder basis.

In principle, health professionals should be aware of their stereotyped and negative image of old age by means of good gerontology training stressing the normal aging process, and teaching techniques with a community approach so that they may be better prepared to fulfil their function as educators.

References

1. Appropriate levels for continuing care for the elderly (1980). WHO Report, 11–14 November. WHO, Berlin (West).
2. Schmachtenberg, W. (1980). Modelle ehrenamtlicher Mitarbeit in der Altenhilfe; Schriftenreihe des Bundesministers für Jugend, Familie, und Gesundheit, Band 79, Stuttgart.

3. WHO (1984). *Self-health/care and older people. A manual for public policy and programme development.* WHO, Copenhagen.
4. Population development and social security (1981). *Aging in developing countries, final report.* Carl Duisberg Gesellschaft, eV, Hamburg.
5. Coppard, L. C. (1985). Self-health/care and the elderly. In *Toward the well-being of the elderly.* PAHO, Washington DC.
6. DeFriese, G. H. and Woomert, A. (1983). Self-care among US elderly. Recent developments. *Research on Aging,* **5** (1), March.
7. Contreras de Lehr, E. (1985). Apuntes para la evaluación de la situación del anciano en América Latina. *Seminario interregional para la implementación del plan de acción sobre el enve jecimiento.* 9–22 septiembre, ONU, Kiev.
8. Shanas, E. (1979). Social myth as hypothesis: the case of the family relations of old people. *Gerontologist,* **19**, 3.
9. Contreras de Lehr, E. (1987). Long-term services in Mexico: homes for the aged. *Danish Medical Bulletin,* No. 5.
10. Almind, G., Freer, C., Muir Gray, J. A., and Warshaw, G. (1985). The contribution of the primary care doctor to the medical care of the elderly in the community. *Danish Medical Bulletin,* **32** (2).
11. Rosenmayr, H. and Rosenmayr, L. (1983). Gesellschaft, Familie, Alternsprozess. In *Das Alter. Einfuhrung in die Gerontologie.* Ferdinand Enke Verlag, Stuttgart.
12. Checkoway, B. (1988). Community-based initiatives to improve health of the elderly. *Danish Medical Bulletin,* No. 6.
13. House, Js. (1981). *Work stress and social support.* Adison-Wesley, Reading, MA.
14. Israel, B. (1988). Community-based social network interventions. Meeting the needs of the elderly. *Danish Medical Bulletin,* No. 6.
15. Tout, K. (1988). Aging: social supports and community interventions in developing countries. *Danish Medical Bulletin,* No. 6.
16. Contreras de Lehr, E. (1984). *Zum Altenbild in Mexiko und Deutschland. Eine interkulturelle Vergleichsstudie.* Latein-America Studien, 17. Wilhelm Fink Verlag, Munich.
17. Glendenning, F. (1985). What is educational gerontology?: North American and British definitions. In *Education al Gerontology. International Perspectives.* Croom Helm, London.
18. Denney, N. W. (1982). Aging and cognitive changes. In *Handbook of developmental psychology.* Prentice Hall, New Jersey.
19. Gonzalez Aragon, G. J. (1984). *Aprendamos a envejecer sanos. Manual de autocuidado y educacion para la salud en el envejecimiento.* Costa Amic, Mexico.
20. Rangel Lopez, L. E. Cartilla de autocuidado. 'Yo anciano cuido mi salud'. (Unpublished manuscript.)

35

Educating health professionals
in the care of the elderly

CHRISTINE EWAN

INTRODUCTION

Aging of populations is a world-wide phenomenon. Population aging gives rise to a greater need for health professionals and the community in general to provide support for individuals with chronic multifaceted illness and mobility problems.

The need for teaching both gerontology and geriatrics is evident, not only for demographic reasons but also because the existing deficits in attitudes, knowledge, and skills in dealing with the elderly are so great. An American study,[1] for example, found that among social work, law, and medical students there was a striking absence of knowledge of the most basic facts about the elderly. None of the students surveyed indicated any interest in working with the aged. This situation appears to be improving in some countries but much remains to be done.

Different cultures may recognize different priority problems in caring for their aged populations. For example, in industrialized Western cultures social isolation of the aged can be as significant a problem as physical illness, while in rural or traditional communities the major problems may be related to the provision of adequate diagnostic facilities to recognize and treat reversible physical illness. For these reasons, and others, descriptions of training programmes for care of the aged can provide only general guidance and basic principles. Each community and each training facility must base its training programmes on its own needs, values, and resources. This paper provides a framework for programme design which allows for local adaptation. General principles are illustrated by specific examples taken from the literature.

PRINCIPLES OF EDUCATIONAL PROGRAMME DESIGN

Educational programme design can be approached in many ways. However, the model which has been most acceptable and has had greatest utility in the health professions is based upon the identification of learning

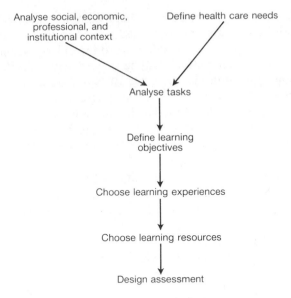

Fig. 35.1 Instructional design process.

objectives derived from an analysis of the health care tasks that need to be done. Once learning objectives have been identified, methods and resources are determined which assist students to achieve those objectives, and assessments are designed which are appropriate for testing their achievement. Fig. 35.1 summarizes the instructional design process. Detailed guidance in the principles and practice of instructional design are available elsewhere.[2–4]

A further consideration which is particularly relevant to designing programmes in care of the aged is the need to take account of the institutional and social context in which the training programme will operate.

Context

Community attitudes to the elderly are an important part of the *social context* which must be taken into account in educational programme planning. In some cultures youth and physical attractiveness are valued more than age and life experiences. In a context such as this students are likely to hold negative attitudes towards aging and possibly towards working with the aged. Personal feelings towards the elderly arise, at least in part, from general social attitudes. In a review of the attitudinal impact of training in gerontology/geriatrics, Coccaro and Miles[5] concluded that the development of desired attitudes or behaviour in students depends on whether those behaviours are supported by the institution and the community. Fostering a positive attitude toward the elderly within the society is essential before training efforts will be fully effective. At the same time, however, training institutions can influence the attitudes of the communities they serve. For example, innovative programmes in care of the aged can be publicized by the local media. Institutions can also provide public education programmes, such as short-term courses for carers of elderly relatives, or they can provide outreach programmes which act as a teaching resource as well as a service for the community. Raising public awareness of the rewards and possibilities of working with the aged will also result ultimately in an increased awareness of potential career paths for students and a more positive attitude towards such careers.

A further aspect of social context which is important to consider is the structure and financing of the health care delivery system. In systems such as the British National Health Service, where public funding of health care is based on a capitation fee for the number of patients receiving care rather than on a fee for service basis, there is an incentive for doctors to refer elderly people to other members of the team who may be more appropriate to their needs. There are no fee barriers to prevent free movement throughout the system. In systems such as the American and Australian Medicare system, which provide free or subsidized care for those in need, payments to doctors are based on fee for service but take little or no account of the need for long consultations, frequent return visits, or care by health professionals other than doctors. There is no financial incentive for doctors to provide high-quality care appropriate to chronic illness management since reimbursement is based on fee structures developed around acute illness episodes. Such issues are critical and must be considered in planning training since they will determine the models of practice that students will witness. Apart from the need to address change in systems of financing care for the elderly, teachers must be aware of the need to help students recognize the non-monetary rewards in the task and to counteract the financial disincentives which may be apparent. Discussion of economic and political realities in provision of care for the elderly should be an important component of the training programme.

The *professional context* is also relevant. In Britain, for example, geriatrics was declared a medical specialty in 1949 and thus there is no serious shortage of well-trained teachers. In the United States of America, on the other hand, the current consensus is that creation of a new practice specialty is unnecessary, although development of an academic cadre of teachers and researchers is essential.[6] Estimates of the numbers of teachers required to provide geriatrics training adequately for health professions in the USA are in the thousands. It has been suggested in the American context that, rather than developing a new physician specialty, geriatric manpower needs could be met by delegating responsibility to physician extenders.[7] Similar professional issues are likely to arise in all health professions. Availability or lack of multidisciplinary teams to help deal with the needs of an aging population will obviously determine the requirements for training of any single professional group.

The final critical consideration is the *context of the educational institution*. Educational planning is a political process which involves negotiation among teachers representing different disciplines and sometimes different value positions and philosophies. In medical education, for example, competition for curriculum time can be fierce and the traditional disciplines such as physiology or surgery often exercise greater power in decision making than the 'newer' disciplines such as community medicine or social and behavioural sciences. Access to suitable venues for teaching about care of the elderly may be difficult if services are not yet fully established. Experience in American medical schools has shown the importance of social and government support in increasing the emphasis on geriatrics and gerontology in curricula. Progress has been reported as slow but steady and due largely to initiatives such as the establishment of fellowships by the Veterans Administration and incentive awards to schools by the National Institute on Aging.[8] Government contracts for the production of modules and course materials have also been an important stimulant to the development of curricula and educational resources.[9]

Another example of political support is government financing of offices of geriatrics/gerontology in medical schools whose role is to stimulate incorporation of relevant material into the teaching of other departments.[10] Even given support of this nature, however, finding a niche in already overcrowded curricula is a problem for academics who have been charged with the responsibility to ensure that geriatrics is taught. Most must find ways of working within the constraints imposed by limited access to students' time and to resources. A good compromise may be found in integration of the special features of health care of the elderly with other courses[11] rather than establishment of a separate geriatrics course.

Effective integration depends on identification and communication of clear objectives, and rational planning of strategies which will enhance students' motivation, facilitate their perception of the meaning and relevance of what they are learning, and encourage early, active involvement in learning new skills, knowledge, and attitudes. Integration is particularly applicable to the biological aspects of aging, while the social aspects may need more independent attention because of their experiential requirements.

Objectives

There are many published reports of educational objectives for gerontology and geriatrics (for example see ref. 12). Robbins *et al.*[13] undertook a review of educational objectives in gerontology in which objectives derived from 40 programmes were rated by experts. The result was 33 general objectives and 85 disease-specific or problem-specific objectives. A recent workshop on curricular changes to meet the health needs of the elderly in Malaysia produced a list of objectives for training allied health professionals in that country.[14] The list is reproduced in Table 35.1. The objectives referred to as specific are at a fairly general level. Table 35.2 reproduces a list of learning objectives in gerontology and geriatric medicine published by the World Health Organization. These objectives provide a general basis which can be adapted to suit the training needs of any profession or community.

Table 35.1 Objectives for training allied health professionals in Malaysia

A. General objectives
1. Attitude—to develop caring attitudes for the elderly.
2. Knowledge—to acquire the necessary knowledge in caring for the elderly in the hospital and the community.
3. Skills—to acquire the skills and abilities to promote and maintain physical ability and well-being in the elderly.

B. Specific objectives.
1. To understand the aging process
2. To acquire knowledge of the socio-economic, physical, and psychological factors in maintaining the well-being of the elderly.
3. To demonstrate a positive attitude towards health and aging.
4. To appreciate the contribution of the elderly to society.
5. To recognize and respect the rights of the elderly.
6. To understand common health problems in the elderly.
7. To recognize the role and responsibilities of the therapist in the care of the elderly.
8. To identify the needs of the elderly and provide appropriate care.
9. To communicate effectively with the elderly.
10. To identify and utilize resources available in the community in the care of the elderly.
11. To develop skills to enable the elderly to be as independent as possible in activities of daily living.
12. To develop clinical skills in preventing and reducing disability, pain, and other chronic disorders.

Table 35.2 WHO learning objectives in gerontology and geriatric medicine[15]

1. To encourage a humane and positive attitude towards old people and to demonstrate the satisfaction and fulfilment which comes from professional involvement with the elderly and their families.
2. To produce an understanding of demographic factors and social changes in the aging of societies.
3. To secure an understanding of age-related changes in the context of human development and an appreciation of the causes of disability in old age. Prevention and management of disability should be understood within both community and institutional settings.
4. To teach the special features of presentation of disease in old age and the problems of therapy. The problems associated with drug therapy in old age require special consideration.
5. To indicate the principles of rehabilitation and their application to the elderly, a major objective being the attainment and maintenance of optimum physical, social, and mental function for each individual.
6. To demonstrate the importance of working as a member of a multidisciplinary team, with full understanding and appreciation of the roles and skills of physicians, nurses, rehabilitation therapists, social workers, and other team members.
7. To indicate the importance of acquiring skill in communicating effectively with the elderly and those involved in their care. This should be done in such a way as to lead to fuller understanding of the importance of the family and the social network of care.
8. To ensure an understanding of the importance of protecting the liberty of the individual, so that the elderly may retain maximum choice and control over their own lifestyles and the manner in which they face death.
9. To reach an understanding of services available to old people and their families, with special emphasis on community aspects, and to stress the essential interdependence of these services and the need for effective co-operation between them and families and other carers.
10. To indicate principles and responsibilities of continuing care for elderly patients with irremediable disabilities, and of terminal care of dying patients.

Table 35.3 summarizes the major categories of objectives obtained from a survey of Australian medical schools. They represent a list of general considerations which apply across all professions and levels of training.[16]

Common themes run through all sets of learning objectives. They relate to the need to promote positive attitudes towards aging and the aged, to recognize the special features of disease and illness in the elderly, to adopt a holistic approach, to work with a multidisciplinary team, and to

Table 35.3 General objectives for learning to care for the elderly

---

Knowledge

Biological

Objectives relate to the need for students to be familiar at an appropriate level with:

    theories of aging;

    the biology and physiology of human development;

    processes of normal aging and the problems of defining normality;

    age-related alterations in pharmacodynamics and pharmacokinetics.

Pathological

Objectives relate to the need for students to be familiar at an appropriate level with:

    the principles of preventive geriatrics and screening procedures;

    the altered presentations of common illnesses in the elderly;

    the interactions of acute and chronic disease and multiple problems;

    the characteristics of specific age-related illness;

    the nature and potential of rehabilitation programmes.

Social

Objectives relate to the need for students to be familiar at an appropriate level with:

    the ego factors, needs, life satisfactions, and frustrations of the elderly;

    the effects of social losses and restrictions on the elderly;

    the interactions of physical, social, and psychological factors and their effects on health care;

    the social roles of the elderly in contemporary society;

    models of health care delivery for the elderly, specifically the roles of home care and extended care;

    demographic trends in the context of history and culture;

    organization of health and welfare and welfare services in the community;

    utilization of health and welfare services by the aged;

    the functions of the members of the health team.

Attitudes

Objectives relate to the need for students to:

    examine their own attitudes to aging;

    overcome stereotypes about the capacity of the elderly to lead purposeful lives;

    recognize the need for rational management plans based on accurate diagnosis;

    recognize that potential value of treatment and rehabilitation is significant;

    respect the dignity of the elderly and commit themselves to providing maximum choice and minimum enforcement of health-related measures;

    consider aspects of professionalism such as ethics, confidentiality, legality, continuing education, and accountability for quality of care.

Table 35.3 (*cont.*)

Skills

Objectives relate to the need for students to demonstrate ability in:
communication with elderly people, their families, community groups, the health team, and the health and welfare bureaucracy;
maintenance of effective relationships with the elderly and others involved in their care;
accurate assessment of the elderly patient's physical, social, and psychological needs;
appropriate management of medical problems including safe prescribing.

---

become comfortable with a supportive rather than curative role. For example, a comprehensive curriculum developed for Israeli medical, nursing, and physiotherapy students cites as its general aims to alert students to the need for: (1) a comprehensive approach towards the elderly, (2) a multidisciplinary team, (3) community-oriented continuity of care, and (4) transforming geriatric medicine into an attractive field of specialization.[17]

While there are undeniably special areas of skill and knowledge acquisition which must be addressed in training, it is the social, behavioural, and attitudinal aspects of training for health care of the elderly which invite specific attention. Teaching health professionals to care for the elderly can be regarded as a model for holistic health practice. For these reasons, teaching and learning experiences must provide a context within which attitudes can be explored and students can be afforded adequate opportunities to develop holistic professional skills.

Method and resources

Teaching methods used in geriatrics and gerontology cross the broad spectrum of methods for training health professionals and, once again, offering prescriptions for choice of teaching methods is inappropriate. Choice of teaching methods depends not only on objectives and available resources but also on curriculum context and philosophy. A curriculum which is divided into preclinical and clinical components will approach the topic differently from a curriculum which is based on integrated clinical problem solving. Nevertheless, it is important to be mindful of the advantages and disadvantages of the various common teaching methods. Such information is readily available e.g. [12, 18, 19] but it is important to be aware of the need for caution in the use of both audiovisual materials and lectures in geriatric education.

Audiovisual materials deserve special attention because they may not always be transferable from one culture to another. This is particularly applicable in care of the elderly because of its many social and cultural aspects. Shinar[20] reviewed 200 programmes (mainly videotapes and films produced in America) for use in Israel and concluded that only 15 were appropriate. It is, therefore, important to preview audiovisual materials before buying them or using them.

Lectures are obviously a vital component of most teaching programmes. They have their place in the transmission of factual information which is not readily available elsewhere. Their limitations should, however, be remembered, particularly in an area such as gerontology where the attitudinal component is so important. Lectures on the biology or sociology of aging, for example, when divorced from clinical reality or practical experience, will lack perceived relevance and may even contribute to negative attitudes towards the subject matter of geriatrics. Wherever possible, basic factual information about aging should be integrated with other basic science teaching or introduced as background material to problem solving in clinical work with elderly patients. Students need an opportunity to be sensitized to the issues surrounding care of the aged before they can readily appreciate the importance of what they must learn. This is also true of other areas of health care but it is especially important when, as in gerontology, students' initial attitudes are frequently negative[21] and motivation to learn to work with elderly patients must be actively fostered. Such negative attitudes are rarely encountered in the fields of paediatrics or obstetrics, for example.

The need to motivate students and to help them understand their own attitudes to aging in themselves and others means that education in geriatrics must be predominantly experiential and oriented towards psychosocial as well as technical competence.

All clinical or experiential education should have three main phases: the preparation phase, the experience itself, and the feedback or reflection phase in which students and teachers take stock of what has been learned. Unfortunately, one or more of these phases is frequently neglected. Students and supervisors may be ill prepared for a practicum, they may be unsure of the objectives and what students should be doing, and time may be wasted or spent carrying out routine tasks. During and at the end of the practicum, opportunities are often missed for discussing experiences and attitudes and consolidating what has been learned. The following discussion of teaching and learning methods is based on this three-phase model of experiential education, which is summarized in Table 35.4.

Preparation phase

Motivation.   Merely telling students what they must know is not enough to create in them a desire to learn. Any activity which puts students into

Table 35.4 Experiential education

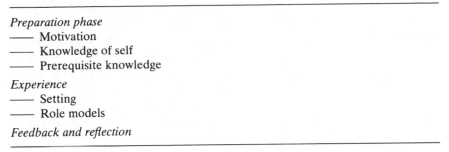

Preparation phase
—— Motivation
—— Knowledge of self
—— Prerequisite knowledge

Experience
—— Setting
—— Role models

Feedback and reflection

direct contact with the lives of elderly people and the contributions of effective health care workers can be used to stimulate interest and motivation to learn. For example, students could be asked to write a brief report on the activities or health needs of an elderly relative or neighbour. Alternatively, elderly people could be invited to attend a class and lead a discussion on their personal experiences of aging.[22] Vicarious experiences such as trigger films or role plays could be used to stimulate discussion and interest, and simulated problems could be used to raise important issues which are to be resolved during the practicum.

These approaches ensure that the students enter their study of care of the elderly having experienced contact with an elderly person as an individual with a personal story to tell rather than as a patient with a medical case history.

Placing students in person-to-person rather than doctor-to-patient relationships with elderly people early in their clinical experience sets a pattern for future relationships. Motivation to learn is enhanced by a desire to contribute to the resolution of general life problems as well as illness problems.

Knowledge of self. Aging, unlike disease and illness, is inevitable and inescapable. It has personal relevance for every student and every teacher. Not surprisingly, many prefer to ignore or deny the aging process, or to treat it as a disease and thus minimize feelings of personal vulnerability. Different cultures will react differently to the personal significance of aging, but until health professionals recognize and come to terms with their own feelings about aging, disability, and death it is unlikely that they will be effective in helping elderly people to cope themselves. It is probable that some students are not suited to this role and it is wise that they come to realize that fact so that they can make appropriate career plans. Most, however, may only need to be provided with opportunities to examine their attitudes and, if necessary, to learn appropriate coping skills and to modify minor aspects of their behaviour.

The most appropriate strategies for addressing these issues involve small group discussion with trusted colleagues and a skilled teacher. Films or personal contact with elderly clients can focus discussion on specific issues such as bereavement, loneliness, personal reactions to aging, or institutionalization; they provide a common stimulus for students to relate to in the first instance, when they may be reluctant to reveal their personal feelings or concerns. As group cohesiveness develops, personal issues can become the agenda. Many trigger films are available to facilitate this process.[23]

Another approach is to reveal to students, in a non-threatening way, the accuracy of their knowledge about aging and their stereotypes of the elderly. Job[24] has described the use of a modified version of Palmore's Facts on Aging Quiz as a way to help students recognize and overcome their inaccurate stereotypes and negative attitudes to aging.

Green[25] reports a similar innovative approach in which nursing students were asked to write down their fantasies in response to questions which dealt with their own aging experience and their anticipated health status, relationships, living conditions, finances, sexuality, and cause of death. Discussion then focused on contributions from these fantasies and known facts about the condition of elderly people. Implications were drawn about health care and negative or stereotypic attitudes that students hold.

Prerequisite knowledge and skills.   All students have some knowledge, from their family experiences, of the aging process and its effects. It is useful to start with the students' existing knowledge and to build from there to what must be learned. Some schools involve students directly in deciding what are the objectives for learning. This is a particularly appropriate strategy for elective courses when students have had some basic training in gerontology. Learners can be helped, through small group discussion, clinical attachments or self-assessment quizzes, to recognize their existing knowledge and skills and their needs for new learning. Once these needs are recognized they can be formulated as learning objectives and used as a basis for a learning contract negotiated between the learner and teacher. Learning contracts specify methods, resources, and assessments which will be employed by the learner in order to achieve the agreed objectives.[26]

Prerequisite knowledge can also be achieved through student projects. Individuals or groups of students can be assigned to research different aspects of the topic of aging. One group could investigate the demography of aging in the community, another the provision of services, another morbidity rates, and another could interview the well elderly to develop a profile of lifestyles. Reports from each group can then be shared to provide a comprehensive picture of the situation of the elderly in the community.

Prerequisite skills, particularly in interviewing and interactions with the elderly, can be developed by similar methods to those used in general clinical training. Role play, with or without video replay, can be a valuable source of feedback for students, provided that feedback is sensitively given and students are afforded the opportunity to make the first comments on their perceptions of the progress of the interaction. It may also be possible to enlist the aid of elderly people who would be willing to help students to practise their skills. These people could also be trained to provide students with feedback on their skill development. Further details of interpersonal skills training are available.[4, 27]

Simulations can also be a helpful way to develop skills in case management or clinical problem solving. The use of printed patient management problems is well established in the clinical fields[28] and computers offer further sophisticated options for simulating reality. At the University of Newcastle (Australia) medical students 'visit' and interact with simulated patients programmed into the computer. The 'patients' are introduced as video-taped patient presentations to help students to identify with the patient. The students keep problem-oriented medical records for each patient for 'visits' which vary across time from several days to 2 years. This allows students to follow the development of the patient's problems, simulating real community practice. The computer simulation is intended to provide a breadth of experience to allow students to practise more thoroughly those management skills they will need in encounters with real patients.[29]

A further aspect of prerequisite knowledge is the need to acquaint students with the environment in which they will be gaining field experience. This can sometimes be done by using audio visual materials or simply by holding briefing sessions in which students are given the opportunity to clarify the objectives of the placement and the expectations of their role. Handbooks which specify the objectives of the field experience and expected outcomes, which suggest activities, guide directions of enquiry, describe models of team functions, and provide useful references, are a support to the confidence of students who are entering unfamiliar situations, with uncertain expectations.

It is also important to make sure that staff and elderly people who will be involved are adequately briefed. Negative attitudes towards working with the elderly are almost guaranteed if the student feels unwelcome or uncomfortable in the field setting. Wherever possible, inclusion of the elderly people themselves in discussions about the purposes of the field experience will not only increase co-operation but may increase their gain from the experience as well. Participation in learning is preferable to being an object of study.

Experience

Setting. Current trends indicate the desirability of broadening the options available for field experience. A survey of American medical schools in 1983 revealed that training sites were expanding to include many non-institutional settings.[30] There is a growing tendency to consider that 'empathically oriented programs that stress the establishment of contact with healthy, functioning older persons...may be twice as effective as cognitively oriented programs that stress the acquisiton of technical knowledge'.[5] Research support for this belief is equivocal. Woolliscroft *et al.*[31] found that students undertaking interviews with elderly people in nursing homes maintained poor opinions about the functional capacity of elderly people in comparison with students who interviewed people in non-institutional settings and whose attitudes significantly improved. Students in all sites demonstrated improved attitudes towards the integrity and personal acceptability of elderly people. Ross[32] reported that nursing students who made home visits to well elderly persons over a 3-month period demonstrated better knowledge and more positive attitudes to aging than did students who worked with the unwell elderly. Ross concluded that the selection of clients is also important, in that students' experiences are more positive with clients who are prepared to reveal facts and feelings about their experience of aging. On the other hand, Greenhill and Baker[33] failed to demonstrate any significant differences in knowledge or attitude between groups of students who worked with the well aged or with hospitalized elderly people.

A broad range of settings for teaching about health care of the aged has been described. These range from students providing routine interviews and physical examinations for the senior citizen residents of apartment complexes[34] to students being assigned to work with elderly clients in community service agencies,[35] and to conducting classes in community facilities for the elderly where local seniors 'served as consumer consultants and models of health and vigour'.[36] Most reports of these types of programmes report high acceptability among students, teaching staff, staff of facilities, and elderly people themselves. While proof of clear superiority of any particular type of venue is lacking common sense dictates that a variety of experience will be beneficial in acquainting students more closely with the realities they will face when they graduate. Sankar and Becker[37] provide an intellectual rationale, should one be needed, when they point out that social, psychological, and environmental factors contribute to adaptation to chronic illness and reduced ability. It is, therefore, essential for students to study the interaction of medical and social factors in the environment in which the patient lives as well as the artificial environment of the hospital which provides acute care.

It is obvious that managing the learning experience in such a variety of settings will be a much more difficult task than that which occurs when teaching takes place within the well-controlled confines of a teaching hospital. That is the reason for the emphasis placed on preparation in the preceding segment of this paper. Effective learning in field settings will occur only if adequate groundwork has been done.

Role models.   Students inevitably learn much of their future habits and style of practice from watching their teachers. They observe and emulate behaviours which are seen to be satisfying and effective in achieving personal and patient care goals. It is, therefore, essential that experiences be provided which allow students to observe instances of satisfying high-quality care of the elderly. One way to do this is certainly within a clinical teaching institution. Jahnigen *et al.*[38] have demonstrated that better patient care outcomes are achieved when people are discharged to intermediate care in a teaching-hospital-affiliated nursing home than to one which is not affiliated. Less medications are prescribed on average and re-admissions are less frequent. This is good practice to which students should be exposed. Similarly, students undertaking a clerkship in a specialist geriatric unit had more favourable attitudes towards care of the aged than did students who had served in a general medical ward.[39] Presumably this occurs because students see models of good practice and satisfying outcomes in an environment which is designed specifically to care for the needs of the elderly. Research suggests that positive orientations after such experiences sag when students proceed to other clinical experiences, but that they are re-activated after graduation when responsibility for patient care is assumed.[40]

Role modelling in relation to working as part of a team is also important. Interdisciplinary courses in gerontology are not uncommon.[23] Croen *et al.*[41] reported a programme in which teams of one medical student and two nursing students conducted patient work-ups and presented cases to an interdisciplinary group of health care professionals. The program significantly increased medical students' perceptions of the nurse's role in working with elderly hospitalized patients. Another approach to incorporating gerontology into the curriculum and increasing the awareness of team capability is the provision of a non-physician gerontologist as consultant to clinicial teams.[42] The gerontologist, a social scientist, attended rounds and acted as a resource providing reference material relevant to discussions of patient care. She used the patients as 'creator' of the curriculum, arranging relevant input for students and residents as problems arose in management. Her presence provided students and trainees with the stimulus and the opportunity to discuss feelings about the aged and treating older people and to develop more positive attitudes. The impact of the programme was judged to be significant by the increase in the number of referrals to the gerontologist.

Provision of good role models may be difficult in those environments where care of the elderly is not well established and specialist staff training is inadequate. Faculty development activities for those staff should emphasize not only cognitive skills in caring for the elderly but also the necessity to practise holistic care and to encourage development of that approach in students.

Feedback and reflection

Learning does not occur simply by immersing students in the type of experience described above. Field experiences may be complex, charged with emotions, and sometimes bewildering or frightening. Students need an opportunity to reflect periodically on their experiences and to assimilate new insights and recognize gaps in knowledge. Too often this reflection occurs in the study period prior to the final examination, by which time it is too late to be of much use. Opportunities for consolidating learning are, by then, long past. Teachers and curriculum planners must recognize this need for reflection and consolidation and incorporate it into the curriculum. Sensitive feedback from teachers and fellow students is a valuable aspect of learning and can be achieved by scheduling regular discussion groups during the period of the field experience.

If teachers are in the field with students then they should be a primary resource and source of feedback for the student. More often, however, students may be supervised by a practitioner who is committed to a service rather than an educational role and may have little time or skill for providing students with advice or assistance. As pointed out earlier, client selection, consultation, and preparation may also permit clients or patients themselves to be valuable sources of feedback for students. Ultimately, however, the student will probably carry the major responsibility for evaluating what he or she has learned from the experience and for identifying what remains to be learned. Learning contracts are a helpful way of facilitating this process, as is the practice of students working in teams of two or three who can consult with each other.

Perhaps the most effective way for assimilating and consolidating learning in areas such as care of the elderly, however, is to encourage students to become amateur anthropologists, to encourage them to be observers of what goes on around them and of their place within the interaction. The anthropologist's field notes are replaced by a student diary in which notes are made of events, interesting aspects of services, questions, feelings, reactions, and insights. These notes are then available for reflection and analysis either in private or in the context of group sessions set aside for sharing students' experiences gained in the fieldwork. Such sessions then allow students to set new personal objectives for the next phase of their practical experience. Both students and teachers need the opportunity to take stock of the situation and work out what progress is being made.

Evaluation

For the most part, evaluation of student learning as part of formal course assessments in care of the elderly should follow the same principles which apply to health care education in general. Students should be assessed on their achievement of the objectives which have been specified at the beginning of the programme. Assessment methods should be appropriate to those objectives. To take an extreme example, it is not possible to assess whether students can interview elderly people if they are assessed only by multiple-choice questions. A variety of assessment methods appropriate to the learning objectives should be employed.

Various methods exist for assessing knowledge (multiple-choice questions, essays, short-answer questions); problem-solving ability (modified essay questions, patient management problems, special multiple-choice questions); and clinical skills (short case, long case, simulated patients, checklists, rating scales, critical incident reports). It is not appropriate to address the details of these methods here. They have been reviewed in gerontology education by Stout,[12] in medical education by Cox and Ewan,[18] in nursing education by Ewan and White,[4] and in general health personnel education by Abbatt[2] and Guilbert.[3]

Assessing attitudes, however, is much more problematic. Various standardized tests for attitudes to aging do exist, although their use outside the culture in which they were developed and validated is dubious. For those without the extensive resources required to develop, test, and validate their own attitude scales a better approach to assessing attitudes is to observe the students in their field experience. Unobtrusive observation may be difficult but, nevertheless, experienced teachers can probably assess with acceptable accuracy whether a student's approach to elderly people is sincere and appropriate.

When blatantly inappropriate attitudes and behaviour are identified in the course of field work or group discussions it raises the question of what should be done. The answer to that question depends on local circumstances. In most cases students should be counselled privately, given specific feedback about areas in which they could improve, and offered assistance in making the necessary adjustments. Frank discussion should address the consequences of failure to adjust to more desirable patterns of behaviour. The decision to fail a student on the basis of undesirable attitudes may or may not be an option, depending upon local philosophy and circumstances. Less serious displays of inappropriate attitude development can be handled more subtly, perhaps by involving the student in special projects during the course of which role modelling can be attempted and feedback on attitudes given as appropriate. In some cases, of course, the decision may be made that a particular student is not suited to work in care of the elderly but this may not necessarily prejudice their ability to work in dissimilar areas. All of these decisions, it must be emphasized, must depend on the objectives of the curriculum and the tasks which the health professional will be expected to perform on graduation. These conditions will vary from context to context.

In summary, the most effective form of assessment of professional attitudes, skills, and behaviour is that which is carried out in the workplace and forms part of the learning experience itself. The use of assessment as feedback is the only sensible approach to accomplishing the transition from student to mature professional.

CONCLUSION

Published reports of training programmes emanate mainly from Western industralized countries. A review of programmes in Asia and Oceania[23] revealed an awakening to the importance of providing training in this area and a growing emphasis upon developing sufficient numbers of adequately trained people to care for the elderly. This paper has reviewed some trends mainly as reported in Western literature but which should also be applicable given appropriate implementation in a variety of cultures for a variety of professions.

In summary the social, cultural, professional, and institutional context must be favourable for the development of adequate training programmes. Community action, professional awareness, and government initiatives can stimulate favourable environments for the development of training programmes. Objectives for training must be identified which are based on the analysis of local tasks and needs. Teaching and learning methods must be integrated with the mainstream of health professions education but must emphasize experiential, practical learning rather than abstract or theoretical learning. Experiences should allow familiarity with the broadest possible range of situations which professionals encounter. Parts of training can certainly be carried out in teaching hospitals but this is no longer a sufficient model as it is no longer sufficient for other aspects of primary care. Resources and audiovisual aids can be very useful, particularly with broadening students' experience and 'unfreezing' their attitudes, but few are appropriate outside the culture in which they were made. Caution should be exercised in their use. Assessment of student performance should emphasize holistic approaches and appropriate behaviours—it is best carried out 'on the job' as part of learning rather than at the end of the course. Knowledge and some skills may be tested in final examinations but attitudes and professional behaviours cannot be tested in that context.

Finally, it is important not to lose sight of the valuable input of the person who is central to the entire effort—the elderly individual. He or she has much to offer, not as a patient or client who needs to be served nor as an object we use to teach students, but as a human being who has much to share from the experience of living through a full lifespan. The elderly person is an expert in the business of living.

References

1. Geiger, D. L. (1978). How future professionals view the elderly: a comparative analysis of social work, law and medical students' perceptions. *Gerontologist*, **18**, 591–4.
2. Abbatt, F. R. (1980). *Teaching for better learning. A guide for teachers of primary health care staff.* WHO, Geneva.
3. Guilbert, J. J. (1981). *Educational handbook for health personnel.* WHO, Geneva.
4. Ewan, C. E. and White, R. H. (1984). *Teaching nursing: a self-instructional handbook.* Croom Helm, London.
5. Coccaro, E. F. and Miles, A. M. (1984). The attitudinal impact of training in gerontology/geriatrics in medical school: a review of the literature and perspective. *Journal of the American Geriatrics Society*, **32**, 762–8.
6. Reichel, W. (1981). Geriatric medical education: developments since the American Geriatrics Society Conferences on Geriatric Education, 1976–1977. *Journal of the American Geriatrics Society*, **29**, 1–9.
7. Romeis, J. C., Schey, H. M., Marion, G. S. and Keith, J. F. (1985). Extending the extenders. Compromise for the geriatric specialization-manpower debate. *Journal of the American Geriatrics Society*, **33**, 559–65.
8. Schneider, E. L. and Williams, T. F. (1986). Geriatrics and gerontology, imperatives in education and training. *Annals of Internal Medicine* **104**, 432–5.
9. Raber, P. E. (1980). Teaching geriatrics: making room for the future. *Geratrics*, July, pp. 18–22.
10. Campbell, E. W. Shanahan, P. M., and Mulrow, P. J. (1982). Establishment of a geriatrics curriculum. *Journal of the American Geriatrics Society*, **30**, 473–4.
11. Stout, R. W. and Irwin, W. G. (1982). Integrated medical student teaching. *Medical Education*, **16**, 143–6.

12. Stout, R. W. (1985). Teaching gerontology and geriatric medicine. *Age and Aging*, **14** (Supplement).

13. Robbins, A. S., Fink, A., Kosecoff, J., Vivell, S., and Beck, J. C. (1982). Studies in geriatric education: I. Developing educational objectives. *Journal of the American Geriatrics Society*, **30**, 281–8.

14. WHO workshop report (1986). *Workshop on curricular changes to meet the health needs of the elderly*. 8–10 July, 1986. WHO Regional Office for the Western Pacific and the Government of Malaysia.

15. World Health Organization (1982). *Teaching gerontology and geriatric medicine*. Report on a workshop, 5–7 April, Edinburgh. WHO publication no. ICP/ADR 045(2).

16. Ewan, C. E. (1983). Teaching gerontology in Australia. *Medical Teacher*, **5**, 132–6.

17. Galinsky, D. (1985). Ten years' experience teaching geriatric medicine. *Israeli Journal of Medical Science*, **21**, 249–53.

18. Cox, K. R. C. and Ewan, C. E. (ed.) (1982). *Medical teacher*, (1st edn). Churchill Livingstone, Edinburgh.

19. Cox, D. R. C. and Ewan, C. E. (ed.) (1987). *Medical teacher*, (2nd edn). Churchill Livingstone, Edinburgh.

20. Shinar, D. (1981). *The use of participatory communications in community work with the elderly*. An interim report paper presented at the XIIth International Congress of Gerontology, Hamburg.

21. Mulder, J. D. (1984). Gerontophobia and medical education. *Tijdschrft Gerontologie Geriatrics*, **15**, 227–9.

22. Radford, A. J. (1981). A multidisciplinary learning exercise in care of the elderly. In *Education in aging: issues and approaches*. National Research Institute for Gerontology and Geriatric Medicine Occasional Paper no. 3. Melbourne.

23. World Health Organization (1985). *Health care of the elderly*. International Meeting on Education and Training in Health Care of the Elderly, 10–11 July, New York.

24. Job, E. M. (1983). Teaching medical students about old age. *Proceedings of the 18th Annual Conference of the Australian Association of Gerontologists*.

25. Green, C. P. (1981). Fostering positive attitudes towards the elderly: a teaching strategy for attitude change. *Journal of Gerontological Nursing*, **7**, 168–74.

26. Knowles, M. (1975). *Self-directed learning—A guide for learners and teachers*. Follett Publications, Chicago.

27. Brodaty, H. (1987). Teaching interpersonal skills. In *The medical teacher* (2nd edn). (ed. Cox, K. R. C. and C. E. Ewan), pp. 90–101. Churchill Livingstone, Edinburgh.

28. Marshall, J. R. (1987). Patient management problems. In Cox and Ewan (1987). *op. cit.*

29. Reid, A. L. A. (1983). Faculty of Medicine, University of Newcastle, NSW, Australia. Personal communication.

30. Barry, P. P. and Ham, R. J. (1985). Geriatric education: what the medical schools are doing now. *Journal of the American Geriatrics Society*, **33**, 133–5.

31. Woolliscroft, J. O., Calhoun, J. G., Massim, B. R., and Wolf, R. M. (1984). Medical education in facilities for the elderly. Impact on medical students,

facility staff and residents. *Journal of the American Medical Association*, **252**, 3382–5.

32. Ross, M. (1985). The impact of client selection on clinical teaching. *Journal of Advances in Nursing*, **10**, 567–73.
33. Greenhill, E. D. and Baker, M. F. (1986). The effects of a well older adult clinical experience on students' knowledge and attitudes. *Journal of Nursing Education*, **25**, 145–7.
34. Cotton, G. E. (1984). Clerkship rounds involving senior citizens at a high rise apartment complex. *Journal of Medical Education*, **59**, 135–7.
35. Ullmann, A. and Ruchlin, H. S. (1985). A gerontology internship program for medical students. *Social Work and Health Care*, **11**, 101–11.
36. Stark, R., Yeo, G., Fordyce, M., Grudgen, M., Gopkins, J., McGann, L., and Shepard, K. (1984). An interdisciplinary teaching program in geriatrics for physicians assistants. *Journal of Allied Health*, **13**, 280–7.
37. Sankar, A. and Becker, S. L. (1985). The home as a site for teaching gerontology and chronic illness. *Journal of Medical Education*, **60**, 308–13.
38. Jahnigen, D. W. Kramer, A. M., Robbins, L. J., Klingbeil, H., and DeVore, P. (1985). Academic affiliation with a nursing home. Impact on patient outcome. *Journal of the American Geriatrics Society*, **33**, 427–8.
39. Peach, H. and Pathy, M. S. (1982). Attitudes towards the care of the aged and to a career with elderly patients among students attached to a geriatric and general medical firm. *Age and Aging*, **11**, 196–202.
40. Arie, T. H. D. (1985). Education in the care of the elderly. *Bulletin of the NY Academy of Medicine*, **61**, 492–500.
41. Croen, L. G., Hamerman, D., and Goetzel, R. Z. (1984). Interdisciplinary training for medical and nursing students: learning to collaborate in the care of geriatric patients, *Journal of the American Geriatrics Society*, **32**, 56–61.
42. Hall, G. G. and Starkman, M. N. (1979). Incorporation of gerontology into medical education. *Journal of the American Geriatrics Society*, **27**, 368–73.

36

Planning for health personnel needed to serve elderly persons

DANIEL I. ZWICK and T. FRANKLIN WILLIAMS

Planning for health professionals and other personnel needed to serve older persons must combine hard facts about the present with creative thinking about the future. This work must be based on up-to-date information concerning existing conditions with respect to elderly populations and their caregivers. It must also be extended and enriched by very careful consideration of potential changes which may affect their status and needs in future years.

Planning for health personnel to serve older persons starts with a quite thorough understanding of the present—or 'what is'. We need to learn as much as practical about the current generation of older persons—especially their health status and experiences, including strengths as well as problems. Information about the types of available health care services and how they are being utilized is just as important as data on education and training of health care practitioners serving older adults, including the capacities and deficiencies of preparatory activities for these responsibilities.

The next phase of the planning process focuses on the future, or 'what may be'. Because changes are inevitable, we must try to anticipate and project the numbers, health status, and other characteristics of older populations to come. Estimates of the types and scope of health services likely to be needed in decades ahead should be developed and reviewed. The potential impact of future developments on requirements and educational experiences for health care personnel should be carefully analysed.

Flexibility and creativity are essential ingredients of the planning process. Planners must be willing—even eager—to accept and apply new information and ideas about 'what is' and 'what may be'. Planners must recognize that today's understandings are only the initial steps toward a better view of tomorrow's realities.

In this paper we present information on recent national activities in the United States. Only limited information is available on similar efforts in other countries. While the US experiences cannot be extrapolated to other situations, we hope that the approaches and principles set forth may be helpful in the consideration of related endeavours by other countries.

IMPORTANCE OF PLANNING

Long-term planning for personnel to provide health care to older persons is especially important because of the unusually long time frame for these efforts and the scope of investments that must be made before results are evident. Such time horizons usually encompass many decades. The development and deployment of education and other resources and activities require extended concentration of efforts to achieve the important effects which subsequently extend over many years. Persistence and patience are essential in achieving meaningful results.

For example, the expansion of the activities in the United States to increase the number of primary care physicians which was undertaken in the 1950s did not produce substantial results until the 1970s and 1980s. Similarly, efforts to introduce new types of personnel, such as physician assistants and nurse practitioners, are still in the developmental stages after decades of effort.

Planning activities provide opportunities to bring together the many agencies and groups concerned with these issues. They should include professional, voluntary health, and consumer associations as well as public bodies. Leaders from service and research programmes as well as eductional institutions should also participate actively. Moreover, effective planning approaches can demonstrate the importance and value of involving the many different disciplines necessary to provide high-quality care to older persons.

Planning for health personnel must consider education and training needs over the lifetime careers of professional and other practitioners. There must be adequate in-service education and continuing education for all types of health workers to ensure that they are prepared to apply new knowledge and practices. For instance, the current supply of practising physicians in the USA will compose over half the number of medical practitioners until after the year 2010.

The importance of long-term planning is also emphasized by the extended period of development of many chronic diseases and disabilities. Scientific findings in recent years have indicated that while much disease and disability are age related, they are not age determined. Rather, many health problems of later life are the results of exposure to risks over many years—not the fixed process of aging—and may be prevented or ameliorated if sound health practices are adopted and followed throughout the lifespan. These include practices related to smoking, diet, exercise, alcohol, and dental care. Health caregivers and the public must be prepared and encouraged continuously to promote appropriate health promotion and disease prevention activities among both current and future generations of older persons.

Long-term planning can also ease the adjustments that are certain to be encountered in almost all countries owing to the increasing number of older persons. The unprecedented growth of elderly populations will present conditions that are new to all of us. Furthermore, research advances promise to provide new knowledge and technologies that will call for changes in everyone's daily practices. Many different types of health care personnel will be required to contribute to these services, often in new ways and in new team arrangements. Systematic approaches and careful forethought can help individuals, institutions, and societies to deal more effectively with these evolving challenges.[1]

DETERMINING 'WHAT IS'

Planning must be based on a solid foundation of facts about current conditions. In order to prepare for tomorrow, we must undestand as much as possible about the status of older persons today. While the future will certainly differ from the present, sound evaluation of existing conditions and needs makes it possible to be more realistic about what is feasible and probable in coming years.

Accurate and complete information about the present situation is often difficult to obtain, even in countries such as the United States where there are well-established data-reporting systems. There are frequent gaps in available information about the older population, available services, and educational activities. It is critical to bring together pertinent facts from many different sources, including data available through health care financing programmes as well as from public health and educational agencies. In addition, special surveys are often needed to provide essential supplementary information specifically about the older population and aging issues.

The United States experience has been that, in the past, inadequate attention has been given to specific data about the older population. Data may not have been collected or analyzed specifically for persons in older age categories, or all older persons may be classified together. We are increasingly recognizing that the heterogeneity of the elderly population is one of its most important characteristics; for example needs for and utilization of services by the younger elderly (under 70 years of age) are very different from those experienced among the oldest old (85 years of age and older). Furthermore, there are usually wide variations in conditions of individuals within specific age categories.

An earnest effort to document the current status of older persons can provide an important set of facts, none the less, when pertinent data are collected from all available sources. By identifying deficiencies in existing data, this approach may stimulate additional activities to produce further information about the older populations and their conditions and experiences.

The United States has recently undertaken a national study concerning personnel and training needs to serve its elderly population through the year 2020. In 1985, there were about 29 million persons aged 65 years and more (Table 36.1)—almost 12 per cent of the national population. This group is estimated to utilize about 20 per cent of ambulatory physician visits, over 40 per cent of short-stay hospital days, and almost 90 per cent of nursing home services (Fig. 36.1). Persons aged 65 years and over may soon use over half of the health care services in this country.

On the other hand, the large majority of older persons in the US are healthy and able to function independently. Special surveys have found that more than 90 per cent of individuals 65 years and older are living in the community. About two-thirds of that groups indicate their health is good to excellent.[2]

Many older adults report some difficulties in carrying out their activities of daily living. These problems vary from relatively minor difficulties which require only modest changes in lifestyle to severe difficulties which may necessitate substantial medical care. In 1984, about one-third of those aged 65 years and over living in the community were reported to experience functional difficulties; almost two-thirds of those of 85 years and over had such problems (Table 36.2). About 10 per cent of the total group—more than 25 per cent of the oldest old—experienced three or more such difficulties. Among those with multiple problems, about half received assistance from another person, usually a family member or

Table 36.1 Projected population (in millions)

	1985		2000		2020	
	No.	%	No.	%	No.	%
Grand total	247.4	100.0	277.1	100.0	307.7	100.0
Total 65+	*29.1*	*11.8*	*36.4*	*13.1*	*54.5*	*17.7*
65–74	17.0	6.9	18.5	6.7	31.7	10.3
75–84	9.2	3.7	12.7	4.6	15.4	5.0
85+	2.9	1.2	5.2	1.9	7.3	2.4

Source: Social Security Administration (1985).

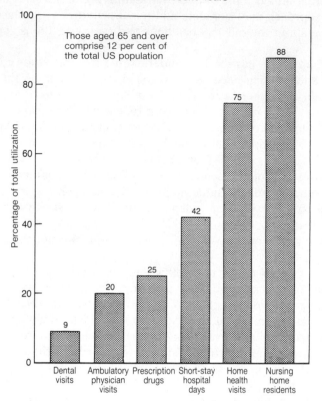

Fig. 36.1 Utilization of health services by persons 65 years and older in recent years.

friend. Assistance was received from a health professional caregiver in only a minority of cases.

The use of health care services has changed in the USA in the last few years. The number of days that older persons stayed in short-term hospitals decreased by about 15 per cent between 1981 and 1985. During the same period, the use of physician services on an ambulatory basis and home health services by nurses and other personnel has increased markedly.

For example, the number of ambulatory visits to physicians by persons aged 65 years and over has increased about 20 per cent between 1981 and 1985 (Table 36.3). The proportion of such visits to all types of medical specialists has also expanded in recent years (Table 36.4).

Table 36.2 Persons with functional difficulties living in the community, 1984[2]

Condition	Total 65+		65–74		75–84		85+	
	No.[a]	%[b]	No.[a]	%[b]	No.[a]	%[b]	No.[a]	%[b]
Total persons with difficulties with 1 or more ADLs or IADLs:	8.6	33	4.2	26	3.2	39	1.2	62
male	2.7	25	1.5	21	0.9	30	0.3	52
female	5.9	38	2.7	30	2.3	45	0.9	66
Total persons with difficulties with 3 or more ADLs:	2.3	9	0.9	5	0.9	11	0.5	25
male	0.7	7	0.3	5	0.2	8	0.1	18
female	1.6	10	0.6	6	0.7	13	0.4	29
Total persons with difficulties with 3 or more IADLs and receiving help:	1.0	4	0.4	2	0.4	5	0.3	14
male	0.3	3	0.2	2	0.1	4	0.1	10
female	0.7	4	0.2	2	0.3	6	0.2	16

[a] In millions.
[b] Percentage of total population living in the community in age category.

Table 36.3 Ambulatory visits to physicians by persons 65 years of age and over (in millions)

	1978		1981		1985		% increase	
	No.	%	No.	%	No.	%	78–85	81–85
Total visits	93.9	100	107.4	100	130.5	100	39	22
Gen'l practice/ family practice	36.0	38	36.7	34	37.9	29	5	3
Internal medicine	21.3	23	25.7	24	28.9	22	36	12
Other specialities	36.6	39	45.1	42	63.7	49	74	41

Source: National Ambulatory Medical Care Survey, National Center for Health Statistics.

Table 36.4 Percentage of total ambulatory visits to various medical specialties by persons 65 years of age and over

	1978	1981	1985
All specialities	*16.1*	*18.4*	*20.1*
General practice/family practice	17.1	19.3	19.6
Internal medicine	31.1	34.4	39.2
Cardiology	39.1	46.1	47.2
Ophthalmology	30.0	39.3	43.8
Urology	29.9	37.6	39.6
Gen'l surgery	21.9	20.1	27.2
Neurology	13.2	17.7	21.0
Dermatology	12.2	13.4	18.3
Otolaryngology	14.1	16.9	17.0
Orthopaedic surgery	10.9	13.7	13.9
Psychiatry	4.5	4.6	6.5
Obstetrics/gynaecology	2.2	2.6	3.3
Other	5.0	6.0	10.2

Source: National Ambulatory Medical Care Survey, National Center for Health Statistics.

Other health professional personnel are also devoting more of their efforts to the care of older persons. Estimates are that about one-third of the current efforts of registered nurses, about 45 per cent of the work of licensed practical nurses, approximately 40 per cent of the services of podiatrists, and 25 per cent of the activities of physical therapists are focused on the care of older persons. As in the case of physicians, almost all of these services are provided by caregivers who also serve younger persons as part of their daily practices.

A small cadre of leaders in medicine and other health disciplines are concentrating all of their efforts on aging and geriatric issues. These individuals are usually educators, researchers, and consultants.

These facts have important implications for the education and training of current and future physicians and other health personnel. Recent studies have confirmed that information on aging, geriatrics, and gerontology has been expanded in the curricula of most health professional schools in the last decade or so. In some cases, more material on these topics has been integrated into established courses; in other instances, distinctive courses on these subjects are being offered, usually on an elective basis. Nevertheless, these studies also indicate far less incorporation of such material into the *required* education of health professionals than is needed.[3]

Community settings (outside hospitals) are increasingly being used as training sites in the USA. Many students are working with the well elderly in senior centres, day care programmes, and similar settings as well as with ill patients at home and in nursing homes. Multidisciplinary approaches, involving medical, nursing, dental, rehabilitation, and other students, are also being expanded in different situations such as geriatric assessment and evaluation programmes. Even more emphasis will need to be devoted to these types of activities in light of recent trends in health care.

The scope and intensity of education and training activities in aging and geriatrics are still relatively modest, however. Expansion has been limited by severe shortages of faculty members who are adequately prepared to conduct and guide programmes. It is estimated that there are only 5 to 25 per cent (depending on the field) of the number of faculty members and investigators who are currently needed for the development of such activities. Thus, the preparation of additional faculty leaders is a priority.

The development of education and training programs to prepare personnel to serve older persons is primarily the responsibility of educational institutions in the USA. In addition, many hospitals and other providers contribute significantly to these efforts for both currently employed and new personnel. State governmental agencies in the education, health, and aging fields are providing encouragement and some supplementary funding for these purposes in many parts of the country. A number of national governmental agencies in these fields are also making available limited targeted support. The US Veterans Administration has been a leader in this regard; about 20 per cent of the veteran population is 65 and older. This ratio may increase to almost 50 per cent by the year 2020.

Coordination of efforts among agencies and institutions responsible for educational programmes and those responsible for the development and provision of services to older persons has been strengthened in the USA in recent years. For example, the national planning study cited earlier was guided by a committee composed of representation from federal government agencies concerned with health professions education, health services delivery, health care financing, aging services, other social services, and aging research and training. In many local communities, joint planning councils have been established to bring together the numerous interested groups, often including faculty members from health education schools.

Co-ordination of education and research programmes in aging is generally at an advanced stage in the USA. At the national level, the National Institute on Aging and the National Institute of Mental Health, which provide leadership and funding for research and research training in their respective fields, are actively involved in planning educational activities. At the institutional level, faculty members in medical, dental, nursing, and other health schools are usually concerned with both teaching and research.

Private philanthropic foundations and other private groups are also contributing in important ways to the planning and development of education and training programmes in geriatrics and gerontology in the USA. Foundations have helped to finance innovative approaches to preparing new faculty and clinical personnel. Professional associations of physicians, dentists, nurses, and allied health personnel are also increasingly interested in these issues and have expanded their efforts, especially in the development of curricula guidelines and the conduct of continuing education for their members.

In the implementation of the recent national planning study, numerous private groups participated by providing information on current activities and view on future trends and needs. A public forum was conducted to solicit their ideas and insights and to discuss outstanding issues. Altogether over 100 public and private agencies contributed to the planning effort.

Available information on geriatric and gerontological education and training activities in other countries indicates both noteworthy similarities and differences. For example, a 1984 survey of the status of clinical education in these subjects in 22 European countries reported that, in 14 countries, related materials were included on a compulsory basis in undergraduate medical curricula; in 17 countries such material was part of postgraduate programmes (Table 36.5). Academic chairs had been established in 15 countries, and medical specialization was reported in 14 countries.[4]

A study of educational programmes concerning health care of elderly persons was also updated in 1984 for 18 countries of Asia and Oceania. As indicated in Table 36.6, multidisciplinary approaches are being undertaken in some situations.[5]

CONCERNING 'WHAT MAY BE'

A starting point for considering potential future needs for services and personnel who will be required to serve the older population is the review of projections about the size and composition of elderly populations in the decades ahead. As indicated in Table 36.1, it is anticipated that there may

Table 36.5 Gerontological medical education in Europe[4]

	Chairs	Undergrad.		Postgrad. Curriculum	Specialization
		Vol'y	Req'd		
Austria		×			
Belgium	1		×	×	
Czechoslovakia	3		×	×	×
Denmark		×		×	×
France	6		×	×	×
Finland	1		×	×	×
West Germany	3				
East Germany			×	×	
Greece		×		×	
Hungary			×	×	
Israel	2		×		×
Ireland					×
Italy	7	×		×	×
Netherlands	1	×			×
Norway	1		×	×	×
Poland	1		×	×	×
Romania	1		×	×	×
Spain				×	×
Sweden	5		×	×	×
Switzerland	2		×	×	
USSR	2		×	×	
United Kingdom	15		×	×	×

Table 36.6 A review of training programmes in health care of the elderly in Asia and Oceania survey of course descriptions by professional discipline[5]

	Medical	Nursing	Allied	Aides	Interdisciplinary
Australia	×	×	×	×	×
Burma	×				
Egypt	×	×			
Fiji	×				
Guam		×			
Hong Kong	×	×		×	
India	×				
Indonesia	×				
Japan	×	×			
Republic of Korea	×				
Malaysia	×	×			
New Zealand	×	×		×	×

Table 36.6 (*cont.*)

	Medical	Nursing	Allied	Aides	Interdisciplinary
Papua New Guinea	×			×	
China (PRC)	×	×			
Singapore				×	
Taiwan	×				
Thailand	×				

Table 36.7 Alternative population forecasts, USA, 2020

	Alternative II[a]	Alternative III[b]	Percentage Difference
Total 65+	*54.5*	*58.3*	*7.0*
65–74	31.7	32.6	2.8
75–84	15.4	16.6	7.8
85+	7.3	9.1	24.7

[a] Assumes mortality will decrease at an average annual rate that equals about half the average annual reduction observed during 1900–1983.
[b] Assumes mortality will decrease at an average annual rate that is about the same as the average annual reduction observed during 1900–1983.
Source: Social Security Administration (1985).

be 54 million older persons in the USA in the year 2020—almost twice the current cohort. The proportion of the national population aged 65 years and older is likely to increase from about 12 to 18 per cent; the proportion aged 75 years and older may expand from about 5 to more than 7 per cent.

A more optimistic assumption about mortality rates produces a higher estimate of the potential size of the older population in the future. Under these conditions, there might be more than 4 million more older persons in the USA in the year 2020 (Table 36.7). About half of the added group might be 85 years of age and older.

Needs for services and personnel by elderly persons in the future are usually first estimated on the basis of the impact of anticipated changes in the size and age composition of the older population, assuming current patterns of utilization of services are maintained. Three assumptions are critical to these calculations: (1) current levels of services are generally adequate, (2) the health status of specific age groups will not change

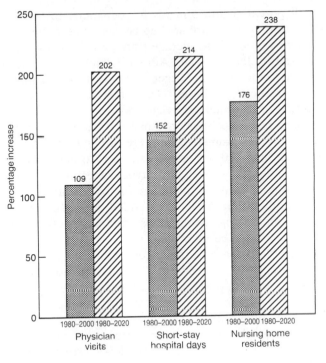

Projected Percentage Increase in Use of Health Services
in Persons 65 Years and Older, 1980-2000 and 1980-2020

Source: Rice and Feldman, 1983.

Fig. 36.2 Projected percentage increase in use of health services in persons 65 years and older, 1980–2000 and 1980–2020.[6]

significantly, and (3) past rates of utilization of services by age group will not alter greatly.

However, all three of these assumptions are very uncertain and are almost certain to require modifications over the years. While this approach provides a useful base for preliminary analyses and discussions, alternataive conditions and developments must also be considered during the planning process. Furthermore, periodic assessments of changing requirements are essential to adequately consider and incorporate new circumstances, knowledge, and practice.

A 1983 estimate of potential future needs for services by older persons in the USA, based on these types of assumptions, identified potential requirements for substantial increases. The estimate highlighted the fact that, by 2020, needs for physician services, short-stay hospital days, and nursing home care by older persons may all more than double (Fig. 36.2).

The projections illustrate the general level of magnitude of potential future needs.[6]

A review of potential future needs for personnel to serve the elderly veteran population in the future applied current staff–patient ratios of the Veterans Administration. The average staff–patient ratios within facilities directly operated by the Veterans Administration in 1986 for physicians were 1:10 in medicine, 1:13 in surgery, and 1:114 in nursing home care units. Ratios for social work staff were 1:45 for medical and surgical patients and 1:30 for psychiatry services. Assuming these ratios are maintained, increased needs for these personnel to care for veterans directly served by the Veterans Administration are projected to increase from 65 per cent to more than 100 per cent between 1986 and 2000.

However, as indicated above, these types of estimates must be considered as only initial steps in planning for the future. They must be reviewed and modified on the basis of added data and creative thinking concerning the underlying assumptions. Let us briefly consider some modifications which may be indicated.

The first assumption concerns the adequacy of current levels of service. A study of future geriatric needs in the USA found that the average period of contact between physicians and older patients in the USA in the mid 1970s was several minutes shorter than for middle-aged patients and that older persons underutilized services when their level of illness was considered. Accordingly, an alternative projection of future personnel needs analysed the increased use of physician services that would be necessary to equalize the length of encounters.[7]

Similarly, a recent study in the USA among nursing home residents found that only 10 per cent received occupational therapy, whereas about 35 per cent would have benefited from such services. Accordingly, estimated needs for rehabilitation personnel based on current practices must be modified if the identified deficiencies are to be overcome in the future.[3]

The second assumption concerns the future health status of the older population. A number of different views concerning this issue have been expressed:

1. There may be a high prevalence of chronic illnesses and mental illness among the very old as the length of life increases. Thus, needs for care are likely to increase substantially.

2. Healthier lifestyles among the future older population may result in declines in the average period of illness and reduced capacities. Accordingly, needs for medical care may decrease.

3. The severity and progression of chronic diseases among older persons may decline in line with related decreases in mortality, research ad-

vances, and the capacities of individuals and caregivers to manage disabilities may extend the length of independent living.

4. The proportions of older persons in relatively good health until death and of older persons with prolonged severe functional limitations may both increase, resulting in fewer elderly persons having moderate degrees of infirmity.

Alternative analyses might consider the potential impact on needs for services of these various scenarios. For example, it has been estimated that needs for services and related personnel might decline at the same rate as potential declines in mortality rates.[8]

A third critical assumption relates to patterns of utilization of health care services. Many future developments—within the national society as well as within the health care system—may affect these practices. Some changes may increase utilization while others may decrease demands for organized health care services. Table 36.8 presents a listing of potential changes which have been identified as factors which may influence future conditions in the United States. Projections of personnel required for long-term care are especially difficult because of the variety of potential organizational and financing arrangements and the important role of informal caregiving by families and friends.

Changing attitudes toward the use of certain health care services—among both the public and health professionals—may be especially important. For example, future older generations may be more interested in health promotion and disease prevention services and in mental health services as the result of experiences earlier in their lifetime. In the USA, there is increasing interest in the development of more extensive community-based services and decreased use of institutional care. Further, the expansion of multidisciplinary approaches at critical points, such as in geriatric assessment activities, may alter demands for different types of personnel and aspects of their preparation.

Likewise, alternations in health care financing programmes may have a major effect on both the provision of care and the education of health personnel. Not only do these policies have a major influence on the extent of interest in certain services and skills, but they also may help to finance many educational activities, particularly in-service training for current staffs. Greater emphases within these programs on health prevention and geriatric assessment practices, for example, would greatly increase needs for personnel with specific preparation in these subjects, and could also be expected to reduce needs for service personnel in certain other aspects of health care.

In order to help evaluate the impact of the many potential developments that may affect future health care utilization, the planning process

Table 36.8 Potential changes that may affect needs for health services and personnel

Societal changes likely to influence demands:	Increase	Decrease
1. Increased availability of national wealth	×	
2. Larger incomes among some older persons	×	
3. Higher expectations concerning quality of life	×	
4. Greater expectations regarding the availability of service	×	
5. Rise in educational levels	×	
6. Greater workplace participation by women	×	
7. Increases in childlessness	×	
8. Larger number of persons living alone	×	
9. New residential and living arrangements		×
10. Limited incomes among some older persons		×
11. Increasing efforts of the younger old in working with older persons		×
12. Expansion in volunteer efforts		×
Health system changes likely to influence demands:		
1. Greater technological capabilities to detect, diagnose, and treat diseases and disabilities	×	
2. Increased health insurance benefits	×	
3. More emphasis on rehabilitation	×	
4. Larger supply of physicians and some other health care personnel	×	
5. Concentration of sickest patients in hospitals	×	
6. Increased levels of illness among patients discharged from hospitals	×	
7. More interest in community-based services	×	
8. New health benefits for low-income groups	×	
9. New research advances to prevent and manage diseases and disabilities		×
10. Greater technological capabilities for prevention and rehabilitation		×
11. Development of professional standards to reduce variations in care practices		×
12. Greater emphasis on health promotion and disease prevention		×
13. Expansion of integrated systems of care		×
14. Closer coordination of health, social, and other human services		×
15. More stringent cost-containment measures		×

might include the deliberations of an expert group convened to focus on these issues. Such an approach has been used in the USA in considering future needs for nursing personnel.[9] Groups of experts in various areas of nursing education and practice and of representatives of several health care associations were assembled to develop and revise potential staffing criteria in light of possible future developments and goals. These groups have given special attention to personnel for nursing homes in view of prospective increases in the numbers of older persons and complexities of their conditions in these facilities.

Uncertainties about future conditions pertain to estimates of the future supply of health personnel as well as projections of needs and demands. For instance, analyses of the supply must consider changes in the number of younger persons who are likely to receive and complete advanced education as well as possible patterns of re-entry by experienced workers, such as nurses, who leave the working population but return later.

In light of the many uncertainties concerning future conditions, estimates of future needs for personnel within specific disciplines and subgroups are usually best presented as a range, rather than a specific figure (e.g. between 100 000 and 120 000). In this way, an indication of the general level of magnitude of future requirements may be provided to help guide recruitment and educational efforts. As emphasized above, ongoing assessments and re-evaluations should consider adjustments which will almost certainly be necessary in light of new information and developments.

The recent national study of potential future needs in the USA, which was cited earlier, concluded that most health care of older persons will probably continue to be provided by physicians and other personnel who also serve younger persons. It is estimated that between one-third and two-thirds of the future practices of most health care practitioners are likely to be devoted to the care of older persons. The substantial increases in the total supply of physicians and certain other health care personnel which are anticipated will provide substantial resources for meeting projected needs if they are specifically and adequately prepared for these responsibilities as part of undergraduate, graduate, and continuing education programmes.

Accordingly, the planning committee emphasized that the preparation of three groups of health personnel in the various health professions be enhanced in order to meet anticipated future health needs of the increasing older population:

1. Essentially all health care personnel should be educated specifically about the special conditions and needs of older persons and have up-to-date knowledge concerning the most effective means of prevent-

ing and managing diseases and disabilities experienced by older persons.

2. A relatively small group of clinicians should be prepared to provide specialized consultation and guidance to other personnel and to provide limited amounts of direct service for special problems.

3. A cadre of full-time faculty members and investigators should be developed to provide leadership in the development and conduct of teaching and research efforts.

CONCLUSION

Planning for professional and other personnel to meet the health care needs of the population of older persons must be an ongoing process. Important increases in requirements are likely during the coming decades, not only because of the much larger number of elderly individuals, but also because of potential alterations in other critical factors such as health status, scientific capacities, and financing arrangements. Initial estimates of prospective needs, based on current practices and knowledge, provide starting points for further analyses and deliberations.

Planning for high-quality care must address the entire range of required services and related personnel. The scope of such efforts must encompass preventive, primary, acute, long-term, rehabilitative, and hospice care services. Participating personnel will range from aides and volunteers to various medical specialists.

Studies of prospective requirements should be closely co-ordinated with other activities that are likely to have a major impact on needs and demands for health services. These programmes include activities focused on health care delivery and financing generally, social services, other aging services, and veterans affairs. They should also be linked on a continuing basis with scientific research and developmental activities so that opportunities for improved prevention and management of diseases and disabilities are promptly incorporated into established educational and service practices.

The organization and conduct of these types of activities must reflect the special character of the educational and health systems of particular countries. In the United States a large number of governmental, private, and professional agencies are involved in the preparation of personnel and the provision of services. Thus, the planning process has been designed to obtain the active participation of the many concerned parties. While US approaches cannot be extrapolated to other countries and conditions, they may be helpful in illustrating some of the issues that may be experienced in these types of efforts.

Experiences in the USA confirm the continuing relevance and importance of the six recommendations pertaining to training and education that
were adopted as part of the International Plan of Action by the United
Nations World Assembly on Aging in Vienna in 1982,[10] namely:

1. Education and training programmes should be interdisciplinary in
   nature because aging and the aging of the population are multidisciplinary issues. Education and training in the various aspects of
   aging and the aging of the population should not be restricted to high
   levels of specialization, but should be made available at all levels.
   Efforts should be made to regulate the training skills and educational
   requirements for different functions in the field of aging.

2. Intergovernmental and non-governmental organizations should take
   the necessary measures to develop trained personnel in the field of
   aging and should strengthen their efforts to disseminate information on
   aging, particularly to elderly people themselves.

3. Retirees' and elderly people's organizations should be involved in
   planning and carrying out exchanges of such information.

4. The implementation of several (other) recommendations will require
   trained personnel in the field of aging. Practical training centres should
   be promoted and encouraged where appropriate facilities already exist
   to train such personnel, especially from developing countries, who
   would in turn train others. These centres would also provide updating
   and refresher courses and act as a practical bridge between and among
   developed and developing regions; they would be linked with appropriate United Nations agencies and facilities.

5. Training in all aspects of gerontology and geriatrics should be encouraged and given due prominence at all levels in all educational programmes. Government and competent authorities are called upon
   to encourage new or existing institutions to pay special attention to
   appropriate training in gerontology and geriatrics.

6. Medical, nursing, and social work students should be trained in principles and skills in the relevant areas of gerontology, geriatrics,
   psychogeriatrics, and geriatric nursing; and those who work with elderly persons at home or in institutions should receive basic training for
   their tasks.

Under any conditions, planning depends upon the availability of reliable information about both current and prospective developments. The
presentation and review of pertinent facts can lead to a better understanding of both 'what is' and 'what may be'. As additional data become
available on the changing status and circumstances of older persons,
estimates must be adjusted and modified to incorporate evolving experiences. As a result, all interested individuals and institutions will be in a

better position to understand and deal with the health needs of older persons at the present time and in future years.

References

1. World Health Organization (1986). *Investigating practices in health manpower planning: report on a country case study*. World Health Organization Regional Office for Europe, Copenhagen, Denmark.
2. National Center for Health Statistics (1986). *Current estimates from the National Health Interview Survey*. DHHS Publication no. (PHS) 86–1588, September. Hyattsville, MD.
3. National Institute on Aging (1984). *Report on education and training in geriatrics and gerontology*. February. National Institute on Aging, Bethesda, MD.
4. Beregi, E. (1985). The situation of clinical gerontology in Europe. Training in health care of the elderly, international congress of gerontology, New York, July. *Zeitschrift für Gerontology*, Berlin–Bonn. (Submitted for publication).
5. World Health Organization (1986). *Aging in the Western Pacific*. World Health Organization Regional Office for the Western Pacific, Manila, Philippines.
6. Rice, D. P. and Feldman, J. J. (1983). Living longer in the United States: demographic changes and health needs of the elderly. *Milbank Memorial Fund Quarterly/Health and Society*, **61** (3), 362–96.
7. Kane, R. L., Solomon, D. H., Beck, J. C., Keeler, E. B., and Kane, R. A. (1981). *Geriatrics in the United States: manpower projections and training considerations*. Lexington Books, Lexington, MA.
8. Manton, K. and Saldo, B. (1985). Dynamics of health changes in the oldest old: new perspectives and evidence. *Milbank Memorial Fund Quarterly/Health and Society*, **63** (2), 206–85.
9. Health Resources and Services Administration (1986). *Fifth report to the President and Congress on the status of health personnel in the United States*. DHHS Publication HHS-P-OD-86–1, March.
10. United Nations (1982). *Vienna international plan of action on aging*. UN World Assembly on Aging, July–August. UN, New York.

Part V

Health and social policy issues in aging

37

Introduction

D. MACFADYEN

DETERMINANTS OF HEALTH IN OLD AGE

The most important single factor affecting the health of older people is the economic condition of elderly individuals. Other important factors are nutrition and the level of education, although there are less data on these. Marital status influences health: death of a spouse prejudices the health of the survivor.

The association noted in Japan between *per capita* resources allocated to government expenditure on medical care and life expectancy at age 65 years suggests that extension of medical care to elderly people is associated with measurable health benefit.

MULTIGENERATIONAL HOUSEHOLDS

In a developing country such as Thailand, 39 per cent of households live in multigenerational arrangements. In Japan the figure is 47 per cent, whereas in the United Kingdom, the United States, and France the corresponding percentages are less than 1, 2, and 4 per cent respectively. It is likely therefore that Asian countries such as Singapore, the Republic of Korea, and China will parallel Japan's policies on aging, since they have comparable traditions and family support systems. Bedridden and senile dementia patients in Japan are increasing at a rate of 2.7 per cent per annum (Fig. 37.1) and a projection to the year 2008 predicts that the numbers in these two categories will equal that of full-time housewives—assuming levels of female participation in the labour force remain at their present levels.

The urbanization process leads to increase in new nuclear families, poses geographical obstacles to family mutual aid, and results in elderly people having relatively weaker economic positions.

INSTITUTIONAL LONG-TERM CARE

An appreciable proportion of elderly men and women in the developed world live in single-person households, often having outlived their rela-

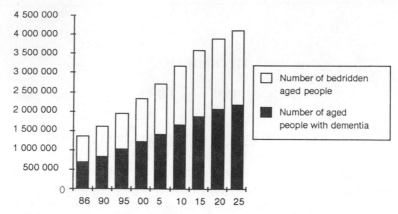

Fig. 37.1 Projected number of aged people with senile dementia and of bedridden elders, Japan 1986–2025.

tives. A small but growing number of these transit to institutions when they need special care. All countries, including developing countries, face severe problems of quality control in nursing homes and residential homes. The dignity of older people in these environments can be assured only in a moral climate which places individual autonomy at the centre of care. In no circumstances should competent elders cede control of their lives to attending staff.

EXIT FROM THE LABOUR MARKET

In developing countries, most elderly persons are in the informal or formal labour market because they cannot afford to withdraw from it. The situation is different in the developed world where the organized urban economy tends to push out aging workers from the labour market, leaving increasing numbers to be supported from a diminishing economic pool. Social security, as a system of enforced saving for old age, exists in the form of the provident funds of some developing countries. Elsewhere, social security has become a welfare benefit in which pensions are paid to the active population from funds generated largely by the working population. Such benefits have become the main component of older peoples' resources and allow them, more and more in developed countries, to enjoy a way of life comparable to that before retirement.

Government intervention in the provision of health and social care for the aged population is increasingly needed as a country proceeds on her modernization path. In establishing or reforming such services for elderly people, a major policy option is between service-based or cash assistance programmes. In the former, the emphasis is on efficiency in matching resources to need; the latter is centred on the equitable distribution of income.

ACCESS AND CONTINUITY OF HEALTH CARE

Health care provision for elderly persons in developing countries is of recent origin, although in Latin America health-insurance-based schemes have been in place for several years. In some Asian and African countries, the extension of health care coverage in such schemes to elderly as well as to young dependents is being established as a principle. However, the population covered by such health-insurance-based schemes is very small outside of the developed world.

Length of stay of elderly patients in health facilities is unnecessarily long and shows very great variation from country to country. Provision of continuity of care with integrated home-based nursing and social support allows more efficient use of health facilities.

IMPROVING QUALITY OF LIFE

Health and social policies for older people are concerned not only with increasing length of life, but also with improving the quality of life. The achievement of these objectives is now measured by the concept of quality-adjusted life years (QALY). Two components of this measure are freedom from disability and from pain and distress. In the present state of this experimental methodology, older people tend to fare worse relative to younger groups.

In the hierarchy of human needs, elderly people in developed countries are aspiring to the level of 'becoming' while, in developing countries they are struggling at the more basic level of 'being'. Thirteen out of 45 responding developing countries reported to the United Nations the unsatisfactory state of housing for elders, and 8 out of 47 reported that they were implementing nutrition policies for poor and underprivileged elders.

AGISM AND RESOURCE ALLOCATION

One of the responses to the massive growth in health care consumption in developed countries has been to ration services. A major debate in medical ethics has been provoked by age-based rationing, that is, restricting access to services or health technology on age-based criteria. This practice is unlikely to be accepted by future birth cohorts who will enter the aged category better educated and in better health than preceding cohorts.

TECHNOLOGY FOR INDEPENDENT LIVING

Advancing technology will provide opportunities to future cohorts of elderly people to adapt to the environment as they become more frail, for example by facilitating home care and through communication technology and intelligent prostheses. However, in the short term there is more scope for improving the quality of life of elderly people through social interventions.

38

Planning more suitable environments for the elderly

BRUNO VELLAS, PATRICK VELLAS, and JEAN-LOUIS ALBAREDE

The course of life is characterized first by an extension and then by a reduction in the sphere of social and vital activity. The process of aging is accompanied by progressive reduction in vital activity, as the space in which elderly people move on leaving the house becomes restricted.

The living space perceived by the child from birth until the moment he (or she) begins to walk is limited to the arms of his mother, to those who carry him to his cradle, and to the park to which he is taken. It is extended when he begins to walk and discovers the world around him, when he goes to school, to the parks, to play games, or to walk with his friends. It becomes maximally extended when he begins his professional life with the activities and travel which that involves. After retirement, that is to say on the cessation of professional activity, the living space becomes constricted. It is limited, usually, to the neighbourhood in which he lives and does the shopping, and to the few visits made to friends or relatives.

Later, with 'aggravated' aging, that is to say with the handicaps of advanced age, the living space becomes reduced even more. The aged or the very aged person may traverse his room only as far as the door. He may take a few steps on the pavement close to the house when the weather is fine. Then the circumference of vital activity shrinks even further, extending from the armchair to the bed and back, and finally to the bed alone.

In attempting to prevent the pathology associated with aging or to postpone the process of aging, the focus for action has been on the person. Preventive medicine, psychology, and social psychology continue to achieve progress through this approach.

But can one also act on the living space? The links between the living being and his sphere of vital activity are so close that all action on the environment directly influences the person. One can focus on the sphere of vital activity of the elderly person in two ways: managing the limited space of the bedroom which he occupies, or enlarging the space in which he lives.

What can one do about the elderly person who is severely handicapped and dependent, who is able to use only the limited space of the room, armchair, or bed? It is necessary to manage the limited space by making it as dense as possible and as bright as possible, and to open up and enlarge the sphere of activity, despite the limited facility in moving about and loss of autonomy. The bedroom space must be re-arranged with the goal of 'diversifying' and of 'densifying'. Diversifying is distinquishing by:

—— a *private space*, which is the area around the bed and the night table. In this are gathered together intimate familiar objects which are strictly personal;

—— the *semi-public space*, which is the area around the armchair to which the person goes to pass a few moments and in which she receives visits, plus that of the table at which she takes her meals when unable to leave the room.

Densifying means enriching the limited space of the bedroom by objects which are rich in memory. These are particularly useful around the bed, that is say in the private space where most personal objects would be arranged. In the semipublic space objects that evoke memories— photographs, landscapes, and pieces of art—may be placed.

Plants or flowers should occupy particularly important places, not only for decoration and for defining the space, but because they bring a balance of natural lively colours, in contrast to the inert wall and the cold wallpaper. Plants also need to be taken care of: it is necessary to water and trim them; you can also breath the scent of flowers, and hold them in your hand.

Familiar animals have an important role in the environment of the room, provided these are compatible with the hygiene and the management of the house. Fish in an aquarium, or canaries singing happily in a cage, convey a sense of vitality. Naturally, the limited space of the bedroom can be enlarged by means of communication that opens the environment to others in the world, for example, telephone, radio, television, newspapers, periodicals, and books.

In homes for dependent elderly people in whom mobility is severely reduced, it is essential to improve on the view of the world seen from the bedroom. Here, the concern is about the environment of the home itself. A transparent architectural structure permits the bed-bound elderly person to access, visually, the interior of the establishment, so that he can follow and perceive and listen to the comings and goings of the caring personnel, the volunteer workers, and visitors.

It is important that the rooms be divided around a common area to which they all give direct access. The separating walls between rooms should be removable by telecommand of the elderly person to be opened or closed according to the need for rest and solitude or for seeing, hearing, and participating in the life of the establishment.

Those who can move around could help to maintain a garden. This might be organized as an atrium, comprising a living garden with birds in their cages and fish in the pool with fountains and lights. This should be a particularly bright place with pathways, with spots for rest or places to meet and hold conversations.

For those who can leave the establishment, paths in the exterior should facilitate entry and departure. Toilets should be sited at the entry hall.

The sphere in which elderly people move must be extended as widely as possible if we are to postpone the process of aging, which expresses itself as a progressive reduction in living space. It is necessary, therefore, to support arrangements that extend the living space and facilitate elderly people getting about, and that motivate them to go from place to place. The following measures are proposed:

Organized excursions to local areas or further afield

These have the advantage of changing habits and behaviour, of widening the living space, and even improving morale through their encounters with others and by raising their curiosity. These measures, the local visit and the longer excursion, are essential elements in preventing the pathology of aging because they constitute a form of adaptation to change, a stimulant for physical, mental, and social activities. Such changes of scene and participation in social life offer the best opportunity for enlarging the boundaries within which people have to live.

The means of transport should correspond to the needs of the elderly person, for example by providing preferential fares, or by avoiding hours of departure and arrival at night or during busy traffic. Transport should be designed with steps that are easy to climb up, support ramps, and an easily accessible toilet, etc.

Ease of movement around the city

An essential task of the urban planner is to take account of the aging of the population. Elderly persons feel comfortable in the urban environment to which they are accustomed, that is to say the neighbourhood or street with which they are familiar. It is a feeling which they share with the young, but it affects the old in a much more accentuated fashion. They have a profound sense of belonging to the place in which they live. The location gives them an identity. They project this to where they have matured and developed personal relationships. This public space with which they are familiar provides security. Their roots are there.

The bulk and surface areas of the environment must remain on a familiar and human scale. Elderly people do not appreciate space that is too extensive, open to the prevailing winds and to the vagaries of climate, or which makes it difficult for them to integrate themselves naturally within the social life of the town.

To facilitate elderly people getting about, it is necessary to take account of the progressive reduction in their mobility. The distance between their homes and neighbourhood shopping centres, administrative services, and bus stops should not exceed 400 to 500 metres.

Pedestrian ways between their apartments and the centre of the neighbourhood must not present obstacles or risks of falls or other accidents. What has to be avoided particularly are raised doorsteps and floor surface that are slippery when wet. Paths and pedestrian crossings that are badly marked and badly maintained are a further risk. Neighbourhood pathways and pedestrian areas should have wide pavements and be as attractive as possible.

Public space should be set aside and gardens set up featuring promenades, with resting places with benches or seats, plus sports areas for use by children, young people, and adults. Favourable orientations should be chosen to provide natural sunlight, shade, and shelter from the prevailing winds. Decorations of trees and bushes, flowers, lawns, and fountains, etc. provide a place that will be frequented. Public space gives a focus for social life and for spending free time or space hours during the day. Such spaces provide the environment for the meetings that are essential to elderly people. They favour their integration within social life and are generally recognized as partly everyone's property and partly one's own domain.

Particular importance is attacted by elderly people to sensory perceptions within the town. Despite their reduced visual, auditory, and olfactory capacity, these senses associate places and objects with distant memories which are rendered immediate by the sensory perception. They contribute to the identification of familiar places. The urban planner should facilitate the sensory perception of the town by measures to which elderly persons are particularly sensitive, namely:

—— floor coverings that give the impression of depth as opposed to plasticity;

—— the texture of light appropriate to the different times of the day, the seasons, the architecture, and vegetation;

—— the harmony between the bulk and the surface area of buildings, the colours of the roofs and facades, the design of streets and pavements, the ornamentation of the lawns, the charm of fountains, or the beauty of sculptures.

The partition of space in an urban setting should be on a human scale. Limitless space gives an impression of emptiness. Space defined by corners and angles, with a small park for example, favours social life by:

—— creating a scenic place;

—— giving a sense of neighbourliness.

It is at the corner that a group likes to meet. It defines the space for playing games, for kiosks, for resting places, etc.

The definition of space to encourage social life must not be exclusively one of perspective and panorama. The urban or architectural environment must render these compatible. A panoramic view which unfolds beauty and a sense of wonder provides stimuli which link the elderly person to the outside world and avoids the tendency to withdraw into oneself into a space that is too restricted and too isolated.

The relationship that the elderly person has established over time, between the urban space and a particular phase of her life, captures memories and embellishes imagination and feeling.

The collective memory of the town is preserved by facts that record history with commemorative plaques, statues in squares, and other monuments. All are architectural witnesses of past years, but are equally links that identify the elderly person in space and time in regard to the urban environment in which she lives.

The streets and districts are rendered familiar by the architecture, by the art, sculpture, fountains, paintings, decorations, facades, publicity posters, and billboards that they pass by during their walks.

The urban landscape must therefore be perceptible to elderly people, familiar, and easy to read. It must enrich life.

Analysis of existing public buildings and public spaces in the town allows one to judge if their utilization and accessibility are sufficient for elderly people. They are sufficient if they have appropriate facilities for getting around without risk of fall by eliminating doorstep entries, by the provision of ramps with bilateral support, and with satisfactory lighting, etc. If this analysis identifies gaps or incompatibility with the needs of elderly persons, all measures must be taken to remove obstacles. This will not only contribute to making the town more human, but will benefit everyone. The re-arrangement of living space to take account of the specific needs of elderly people will contribute directly to improving the condition of life and health of elderly people. It will also help the whole population.

Further reading

Acheson Cooper, B. (1986). The use of color in the environment of the elderly to enhance function. *Clinics in Geriatric Medicine.* **2**, 151–7.

Brinck, C. A. and Wells, Th. J. (1986). Environmental support for geriatric incontinence. *Clinics in Geriatric Medicine,* **2** (4), 829–36.

Feller, B. (1983). Americans needing help to function at home. *Vital and health statistic of the National Center for Health Statistic.* 14, 92, Sept. 1–72. USDHHS, PHS, Hyattsville.

Fornarini, G. (1986). Gli aspetti urbanistici et d'ambiente. *Giornale di Gerontologia (Societa italiana di Gerontologia i Geriatria)*, Nov. 867.

Foundation Nationale de Gerontologie (1985). *Démence du sujet âgé et environment.* Maloine, Paris.

Foundation Nationale de Gerontologie (1986). *Maladie de type Alzheimer et autres demences séniles.* Maloine, Paris.

Jimenez Herrero, Fernando (1984). Algunos factores ecologicos del habitat del anciano. *Revista Espanola de Geriatria y Gerontologia*, 66.

Ouslander, J. G., Kane, R., and Abrass, I. (1982). Urinary incontinence in elderly nursing home patients. *Journal of the American Medical Association,* **248**, 1194–8.

Vellas, P. (1987). Architecture et logement des personnes âgées, réduction des capacités fonctionnelles, logement thérapeutique maladie d'Alzheimer. In *Année Gérontologique,* (ed. Vellas, P. and J. L. Albarede) Ch. II, pp. 229–56. Editions Maloine, Paris.

Vellas, P. (1987). Architecture, Urbanisme et Vieillissement. *Editions du Centre International de Gérontologie Sociale*, p. 119.

Vellas, P. (1987). Urinary incontinence and architecture. *Collogue du Kellogg International Program on Health and Aging de l'Université du Michigan*, Toulouse.

39

Economic factors affecting the health of the elderly

NAOHIRO OGAWA

INTRODUCTION

The urbanization process, which is both an antecedent and consequence of development, tends to contribute to an increase in new nuclear families and to a decrease in traditional joint families. Urbanization also brings about various lifestyle changes not only among the young but also among the aged. In parallel with such changes in the family structure and lifestyles, development induces a rise in rural–urban mobility, which in turn poses geographical obstacles in the way of family mutual aid. Moreover, in societies experiencing rapid development, the economic value of the aged is diminished as a result of changing production systems and technological requirements, thus leading to a relatively weaker position of the elderly.[1]

These interactive processes between development and demographic factors point to the fact that the government intervention in the provision of health care for the aged population is increasingly needed as a country proceeds on her modernization path. Reviews of health programmes and planning in world perspective document pronounced differences in approaches.[2] In the United States, for instance, market forces are stressed in the development and allocation of health resources. In contrast, the welfare of socialist states hinges upon centralized national health planning. Between these two extremes lie most countries in both developing and developed regions; the extent to which these considerations are reflected in the health programme of each of these countries is heavily dependent upon not only her economic and demographic development but also cultural, historical, and ideological factors.

Despite such intercountry differences in the provision of health care, an attempt has been made in this paper to analyse how economic factors affect the allocation of national resources for health care, particularly for the elderly population. In the next section, the impact of economic development upon the health of the aged is examined, using intercountry cross-sectional data. The third section deals with a simulation analysis for Japan in an attempt to show quantitatively how and to what extent the health of the elderly is influenced by a change in the price of medical services under the social insurance scheme. In the fourth section, the economic role of the family support system in maintaining the health of the aged is considered by heavily drawing upon the simulation model employed in the previous section. In the final section, some policy implications of the present study are briefly discussed.

Although the scope of this paper is confined substantially to the Japanese context, Japanese experiences of providing health care for the elderly in her dynamic economic and demographic process seem to be useful in formulating appropriate health programmes, particularly in developing countries currently undergoing rapid demographic changes. Furthermore, in the face of her fast economic development, Japan has retained some of the traditional cultural values, so that the Japanese model may be of relevance to policy makers in the developing region interested in combining the best of traditional and modern approaches in order to provide health services to the elderly.[3]

IMPACT OF ECONOMIC DEVELOPMENT UPON THE HEALTH OF THE ELDERLY

Regardless of whether a country is developed or not, health is an essential prerequisite for achieving and maintaining the individual and societal well-being. There are, however, marked differences in the pattern of causes for mortality and morbidity between developing and developed regions; infectious disease and malnutrition are the leading causes of death in the former, and heart disease and cancer in the latter.[2] In addition, although it is the case in virtually all populations that older age groups experience more illness and need considerably more health services than younger age groups, the health condition of the elderly in developing nations is generally less favourable than in developed nations, owing to limited access to health care services in both public and private sectors.

It is generally observed that, because resources for health compete with resources for other socio-economic development goals,[2, 4] *per capita* national resources allotted to health care programmes differ pronouncedly with stages of development. It is also considered that the amount of the government budget directed to health services is affected by the age composition of the population.[5, 6] With these general observations borne in mind, we have gathered intercountry data on the following three variables: (i) *per capita* public medical expenditure (*MED/POP*), (ii) *per capita* gross domestic product (*GDPPC*), and (iii) the percentage of those aged 65 and over in the total population (*AGED*).

The data for these three variables cover 39 developing and developed countries in 1975, and the list of these countries is shown in the appendix. The data for *MED/POP* have been compiled by the International Labour Office (ILO),[7] those for *GDPPC* by the World Bank,[8] and those for *AGED* based upon the 1984 United Nations population projections.[9] As regards *MED/POP*, the minimum value was US$0.763 for Ethiopia, while the maximum was US$656 for Sweden. The range of *GDPPC* was from US$77.8 for Ethiopia to US$8455 for Sweden. In so far as *AGED* is concerned, Nicaragua takes the lowest value of 2.4 per cent, and Sweden the highest value of 15.1 per cent. The pattern of the relationship between *MED/POP* and *GDPPC* is depicted in Fig. 39.1, while that for *MED/POP* and *AGED* is plotted in Fig. 39.2. These illustrative comparisons reveal that there are wide intercountry variations among these variables. The simple correlation between *MED/POP* and *GDPPC* is 0.918 and that between *MED/POP* and *AGED* is 0.742.

Using this data set, let us first examine to what extent the amount of the *per capita* government medical expenditure is affected by such factors as the level of economic development and the proportion of the aged in the population. For this purpose, *MED/POP* has been regressed on *GDPPC* and *AGED*, and the computed result is as follows:

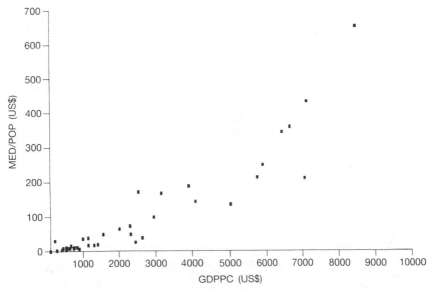

Fig. 39.1 Observed relationship between *per capita* GDP and *per capita* medical care expenditure among 39 countries in 1975.

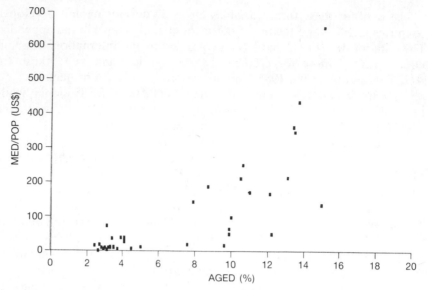

Fig. 39.2 Observed relationship between percentage of population aged 65 and over and *per capita* medical care expenditure among 39 countries in 1975.

$$MED/POP = -0.04041 + 0.05512\ GDPPC + 0.00057\ AGED \qquad (39.1)$$
$$(0.0192) \quad (0.0073) \qquad\qquad (0.0040)$$
$$\bar{R}^2\ 0.834$$

where the values in the parentheses represent standard errors. The estimated coefficient for each explanatory variable is in agreement with *a priori* expectation. That is, the higher the *per capita* income level or the proportion aged, the larger is the amount of *per capita* government resources committed to medical expenditures. The estimated coefficient for *GDPPC* is several times larger than its standard error, thus being statistically significant at the 1 per cent level with a one-tail test. It should be stressed, however, that the coefficient for *AGED* is statistically insignificant. In other words, among the sampled countries, the size of *per capita* national resources is the main determinant of the amount of *per capita* government resources allocated to medical care services.

It should also be added that in equation (39.1), the elasticity of *GDPPC* evaluated at the mean value is 1.365, which indicates that if *per capita* GDP increases by 10 per cent the amount of the *per capita* government medical expenditure in these sampled countries rises, on the average, by approximately 14 per cent.

By using the same data set, let us now analyse the magnitude of the impact of *per capita* resources channelled into the medical care program-

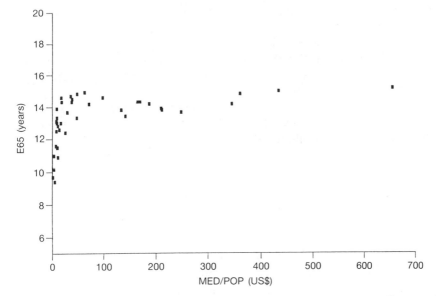

Fig. 39.3 Observed relationship between *per capita* medical care expenditure and life expectancy at age 65 among 39 countries in 1975.

me upon the health condition of the elderly. To accomplish this, we have regressed life expectancy at age 65 (*EXP65*) on *MED/POP*. Because the data on *EXP65* are not readily available, we have first collected the data on life expectancy at birth from the 1984 UN population projections, and then have matched them against appropriate UN model life tables[10] to calculate the value of *EXP65* for each country.

The estimated result can be expressed as below:

$$\ln EXP65 = 2.7640 + 0.05312 \ln MED/POP \qquad (39.2)$$
$$(0.031) \quad (0.0082)$$
$$\bar{R}^2 = 0.520$$

where ln denotes the natural logarithm. This non-linear functional specification has been chosen by inspecting the scattered diagram on these two variables, as presented in Fig. 39.3. It should also be observed in Fig. 39.3 that the variance in *EXP65* is relatively small. One of the primary reasons for this pattern is that the average remaining years of life for individuals who survive to age 65 in both developing and developed nations are about the same due to the principle of survival of the fittest.[?]

Despite the relatively limited variance of the dependent variable, the computed coefficient for *MED/POP* is not only statistically significant but also positive as theoretically expected; the greater the *per capita* resources allocated to the government medical care programme, the longer is the life expectation of the elderly at age 65. It should also be noted that the elasticity of *MED/POP* with respect to *EXP65* is 0.0531, which implies that a 10 per cent increase in *MED/POP* leads to a 0.53 per cent extension of life for the elderly at age 65.

It is also interesting to observe that the elasticity decreases considerably when another regression is estimated for the countries at comparatively advanced stages of economic development. For example, the estimated result for 23 countries showing the value of *GDPPC* greater than US$1000 is as indicated below:

$$\ln EXP65 = 2.6859 + 0.01607 \ln MED/POP \qquad (39.3)$$
$$ (0.023) \quad (0.0091)$$
$$\bar{R}^2 = 0.087$$

The computed elasticity of *MED/POP* falls to 0.0161, which is almost one third of that for equation (39.2). It appears to be reasonable to conclude from these results that the magnitude of the effect of *per capita* government resources for medical care services upon the extension of life for the aged declines with economic progress. This points to the presence of the law of diminishing marginal returns to allocating additional national resources to medical care services. (Note that the marginal returns are still positive, and are neither zero nor negative.)

Of resources spent on health, it is often argued that developed countries are prone to channel most of their resources to medical care and its related technology, while developing countries devote them largely to such basic health inputs as clean water and sanitation.[2] To test whether or not this view is valid, we have estimated a modified version of equation (39.2), by including an additional term (i.e. the percentage of the population having access to safe water (*WATER*)). However, due to the paucity of data on this added variable, we were able to include only 22 low-income developing countries in the regression analysis as listed in the appendix. The source of data for WATER was the *World tables* published in 1980 by the World Bank.[8]

The fitted regression result is:

$$\ln EXP65 = 2.8733 + 0.08662 \ln MED/POP + 0.01179 \ln WATER$$
$$ (0.364) \quad (0.0354) (0.0554)$$
$$\bar{R}^2 = 0.488 \qquad (39.4)$$

The estimated coefficients for both *MED/POP* and *WATER* conform to theoretical predictions, but only the coefficient for the former is statistically significant at the 5 per cent level with a one-tail test: The result does not support the view pertaining to the availability of safe water. The poor predicability of *WATER* may imply that the basic health inputs such as safe water contribute mainly to an improvement in infant and child mortality rather than the health status of the elderly. It should also be noted that the computed elasticity of *MED/POP* in equation (39.4) is considerably larger than that in equation (39.2), thus reinforcing the validity of the conclusion reached on the basis of equation (39.3).

The above findings derived from the four estimated regressions appear to suggest that, although economic development tends to induce a larger amount of *per capita* national income spent on medical care, the marginal gain in the extension of life among the elderly decreases as a country develops. In other words, macroeconomic factors play an essential role in improving the health condition of the aged, but the additional cost for inducing an equiproportionate increase in the life expectancy of the elderly rises pronouncedly as the process of development proceeds.

Attention should also be drawn to the fact that the above regressions show that approximately one-half of the variance in the health status of the elderly is explained by the economic factors. Evidently, a number of non-economic factors affect the health conditions of the elderly.[2] For instance, the level of educational attainment, the nutritional intake pattern, and the help-seeking behaviour of the elderly are typical of these non-economic factors. Due to the limited availability of data on these variables, however, these considerations have been excluded from the above regressions.

EFFECT OF PRICE CHANGE IN MEDICAL CARE UPON THE HEALTH OF THE ELDERLY

In the recent past, the escalating cost of health care has been a growing concern among government policy makers in both developing and developed nations. Although there are a number of future projections of demand for health and medical care for various countries,[11] most of them show an extremely fast growth of financial resources required for health services in the next several decades. Japan is one of the salient examples.

Because of the unprecedentedly rapid aging of her population and the maturity of public old-age pension schemes, Japan's social security system is expected to call for more than 25 per cent of national income at the beginning of the next century.[12] To cope with such serious financial problems, the government of Japan has recently implemented a wide range of policy measures to modify numerous components of the social insurance system. As regards medical schemes, the free medical care service programme for old people aged 70 and over was abolished in

1983. Starting from October in 1984, all insured persons have been required to cover 10 per cent of their medical care costs. In addition, an increase in the price of medical care services has been severely suppressed by the government since the early 1980s. As a consequence, the proportion of the gross national product (GNP) allocated to medical care declined from 5.12 per cent in 1983 to 4.97 per cent in 1984. In view of the fact that it rose from 2.53 per cent in 1960 to 4.98 per cent in 1980, the recent trend suggests a major change in policies on the allocation of economic resources for the medical care programme in Japan.

It is also important to note that life expectancy at birth for Japanese males was 65.32 years in 1960, but it increased to 74.84 years in 1985. During the same period, male life expectancy at age 65 rose from 11.64 to 15.43 years. The comparison of these figures indicates that the extension of longevity of the elderly has substantially contributed to an increase in life expectancy at birth in the past 25 years.

Such a rapid rise in the expectation of life is largely attributable to the increased economic resources for the medical programme. Quantitatively, the effect of the availability of *per capita* economic resources for medical care upon life expectancy at birth can be expressed as below:

$$\ln ((78.12 - EM)/EM) = -1.5031 - 1512.8 \, RMEDPC_{-1} \qquad (39.5)$$
$$ (0.023) \quad (36.52)$$
$$\bar{R}^2 = 0.989$$

$$\ln ((83.58 - EF)/EF) = -1.5189 - 1584.8 \, RMEDPC_{-1} \qquad (39.6)$$
$$ (0.031) \quad (48.53)$$
$$\bar{R}^2 = 0.982$$

where EM = male life expectancy at birth, EF = female life expectancy at birth, and $RMEDPC_{-1}$ = 1-year lagged medical expenditure *per capita* (100 million yen of 1980 constant prices). It should be noted that, to keep predicted values within a reasonable range, each equation has been estimated on the basis of a logistic curve with its ceiling imposed. The ceiling values for both sexes have been utilized directly from one of the hypothetical life tables compiled by synthesizing the best age–sex-specific mortality rate in the contemporary world.[13] The ceiling value for males is 78.12 years, and for females 83.58 years. Both of the above logistic regression equations have been estimated on the basis of annual time-series data over the period 1964–1984.

These computed results appear to imply that an increase in *per capita* economic resources allocated in the previous year by the government of Japan leads to a further improvement of the life expectation for both sexes in this year. Hence, although Japan's life expectancy is presently at the world's highest level, the pace of its further improvement might be adversely affected by government control on the price of medical care. To examine the impact on life expectation for the aged due to the changes in the price of medical treatment, we have conducted a few numerical experiments, by using a long-term macroeconomic–demographic–medical simulation model formulated in 1986 by the Nihon University Population Research Institute (NUPRI). This NUPRI model contains approximately 800 variables in the following three submodels: the population submodel, the economic submodel, and the social security submodel. These three submodels are interactive and interdependent with each other; the population submodel is first determined by a set of economic and social security variables with a 1-year time lag, and then the variables in both economic and social security submodels are simultaneously determined, employing the computed demographic variables. In the demographic submodel, the fertility function is based upon a variant of the new home economics approach, while the mortality level is computed from the above equations (39.5) and (39.6). Because a detailed framework of the model has been described elsewhere,[14] no further explanation of the mechanism of the model seems to be in order here.

For expository purposes, let us call the simulation exercise based on the above-mentioned model the 'standard case'. The price equation for medical care services incorporated in the standard case has been estimated on the basis of data observed from 1973–1984. Table 39.1 presents such simulation results for selected variables over 1986–2025. The total medical expenditure is expected to increase monotonically from 17.4 trillion yen in 1986 to 113.9 trillion yen in 2025. The financial burden of the medical expenditure on the national economy, as measured in terms of the proportion of GNP allocated to medical care services, rises from 5.04 per cent in 1986 to 6.12 per cent in 2020, after which it falls slightly. Furthermore, the proportion of the total medical expenditure allotted to those aged 65 and over is 34.79 per cent in 1986, but it increases to 41.86 per cent by 2000, and to 51.15 per cent by 2025.

Demographically, male life expectancy at birth improves continuously from 74.72 to 77.51 years over the entire simulation period. Similarly, the expectation of life for males at age 65 grows from 15.56 to 17.12 years during the corresponding period. Total population size, which is 121.68 million persons in 1986, continues to expand to 131.64 million persons in 2010. After reaching this peak, Japan's future population is likely to decrease to a level of 127.06 million persons in 2025. The proportion of those aged 65 and over is projected to rise monotonically from 10.56 per cent in 1986 to 24.10 per cent in 2020; this result implies that the Japanese population is likely to become the world's most aged population in the early part of the next century.[15]

In addition to the standard case, the following two alternative simula-

Table 39.1 Future changes in selected variables under standard case projection

Year	Total medical expenditure (trillion yen)	Share of total medical expenditure in GNP (%)	Proportion of total medical expenditure allocated to those aged 65+ (%)	Male life expectancy at birth (years)	Male life expectancy at 65 (years)	Total population (million persons)	Population aged 65+ (%)
1986	17.4	5.04	34.79	74.72	15.56	121.68	10.56
1990	21.3	5.25	36.68	75.14	15.79	123.84	11.87
1995	30.4	5.55	39.61	75.94	16.24	126.40	14.01
2000	44.6	5.80	42.66	76.81	16.73	129.25	16.21
2005	55.7	5.97	45.64	77.10	16.89	131.28	18.13
2010	66.8	6.06	48.67	77.18	16.93	131.64	20.22
2015	83.5	6.10	52.37	77.38	17.05	130.65	22.95
2020	98.9	6.12	54.22	77.48	17.10	128.94	24.10
2025	113.9	6.02	53.95	77.51	17.12	127.06	24.00

tion runs have been carried out for comparative purposes: the 'high case' and the 'low case'. In the former, the price equation has been estimated on the basis of data reflecting the time period when the price of medical services increased very rapidly (i.e. from 1973 to 1978). In the latter, it has been assumed that the tempo of the price increase is half as fast as the standard case.

Tables 39.2 and 39.3 display simulated results for these two additional experiments. In the high case, as presented in Table 39.2, the total medical expenditure is considerably higher throughout the simulation period than in the standard case; in 2025, the difference between these two cases amounts to slightly more than 50 per cent. Similar observations are applicable to the results for both the share of the medical expenditure in GNP and the proportion of the total medical expenditure allocated to the aged population. In addition, both the total population and the proportion of those at ages 65 and over are also comparable between the two cases. As regards the expectation of life for males at birth and at age 65, however, the high case yields only marginally larger values than the standard case. This result reflects that in both cases, the projected levels of life expectancy gradually approach very close to the ceiling value incorporated in equations (39.5) and (39.6).

As compared with both the standard and high cases, the low case shows substantially lower projected values for all the variables under consideration. As presented in Table 39.3, for example, the total medical expenditure is expected to amount to 72.3 trillion yen in 2025, which is 36.5 per cent lower than that for the standard case, and 58.0 per cent smaller than that for the high case. The ratio of the total medical expenditure to GNP falls continuously throughout the simulation period. In 2025 it is 3.97 per cent in the low case, as opposed to 6.02 per cent in the standard case, and 8.72 per cent in the high case. The share of the medical cost for the elderly in the total medical expenditure shows an increasing differential over time between the low case and the two other cases; in the final year, it is 51.15 per cent for the low case, thus being 2.80 per cent lower than the standard case and 4.36 per cent smaller than the high case.

In terms of life expectancy at birth for men, it grows from 74.16 to 76.19 years during the simulated period. In the year 2025 it is 1.32 years shorter than the standard case, and 1.80 years short of the high case. Similarly, male life expectancy at age 65 for the low case is 0.74 years and 1.01 years shorter than the standard case and the high case, respectively. As a consequence of such shorter longevity, the low case has a smaller total population size and a lower aging level than both the standard and high cases.

It is also important to stress that, by controlling the price of medical services, the government would be able to save its financial resources to a

Table 39.2 Future changes in selected variables under high case projection

Year	Total medical expenditure (trillion yen)	Share of total medical expenditure in GNP (%)	Proportion of total medical expenditure allocated to those aged 65+ (%)	Male life expectancy at birth (years)	Male life expectancy at 65 (years)	Total population (million persons)	Population aged 65+ (%)
1986	18.2	5.26	34.79	74.85	15.63	121.17	10.56
1990	24.2	5.82	36.73	75.63	15.83	123.94	11.90
1995	37.9	6.67	39.94	76.71	16.14	126.73	14.13
2000	59.8	7.44	43.40	77.52	16.38	129.83	16.41
2005	76.7	7.93	46.65	77.74	17.25	132.06	18.41
2010	94.7	8.26	49.89	77.82	17.29	132.56	20.55
2015	122.3	8.55	53.82	77.93	17.35	131.67	23.31
2020	147.5	8.74	55.77	77.98	17.38	130.00	24.45
2025	172.2	8.72	55.51	78.00	17.39	128.13	24.34

Table 39.3 Future changes in selected variables under low case projection

Year	Total medical expenditure (trillion yen)	Share of total medical expenditure in GNP (%)	Proportion of total medical expenditure allocated to those aged 65+ (%)	Male life expectancy at birth (years)	Male life expectancy at 65 (years)	Total population (million persons)	Population aged 65+ (%)
1986	16.8	4.87	34.79	74.61	15.49	121.67	10.56
1990	19.4	4.84	36.63	74.74	15.56	123.76	11.84
1995	25.4	4.75	39.32	75.21	15.83	126.11	13.91
2000	34.3	4.61	41.86	75.87	16.20	128.67	16.00
2005	41.0	4.52	44.39	76.07	16.31	130.38	17.80
2010	47.1	4.41	47.00	76.05	16.30	130.43	19.76
2015	56.2	4.26	50.16	76.18	17.37	129.15	22.37
2020	64.3	4.14	51.65	76.23	16.40	127.20	23.41
2025	72.3	3.97	51.15	76.19	16.38	125.12	23.24

considerable extent. If the government should select the low case rather than the high case scenario, it could save financially a total of 660 trillion yen (1980 constant prices) over the period 1986–2025. In view of the fact that GNP for 1980 was 245 trillion yen, the amount of government savings to be generated in the long run by the choice of the low case rather than the high case is quite substantial. As compared with the high case, however, male life expectancy at 65 is 1.01 years shorter in the low case, so that a considerable part of these financial gains is made at the sacrifice of the well-being of the elderly.

The above illustrative analysis points to the importance of economic considerations on the part of the Japanese government in improving the health of the elderly through the provision of its medical insurance schemes. It is quite possible, however, that if similar simulation analyses were conducted for developing countries where mortality risks are much higher, the importance of economic considerations might be substantially greater, as compared with a low-mortality country like Japan. In the next section, our discussion will be shifted from the government support system to informal kin support and services.

FAMILY SUPPORT AND THE HEALTH OF THE AGED

Because of the high cost of use of hospitals and technology in the care of ever-increasing population of older persons, growing attention has recently been directed toward the role of families in supporting the health of their aged parents in both developing and developed countries.[15] It is worth noting, however, that owing to the intercountry differences in the family structure the extent to which aged parents have access to their informal family support varies substantially between developing and developed nations. According to one of the international comparative surveys conducted in 1981 covering five countries,[16] in a developing country like Thailand, 38.9 per cent of the elderly aged 60 and over were living in three-generation arrangements. In contrast, it was only 0.6 per cent in United Kingdom, 1.6 per cent in the United States, and 3.5 per cent in France. Although highly industralized, Japan showed a high percentage of extended families; 36.9 per cent of the elderly sampled were living in three-generation households.

Despite their unique pattern by international standards, the Japanese families are likely to face in the next few decades an extremely fast growth of the number of their aged parents who need intensive human care. Among elderly parents in need of such care are those suffering from senile dementia and those who are bedridden. Given the assumption that the age–sex-specific incidence of senile dementia and bedridden cases observed in recent years will remain unchanged, the total number of aged people with senile dementia and the total number of bedridden elderly people have been projected from 1986 to 2025, by drawing upon the simulation model used for analysis in the previous section.

As presented in Table 39.4, the number of senile dementia cases among the population aged 65 and over rises phenomenally from 691 000 in 1986 to 2 165 000 in 2025. The average growth rate during this period is 2.97 per cent per annum. Similarly, the total number of bedridden patients among the population at ages 65 and over grows from 681 000 in 1986 to 1 960 000 in 2025. The average annual growth rate of these patients is 2.74 per cent.

Due to the wide prevalence of extended families and the limited availability of institutional care, the majority of these aged persons are looked after at home in contemporary Japanese society. More importantly, middle-aged women outside the labour force usually assume this responsibility. In view of this, the ratio of the bedridden or senile elderly persons compared with non-working women at ages 45–54 has been projected over the period 1986–2025, as depicted in Fig. 39.4. As can be seen from this graphical exposition, the ratio of these types of patients to housewives is 0.43 in 1986, but rises to 0.62 in 2000 and to 1.20 in 2025. In the year 2008, the number of the aged population suffering from senile dementia or being bedridden is equal to that of full-time housewives.

In an aging society like Japan, however, it is conceivable that, owing to a growing scarcity of the overall supply of labour, labour demand for women at ages 45–54 might increase gradually. Although the labour force participation rate for this age group is assumed to remain at a level of 61.3

Table 39.4 Projected number of aged people with senile dementia and that of bedridden elderly people, 1986–2025

Year	Number of aged people with senile dementia (1000 persons)	Number of bedridden aged people (1000 persons)
1986	691	681
1990	824	797
1995	1004	957
2000	1191	1132
2005	1399	1335
2010	1635	1543
2015	1869	1736
2020	2046	1870
2025	2165	1960

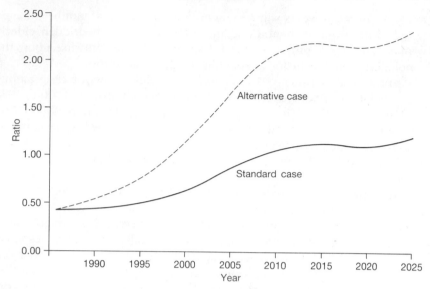

Fig. 39.4 Change in the ratio of aged population suffering from senile dementia or being bedridden to non-working housewives, 1986–2025.

per cent in the standard case, an alternative scenario has been considered in order to analyse the effect of the possible rise in labour demand for women of this age group upon the provision of home care for these aged patients. In the alternative case, it has been assumed that the labour force participation rate for this age group would increase linearly to 80 per cent by the year 2000 and remain unchanged at this high level for the rest of the simulation period.

As represented by the dotted line in Fig. 39.4, the ratio of these patients to housewives caring for them at home rises at a much faster rate than in the standard case. It increases from 0.43 in 1986 to 1.20 in 2000, and to 2.33 in 2025. These simulated results indicate that, compared with the standard case, the ratio of aged patients to be attended to at home by their daughters or daughters-in-law at ages 45–54 is approximately twice as large in the long run for the alternative case. These computed results also imply that the need for institutional care as an alternative to home care would be substantially greater in the alternative case than in the standard case.

It is also worth noting that, owing to the greater participation of women in the labour force, the level of real GNP is expected to be higher in the alternative case compared with that for the standard case. The cumulative difference between these two cases over the period 1986–2025 amounts to 166.1 trillion yen as measured in terms of 1980 constant prices. Although part of such sizable economic gains could be used for providing additional facilities for institutional care, the psychological and emotional well-being of the elderly sick might deteriorate more seriously in the alternative case than in the standard case.

CONCLUDING DISCUSSION

In the present chapter we have discussed, by referring to the intercountry data analysis and the Japanese experience, the impact of a few selected macroeconomic changes upon: (i) the government medical expenditure in relation to the national productive capacity, (ii) an extension of longevity of the elderly, and (iii) the role of the informal family support system in caring for the sick aged. The numerical results obtained in the present study seem to suggest that economic development, coupled with a greater allocation of economic resources for medical services, tends to contribute to higher life expectancy for the elderly, thus leading to a further advance of the process of population aging and imposing a heavier burden upon both formal government and informal family assistance in supporting the elderly in retirement.

To alleviate the adverse effects of improved longevity among the elderly, a set of appropriate policies should be formulated and implemented. These policies include offering not only older workers but also their employers stronger incentives to delay retirement. Policies of this nature, though not directly related to health, are quite consistent with improvements in longevity and the health of the aged.

In spite of the desirability of such policies, their implementation has been extremely slow in the case of Japan. For instance, Japan's average retirement age for male workers employed by large businesses increased only 2.6 years during 1965–1983, from 55.5 to 58.1 years of age. In contrast, male life expectancy at birth improved from 67.74 to 74.20 years over the corresponding period. Considering the unprecedented aging of the Japanese population which will almost certainly occur in the next few decades, a wide range of institutional factors operating in the labour market should be modified immediately to facilitate a more rapid extension of retirement age. In this way, the improved health of the elderly can be used constructively, rather than unproductively by shunting the elderly away from mainstream society.

In closing, it should also be mentioned that other societies, notably some of the Asian countries such as Singapore, Hong Kong, the Republic of Korea, and China, will most likely face various problems of aging parallel to Japan in the early part of the next century, owing to their rapid fertility declines in the 1960s and 1970s.[17] Because these developing countries in Asia have cultural values and family support systems comparable to those for Japan, the Japanese experience may prove a model for them in the years ahead.

References

1. Cogwill, D. O., and Holmes, L. (1972). Aging and modernization. Appleton-Century-Crofts, New York.
2. Maddox, G. (1982). Challenges for health policy and planning. In *International perspectives on aging: population and policy challenges* (ed. Binstock R., W. S. Chow, and J. Schulz) pp. 127–58. United Nations Fund for Population Activities policy development studies no. 7. United Nations, New York.
3. Petri, P. A. (1982). Income, employment, and retirement policies. In *International perspectives on aging: population and policy challenges* (ed. Binstock R., W. S. Chow, and J. Schulz). pp. 75–125 United Nations Fund for Population Activities policy development studies no. 7. United Nations, New York.
4. Jones, G. (1975). Population growth and health and family planning. In *Population and development planning* (ed. Robinson, W.). pp. 107–33. The Population Council, New York.
5. Ogawa, N. (1985). *Population growth and the costs of health care: the case of Malaysia.* Economic Planning Unit discussion paper no. 13, pp. 1–30. Kuala Lumpur, Malaysia.
6. Ogawa, N., Poapongsakorn, N., and Mason, A. (1987). *Population change and the costs of health care in Thailand.* pp. 1–52. Asian Development Bank. Manila, Philippines.
7. International Labour Office (1985). *The cost of social security.* Geneva.
8. World Bank (1980). *World tables.* The Johns Hopkins University Press, Baltimore and London.
9. United Nations (1986). *World population prospects: estimates and projections as assessed in 1984.* United Nations, New York.
10. United Nations (1982). *Model life tables for developing countries.* United Nations, New York.
11. Heller, P., Hemming R., Kohnert P. *et al.* (1986). *Aging and social expenditure in the major industrial countries,* 1980–2025. International Monetary Fund, Washington DC.
12. Ogawa, N. (1986). Consequences of mortality change on aging. In *consequences of mortality trends and differentials.* United Nations, New York. pp. 175–84.
13. Kamagata, K. and Hishinuma, S. (1982). Heikinjumyo no hendo no yoin bunseki oyobi shoraiyosoku ni kansuru kenkyu (A study on the determinants of changes in life expectancy and on its improvements in future). In *Raifu supan (Life span),* pp. 1–34. The Group for the Study on Longevity, Tokyo.
14. Ogawa, N. *et al.* (1986). *Jinko keizai iryo moderu ni motozuku choki tenbo: feisu II (Long-term prospects based upon the population-economic-medical model: phase II).* Nihon University Population Research Institute, Tokyo.

15. Ogawa, N. (1988). Population aging and medical demand: the case of Japan. In *Economic and Social implications of population aging*. United Nations, New York.
16. Office of the Prime Minister, Government of Japan (1982). *Rojin no seikatsu to ishiki: kokusai hikaku chosa kekka hokokusho (Life and awareness of the elderly: report of the results on the international comparative survey)* pp. 254–75. Tokyo.
17. Ogawa, N. (1988). Aging in China: demographic alternatives. *Asia-Pacific Population Journal*, **3**(3), 21–64 United Nations, Bangkok.

APPENDIX

Name of country	Used in equations		
	(39.1) and (39.2)	(39.3)	(39.4)
Argentina	Yes	Yes	Yes
Austria	Yes	Yes	No
Barbados	Yes	Yes	Yes
Bolivia	Yes	No	Yes
Chile	Yes	No	Yes
Colombia	Yes	No	Yes
Costa Rica	Yes	No	Yes
Denmark	Yes	Yes	No
Dominican Rep.	Yes	No	Yes
El Salvador	Yes	No	Yes
Ethiopia	Yes	No	Yes
Fiji	Yes	Yes	Yes
Finland	Yes	Yes	No
France	Yes	Yes	No
Greece	Yes	Yes	No
Guatemala	Yes	No	Yes
Guyana	Yes	No	No
Ireland	Yes	Yes	No
Italy	Yes	Yes	No
Japan	Yes	Yes	No
Luxembourg	Yes	Yes	No
Malaysia	Yes	No	Yes
Morocco	Yes	No	Yes
New Zealand	Yes	Yes	No
Nicaragua	Yes	No	Yes
Norway	Yes	Yes	No
Panama	Yes	Yes	Yes
Portugal	Yes	Yes	Yes
Senegal	Yes	No	Yes
Singapore	Yes	Yes	Yes
Spain	Yes	Yes	No
Sri Lanka	Yes	No	Yes
Sweden	Yes	Yes	No
Togo	Yes	No	Yes
Trinidad and Tobago	Yes	Yes	No
Turkey	Yes	No	Yes
United States	Yes	Yes	No
Uruguay	Yes	Yes	Yes
Venezuela	Yes	Yes	No

40

The role of aging in establishing social priorities: an economic perspective

KEN WRIGHT

INTRODUCTION

Economics is all about allocating scarce resources to competing ends, to maximizing the outcome of the use of any set of resources. However, there are usually two competing objectives in this process: one concerned with efficiency, which is the maximization of outcome or the minimization of costs, the other with equity, which is concerned with how the outcomes and costs are distributed amongst different sectors of society. Although the efficiency calculus is mainly technical, involving the measurement of costs and outcomes, it also contains a number of elements requiring judgement and valuation. Equity considerations are judgemental; they involve assessing the fairness of the burden of costs and the benefits of outcomes that accrue to specific groups in the population. Decisions on social priorities from an economic viewpoint require the consideration of the achievement of both objectives.

Since it is necessary to know what the costs and outcomes of various policies are before it is possible to assess their impact on society, the efficiency calculus is logically prior to the equity judgements. This chapter follows this logic. The following sections deal with the main efficiency-related concepts of the measurement of costs and benefits and highlight some of the valuations which are related to effects of aging on the decisions or priorities. Questions about the equitable distribution of costs and benefits are then discussed before summing up the points which economic analysis makes in decision making on social priorities.

THE EFFICIENCY OF ALTERNATIVE POLICIES

In the consumption of private goods and services it is not necessary to measure costs and outcomes explicitly because consumers choose between all those goods and services by weighing up costs against the statisfaction or benefit gained from their consumption. Consumers can, therefore, use a given budget to maximize their consumption benefits. In the case of public policies, consumers are not working in the same choice framework; the goods and services are frequently available below their cost and the consumers often act as passive recipients of the services provided instead of making choices for themselves. The choice of services to be made available and the quantity allocated to individuals is the responsibility of an intermediary person or agent. Public economics faces the challenge of following the analogy of the private consumer in deciding how to maximize the benefits to be produced by public services within a given budget constraint. This decision requires information on the costs and outcomes of various services.

Economists have developed several approaches to providing information about alternative forms of service delivery with varying degrees of sophistication:

1. *Cost–benefit analysis* is concerned with the maximization of net social benefit (social benefits minus social cost). This analysis requires that the costs and outcomes (benefits) of the services under accommodation are both measured in terms of cash. While it is usual to measure costs in money terms, it has so far proved impossible to measure benefits of health and social services in this way. Thus, cost–benefit analysis is not yet well enough developed to help make decisions about priorities in health and social care.

2. *Cost–utility analysis* is the technique used where benefits are measured in standardized units (not cash) and alternative policies can be assessed according to their cost per unit. Early detection of illness or screening programmes can be assessed in terms of the cost per positive case identified, or some treatments may be assessed in terms of their cost per extra year of life expectancy generated. Cost–utility analysis can be used to assess priorities across policies which produce appropriate standardized outcomes of benefits.

3. *Cost–effectiveness analysis* is used to measure the relative efficiency of alternative policies which have either the same costs and different outcomes or the same outcome with different costs. While this technique is useful in guiding decisions about closely related alternative forms of service provision (e.g. alternative day care services, alternative forms of domiciliary care) it has very limited usefulness across main programmes because it cannot determine efficiency when one alternative is more costly but more effective than another.

Given that cost–benefit analysis requires considerable methodological advances before it can be used to determine priorities in health and social welfare policies and that cost–effectiveness analysis has a narrow focus, the most promising aid to decisions on priorities would appear to be the development of cost–utility analysis. The crucial question here is whether it is possible to standardize the outcomes of health and social services.

Measuring outcomes

Health and social care policies are concerned with increasing the length and improving the quality of life. A methodology of measuring the way in which alternative treatment regimens achieve these objectives has been developing slowly over the last 15 years or so. Its main product has been the concept of the quality-adjusted life-years (QALY). This concept raises several important practical and evaluative problems:

(1) the valuation of life-years gained;
(2) the quality adjustment;
(3) the evaluation of life and quality gains brought about by different treatment and care regimens.

Each of these issues is examined in turn.

Increased life expectancy

If quality adjustment is ignored temporarily and it is assumed that an extra year of life gained is the same value for everyone, health care priorities could be determined according to the cost per life-year gained. Since younger people will tend to gain the most extra years, this allocation rule would discriminate against elderly people.

Thus, one question which arises immediately is whether or not it is valid to assume that 1 year of life gained is the same for a 20-year-old as a 40-year-old or a 60-year-old person. This is not a judgement for economics to make. Economics can follow the logic and show how this judgement affects priorities. The priorities implied by other valuations of life-years gained could also be used in cost–utility analysis. The main point is that the outcome measure is made explicit, as are the priority rankings which follow from it.

Quality adjustment

Quality adjustment raises three important issues:

1. What are the relevant qualities?
2. How is each of these qualities to be measured?
3. Can different aspects of quality be combined into an overall 'quality adjustment'?

Each of these issues requires considerable social experimentation to develop appropriate constructs, to test them for validity and reliability, to develop measures of quality, and to test the relative valuation of one quality against another. It is worthwhile to consider how the QALY methodology has tackled these issues.

The QALY methodology grew out of attempts to measure the output of hospitals. The main two components which stood the tests of construct validity and reliability were freedom from disability and freedom from pain and distress.[1] The categorization of each of these two major components is set out in Table 40.1.

Scaling work has subsequently tackled two main problems. The first of these was to develop a ranking of states of disability and states of distress or pain. The ordering of these categories is set out in Table 40.1. The second problem was to develop a scale which combined these two separate dimensions into a composite measure of health status. This was and remains a complex exercise. Those people who have undertaken to join the experimental scaling work have had to order, in terms of increasing severity, all the logical combinations which occur from putting together the eight statements on disability with the four statements on pain or distress. Although this would yield 32 states to be compared, three were

Table 40.1 Rosser and Watts' classification of states of illness[1]

Disability	Distress
1 No disability	1 No distress
2 Slight social disability	2 Mild
3 Severe social disability and/or slight impairment of performance at work. Able to do all housework except very heavy tasks	3 Moderate
4 Choice of work or performance at work severely limited. Housewives and old people able to do light housework only, but able to go out shopping	4 Severe
5 Unable to undertake any paid employment. Unable to continue any education. Old people confined to home except for escorted outings and short walks and unable to do shopping. Housewives able to perform only a few simple tasks	
6 Confined to chair or to wheelchair or able to move around in the home only with support from an assistant	
7 Confined to bed	
8 Unconscious	

subsequently regarded as inapplicable since people who were on point eight of the disability ranking (unconscious) would not feel the states of mild, moderate, or severe distress. After having ranked these statements, the next stage was to value each of these states on a scale in which death was given a fixed value of 0 and full, pain/distress-free functioning was given a fixed value of 1.

People from different backgrounds (clinicians, nurses, general members of the public, patients) were able to complete this task in a series of small experiments; the results of their labours are summarized in Table 40.2, which is a valuation matrix in which the eight rows are the disability categories and the four columns are the distress categories from Table 40.1. Further work is needed on a larger scale to see how well the values set out in Table 40.2 are representative of general population valuations of states of health.

In further developments, the values in Table 40.2 have been used as a quality of life weighting to be applied to extra years of life expectation generated by different treatments and estimates have been made on how different treatments rank in terms of the cost per quality of life-year (cost per QALY) produced.[2]

If cost per QALY is to be used as a major guide to setting social priorities, the quality adjustment (and cost measurement) should be applicable to all users and potential users of the relevant services. Given the origins of the work in measuring the outcome of hospitals, it has to be determined whether other forms of treatment or care produce similar qualities. In particular it is worthwhile to focus on the pain/distress aspect of quality and ascertain whether this can encompass the benefits produced by services which are important to the long-term care of the elderly (e.g.

Table 40.2 Valuations of pairwise combinations of disability and distress[2]

Disability \ Distress	1	2	3	4
1	1.000	0.995	0.990	0.967
2	0.990	0.986	0.973	0.932
3	0.980	0.972	0.956	0.912
4	0.964	0.956	0.942	0.870
5	0.946	0.935	0.900	0.700
6	0.875	0.845	0.680	0.000
7	0.677	0.564	0.000	−1.486
8	−1.028			

Sample size = 70.

domiciliary or nursing home care) where the main objective may well be the nurture of the person rather than increasing life expectancy or the improvement of social functioning.

The provision of long-term care, whether at home or in residential, nursing home, or hospital, is most likely to affect the pain/distress aspect of quality. It is not clear from the work published so far whether this dimension can cope with the relief of loneliness, improvement in morale, self-esteem, or general psychological well-being. Certainly, the distress aspect was designed to show the relief of anxiety, depression, and mental distress brought about by psychiatric treatment. How far these other factors are related to the distress category is a matter for further experimentation.

So far the QALY methodology has been used in a fairly restrictive framework and its application has been illustrative of its potential in determining priorities in resource allocation rather than for formal policy making. Even in its present relatively under developed form, the methodology has the advantage of provoking answers to questions about how various services produce extra life-years and improved quality of life. Its disadvantage is that people may use the methodology inappropriately to make decisions about resource allocation across different preventive, curative, or caregiving regimens where the quality adjustment has not been tested for validity, reliability, or sensitivity. In the present state of the methodology, elderly people will tend to fare worse than other groups because their life expectancy is lower and it is not at all clear how some of the outcomes of the major policies on long-term care can be built into the quality adjustment.

It must be emphasized, however, that the methodology is still very experimental, that it is used to guide not make decisions, and that it has been used in the cost–utility analysis of the treatments of acute conditions.[2] Its great merit has been to make the criteria on which priorities can be made more explicit and has opened up debate about priorities which previously never took place in public. Obviously, there is much more work to be done on this type of approach, particularly in its application to chronic conditions. Other methodologies may well develop, or people may decide that efficiency is not a good criterion on which to base priorities. An appropriate basis is a matter for general discussion and consensus. However, the resource implication of the criteria will be important and this is where the economist would have an important role to play. No debate, no consensus, and no calculation of resource implications can take place unless the criteria are explicitly stated.

Evaluating the outcome of alternative treatments

Evaluating the outcome of alternative treatments is necessary, whether or not the QALY methodology is used, if priorities are to be based in any way on the efficient use of resources. Information on increased survival and/or improved social functioning has become available for many curative and rehabilitative regimens for conditions such as heart transplants, renal failure, coronary artery bypass grafting, hip replacements, and breast cancer.[2,3] Very little is known about survival or quality of life in other areas such as palliative treatment for cancers and in major policy concerns such as alternative forms of long-term care for chronically disabled people of all ages.

This is a further reason for the limited role that economics is playing in determining priorities. Some of the major decisions about developing hospital, nursing home, or domiciliary care are ill informed about the relative outcomes of these alternatives. At present this decision making is aided by cost–effectiveness analysis, which has given some general indications of the circumstances in which one form of care become more efficient than another[4] and is reinforced by other social research[5] indicating how policies to maintain the elderly in their own home need to give priority to:

(1) relieving the burden on principal helpers;
(2) reducing poverty and maintaining a satisfactory domestic environment;
(3) preventing social isolation and relieving loneliness;
(4) reducing disability.

Thus, until more knowledge is available on all outcomes, it will be impossible to decide on priorities across all groups in the population in terms of efficiency criteria. Even allocating priorities in the care of elderly people requires the input of a considerable effort into policy, care, and service evaluation.

The measurement of costs

The measurement of costs is generally more straight forward than the measurement of outcome for health and social services, although it does present some interesting if difficult technical problems to the practising economist. The main point about economic costs is that, first, they are comprehensive, and cover all resource use, irrespective of the agency paying for it. Secondly, they differ at times from accounting conventions. This is because the economic cost of a resource depends upon its value in other uses which may not at times reflect the cash that is paid for it. In many instances there is no need to worry about such notions, but occasionally a major difference occurs. One of these instances occurs regularly in the care of elderly people. This is the treatment of the help provided by families and friends, which is often not paid for by cash but uses their time which has value in other uses either for productive purposes or for the enjoyment of leisure.

If priorities are to be assessed on efficiency grounds, costs must be comprehensive. The informal care given by families and friends often substitutes for public care, and home-based care will appear cheap if these resources are not counted. Of course, it is difficult to cost these inputs because people have distinctly different attitudes to the time they devote to caring for others. For some people the benefits of care exceed the costs of lost opportunities either of working or leisure time. For others the costs of lost opportunities exceed the benefits of caring and the costs of care for these people may be regarded as the compensation they require to ensure that this difference between costs and benefits is eliminated. This compensation might take the form of a cash payment or the provision of a set of substitute services which restore the opportunities forgone.

Although economists have concentrated on the measurement of all costs irrespective of who is paying for them, it is widely recognized that the way in which services are financed is likely to affect priorities. Budget-constrained public services have a major incentive to push costs on to other organizations or individuals. Hence there is a need to recognize the costs falling on informal carers. But public agencies will also pass on responsibilities to each other if they see an opportunity to do so. A good example of this has been the way in which public agencies in the United Kingdom have exploited the development of private care for the elderly because it can be financed from central government's social security fund.[6] Whether or not this has been an efficient development is as yet unclear, but it has shown how budget-constrained agencies will shunt costs on to other unconstrained budgets without regard to priorities. Generally, then, policies which identify groups to receive priority service or treatment provision need to ensure that the financing of the agencies concerned encourages them to follow the declared policy objectives. Since social care often involves a multiplicity of agencies, an important development in public economics has been the design of systems which ensure that priority needs are identified and satisfied. These systems are closely related to the concept of equity as well as efficiency and are taken up in the next section.

EQUITY IN THE ALLOCATION OF RESOURCES

Equity in the distribution of resources involves two sets of decisions. One is concerned with ensuring the equal treatment of people in the same circumstances and is usually defined as *horizontal equity*. The other is *vertical equity*, which is ensuring that people are treated according to their particular circumstances. These concepts are two sides of one coin since if people with equal needs are treated equally and needs differ over the population, people with different needs will be treated differently. The implication of all this for determining priorities is the development of systems which can assess needs and ensure that resources are used to meet them. This, in turn, raises an agenda of issues:

—— what needs are to be taken into account;

—— who is to assess the intensity of these needs;

—— which forms of help best meet these needs;

—— how the help is to be provided.

All these issues call for information which is at present largely unavailable. Very little is known about the benefits of channelling help to people while they are fairly independent to prevent further deterioration in their health status, as against concentrating help on very disabled people. Similarly, very little is known about the benefits of alternative forms of care for very disabled people. A considerable amount of evaluation of service or treatment outcomes as well as experimentation with different methods of case finding and assessment systems is needed before this type of information will be available. Thus, heavy reliance is now placed on professional judgement to identify priorities.

This lack of information has forced the use of a piecemeal approach. In order to make progress in priority allocation of resources it has been necessary to single out groups who are likely to be in the greatest need of care. A good example of this is the case management approach used to match resources to needs in community care in parts of the United Kingdom. For this exercise it was decided that frail elderly people who were at risk of admission to full-time institutional care formed a priority group.[7] The process of case management involved assessing the need for health and social care required by both the old people and the principal helpers and the mobilization of a suitable set of services subject to a budget constraint.

The characteristics of this approach are that needs of individuals are assessed by an appropriate professional, that resources are matched to need, that a responsible professional has command over the prescription and delivery of services, and that the budget constraint encourages the delivery of the least cost mix of services. The factor which called forth this priority response was the physical and mental frailty of the old people concerned. Other factors could be used in other work to single out other groups for priority treatment, for example people on low incomes or those in poor housing accommodation. The targeting of a suitable set of services would use the principles outlined above to ensure an efficient and sensitive solution to the problems identified.

The role of the professional case manager is crucial in this system. Alternative systems might test whether similar results could be obtained using a budget that is spent by either the old people themselves or advocates acting on their behalf. No definite answer could be given without putting such approaches to the test, although it is easy to visualize the difficulties which would arise, particularly where people are suffering from mental infirmity. Developing a system based on cash allowances paid to the elderly themselves would raise considerable problems about whether people would be able to choose those services which would offer them the greatest benefits or whether a lay person acting as advocate could make such a judgement for another person. Obviously, this approach would be open to scandalous misappropriation of monies if unscrupulous people were allowed to act as advocates or set up agencies to provide inefficient services.

One way of avoiding some of the risks of such behaviour would be to issue vouchers which could be exchanged only for approved services. The use of vouchers is less flexible than that of cash but is more flexible than using professional assessment.

All these systems are aimed at reproducing the principles of the purchase of private goods and services as outlined at the start of the previous section. They are attempting to acquire or encourage people to acquire for themselves that set of social services which produces the greatest satisfaction. The choice of an appropriate system depends upon whether it is believed that people have the ability to decide for themselves which services will yield them the greatest benefits. Traditionally, it has been held that people need very specialized knowledge to make choices about health and social care and that an appropriate professional is the best agent to aid people with their decision making.[8] While this may be true for specialized diagnosis and treatment of disease and trauma, it may not hold for choices about domiciliary care or a full-time stay in a residential home or a nursing home. The point has to be made that unless people are suffering from severe mental infirmity they may well be able to buy in their own social care services provided that they have an adequate income. If this point were accepted politically it would imply a general switch from service-based to cash-based assistance, although there would be a need to develop advisory services which would help people to choose between competing services and to set up regulatory agencies who would control the standards of service.

At present there is very little evidence about people's preferences for help in the form of cash or kind. If there is a move to developing cash-based help the discussion on social priorities will focus on the distribution of income and how increases in income might compensate for increasing disability. If it is found preferable to stay with a service-based system, the discussion on priorities will revolve around the development of an efficient mix of services and systems which facilitates the identification, assessment of needs, and the organization of resources to match those needs.

THE GENERAL APPLICABILITY OF ECONOMIC PRINCIPLES

The points made in this paper arise from the economist's basic premise that resources are always scarce. The ideas and methods that are brought to bear on the allocation and distribution of resources are therefore applicable to all types of economies. The principles apply to other groups in the population as well as old people. Thus, all health and social policies can benefit from using the framework of economic appraisal to set out options, to analyse tentative ways of achieving objectives and following through the resource implications of decisions on priorities about who is to receive help, where, when, and how.

SUMMARY POINTS

1. Economic perspective of setting social priorities is concerned with efficiency in the allocation of resources and equity in the distribution of the benefits and costs of services. Both aspects require considerable judgement to be used in the valuation of costs and benefits of services and in determining the distribution of services.

2. In the present state of the art of economic appraisal, the most useful aid to decision making is cost–utility analysis, which involves assessing the cost per unit of output for alternative services.

3. A considerable effort is now being made to measure the output of health and social programmes in terms of the cost per quality-adjusted life-year produced which entails making judgements about the value of extra years of life and the quality of life produced.

4. The measurement of costs of service provision is mainly technical, but costing the inputs of services provided by families and friends requires more development work.

5. Equity rules require the equal treatment of people in the same circumstances. If equity in the allocation of social priorities is to be achieved, judgement is needed on the way in which needs are to be identified, assessed, and met.

6. There are several different systems for ensuring that people receive the help they need. At present professional judgement is used, but special systems may have to be developed to ensure the delivery of the most appropriate care to people who need it.

7. If professional judgement is not considered to be appropriate, there is a need to switch to benefits in cash instead of the provision of public services.

8. The main point of the economic perspective in the setting of social priorities is the clarification of the criteria on which priorities are determined. If this is done it is possible to debate the priorities identified and their resource implications. If the criteria remain secret and undisclosed it is not possible to discuss either their social or their economic consequences for elderly people or for any other group in the population.

References

1. Rosser, R. M. and Watts, V. C. (1972). The measurement of hospital output. *International Journal of Epidemiology*, **1**, 361–8.
2. Williams, A. (1985). The economics of coronary artery by-pass grafting. *British Medical Journal*, **291**, 326–9.
3. Forrest, P. (1986). *Breast cancer screening*. A report of a working group to the Health Ministers of England Wales, Scotland and Northern Ireland. HMSO, London.
4. Knapp, M. (1984). *The economics of social care*. MacMillan, London.
5. Sinclair, I. (1986). The residents: characteristics and reasons for admission. In *Residential care for elderly people* (ed. Judge, K. and I. Sinclair), pp. 21–34. DHSS, London.
6. Day, P. and Klein, R. (1987). Residential care for the elderly 'a billion pound experiment in policy-making'. *Public Money*, March 1987, 19–24.
7. Challis, D. and Davies, B. (1986). *Case management in community care*. Gower Press, Aldershot.
8. Culyer, A. J. (1976). *Need and the National Health Service*. Martin Robertson, London.

41

Contribution of social security to the well-being of the elderly

J. JLIOVICI

Social security plays an essential role in the maintenance of income during old age and more generally contributes in a large number of ways towards improving the conditions of health and life for the elderly.

Describing the contribution of social security to the well-being of the elderly is really a description of a nearly universal experience, applying to socialist as well as to market economy countries and to developing as well as to industrialized countries. It is also a description of tried and tested arrangements which until recently have provided ever-improving protection to a growing proportion of the population in each country. On the latter point, however, one should add that in a number of countries social security systems appear to have reached a turning point and we are now on the threshold of changes in the arrangements and the extent of protection they provide.

OLD-AGE BENEFITS: AN ESSENTIAL FACTOR FOR THE STANDARD OF LIVING OF THE ELDERLY

Social security pension schemes were originally designed as a form of compulsory saving, with contributions taken from a worker's salary (and in most cases supplemented by a contribution from the employer) being fed into an individual account and forming a capital sum to finance the retiree's future pension. Today very elaborate social security systems have replaced this form of capitalization with a sharing mechanism, whereby the pensions paid to the inactive population are in fact funded by payments by the working population, whether in the form of contributions or taxes. However, arrangements to increase the income of the elderly by supplementing basic pensions, either in the framework of social security (addition of a 'second level' pension) or outside that framework (supplementary occupational pensions) are usually based on capitalization.

In the socialist countries, financing of social security schemes is to a large extent ensured by the state, although certain contributions are required from employers and, in certain countries only, also from employees.

In some developing countries (English-speaking Africa, Asia, and the Caribbean), capitalization methods are applied in a still rudimentary form of social security: the provident funds. These are simply a form of compulsory individual saving whereby the period of saving ends with the payment of a lump-sum corresponding to the contributions plus interest. Pension schemes similar to those of industrialized countries do, however, exist in many developing countries, but there is a marked contrast between these two groups of countries as regards the proportion of the population covered by the schemes. In the pattern of development of such schemes in the Third World, civil servants and military personnel are among the first to be covered, followed by employees in the modern sector of the economy; extension to other categories of the population is often slow because of the economic and administrative difficulties that have to be overcome. Today, pension schemes covering employees as a whole are in operation in the great majority of countries in Latin America and the Carribean, in the majority of African countries, and in about one-third of Asian countries; progress in extending coverage to the self-employed has been considerable in Latin America, but is still slow elsewhere; the same is true of rural populations, with some significant exceptions, particularly the countries of north Africa.

In the industrialized world, existing pension schemes now cover nearly the whole of the national population in cases where they are financed by taxes; where they are financed by contributions from workers and employers and are hence intended essentially for the working population, there may still be cases where coverage is inadequate—particularly for women and for certain part-time workers. But universal coverage is close to being achieved nearly everywhere, and that is only one aspect of the spectacular progress made over the last quarter of a century in the way of old-age insurance both in market economy countries and in socialist countries.

With the weakening of traditional ties of solidarity, modern conditions of economic activity, and the risks of inflation, the individual is able to count less and less on saving and mutual aid to subsist after retirement from working life. Hence social security benefits have become the main component in resources for the elderly. This trend, as well as the increase in life expectancy and a more positive attitude towards retirement, seen as a stage in life that one should be able to enjoy, have increased people's demands with regard to the level of pensions; more and more the improvement of pensions has enabled the elderly not only to be shielded from want but also to maintain a way of life comparable to that before retirement. It is not unusual today for pensions to provide over three-quarters of the income received during the working life—at least for those with modest incomes who receive relatively better treatment from most of the schemes than those in a higher social position. The last few decades have also witnessed the establishment or refinement of arrangements to protect future pensions from monetary erosion (this is one of the main reasons for the changeover from capitalization to 'pay-as-you-go' systems as a basis for financing of the schemes) and periodically to adjust current pensions in order to maintain their purchasing power.

Because of these trends, combined with the increase in the proportion of the elderly in the population, it is not surprising that old-age pensions are becoming the most important category of social security expenditure. Moreover, if account is also taken of health care coverage for the elderly, discussed below, the share of social security expenditure allocated to the elderly is even greater.

QUALIFYING REQUIREMENTS FOR PENSIONS: IMPLICATIONS FOR LIVING CONDITIONS OF THE ELDERLY

Because of the fact that old-age pensions are intended to replace the income that a person retiring from active life used to derive from work, the influence of old-age insurance schemes on the living conditions of the elderly stretches far beyond the area of income maintenance. Depending on the requirements governing pension entitlement, even the employment of older workers or the elderly can be directly affected.

For a long time, there was a rigid interdependence between employment and pensions. Obviously, social security administration could not take account of the extreme diversity in the aging process without coming up against insurmountable problems, hence when the first social security schemes were established, the entitlement to a pension was acquired, other than in exceptional circumstances, or reaching a given age. This restriction on the freedom of choice of those concerned was further reinforced by the tendency to regard entitlement to a pension as an obligation to retire, even though such an obligation has no basis in law or contractual labour agreements.

However, most national legislations have always included provision for retirement before the normal age when justified by circumstances related to the person's health. Either it is recognized that the performance of certain strenuous jobs (in the mines, for instance) involves a presumption of disability by a wearing down of the body at a given age—hence the granting of a pension; or it is recognized that the performance of any job over a long period entails a similar presumption; or again this presumption is applied to workers suffering from certain disabilities. Furthermore;

a similar reasoning has led many countries to lower the age of retirement for women; while in most cases this age is 65 years for men (or usually 60 or even 55 years in the developing countries) it is often 5 years earlier for women, although this differentiation is challenged according to the principle of equality of treatment for both sexes.

In situations where a reduction in the working capacity is medically confirmed and not merely presumed, and where older workers are concerned, there may be provisions allowing the award of an old-age pension before the normal age of entitlement in place of a disability pension.

While exceptions to the retirement age have for many years been limited, a number of recent reforms reflect a reaction to rigidity concerning the retirement age in favour of flexibility considered to be in keeping with the desire for greater freedom of choice for the elderly. This is what is often referred to as retirement 'a la carte': rather than having to accept a 'fixed menu' which may not suit him, the worker has the possibility, by paying a certain price—either in the form of a reduced pension, or in the form of later departure from the job—of choosing within certain limits the time at which he will receive his pension and its amount. Still more favourable would seem to be the arrangements that allow a transition between full-time work and retirement by giving older employees the possibility of gradually reducing their working day, with the resulting reduction in wages being compensated by a partial pension.

For some years, a new trend has emerged in the linkage between pensions and employment in the market economy industrialized countries: under the impact of the economic crisis, various steps have been taken to encourage early retirement in the hope of reducing unemployment. In some cases the aim is more specific in that, for award of an early pension, there must be evidence that the beneficiary has been replaced in the company by a young unemployed person. The same philosophy lies behind measures prohibiting the cumulation of a salary and a retirement pension and other measures in way of heavy financial penalties to discourage the retired from working.

In this respect the situation is quite different in the socialist countries where the combined effect of demographic aging and the employment situation has led governments to encourage work by the elderly. On the one hand, there is every possibility for older workers to put off the age of retirement and thereby receive higher pensions. On the other hand, a whole series of measures has been taken to encourage the employment of pensioners: in recent years, many socialist countries have further expanded the list of employment sectors where it is possible to work while continuing to receive a full or partial pension, or have raised the ceiling of employment income that may be received concurrently with a retirement pension.

OTHER SOCIAL SECURITY MEASURES
IN FAVOUR OF THE ELDERLY

The social security contribution to the health of the elderly is a very important aspect of the role played by social security in maitaining living standards during old age. At the same time, care of the elderly represents a considerable and growing proportion of social security expenditure on health.

In countries with a national health service or a universal health insurance system providing free or readily accessible care to the population as a whole, health care for the elderly is provided in the same way as for the rest of the population. This is the case particularly in the socialist countries, as well as some market economy industrialized countries and developing countries. The situation is different in most of the market economy countries where health insurance schemes cover all or part of the working population using contributions paid by or on behalf of the beneficiaries. In these countries, extension of health care under social security to the elderly implies that one must reconcile the fact that the elderly are major 'consumers' of health care with their very limited possibility of making contributions—a problem further aggravated by the impossibility, where the non-working population is concerned, of obtaining contributions from employers. In general, the elderly receive the same health care as the rest of the population but make lower or nil contributions in return—although this preferential treatment has recently been called into question in several countries, owing to the unfavourable economic climate and the crisis specifically affecting the health sector of social security.

As for the developing countries, more than half of them have introduced certain forms of health care and coverage of health costs under social security. However—except in various Latin American countries— the systems are of recent origin and in most cases cover only a limited proportion of the population. Where health insurance exists, the situation of retirees in this respect is more favourable if the insurance is part of a social security system with several branches including an old-age scheme; with few exceptions, health coverage then extends beyond life subject to payment of a small contribution, or even no contribution by the retiree. Retirees tend to be less well treated when social security schemes do not yet include the payment of regular old-age benefits, since in this case the health insurance institutions do not always have the necessary administrative capacity to keep in contact with a now inactive elderly population. In several African and Asian countries, the elderly may be indirectly protected by the extension of health coverage to individuals—parents as well as children—who are dependants of the insured person.

Helping the elderly to maintain a satisfactory level of health is in fact only one aspect of a broader goal of policies for the elderly—namely to strengthen, and to prolong as far as possible, the capacity of the elderly to live independently despite the adverse effects of physiological aging. The health of the elderly and the maintenance of their capacity to live independently are inextricably linked; it is therefore not surprising that both are reflected in the action taken by social security institutions with regard to the elderly.

The social security institutions help to maintain the elderly's capacity for living independently by meeting the costs of home care and including in them the cost not only of health care but also of social welfare services such as home helps. To meet the needs of elderly people who are unable to continue living at home unless they receive full- or part-time assistance from a third party, social security benefits have been established to cover such costs and thereby help the elderly to remain at home. Such arrangements have also proved effective in encouraging families to take in elderly relatives; in some countries they have been strengthened by offering direct monetary support to families who take care of elderly or disabled relatives.

For elderly people who no longer have the possibility of living at home or with their family, and for whom placement in an institution becomes necessary, social security measures differ, depending on whether the care required is predominantly medical or otherwise. In the first case, the elderly person's hospital costs are reimbursed under social security. Where it is a question of accommodation rather than medical care, and where the costs exceed the financial possibilities of the person, a number of social security schemes have developed special arrangements, such as paying a pension supplement or meeting the cost of the accommodation in place of a pension.

Social security measures in favour of the elderly are sometimes compromised by the inadequacy of existing social and health facilities—a phenomenon that can indeed be observed in countries at all levels of development—inadequacy of basic medical and social institutions in the less-developed countries, and inadequacy of specialized geriatric facilities in the others. Under these circumstances, the social security institutions are required to adopt approaches (construction, management of institutions, subsidies, etc.) which are quite different from their usual ones. Participation in strengthening the health and geriatric infrastructure is by no means the smallest contribution by social security to the well-being of the elderly.

TRENDS AND PROSPECTS

The social security schemes of which we have described some aspects have assumed such importance in society today that they cannot fail to be affected by the socio-economic climate in which societies develop. Thus they have everywhere been affected by the world economic recession which started at the beginning of the 1970s and is still with us. In the market economy countries particularly, continuing unemployment is taking a heavy toll from the workers concerned, their families and the community; this is also a source of major difficulties for social security, in that unemployment brings an increase in expenditure in respect of different types of benefits while reducing the resources anticipated from contributions based on salaries of the employed. Financing of social security is also adversely affected by the aging of the population—a long-term trend which applies to the industrialized countries as a whole.

Up to now, the need to balance the financing of social security has in most cases prompted cautious responses of limited scope. Hence, as far as pensions are concerned, rather than directly reducing the amounts, the preference has been for indirect measures relating to the method of calculation of benefits (e.g. stricter computation of reference salaries) or the conditions governing their award (duration of contributions, length of residence for certain universal benefits). In general, the same caution has been shown with regard to resources, taking only indirect measures to increase them such as no longer exempting pensioners from health insurance contributions. A similar approach has been (without calling into question the present level of old-age benefits) to draw up long-term plans, sometimes extending well beyond the year 2000, so as to bring future pension payments and age of retirement into line with demographic forecasts.

In the developing countries, the internal dynamic of programmes set up with the perspective of expansion—and still far from achieving their objectives—has continued to operate. The persistence of health and nutritional deficiencies, the aggravation of risks of all kinds as part of industrialization, and the weakening of traditional solidarity due to the processes of modernization and urbanization have all been reasons for the developing countries to attain higher levels of social support despite an unfavourable economic environment.

It is difficult to say whether the future course of social security will be one of new progress along the established paths or, on the contrary, one of re-assessment and more or less radical re-orientation. Today there is much talk of reform. For some, the trend to provide universal coverage and to guarantee to each person a standard of living approximating that enjoyed while working, rather than ensuring the bare necessities, have imposed on the social security systems a role and a dimension that are no longer appropriate in societies where hard times have brought a lessening of solidarity. Concentrating social support on certain categories of the population only by applying resource criteria, limiting the commitment to the provision of minimal and uniform basic support, encouraging a sense of individual responsibility, and trusting to spontaneous forms of solidarity—these are some of the approaches suggested in the current debate on reform of the 'welfare state'.

In any case, one must hope that the social security institutions retain the necessary means to continue supporting policies for the elderly as effectively as they have up to now. It is through social security that solidarity between the generations has its most direct expression and it is on this solidarity that the place of the elderly in societies, from the most traditional to the most advanced, depends.

Further reading

As it is impossible to give all of the sources of information used for this article, we have preferred to refer readers to two documents of the International Social Security Association which provide an overview of the situation as well as recent information concerning social security for the elderly in different countries:

International Social Security Association (1982). Sécurité sociale et troisiéme âge: document d'information préparé pour l'Assemblée mondiale sur le vieillissement. *Revue internationale de sécurité sociale*, **4**, 539–82.
International Social Security Association (1986). Développements et tendances de la sécurité sociale 1984–1986. *Revue internationale de sécurité sociale*, **4**, 415–512.

42

Ethical issues and the care of the elderly

ARTHUR L. CAPLAN

THE ELDERLY OCCUPY CENTRE STAGE

The field of bioethics has grown almost exponentially during the past two decades. Health care ethics was once terrain where only a few intellectually daring theologians and physicians were willing to explore. Today the intellectual landscape is flush with hordes of philosophers, lawyers, social scientists, historians, and all manner of health professionals. They are dragging along with them all of the accoutrements requisite for comfort in alien intellectual environments—journals, yearbooks, encyclopedias, conferences, anthologies, textbooks, professional societies, etc.

Early work in bioethics had a rather narrow focus. The clinical encounter and the norms and values appropriate or inappropriate to it constituted the boundaries of bioethical discourse. Issues of the desirability of truth telling, the duty of informed consent, the legitimacy of paternalism, and the right to privacy were the major themes. That too has changed.

Today, a rather different set of issues has come to the fore. Questions of resource allocation have replaced concerns about the nature of the health care provider/patient relationship. The escalating cost of medical care, doubts about the desirability of the quality of life conferred by various kinds of medical interventions, and the decision of many nations to place higher priorities on defence, the provision of housing and other social services, agriculture, and other social goals, has put enormous burdens on health planners and providers to make hard choices about how the funds that are available for health care should be spent. Constraints on resources have brought new ethical pressures to bear on physicians as they try to decide how to allocate scarce but needed forms of health care at the bedside.

In the early days of bioethics discussions and debates viewed all segments of society with equal interest. Whether patients were young or old was more or less irrelevant in thinking about whether or not doctors should tell them the truth or obtain informed consent for procedures.

Age has come to matter a great deal in contemporary discussions concerning resource allocation. Those who are old are now centre stage. Their common bond appears to be that they are higher than average consumers of medical care. In fact, the elderly, especially the very elderly, consume a far larger proportion of resources in Western nations than any other age group.[1]

Resource allocation has moved to the front burner of bioethical concern. The elderly, for a variety of reasons, are most at risk of being burned.

RATIONING BY AGE: PRUDENT CONSUMERS AND NATURAL DEATH

A major emphasis in recent discussions in the literature of medical ethics concerning matters regarding the elderly is the appropriateness of using age as a criterion for allocating health care resources.[2-3] The interest in allocation includes both debates about the legitimacy of using age in making decisions about the duty to provide access to health care[3-5] and about providing access to particular forms of care that are scarce and expensive, such as organ transplantation or renal dialysis.[5]

The primary motivation for the current concern with resource allocation is not simply that health care costs, at least in Western nations, have escalated enormously over the past 20 years. Costs have spiralled in the United States, the United Kingdom, the Scandanavian countries, Japan, Canada, France, Israel, and Australia. In each of these countries political pressures have been brought to bear to do something about reining in these costs. Moreover, those who argue most vociferously for containing costs[3, 7-8] do so from a conviction that there are no public policy options other than to deny access to care to certain individuals or groups. Rationing is an unavoidable reality if costs are to be contained.

Those who believe that rationing is an inevitable consequence of the high costs associated with modern medicine have tended to target the elderly as the group most eligible for bearing the burden of cost containment. The ethical justifications for arriving at this position are varied.

One school of thought argues that, since rationing is inevitable, the elderly ought be denied access to various forms of life-extending care on the grounds that this is what rational consumers of health care would choose as a just policy. If confronted with the need to make choices about how to spend limited health care dollars, prudent consumers would decide to allocate more of their resources to health care needs occurring early in life.

Inspired by the work of the philosopher John Rawls, many scholars[3-4, 8] argue that each one of us, were we ignorant of our station in life and our medical needs, would adopt a strategy of investing our health care dollars so as to maximize our chances of reaching old age. In order to maximize our chances of a long life, we would want to live in a society that gave priority to the health care needs of those in early or mid life.

In order to see what fairness is in the distribution of scarce resources we must, on the prudent consumer view, imagine what would be in our individual interest not knowing whether in fact we would be rich or poor, healthy or unhealthy, old or young, disabled or not. In other words we must try to imagine what we would want in the way of the distribution of health care resources behind a veil of ignorance concerning the details of our particular lives. We will, as prudent consumers, agree that the wisest and fairest strategy to follow in terms of both general health policy and allocation decisions that ought to guide health care providers at the bedside, is to favour the young as against the old.

The other school of thought leading to public policies and clinical attitudes that would discriminate against the elderly arises from the view that there is a natural limit to each human lifespan. Once one has completed one's major projects in life—raising a family, engaging in a career, forming friendships, etc.—one has accomplished what one can legitimately expect from life. The goal of medicine and health policy should be to try and assure each person the opportunity to live a reasonable lifespan and to die what is sometimes termed a 'natural death'[2]

On this view there is no sense devoting resources to the extension of lives in society beyond the 'natural' end point defined by the attainment of the basic goods and social roles of human existence. This is especially so if there are members of society who are not likely to attain a natural lifespan because social resources are being allocated to the extension of the lives of others beyond the point of 'natural death'.[2]

The elderly must be excluded from access to life-extending medical care in favour of allowing younger persons an opportunity to enjoy what all members of a society would agree is a reasonable or natural lifespan. Moreover, on this view, the proper aim of medicine is not to strive for the attainment of immortality, but rather to develop interventions and techniques that can enhance the quality of life across a reasonable conception of the lifespan.

Both of these views provide provocative reasons for ethically justifying the denial of certain kinds of medical resources to the elderly. The 'prudent consumer' view argues that rational consumers would impose a system of age-based rationing upon themselves as a fair and equitable response to the problem of what to do about limited resources for health care. The 'natural death' approach argues that the proper goal of medicine is to maximize the quality of life of the normal lifespan—not to seek its infinite extension. Moreover, if some members of society are being denied an opportunity to enjoy a minimally normal lifespan, then there is a strong obligation to redress this inequity by re-allocating resources away from medical interventions—transplants, artificial organs, chemotherapies, etc.—whose goal is to add years of life to those who already have completed the projects of a normal human life.

Both of these schools of thought—the 'prudent consumer' view and the 'natural death' view—are provocative responses to the question of what would be fair and equitable in allocating resources. Both, however, appear vulnerable to serious criticisms.

The primary flaw with both views is that it is not clear that everything that could be tried has been tried in the attempt to avoid or stave off the need to ration health care resources. Certainly, the fact that the United States is spending nearly 12 per cent of its gross national product on health care costs is startling. But there are many nations spending far less money without appreciable differences in either the length or quality of life enjoyed by their citizens.

The stakes involved in talk of rationing in the arena of health care are enormous. If policies favouring any sort of rationing are adopted, either explicitly or tacitly, lives will be lost as a direct result.

Rationing presumes that some persons who might benefit by access to life-saving resources will be denied access to them. Certainly, the first obligation any society has in confronting the issue of rationing health care resources is not to debate the niceties of which group or sub-group of the population should be asked to jump out of or be pushed over the side of the health care lifeboat. Rather, it is to make every possible effort to insure that resources are being utilized in as efficient manner as is possible in order to provide the greatest access to all who might benefit from and desire access to health care.

No nation has yet undertaken the kinds of efforts that would be needed to justify the implementation of any sort of rationing policies, age based or otherwise, at this point in time. There is simply too much waste and too little known about the efficacy of various kinds of medical interventions to state with assurance that the time for rationing has come or is even on the horizon.

It is true that many Western nations spend enormous sums of money on health care. But there is no established consensus on the part of the public in these nations that too much is being spent. Rather, there is a general concern that the high cost of delivering sophisticated medical services be justified in terms of benefits to those receiving care.

And this is where much remains to be done in the formulation of health policy. There is simply too little effort being made to collect and analyse in a systematic fashion data on the benefits that are associated with surgical, medical, nursing, psychological, palliative, rehabilitative, preventative, and pharmacological interventions. The variations that exist in the utilization of medical services from region to region in various countries and from nation to nation are so large as to raise obvious questions about the desirability of paying for them. Too little attention has been given over to the assessment of outcomes in medical care to justify claims that nothing except rationing can be instituted in the way of a response to the high cost of medical care.

Talk of rationing can only follow upon rigorous and systematic efforts to assure that real and significant benefits can be derived from the provision of all forms of health care services. Every effort must be made to insure that health services are being provided in the cheapest possible manner with a reasonable chance of benefit. Rationing in a situation where inefficiency or worse, ineffectiveness, exists is immoral.

The other major problem confronting those who arrive at positions entailing the denial of access to health care benefits to the elderly as the only fair response to the high cost of health care services is that it is not clear that such arguments work equally well for both micro and macro choices. It may be that prudent consumers of health care would want to create policies in hospitals or clinics such that limited and life-saving medical resources would be devoted to the young or middle aged rather than the old. If forced to choose most people would agree that it makes more sense to give a scarce heart transplant or intensive care bed to someone who is 13 or 30 rather than to someone who is 70 or 80. And they would also choose to exist in a system that followed such normative policies if they did not know anything more than that they might require life-saving medical care at 13, 30, or 80.

A similar conclusion follows from the notion that there exists a natural lifespan. Someone who has yet to enjoy the opportunity of a full life ought get a transplant or heart operation ahead of someone who has already lived many many years.

But arguments concerning the ethical norms that should guide health care providers in making hard choices about the allocation of scarce, life-saving resources in clinical settings say nothing about our obligation to insure that the resources are not and will not in the future be scarce. It may be just to deny access to kidney dialysis on the basis of age to those who are old when the doctor has only a few machines available. It is not just to avoid the question of how many such machines ought exist by allowing social complacency about the existence of scarcity because consensus exists about what to do when scarcity exists.

This leads to the question of whether either a prudent consumer view of justice in health or one grounded in a view of a natural lifespan would lead to age-based rationing policies for overall expenditures in health care that would give priority to youth or middle age as against old age. Here the question of what is fair is not so simple as the proponents of either of the above views would have us believe.

Prudent consumers might be inclined to avoid expenditures which extend life because they have attitudes and views of aging which are based upon the recognition that, in most societies, the lot of the aged is not pleasant. Those who think that one's projects and activities reach a natural completion point in old age are also committed to a view of old age that sees old age as a time of retirement, institutionalization, social isolation, and loss of self determination—a time of life of especially low quality. But, of course, such views are entirely a function of how individual societies and groups define the roles and responsibilities of old age.[9] If we expand our view of what old age should be in terms of projects and plans then what seems natural today in terms of our lifespan will not seem natural tommorow.

In fact this is to a degree what has been happening in the developed world as medical interventions have succeeded in extending the lifespan of individuals. In the fourteenth or fifteenth centuries, or in many poor societies in the twentieth century, few people lived beyond middle age. The chance of surviving beyond early childhood was, and still is in all too many countries, low. But, as medical interventions and public health measures increase individual life expectancy, our self-conceptions of what is natural *vis-à-vis* life and death drastically alter.

Where once child bearing and the raising of a family were tasks to be completed in one's teens or twenties, they are now, in the developed world, undertakings that occupy the lives of many in their thirties, forties, and fifties. Where once persons were happy if they could enjoy a single career, a longer lifespan raises the opportunity of enjoying two, three, or more complete careers or occupations. The concepts we bring to our view of old age are very much a function not of biology, but of the social, economic, and cultural climates in which we live. And if this is so, it is not at all evident that the fairest or most just approach to the distribution of health care resources at the level of societal expenditure leads only and inevitably toward the exclusion of the elderly on grounds of either prudent choice or the naturalness of mortality and death.

The issue is whether life can be made meaningful and useful by social arrangements that afford opportunities and choices to all citizens regardless of age. If we make the lives of the elderly miserable by making pariahs of them then no prudent consumer would choose to spend social resources to extend their lives. If we view ourselves as having of necessity only 70 or 80 years on this globe, then we will adjust our expectations concerning the nature of our projects and plans accordingly. But if medicine can discover techniques that will permit the extension of life for years or decades beyond what is now possible, then it is not clear what justice or fairness would dictate in terms of the allocation of resources toward the achievement of various policy options.

Views of fairness and equity concerning the allocation of medical resources are very much a function of our views concerning the desirability of living to an old age. It is important to examine the ways in which our existing health care system, at least in the developed countries which can afford to provide care that allows the possibility of extended life, permit persons to exercise self-determination and autonomous behaviour with respect to their medical care.

The elderly, especially the very old, often fear the loss of personal control over their lives, or the prospect of placement in an institutional setting, more than they fear the loss of access to a hospital bed or some form of technological gadgetry. Yet in many Western societies it is the debates about access to acute care and life-saving medical interventions that have dominated discussions of resource allocation. If autonomy and self-determination are critical components of our view of what it is that makes life meaningful at any age, then we need to examine the ways in which our present health care system enhances or discourages the attainment of these goals.

Similarly, in those nations where the care of the elderly is seen as primarily a matter of family responsibility, there has not been much discussion of the limits of responsibility for family members. Nor has there been much attention paid to the ways in which personal habits and customs of older persons must yield in the face of familial or communal requirements. The ability to strike a balance between personal choice and social requirements is an ethical issue that touches the lives of elderly persons, families, and health care providers in an ongoing and pervasive manner.

The need to attend closely to the problem of autonomy where elderly patients are concerned is made all the more acute by the fact that so many of those with moderate or severe illnesses or impairments receive care in institutional circumstances. Such settings may hinder or impede the ability to be autonomous. Institutional requirements are often at odds with personal freedom despite rhetorical claims to the contrary.[10]

How important is autonomy for older patients? How hard ought societies strive to deliver care in settings that respect and enhance the possibility for autonomous behaviour? In order to answer these and other questions related to autonomy, it will be necessary to examine why it is that autonomy has come to occupy such a central role in the writings of those concerned about ethics in health care.

THE IMPORTANCE OF AUTONOMY

Prior to the Second World War relationships between health care providers and their patients were characterized by a model often referred to as 'paternalistic'.[11-13] Health care providers believed themselves capable of both determining the needs of patients and of deciding what course of treatment was necessary in light of those needs.

Healers, at least those trained in Western nations, saw themselves as able to discern both the interests of their patients and the medical steps that could be taken to protect or enhance those interests. Their motives in acting paternalistically toward their patients were not evil. On the contrary, the desire to do good, to benefit the patient through the use of special knowledge and skills, was the linchpin of medical morality. The obligation of beneficence, to help those who sought medical care, and as a corollary to avoid harming patients, was seen as overriding all other considerations, personal and professional.[14]

Matters changed significantly regarding the ethics of provider—patient relationships after World War Two. The revelations that many physicians had participated in barbarous experiments upon those confined in concentration camps in Germany, Eastern Europe, and China, or had aided and abetted torture and murder through the use of their knowledge of the body and its physiological requirements,[15] weakened societal willingness to trust in the benevolent motives of health care providers. Beneficence no longer seemed an adequate ethical protection for those seeking or requiring medical care.

Trust in health care providers was further weakened by the arguments advanced by German medical officials in defending their conduct in the concentration camps. During the Nuremburg trials, these physicians denied that what they had done was evil, much less morally wrong. They insisted that their conduct was morally defensible in that it was reasonable to sacrifice a few so that the majority might be benefited.

A number of medical societies enacted resolutions condemning the abuse of patients at the hands of physicians in the post World War Two era. The World Medical Association, at various conferences held during the 1950s and 1960s, articulated codes of conduct which explicitly rejected both paternalism and utilitarianism as adequate ethical foundations for governing physician–patient relationships. Courts in numerous nations also found paternalism and utilitarianism to be an inadequate basis for the practice of health care.[14, 16]

During the past two decades, many physicians, lawyers, and philosophers have argued that the dignity of patients can only be assured in a moral climiate which places individual autonomy at the centre of medical care.[17] Patients, whether serving as subjects in medical research or as the recipients of therapy, ought to have the right of self-determination. Each patient, regardless of sex, race, or socio-economic standing, ought be allowed to decide whether or not they wish to receive medical care and the circumstances under which such care should be stopped.[6,13]

INFORMED CONSENT AND THE ELDERLY

There are large numbers of persons who are not capable of asserting personal autonomy. Some cannot do so as a consequence of severe cognitive impairments. Some cannot as a consequence of their status as prisoners or in other types of institutional environments in which privacy and freedom are severely constrained. And some cannot do so as a consequence of age.

Obviously very young infants and children are not capable of self-determination. Adolescents may be capable of self-determination with respect to some decisions but not others. However, it is the elderly who have posed some of the most vexing questions about autonomy, self-determination, and informed consent within medical relationships.

There is a marked tendency in many societies to stereotype those who are elderly as incapable of autonomous behaviour. The elderly are sometimes seen as mentally limited, emotionally unstable, and physically inadequate.[9]

Such stereotypes are quite obviously false. Yet it is also true that even in those societies where reverence for the elderly is a long-standing and important cultural norm, there are many elderly persons who, as a result of acute diseases, chronic illness, or the cumulative impact of senescence itself, suffer from limitations in their mental or physical capacities.

The elderly are more susceptible to illness and disability than are other age groups within society. Moreover, in many societies the elderly are not treated with dignity or respect because of bias, ignorance, and prejudice. They often bear a disproportionate burden of poverty and economic disadvantage. And in those societies where there are more women than men represented in the ranks of the elderly, they may have to contend with social biases against women as well as against age.

These realities highlight the importance of addressing the question of the adequacy of informed consent for protecting the rights and dignity of elderly persons who are either subjects in medical experiments or patients receiving care. If autonomy is not enhanced or maintained, old age will lose all of its appeal and those who argue against its extension by means of medical care will not have an especially hard case to make.

The elderly are especially vulnerable to the loss of their personal autonomy and, as a result, their individuality and dignity. There are physiological, social, economic, and cultural forces that have adverse impacts upon the elderly in terms of their personal autonomy. As a result, the elderly are caught in a bitter irony—the less autonomy they have the less they will see their lives as worth living and the easier it will be to invoke social policies that discriminate against them.

Can the elderly utilize the doctrine of informed consent to protect their interest adequately in health care settings? Are they afforded the opportunity to express their views and to choose among the options that are made available to them by health care providers? Do economic considerations limit the degree to which providers and governments are willing to tolerate self-determination as expressed through informed consent in medical settings? And are the elderly, who may feel intimidated, frightened, or coerced by family members or health care providers into making health care decisions that they believe are not in their own best interest, afforded sufficient opportunities under existing policies and practices in nursing homes, hospices, hospitals, long-term care facilities, home care agencies, and psychiatric facilities to express their views? More importantly, can their views be heard by persons in positions of authority?

There is no reason to think that the elderly can be treated as a group where matters of competency to provide consent are concerned. While stereotypes are hard to debunk, the fact remains that the diversity and variation present in this subsection of humankind is so enormous as to defy any simple classification or taxonomy. Old age, in and of itself, is not a sufficient basis for disenfranchising an elderly person, even one who is a patient, as an autonomous agent.

At the same time it must also be recognized that some elderly patients may require special assistance in expressing their desires and wishes relative to what is required where those of other ages are concerned. The elderly often speak in a somewhat quieter voice than do those of other ages. They may be so eager to show respect for their healer or for the practice of medicine that they do not speak out when something is done that they do not believe is correct or do not understand. Some of the elderly who require medical help may have impairments in sensory abilities or emotional capacities that make it more difficult for them to communicate in surroundings which are not familiar to them. Still others may be capable of competency only at certain periods during the day, with the assistance of medication, or with other forms of compensatory assistance.

If it is true, as health care professionals from all nations have insisted since the horrors of the Second World War were revealed, that autonomy ought be viewed as a central value in the ethics of health care, then it would appear that health care professionals and politicians must do more than has been done to date to create the contexts in which autonomy can flourish and grow so far as the elderly are concerned. There are simply too many elderly patients who are not afforded the opportunity for access to and full participation in the determination of their health care or in any other aspect of their lives.

It is not enough to merely present information or to obtain written consent on a piece of paper for a particular medical procedure. Informed consent connotes the fact that patients understand what is being proposed to them in the way of medical care, that they be given time to think about their options, that they not be threatened or coerced in the choices that they make, and that they be able to ask questions about all aspects of medical care.[18] Informed consent is therefore an ongoing process rather than a single event or occurrence.

Every health care provider must take care to assess the competency of each patient. Elderly persons must be actively encouraged to take responsibility for the determination of their own medical care and participation in it. If there are factors which hinder the ability of an elderly person to comprehend information or to make free and voluntary choices among options then it is the health care provider's obligation to do what can be done to minimize the impact of such factors.

Why must extraordinary efforts be made to protect and enhance the autonomy of the elderly as against other groups who may also require or seek health care? First, the elderly may face special obstacles to the exercise of their autonomy. Second, for social and cultural reasons the elderly may not always feel comfortable with behaviour that they may perceive as challenging the authority of a healer or professional. Third, and most importantly, the elderly are simply more likely to be in a position to engage in self-determination simply by dint of their age and experience.

AGE, WISDOM, AND AUTHENTICITY

A truth about aging that is recognized by nearly every society is that, while there may be certain losses associated with aging in terms of physiological capacities, there are certain specific benefits associated with the process of aging. Not the least of these is the fact that those who are older have had the benefit of experience gained over time. Such experience is recognized in many cultures as so deserving of respect that societies are organized with their oldest members in leadership positions. It is not that younger members lack intellectual acumen or training in various arts or skills. Rather, it is that age is commonly thought to bring with it wisdom—the ability to interpret events through the lens of one's own personal experience. Personal experience, other things being equal, is richer in proportion to the amount of time a person has lived.

A case might be made that wisdom does not accrue to any person simply as a function of a long life. But it would be harder to argue that older persons are not in a better position than younger members of society to know their own values and desires.

Experience is a good teacher. Those who are older are more likely to have had the chance to think about their personal values and goals and to decide whether to maintain them or alter them in favour of other values and goals. It might be said that a woman of 20 does not really know what she wants from life. But a woman of 70 can hardly be said to be ignorant or uncertain about her life plans and expectations.

The elderly are in possession, or more likely to be in possession, not perhaps of wisdom but of authenticity. They are more likely than anyone else to know their own minds, feelings, values, characteristics, and aspirations. They are more likely to have had the chance to refine and reform these beliefs—a chance which is very much a function of time.

If it is true that the older we become the more authentic our values are likely to be, in terms of their being chosen by us as opposed to being taught by others or merely the echoes of influential figures in our lives, then it is easy to see why autonomy and informed consent must play a prominent role in the health care of the elderly. For self-determination or autonomy are not merely reflections of the ability to choose. They are powers that can best be exercised when opportunities for uncoerced decision making are given and when those making decisions have the self-knowledge to know what their values and desires actually are.[19] The elderly are often in the best position of all members of society to fulfil these requirements for self-determination and autonomous behaviour. And if autonomy is properly understood, it is the elderly who may be in the most favourable position to enjoy life truly since they have the wisdom to act from real self-determination and autonomy!

Who is better placed to know what they wish from health care relationships than the elderly? Who is in a better position than an older person to know exactly what is and is not a deeply held personal value?

The obligations to heed the choices and wishes of older patients is especially strong since they, among all members of society, are most likely to know reflectively their personal values. If the aim of medical interventions is to serve the welfare and interest of the patient, then who is in a better position than an older patient to understand what conception of welfare or interest is valid from the point of view of his or her care?

It may be difficult to ascertain the wishes or desires of elderly patients, but difficulties in communication ought not be confused with the presence or absence of deeply held, authentic value commitments. The health care provider must presume, if anything can be presumed simply by dint of age, that those who are older are in a better position to know their own values than are others who are younger. The duty of the health care provider is then to try and create an environment in which elderly patients feel free to indicate the values and goals that they wish to guide their care. Similar presumptions ought guide the deliberations of politicians, bureaucrats and others involved in the articulation of public policies.

The obligation of the health care provider where the elderly patient is concerned is to seek informed consent for any and all interventions or changes in the course of care. This is an obligation that has at its foundation the duty to allow individuals to exercise their autonomy in order to respect their dignity as individuals. But if it is true that the elderly are more likely than others to be in possession of the experience and knowledge required to label an autonomous choice as authentic, then health care providers must show extra zeal in attempting to both ascertain the autonomous wishes of the elderly and to comply with those decisions that are expressed. They must also strive to assure that the degree of autonomy afforded the elderly is not such so as to make their exclusion from access to health care resources a foregone conclusion.

CONCLUSION

Access to health care and health care resources is obviously important to the elderly, as it is to all persons. But the elderly, by dint of their life experience, ought to command special attention in matters pertaining to health care, not in terms of access to care but in terms of the authority they are granted to determine the course of their care. Autonomy and self determination are capabilities that the elderly are better positioned to exhibit than other members of society. However, if this is true, those responsible for the provision of health and health related services to the elderly must make greater efforts than have been mounted to date to accord the capacity for self-determination a greater respect.

The case for rationing with respect to health care services has not been persuasively established. To some extent, inefficiencies in the provision of care account for the extraordinary increase in health care costs in the developed nations. Moreover, in all nations too little emphasis has been placed on assessing the outcomes of health care interventions in order to assure that there are benefits associated with the investment of resources in all manner of interventions.

Still there may be situations, now and in the foreseeable future, where the costs of modern medical care will exceed the abilities of societies to pay for them. Considerations of fairness would seem to point in the direction of using age as a factor in deciding how to allocate scarce, life-saving, and efficacious interventions to particular persons in clinical settings. If more than one person is eligible to receive a particular form of life-saving medical care, say a liver transplant or a dose of interferon, and if the supply of such medical resources is limited, then, other things being equal, fairness would seem to dictate providing that resource to the person who stands to benefit the most in terms of both quality of life and years of life added. Inevitably, where bedside rationing decisions must be made this will result in rationing policies that favour the young over the old.

However, it is not so clear that considerations of justice point in the direction of giving priority to the young over the old where matters of general social expenditure for health care are concerned. It is true that each citizen of a society ought to expect an equal chance of living a full and meaningful life. But there may be newborns or young children whose health problems are so severe that they stand almost no chance of attaining a full and meaningful life no matter what medical interventions are attempted. Other children may be so ill that the cost of trying to give them a reasonable opportunity to enjoy a full and meaningful life would so distort the amount of resources available to others that prudent and rational consumers of health care would not want to allocate needed resources owing to the burdens that would be imposed on the other members of society. The age of social groups provides no hard and fast rules of equity as to how best to distribute social resources for health care.

Most importantly, those who argue that either prudent consumers or those committed to a view of 'natural lifespans' have not made an adequate case for age-based rationing that would exclude or give lower priority to the health needs of the elderly. Prudent consumers might be inclined to allocate more resources to their old age if old age were made more attractive than it presently is in many societies in terms of the quality of life to be enjoyed and the degree of self-determination that can be exhibited. Moreover, our sense of what is a natural lifespan, while defined by our sense of our projects and goals, is a highly subjective and culturally dependent notion.

Our distant ancestors could never have envisaged what we would consider natural in terms of years of life to be lived in the twentieth century, and there is no reason to assume that we will do any better a job of prognosticating what is normal or natural for generations to come.

Those who live in developed nations have a very different view of the time span in which death seems 'natural' then those who live in underdeveloped nations where conditions make it unlikely that persons will survive into their seventies, eighties, and nineties or beyond. Whether the view is right or wrong is less interesting than that it is relative to a huge set of social, economic, and cultural variables.

The primary ethical responsibility facing those concerned about the high cost of care for the elderly is to recognize that the elderly are in the best position within our society to articulate their views of what a meaningful and rich life is. Our obligation is to assure that social policies are created which allow each person, old or young, to enjoy the opportunities and benefits of a high quality of life at all points of the lifespan. We have a long way to go in order to achieve this goal. Talk of age-based rationing at this point of time is simply premature. We cannot really know what is prudent or natural until we have done what must be done to allow all persons to have a fair opportunity to exercise self-determination sufficient to allow them to decide what it is and is not that makes life worth living.

References

1. Scitovsky, X. (1984). The high cost of dying: what do the data show? *Milbank Memorial Fund Quarterly*, **62**, 604–13.
2. Daniels, N. (1985). *Just health care*. Cambridge University Press, Cambridge.
3. Daniels, N. (1987). *Am I my parents' keeper?* Oxford, New York.
4. Callahan, D. (1987). *Setting limits*. Simon and Schuster, New York.
5. Wikler, D. (1988). Ought the young make health care decisions for their aged selves?, *Journal of Medicine and Philosophy*, **13**, 57–71.
6. Caplan, A. (1987). Equity in the selection of recipients for cardiac transplants. *Circulation*, **75**, 10–20.
7. Califano, J. (1986). *America's health care revolution*. Random House, New York.
8. Aaron, H. and Schwartz, W. (1984). *The painful prescription*. Brookings, Washington.
9. Butler, R. (1975). *Why survive?* Harper & Row, New York.
10. Caplan, A. Callahan, D., J. Haas, and J. (1987). 'Ethical and policy issues in rehabilitation medicine, *Hastings Center Report*. **17**, (4), 1–20.
11. Veatch, R. (1972). Models for ethical medicine in a revolutionary age. *Hastings Center Report*, **2**, 5–7.
12. Bok, S. (1978). *Lying*. Pantheon, New York.
13. Katz, J. (1984). *The silent world of doctor and patient*. Free Press, New York.
14. Faden, R. and Beauchamp, T. (1986). *A history and theory of informed consent*. Oxford University Press, New York.
15. Lifton, R. (1986). *Nazi doctors*. Basic Books, New York.
16. The President's Commission for the Study of Ethical Problems in Medicine (1983). *Implementing human research regulations*. No. 040–000–00471–8, USGPO, Washington.
17. Caplan, A. (1985). Let wisdom find a way. *Generations*, **10** (2), 10–14.
18. Levine, R. (1986). *Ethics and regulation of clinical research*, (2nd edn). Urban G. Schwarzenberg, Baltimore.
19. Dworkin, G. (1976). Moral autonomy. In *The roots of ethics* (ed. Callahan, D. and H. T. Engelhardt Jr), pp. 29–44. Plenum, New York.

APPENDIX

Diagnosis and classification of dementias in the elderly with special reference to the tenth revision of the international classification of diseases (ICD-10)

A. JABLENSKY

INTRODUCTION

Since the beginnings of scientific psychiatry, age has been recognized as a major variable influencing mental morbidity. In the fifth edition of his classic text,[1] Kraepelin wrote: 'We bring together, as insanity of the involutional age, all those mental disorders which stand in a causal relationship to the general process of aging...it is beyond doubt that quite specific forms of insanity occur in the period of bodily decline, which betray in their clinical picture an origin in the involutional process.' One of the remarkable developments in the decades that followed the widespread adoption of Kraepelin's nosological scheme was the progressive 'downward' revision of this view, which gradually resulted in a practical abandonment of the idea that age *per se* is an aetiological factor in psychiatric morbidity.

Thus, although Jaspers[2] stated that 'the age-epoch gives a specific stamp to every morbid state', he was the first to introduce the important caveat that we should distinguish between illnesses due to old age and those occurring in old age. In the seventh edition (1959) of his *General psychopathology* he concluded: 'The psychoses that can actually be attributed to aging get fewer in number. Perhaps senile dementia is the only disease of age...The other psychic illnesses of old age are "to a big extent hereditary disorders of a particular stamp"'.

Jaspers foresaw a development which is well illustrated in the successive revisions of the chapter on mental disorders in the *International classification of diseases* (ICD). In the eighth revision[3] there were five diagnostic rubrics in which age is a defining feature: senile dementia, presenile dementia, involutional melancholia, involutional paraphrenia, and non-psychotic mental disorder associated with senile or presenile brain disease. The ninth revision[4] no longer contains a rubric for involutional melancholia, and the qualifier 'involutional' was dropped from the rubric of paraphrenia. The tenth revision (now available as a draft for field trials[5]) dispenses altogether with the terms 'senile' and 'presenile', as well as with the notion of 'paraphrenia', thus leaving no provision for identifying any mental disorder as aetiologically linked with aging. The position adopted in another influential classification of mental disorders, the *Diagnostic and statistical manual of mental disorders* (DSM-III, DSM-IIIR) of the American Psychiatric Association,[6] is a similar one; it contains no diagnostic categories specific to old age, and none of its five axes is age related.

In so far as ICD-10 and DSM-IIIR reflect a degree of current consensus on the state of scientific knowledge, it can be said that mental disorders occurring in the elderly are no longer considered to belong in a separate category of morbidity.

This development may appear to be in conflict with the demographic trend of a steady increase of the proportion of the elderly people in many (mainly developed) parts of the world. One would expect that the growth of the number of the elderly, and in particular the marked increase of the size of populations aged 75 and over, would enable the delineation of a mental pathology that is specifically linked to processes of aging of the central nervous system. However, this has not been the case. The main trends of research in the past two decades concern several aspects of aging.

First, although it is now known that many psychosocial factors affecting the mental well-being of the elderly, such as social isolation, cultural uprooting, and institutionalization, are responsible for the high levels of psychiatric morbidity that may be observed in elderly populations, they do not produce specific forms of disorders. In interaction with age-related metabolic, hormonal, and tissue changes which increase the vulnerability of the elderly to a variety of stresses, the environmental factors may facilitate the expression of a genetic predisposition to affective or paranoid disorder.[7,8] Furthermore, such factors, together with the accentuation of personality traits which often occurs with 'normal' aging, are likely to put a characteristic pathoplastic stamp on the clinical manifestations of disorders such as depression, anxiety, or paranoid states. However, the existence of a particular pathoplastic 'colouring' of the psychopathology exhibited in advanced age is not a sufficient reason for classifying such relatively common conditions in a separate group, although the recognition of the psychological and physiological vulnerabilities in the elderly is an important prerequisite for their proper diagnosis and treatment.

Dementia, however, is a problem which merits a special place in a discussion of mental morbidity in the elderly. Although not a single dementing illness described so far is strictly age specific in its occurrence, dementia in Alzheimer's disease, dementia in cerebrovascular disease, as well as a number of other atrophic processes affecting the brain, are much more common in populations aged 65 and over than in younger age groups.[9] The relationship between the pathological changes occurring in Alzheimer disease and those in 'normal' aging is still incompletely understood. It is not known whether the formation of plaques and neurofibrillary tangles, the loss of neurons in particular areas of the brain, and the complex disturbance of cerebral neurotransmission which occur in Alzheimer's disease represent an accelerated form of cerebral aging or are the expression of a morbid process which is qualitatively different from 'normal' aging.[10] For such fundamental issues to be resolved, epidemiological and clinical research will be of crucial importance, and this brings up the question of classification, diagnostic criteria, and rules.

ICD-10: BACKGROUND AND GENERAL FEATURES

In the 1960s and early 70s, the World Health Organization carried out an extensive programme of international seminars and consultations which had the aim of reducing disagreement and improving the reliability of psychiatric diagnosis, classification, and statistics. One of the seminars was specifically devoted to the problem of classification of mental disorders in the elderly. The result of this work was a substantially improved chapter on mental disorders in the eighth revision of ICD, and the first internationally accepted glossary of diagnostic terms.[11] With minor modifications, both the classificatory scheme and the glossary were carried over into ICD-9 (adopted in 1975 and still in force).

Some significant developments took place after the introduction of ICD-9: (1) following a period of relative neglect, psychiatric nosology and the issues of diagnosis and classification became the focus of a renewed interest; as a result, 'operational' diagnostic criteria, new instruments, and research-oriented taxonomies such as RDC and DSM-III were developed and rapidly gained wide acceptance; (2) the new wave of 'high-technology' research into the biological basis of mental disorders expanded considerably the clinical horizon; (3) the major transcultural studies on schizophrenia, depression, and other disorders which were co-ordinated by WHO provided strong support to the notion that the basic forms of mental disorders are very similar in different populations and, hence, could be validly approached by collaborative research.

In response to these developments, WHO and the Alcohol, Drug Abuse and Mental Health Administration (ADAMHA) of the United States initiated in 1979 a joint programme on diagnosis and classification of mental disorders which involved the participation of over 200 experts from 47 countries. One of the products of this programme was an extensive and critical review of the 'state of the art' in the field as well as a list of recommendations and proposals concerning the future redrafting of the classification for clinical and research purposes.[12]

Drawing on this experience, in 1984 WHO commenced work on the 'mental disorders' chapter for the tenth revision of the ICD, in collaboration with some 150 experts from all the geographical regions, representing a variety of research and clinical approaches. A provisional version of the new classification of mental disorders is now available and is currently undergoing field trials in a number of research centres all over the world. The adoption of ICD-10 by the World Health Assembly is scheduled for 1990 and its practical implementation in the member states will start in 1992. However, the informal or pilot use of any portion of ICD-10 prior to that date should be encouraged.

ICD-10 uses a system of alphanumeric codes which appreciably enlarge the space available to accommodate new rubrics and categories. This should make it possible to space future revisions of the classification at longer intervals, because new categories can be added, or obsolete ones deleted, as and when the need arises, without major re-arrangements of the entire structure. Further, ICD-10 represents a 'family' of instruments and classifications rather than a single document. The central part of the system is a 'core' classification which retains its uniaxial character. However, there is sufficient flexibility in ICD-10 to accomodate, when needed, multiaxial schemes or other supplementary instruments, such as the Classification of Impairments, Disabilities and Handicaps.

THE CLASSIFICATION OF MENTAL DISORDERS IN ICD-10

The mental health components of ICD-10 comprise the mental disorders chapter (Chapter V, containing rubrics supplied with the prefix 'F', which identifies mental disorders); a series of Z-codes for psychosocial and behavioural factors related to health; X- and Y-codes for external causes of death and injury, including suicide; and provisions for recording ill-defined behavioural symptoms and signs, especially those encountered in primary health care.

The mental disorders chapter of ICD-10 is a major departure from ICD-8 and ICD-9 in many respects. It has been designed not only as a guide to the statistical reporting on morbidity, but also as a clinical and research manual and, possibly, as a teaching tool. Its features include:

—— an updated list of diagnostic categories which takes into account both recent research developments and nosological concepts;

—— the provision of glossary definitions of disorders and of explicit diagnostic criteria in two formats: (1) clinical diagnostic guidelines for routine use (allowing the flexibility of interpretation that clinicians usually require); and (2) diagnostic criteria for research (providing stringent decision-making rules aiming to ensure a high level of specificity for research purposes);

—— the grouping of all the diagnoses into 10 major blocks, so that disorders exhibiting common features of pathology (e.g. demonstrable brain disease), aetiology (e.g. substance use), clinical manifestations (e.g. mood disorders, schizophrenia and related conditions, neurotic disorders), or age at onset (e.g. developmental disorders) appear in contingent rubrics.

Organic mental disorders in ICD-10

The section of ICD-10 which deals with organic and symptomatic mental disorders and, therefore, is of particular relevance to problems occurring in the elderly, contains 10 major rubrics:

F00 dementia not otherwise specified;

F01 dementia in Alzheimer's disease;

F02 dementia in cerebrovascular disease;

F03 dementia associated with other disorders;

F04 organic amnestic syndrome (Korsakov syndrome) other than alcoholic;

F05 delirium other than alcoholic;

F06 other mental disorders due to brain disease, damage, or dysfunction, or to physical disease;

F07 personality and behaviour disorder due to brain disease, damage, or dysfunction;

F08 other organic or symptomatic mental disorder;

F09 unspecified organic or symptomatic mental disorder.

The subdivisions of these rubrics provide a total of 27 separate codes (each supplied with a glossary definition and diagnostic guidelines/criteria) for identifying specific diagnostic entities. This is a considerable improvement over the ICD-9 provisions for classifying organic mental disorders, which included only 10 diagnostic categories (not counting those related to alcohol and drug psychoses) in sections 290–4 (organic psychotic conditions) and a further four in section 310 (entitled specific non-psychotic mental disorders following organic brain damage').

The structure of this ICD-10 section reflects a conceptual departure from the principles underlying the classification of the organic mental disorders in ICD-9. Although the term 'organic' has been retained as a common denominator, its use no longer implies a sharp dichotomy between 'organic' and 'non-organic' psychiatric illnesses. The term 'organic' in ICD-10 is specified as meaning only that 'the syndrome so classified can be attributed to an independently diagnosable cerebral or systemic disease' but not that 'the conditions in other section of this classification are 'non-organic' in the sense of not having a cerebral substrate'. Another traditional dichotomy which is deemphasized in ICD-10 is that of psychotic versus non-psychotic disorders. In so far as these terms still appear in ICD-10, they are used only descriptively, referring to the presence or absence of symptoms such as delusions, hallucinations, or formal thought disorder. Psychotic and non-psychotic features, however, are not thought to denote a fundamental dichotomy within the domain of mental morbidity, and they do not necessarily provide a valid grading of severity. These are some of the reasons for grouping together, in section F0 of ICD-10, dementing, psychotic, and non-psychotic disorders for which a common aetiological base can be found in identifiable cerebral lesions or dysfunctions, although their symptoms may be heterogeneous from the point of view of classical psychopathology.

When section F0 (organic and symptomatic mental disorders) of ICD-10 is used for clinical diagnostic decision making, the clinician has the choice of five entry points at the level of syndrome: (1) dementia, (2) amnestic syndrome, (3) delirium, (4) 'functional' disorder (affective, delusional, hallucinatory, or other), and (5) personality or behaviour disorder. Once a disorder is identified at this general syndrome level, the next step is suggested by the diagnostic guidelines or criteria which lead into four-character diagnostic categories. The rules of diagnosis in the area of dementing illnesses are of particular interest from the point of view of mental morbidity in the elderly.

CLASSIFICATION OF THE DEMENTING ILLNESSES

The syndrome of dementia is defined in ICD-10 by 'evidence of a decline in both memory and thinking, which is of a degree sufficient to impair functioning in daily living', in a setting of clear consciousness. For a confident diagnosis to be established, such disturbances should have been present for at least 6 months. Deterioration of emotional control, social behaviour, and motivation is included as a criterion but is given less weight than mnestic and intellectual deterioration. Disturbances in higher cortical functions (aphasia, agnosia, apraxia), as well as personality change with conspicuous loss of spontaneity, are regarded as supportive evidence but not as necessary features. The research criteria (but not the clinical guidelines) provide anchor points for a grading of the severity of functional impairment into mild, moderate, and severe separately for memory and intellectual capacity. The overall grading of the severity of the dementia is based on the sphere of functioning which is most severely impaired.

Dementia in Alzheimer's disease (code F01) is defined, in addition to the presence of the syndrome of dementia, by the following criteria:

—— insidious onset with a slow deterioration;

—— absence of clinical or laboratory evidence that the syndrome could be explained by other systemic or brain disease;

—— absence of a sudden, apoplectic onset, and of focal neurological signs.

Several further features are listed as supportive of the diagnosis, without being necessary elements: (1) aphasia, agnosia, apraxia, or other evidence of higher cortical function involvement; (2) amotivation, apathy, aspontaneity, and disinhibition of social behaviour; (3) evidence of cortical atrophy; and (4) parkinsonism, logoclonia, or epileptic seizures.

A diagnosis of dementia in Alzheimer's disease can be definitive only if confirmed by neuropathological examination (evidence of neurofibrillary tangles and plaques in excess of those found in normal aging of the brain). However, it needs to be emphasized that ICD-10 allows for a confident clinical diagnosis to be made if there is clear evidence of cognitive deterioration from a previous level of functioning lasting for 6 months or more (if the period is shorter then the diagnosis is tentative).

It needs to be emphasized that the ICD-10 concept of the diagnosis and classification of dementia in Alzheimer's disease gives a priority to the clinical approach (fortified by neuropsychological investigation) even if ultimate validation in some, but not all, cases can be provided by neuropathology. Problems arise in those instances where the clinical evidence of a dementia of Alzheimer's type is not matched by the neuropathological evidence on postmortem examination, or where the typical morphological changes of Alzheimer's disease develop without the clinical manifestations of a dementia. In the first instance (i.e. dementia exhibiting Alzheimer-type features but lacking the corresponding neuropathological changes) the ICD-10 guidelines allow the condition either to be classified (presumptively) under F01 (dementia in Alzheimer's disease) or to be allocated to F00 (dementia not otherwise specified). In the second instance—that of a positive neuropathological identification of Alzheimer-type change in the brain but in the absence of the clinical picture of dementia—it is recommended to use the code for Alzheimer's disease in the ICD-10 Chapter VI (diseases of the nervous system) but not the code for dementia in Chapter V.

The ICD-10 criteria also contain the option of subtyping Alzheimer's disease dementia on the basis of the age at onset. Code F01.0 denotes dementia in Alzheimer's disease, *senile onset*, or type I; code F01.1 is used for *presenile onset*, or type II. The age dividing the two forms is specified at 65 in both the research criteria and the clinical guidelines, but the latter add the qualification that the senile onset is 'usually in the late 70s or thereafter'. It is assumed, on the basis of research evidence, that the typical clinical presentation of the two forms is different, although quite a few exceptions are known to occur.[13] Thus, the type I (senile) form is characterized by a very slow, gradual onset and progression and by a predominance of memory impairment over any signs of focal cortical dysfunction, while type II (presenile) more commonly exhibits a rapid onset and progression, as well as an early appearance of multiple and severe disturbances of higher cortical functions.

The present version of the ICD-10 criteria gives no specific instruction on how to handle discrepant cases (i.e. those patients in whom no correspondence is found between the age at onset and the configuration of the clinical presentation). By implication, however, the criterion of age should take precedence in such instances.

The definition of *vascular dementia* (F02: dementia in cerebrovascular disease) includes, apart from the requirement that the general syndrome of dementia should be present, a reference to previous ischaemic attacks, cerebrovascular accidents, or stroke. The diagnostic criteria also require:

—— an abrupt onset and/or stepwise deterioration (though periods of clinical improvement are possible);

—— unequal distribution of the deficits in higher cognitive functions;

—— evidence of focal brain damage (e.g. residual symptoms of stroke, unilateral spastic weakness of limbs, increased tendon reflexes, an extensor plantar response, pseudobulbar palsy).

Evidence from special investigations (CAT, PET, MRI) is supportive of the clinical diagnosis, but only the neuropathological examination can provide a confirmation of the diagnosis.

Four subtypes of vascular dementia are distinguished in ICD-10:

(1) vascular dementia of *acute onset* (F02.0): developing rapidly after a succession of strokes;

(2) *multi-infarct* (predominantly cortical) vascular dementia (F02.1): more gradual in onset, and having as its basis the cumulative forma-

tion of lacunae in the cerebral gray matter following a series of ischaemic episodes;

(3) other (predominantly *subcortical*) vascular dementia (F02.2): due to lacunae in the deep white matter (Binswanger's encephalopathy), with relative sparing of the cortex (although the clinical picture may resemble that in Alzheimer-type dementia);

(4) *mixed* cortical and subcortical vascular dementia (F02.3).

It should be noted that, in distinction from DSM-III, the ICD-10 definition does not equate all vascular dementias with the multi-infarct type.

ICD-10 provides codes and diagnostic guidelines or criteria for the identification of four other dementing disorders: in *Pick's disease* (F03.0); in *Creutzfeld–Jacob's disease* (F03.1); in *Huntington's disease* (F03.2); and in *Parkinson's disease* (F03.3). In the case of Parkinson's disease, it is stated that no specific distinguishing features of the dementia occurring in such patients have yet been demonstrated, and that the syndrome may be a manifestation of a co-occurrence of either Alzheimer's disease or a vascular dementing process with Parkinson's disease. However, since dementia is not uncommon in Parkinson's disease, it is considered advisable to record its occurrence separately from that of other dementias.

In addition to the above four diseases, the classification contains a collective rubric for dementia in other specified conditions, such as neurosyphilis, trypanosomiasis, head injury, AIDS, multiple sclerosis, thyroid disease, intoxications, hypercalcaemia, vitamin deficiency (niacin and B_{12}), systemic lupus, and the parkinsonism–dementia complex of Guam.

DEMENTIA IN ICD-10 AND IN OTHER CURRENT CLASSIFICATIONS

In the course of the preparation of the provisional ICD-10 classification of mental disorders, a number of consultations were held with groups and individuals representing other approaches to the classification of organic mental disorders. These exchanges involved also the developers of DSM-III-R, as well as experts involved in the preparation of the criteria for clinical diagnosis of Alzheimer disease proposed by the National Institute of Neurological and Communicative Disorders and Stroke (NINCDS) and the Alzheimer Disease and Related Disorders Association (ADRDA) of the United States.[14] Although the ICD-10, NINCDS-ADRDA, and DSM-IIIR criteria converge in many respects as regards the definitions of syndromes and the diagnostic criteria of the dementing disorders, some important differences remain. For example the DSM-III-R criteria for the general syndrome of dementia are more restrictive than the ICD-10 guidelines and criteria. In addition to a decline of memory and intellectual function in a setting of clear consciousness, DSM-III-R requires evidence for the presence of one or more features such as impairment of abstract thinking, impaired judgement, higher cortical function disturbances, or personality change. Such manifestations, however, may be difficult to ascertain in the early stages of a dementing illness, and may even be absent in advanced stages of the process. By introducing a grading of severity, as well as a provision for qualifying the degree of confidence in the diagnosis, ICD-10 ensures a more flexible approach to the clinical identification of dementia.

As concerns the subtyping of dementia in Alzheimer's disease, the two classifications agree on the criterion of age at onset but disagree on the further subdivision of the disorder. 'Primary degenerative dementia' (in DSM-III-R terms) is subdivided according to the presence of delirium, delusions, or depression—features which, from the point of view of ICD-10, are secondary or accidental. Such complications can be recorded in ICD-10 by using a separate code (there is, for instance, a special code for delirium superimposed on dementia). Similar considerations apply to the classification of multi-infarct dementia in DSM-III-R, which is also subdivided according to possible complications or associated features rather than according to forms and variants of the disease process itself. Thus, DSM-III-R criteria ensure greater specificity at the level of identification of the general syndrome of dementia, but less specificity at the level of diagnosis of the individual subtypes. The advantages and disadvantages of the two approaches are yet to be ascertained.

Perhaps the most debatable issue in the ICD-10 classification of dementia in Alzheimer's disease is the present choice of a criterion for the subtyping of the disorder. While substantial evidence exists of a correlation between the age at onset and the pattern of clinical manifestations and course (i.e. type-I and type-II clinical picture), the proposed distinctions based on age at onset are not universally accepted. For example, to date there is no clear evidence of a bimodal distribution of the age-specific onsets of dementia in Alzheimer's disease, and the male: female ratio does not seem to be different in the new cases occurring in the age groups below 65 and over 65. In the absence of unequivocal evidence for either the existence of a continuum or that of well-circumscribed specific subtypes, the subclassification of dementia in Alzheimer's disease remains a problem that can be resolved only by new research. Such research should be carried out on a much wider geographical basis than before, utilizing comparable and, if possible, standard methods and criteria. By incorporating in its definitions and criteria specific and testable propositions about the nature and manifestations of the dementias, ICD-10 can provide a useful point of departure for such research.

References

1. Kraepelin, E. (1896). *Psychiatrie. 5 Auflage*. Barth, Leipzig.
2. Jaspers, K. (1963). *General psychopathology*. Manchester University Press, Manchester.
3. World Health Organization (1974). *Glossary of mental disorders and guide to their classification for use in conjunction with the international classification of diseases (8th revision)*. WHO, Geneva.
4. World Health Organization (1978). *Mental disorders: glossary and guide to their classification in accordance with the ninth revision of the International classification of diseases*. WHO, Geneva.
5. World Health Organization (1987). *ICD-10: 1986 draft of chapter V. Mental, behavioural and developmental disorders*. Document no. MNH/MEP/87.1. WHO, Geneva.
6. American Psychiatric Association (1980). *Diagnostic and statistical manual of mental disorders*, (3rd edn). (DSM-III). APA, Washington DC.
7. Mechanic, D. (1986). Social factors affecting the mental health of the elderly. In *Mental health in the elderly. A review of the present state of research* (ed. Häfner H., G. Moschel, and N. Sartorius). Springer, Berlin.
8. Häfner, H. (1986). *Psychische Gesundheit im Alter*. Fischer, Stuttgart.
9. Katzman, R. (1986). Alzheimer's disease. *New England Journal of Medicine*, **314**, 964–73.
10. Roth, M. (1986). The association of clinical and neurological findings and its bearing on the classification and aetiology of Alzheimer's disease. *British Medical Bulletin*, **42**, 42–50.
11. Kramer, M., Sartorius, N., Jablensky, A., and Gulbinat, W. (1979). The ICD-9 classification of mental disorders. A review of its development and contents. *Acta Psychiatrica Scandinavica*, **59**, 241–62.
12. Mental disorders, alcohol and drug-related problems: international perspectives on their diagnosis and classification. (1985). Reports and recommendations of the international conference on diagnosis and classification of mental disorders and alcohol and drug-related problems, held at the WHO regional office for Europe, Copenhagen, 13–17 April 1982. Excerpta Medica, Amsterdam.
13. Reisberg, B. (1983). An overview of current concepts of Alzheimer's disease, senile dementia, and age-associated cognitive decline. In *Alzheimer's disease. The standard reference* (ed. Reisberg, B.) pp. 3–20, Collier Macmillan, London.
    The standard reference (ed. Reisberg, B.) Collier Macmillan, London.
14. McKhann, G., Drachman, D., Folstein, M., Katzman, R., Price, D., and Stadlan, E. M. (1984). Clinical diagnosis of Alzheimer's disease. *Neurology*, **34**, 939–44.

Index

academic leadership 560
accelerated osteoporosis 149
access to health services 109, 123
accidents 50, 55, 112, 113, 222, 296, 297,
    308, 311, 320, 321, 329, 330, 566, 624
accreditation of nursing homes 483
acoustics 256
activities of daily living 69, 71, 73, 100, 402,
    421, 530, 531, 599
acute confusional states 263, 265
acute illness 62, 278, 306, 578
acute services 444
ADL 73, 80, 84
adult day care 459
advances in geriatric care 3
adverse reactions to prescribed drugs 231
Africa 24, 363, 366, 619, 660
age dependency 121
age of retirement 662, 665
age structure 22
age-based rationing 15, 619, 669, 680
age-integrated social programmes 469
age-integrated society 372
age-related changes in neurones 131
age-segregated communities 522
age-sex registers 197
age-specific mortality 28, 39, 50
aging and disease 58
aging of the older population 22
aging of the population 613, 623, 665
agism and resource allocation 619
alarms 114, 252
alcohol 307, 329
alpha adrenergic agonist 285
alterations in gene activities 135
altered proteins and slowed cell
    metabolism 134
alternative health services 102
alternatives to nursing homes 400
Alzheimer's disease 1, 60, 131, 133, 134,
    136, 222, 263, 265, 266, 267, 528, 530,
    534, 539, 684, 685, 687, 689, 690, 692
Alzheimer's disease and related disorders
    (ADRD) 265
Alzheimer's Disease and Related Disorders
    Association 541
anabolic steroids 160
ancient Greece 502
anticholinergic agents 285

anticoagulants 181, 218
antidepressants 219
antidepressants and falls 307
antihistamines 219
antirheumatic drugs 221
anxiety 268
areas of functional assessment 73
Argentina 71, 368, 371
arthritis 300, 320
Asia 22, 24, 362, 366, 369, 373, 376, 382,
    448, 617, 619, 643, 660, 663
assessing attitudes 591
assessing health status in the elderly 91
assessing hearing function 243
assessment and rehabilitation unit 443
assessment of mental health 80
assistive devices 530
assistive listening devices 247, 251
at risk 327, 348, 352, 399, 400, 455,
    541, 665, 668
atherosclerosis 56, 213
attitudes toward disability 46
auditory brain 242
auditory brainstem 241
auditory training 254
aural rehabilitation 252
aural rehabilitation programme 239
aural rehabilitation techniques 253
Australia 25, 27, 28, 176, 189, 398, 418,
    440, 443, 444, 520, 578, 581, 587, 668
Austria 477
autonomy 17, 302, 551, 618, 673, 675, 676,
    677, 678
autonomy and self-determination 673, 679

balance control 306
Barbados 71
basic self-care 80, 401, 530
bed rest 235
bed-disability days 402
bedridden elderly 385, 391, 395
Belgium 70
bereavement 586
    counselling 496
binaural test measures 244
biochemical events at the menopause 151
biofeedback 283

biogerontology 128
biology of aging 128
biadder neck suspension 286
bladder training 283
blood lipid 317
boarding homes 404
bone formation promotion 160
Botswana 372, 375
brain imaging 265
brain oedema 180
Brazil 22, 71
Bulgaria 22, 26, 176

calcitonin 158
calcium supplementation 155
Canada 214, 328, 398, 400, 405, 440, 453,
    485, 499, 502, 503, 505, 506, 508, 509,
    520, 523, 524, 625, 668
Canadian 25, 45, 46, 299, 404, 408, 435,
    464, 513, 525
cardiac failure 213, 217, 218, 220, 235
cardiac glycosides 216
cardiogenic cerebral embolism 181
cardiovascular disease 317
care of the patient with acute stroke 178
care planning 403
carotid endarterectomy 185
Carribean 69, 660
case management 102, 103, 398, 399, 400,
    401, 404, 405, 407, 408, 409, 410, 412,
    413, 414, 418, 419, 421, 587, 655
case manager 405
cataract 135, 304
catheterization 287
catheters 287
cell nucleus and the genome 132
cerebral embolism 182
cerebral haemorrhage 180
cerebral infarction 179
cerebrovascular accident 187, 188, 213, 242,
    246, 690
changed pharmacodynamics 216
changes in sensitivity to drugs 216
changing family pattern 370
chewing 321, 322
Chile 71
China 19, 21, 22, 368, 369, 617, 643
cholinergic agonist 286
cholinergic neurotransmitters 264
chronic illness 96, 300, 320, 467, 534, 588,
    608, 675
    management 578
chronological age 15, 16, 17, 103, 130, 498
classification of dementias 683
classification of mental disorders 686
classification of dementing illnesses 688

clonal senescence 128, 133, 136
clubs 443, 459, 566
cognitive function 80, 95, 238, 421, 435, 690
cohort 3, 15, 34
    effects 43, 52
Colombia 71
communication techniques 254
community care 102, 342, 357, 394, 400,
    401, 408, 409, 410, 453, 454, 479, 567,
    655
community control of hypertension 196
community self-help 375, 377
community-based long-term care 458
community-based care 3
complications of hospitalization 233
comprehensive assessment 401
comprehensive health services 346, 351
compression of morbidity 30, 31, 32
computer-assisted tomography 3
concept of lay care 561
concept of self-help 353
confusion 216, 219, 264, 269, 321, 323, 324,
    442
congestive heart failure 278
congregate housing 408, 523, 524
congregate meals 459, 465
consequences of falls 301
contextual scenarios 550
continence 273
continuity of care 349, 350, 357, 359, 360,
    583, 619
continuum of health and social services 469
control of hypertension 187
convulsions 179
coronary artery bypass surgery 99
cost-benefit analysis 648
cost-effectiveness analysis 648
cost-utility analysis 648
Costa Rica 24, 71, 371
cost benefits of treating hypertension 198
costs in hospice 498
costs of stroke 199
counselling 406
cross-cultural comparisons 17
cross-cultural studies 373
cross-national comparison 69, 70, 80, 81, 85
cross-national differences 73, 84
cross-national evaluations 69
cross-national studies 72
cross-sectional data 627
cross-sectional studies 52
Cuba 71
Czechoslovakia 173, 176

day care 5, 102, 352, 353, 355, 356, 376,
    395, 408, 409, 418, 443, 449, 452, 458,
    459, 464, 469, 541, 559, 566, 603, 648

day hospital 417, 418, 443, 457, 458, 459
de-institutionalization 485
death from cancer 318
decline in family role 388
decreased use of nursing homes 434
decreased capability of families 390
defensive use of health services 52
definitions of autonomy 332
definitions of falling 297
degenerative osteoarthritis 531
delirium 265, 278, 687, 688, 692
delivery of primary care 351
dementia 3, 60, 172, 189, 190, 232, 263,
    265, 267, 268, 356, 404, 528, 530, 534,
    539, 540, 541, 684, 687, 690
  in ICD-10 691
  of Alzheimer's type 267, 689
  syndrome 268
demographic transition 21
Denmark 322, 324, 325, 443, 477, 485
dependency 479, 484
dependency ratio 108
depression 1, 95, 162, 185, 218, 219, 262,
    263, 264, 265, 268, 269, 296, 323, 402,
    403, 493, 503, 652, 684, 685, 692
determinants of health in old age 617
determinants of longevity 54
developing countries 107, 346, 362, 381,
    449, 473, 559, 561, 618, 619, 628, 660,
    662
diabetes 56, 99, 135, 190, 195, 213, 476,
    530, 551, 564, 571, 572
diagnostic and statistical manual of mental
    discrders 684
dialysis 99
differences between young and old 51
differences not due to aging 51
difficulties of families 390
diphosphonates 159
disability 18, 31, 32, 33, 35, 36, 38, 39, 43,
    60, 93, 650
  categories 651
  days 81, 84
  expectancy 45
  levels 97
  years 45
  – free life expectancy 38
discharge planning 100
discriminatory attitudes 64
diuretics 217
DNA damage 135
domiciliary care 648, 653, 656
domiciliary services 60, 443, 474
Dominican Republic 371
drug consumption patterns 214
drug-induced disease 214
drugs for high blood-pressure 217

drugs for heart rhythm disturbances 218
DSM-III 684

early mobilization 235
early retirement 662
ease of movement around the city 623
Eastern Europe 26, 176
Eastern Mediterranean 475
economic factors 627
economic perspective 647
economic principles 657
educating health professionals 576
education 81, 108, 119, 358, 367, 373, 377,
    389, 447, 544, 563, 569, 613, 617
educational objectives in gerontology 580
educational programme design 576
effect of price change in medical care 633
effectiveness of geriatric assessment 422
effects of institutionalization 477
efficiency of alternative policies 647
Egypt 475
El Salvador, 71
elderly women 23, 195, 202, 281, 283, 300,
    318, 368, 374
emergence of longitudinal studies of
    aging 358
encouraging autonomy 485
England 53, 113, 172, 178, 440, 499
England and Wales 174, 175, 503
epidemiology 56, 97
  of aging 60
equity in the allocation of resources 654
ethical issues 667
Ethiopia 375, 629
Europe 70, 201, 224, 604
evaluating efficacy 466
evaluating home care efficacy 466
evaluation of geriatric units 446
evaluation of student learning 591
evidence of benefit 467
evidence of reduced disability 40
evolutionary lag theory 56
excessive prescribing 212
exercise 160, 329
exit from the labour market 618
extended family 119, 363, 365, 366, 368,
    369, 370, 371, 372, 376
extension of longevity 643
extracranial-intracranial bypass surgery 185
extrinsic aging 55, 56, 57
extrinsically determined aging 54

fall rehabilitation programme 311
falling risk of 299
falls 296, 302

familial relationship 115
family care 382, 565
family support 119, 374, 376, 377, 541, 566,
    567, 640, 644
family support groups 559
family support services 542
family support systems 617, 628
fertility 19, 21, 475, 643
fibrinolytic agents 183
Fiji 70, 476, 486
Finland 70, 80, 162, 178, 199, 200
foster families 376
frail elderly 324, 331, 356, 394, 406, 410,
    417, 419, 422, 436, 465, 478, 655
France 21, 24, 70, 296, 299, 300, 301, 302,
    412, 502, 617, 640, 668
freedom from disability 619, 650
functional status 93
functional status indices (FSIs) 94
fundamental principle of rehabilitation 17
future geriatric needs 608

genetic potential for longevity 55
genetics of longevity 130
geriatric
    assessment 343, 404
    assessment efficacy 417
    assessment process 420
    assessment programmes 419
    assessment units 101
    care 17, 418
    pharmacology 214, 224
    clinics 356
    consultation services 419
    departments 53
    drug use 213
    drugs 212
    education 583
    health status 94
    hospitals 296
    literature 93
    manpower needs 579
    medicine 324, 325, 417, 440
    nursing 613
    paradigm 341
    pharmacology 211
    pioneers 417
    rehabilitation units 419
    service 442
    specialists 560
    team 407, 444
    units 443
    urinary incontinence 273
geriatrics 16, 222, 223, 324, 343, 417, 440,
    446, 538, 576, 577, 578, 579, 580, 583,
    584, 602, 603, 604, 613

Germany 24, 70
gerontology 15, 16, 444, 568, 576, 579, 580,
    583, 584, 586, 589, 604, 613
    education 591
    training 569, 574
Ghana 367, 369, 371, 372
grading of the severity of dementia 689
granny flat 517, 520
Greece 22, 70
Guatemala 368
Guyana 71

haemodilution therapy 183
handicap 35, 36, 316, 441
hazards 307
head of the household 116
health and social care policies 649
health care 341
health care effectiveness 97
health education 63, 356, 360, 564, 568,
    569, 570, 572
health education-Mexico 571
health education schools 603
health expectancy index 45
health habits 329
health insurance 663, 665
health maintenance organization 436
health promotion 6, 316, 330, 356, 360, 464,
    597, 609
health services 64, 561, 628
healthy lifestyles 328, 332
hearing 321
hearing aids 247, 248, 260
hearing disorders 237
heart failure 98, 217, 264
help for incontinent people (HIP) 280
high blood-pressure 213, 217, 551
hip replacement 99
home care 4, 101, 102, 324, 394, 400, 401,
    408, 452, 453, 454, 456, 457, 458, 460,
    462, 464, 465, 466, 468, 469, 479, 485,
    491, 492, 493, 498, 499, 524, 525, 548,
    551, 554, 582, 620, 642, 664
    technology 551
home help 61, 324, 331, 349, 386, 394, 395,
    408, 444, 664
home monitoring 548, 549
home nursing 407
home nursing foundation 355
home renewal 516
home repairs 516
homemaker programme 525
homemaker services 410
homes for the aged 408
homesharing 517
Honduras 71

Hong Kong 643
hormones 153
hospice 491, 492, 493, 495, 496, 498, 499,
    500, 612, 676
hospice care 418, 491
hospital and home care hospices 497
hostel 514
household composition 113
housing 4, 16, 52, 57, 72, 85, 86, 108, 112,
    113, 330, 332, 341, 348, 358, 372, 376,
    377, 389, 469, 474, 505, 508, 509, 525,
    619, 655, 667
    adjustments 506
    estates 355
    for older people 502
    for the elderly 504
    needs 504
    quality 506
    repairs 331
    technologies 530
human lifespan 130, 669
human warehouse 474
Hungary 28, 176
hypertension 191
hypochondriasis 219
hypostatic pneumonia 235
hypothermia 52, 301, 302

iatrogenic disease 323
iatrogenic disorders 231
ICD-10 683
identification of hypertensives 196
illness in old age 62
imaging devices 181
immune mechanisms 2
impact of economic development 628
impairment 35, 36, 45, 93, 95, 398, 407,
    410, 413, 530, 531, 534, 536
improving quality of life 619
inadequate diagnostic effort 231
incapacity for self-care 44
income and health 107
income tax subsidies to homeowners 513
income-generating projects 378
incontinence 278
incontinence clinics 280
India 19, 108, 109, 110, 111, 114, 115, 116,
    117, 118, 119, 121, 122, 366, 369, 371,
    373, 376
indicators of quality of life 496
indices of disability 44
inequity 669
infections 322
informal support 331, 374, 469
informal support network 457, 458
informal support system 341, 464, 468

informed consent 675
injury 299, 300
institutional care 3, 4, 5, 101, 102, 222, 299,
    324, 342, 352, 356, 377, 391, 394, 400,
    436, 447, 449, 452, 467, 469, 474, 476,
    478, 479, 480, 486, 523, 524, 530, 609,
    617, 641, 642, 643, 655
institutional services 443
institutionalization 234
instruments for government supervision 480
insurance for long-term care 410
integrated care 377
integrated case management 413
integrated care 360
integration of housing and services 523
intensive care 98
intergenerational competition 5
intergenerational contact 371
intergenerational experiences 367
intergenerational living 368
intergenerational shared households 519
intergenerational solidarity 550
International Plan of Action 613
International Social Security
    Association 666
intracerebral haemorrhage 186
intrinsic aging 54, 59
Ireland 176
irreversible dementia 436
Israel 323, 398, 418, 475, 476, 477, 478,
    479, 481, 486, 583, 584, 668
Italy 22, 70

Jamaica 24, 71, 368, 371
Japan 20, 21, 22, 24, 25, 27, 28, 39, 173,
    177, 182, 381, 382, 385, 386, 387, 388,
    389, 390, 391, 392, 394, 395, 396, 484,
    617, 627, 633, 634, 635, 640, 643, 668

Kenya 371, 375
Korea 70, 617, 643
Kuwait 70, 475, 476, 486

lack of autonomy 324, 478
Latin America 22, 23, 108, 362, 366, 369,
    371, 376, 619, 660, 663
laundry 402
    costs 281
    service 444
lay and self care 561
Lebanon 371
legal guardianship 404
length of stay 302, 435, 492, 495, 552, 619
less developed countries 95, 110

life expectancy 24, 25, 26, 30, 31, 33, 34, 38, 39, 40, 45, 95, 107, 200, 475, 528, 633, 635, 637, 643, 652, 660
  and lifespan 33
  at age 65, 617, 631, 640
life table 29, 631
life-care 522
life-sustaining technologies 536
lifelong process 56
lifespan 25, 32, 55, 91, 672
lifespan and disease 129
living space 621
living will 396
long-term care 4, 38, 341, 442, 452, 473, 474, 486, 652
long-term care facility 417, 418
long-term care programmes 400
long-term care services 476
long-term care system 479
longevity 26, 63, 634
  and mortality 91
longitudinal designs 466
longitudinal follow-up 422
longitudinal studies 46, 311, 324
loss of personal autonomy 309

macroeconomic changes 643
maintenance of autonomy 316, 331
maintenance of personal health 328
maladaptive evolution theories 57
Malaysia 70, 580, 581
mandatory screening 401
Manitoba continuing care program 453
marginal returns 632
marital status and health 120
market for retirement housing 522
maximum lifespan 34, 54, 55, 129, 130, 131
meals-on-wheels 61, 113, 418, 444, 459, 465, 525
mechanical presbyacusis 238
medical expenditure 628
medicalization 231
menopause 53, 134, 145, 146, 147, 149, 150, 151, 153, 157, 162, 163, 319
metal health 262
metabolic presbyacusis 238
Mexico 108, 373
model of long-term care 102
models of primary care 355
modernization 372
modified Delphi 1
Morocco 375
motivation 584
motivation to learn 585
multi-infarct dementia 188, 189, 191, 265, 267, 692

multigenerational households 617
myocardial infarction 181, 182, 192, 213, 216, 217, 218, 564

National Health Service 99, 417, 436, 578, 663
National Hospice Study 493, 494
natural lifespan 669, 671, 680
nature of human aging 50
need to be useful 120
needs for physician services 607
needs of the elderly 441
Netherlands 219, 325, 418, 443, 477, 485
neural presbyacusis 238
neuroleptics (antipsychotics) 220
neurotransmitters 2, 131, 266, 267
new technologies for the elderly 544
New Zealand 176, 298, 300, 407, 440, 447, 448
Nigeria 369, 374
non-steroidal anti-inflammatory drugs (NSAIDs) 221
nootropics 266
Northern Europe 326
Norway 418, 523
nursing home 5, 257, 287, 296, 316, 323, 324, 342, 385, 386, 387, 392, 395, 401, 414, 452, 459, 479, 481, 486
  care 101, 473
  industry 477
nutrition 111, 235, 373, 617
nutrition policies 619
nutritional status 111

occupational therapy 355, 444, 459, 608
Office of Technology Assessment 528
old-age benefits 659
older women 391
ombudsman 483
On Lok 412
oral antidiabetic drugs 220
organized excursions 623
origins of geriatric assessment 417
origins of the nursing home 476
osteoarthritis 56, 213, 530
osteoporosis 53, 134, 143, 301, 319
over investigation 231
overflow incontinence 286
overprescribing of psychotropic drugs 222

Pacific 70
Pakistan 369, 374, 376, 475
Panama 368, 371
paraphrenia 262, 269, 270, 683, 684

parathyroid hormone 162
Parkinson's disease 222, 531, 691
parkinsonism dementia complex of
    Guam 691
paternalism 674
pattern of aging 60
pedestrian ways 624
pension 331, 387, 469, 474, 618, 633, 659,
    660, 661, 662, 665
peripheral hearing system 240
persistent incontinence 279
personal care home 462
personnel required for long-term care 609
pharmacodynamic problems 212
pharmacokinetic problems 212, 214
phenothiazines 220
Philippines 70, 366, 486
physician neglect 323
physiotherapy 235, 255, 444, 459, 485, 524
planning for health personnel 596
planning environments 621
platelet anti-aggregants 182
pneumonia 301, 323
Poland 70, 176
population at risk of falling 298
population growth in developing
    countries 19
population pyramid 21
portable living units for seniors 517
Portugal 27
potentially reversible dementia 265
poverty 88, 109, 475, 476, 486, 675
    level 85
    line 505
    reduction 653
premature nursing home placement 461
prerequisite skills 587
presbycusis 238
preventable conditions 317
preventing falls 309
preventing stroke 201
prevention 63, 316
prevention of osteoporosis 145, 152
preventive geriatrics 582
primary aging 54
primary care 341, 343
primary care team 359, 360
primary degenerative dementias 263, 692
primary dementia 263, 266
primary health care 346
primary prevention 316
private space 622
problem drugs 216, 212, 220
promoting self-care ability 485
promotion of independence 508
property tax relief programs 512
proprioceptive disorders 305

prostate 285, 286, 287, 318
prostatic resection 286
protheses 547
provident fund 618, 660
proximal femoral fractures 143
prudent consumers 671
pseudodementia 219, 222, 265, 268
psychogeriatric care 4
psychogeriatrics 613
psychotropic drugs 212, 219, 278
public services 394
public space 624

QALY 201, 649
QALY methodology 650
quality assurance 483
quality control in nursing homes 618
quality of care 479
quality of life 43, 93, 98, 99, 202, 468, 649
quality-adjusted life years 201, 649

randomized clinical trial 446
randomized trial 183, 319, 435
rationing 538, 668, 679, 670, 671, 680
rationing and cost constraints 411
record keeping 483
recoverability of the aged patient 441
recreation 348, 572
    areas 256
recreational activities 355
recreational facilities 376, 377, 518
recreational services 86
rehabilitation 4, 62, 101, 235, 355, 395, 442
    programme 255
    trial 417
reimbursement policies 481
renter programmes 510
resources spent on health 632
respite care 268, 459, 460, 469, 541
restraints 309
retardation of senescence 96
retirement 'à la carte' 662
retirement age 5, 64, 331, 643, 662
retirement communities 518, 522
retirement community planning 518
retirement village 522
rights of the elderly 330
RNA and protein synthesis 132
role of the nursing home 473
role models 589
role of service providers 324
role of the family 362, 381
roles of offspring 387
Romania 70, 72

Scandanavia 668
schizophrenics 269
scope of action of lay persons 562
Scotland 349
screening 163, 178, 195, 197, 198, 318, 319,
   320, 327, 328, 356, 401, 648
screening and case finding 326, 400
secondary aging 53
sedatives, tranquillizers, and hypnotics 219
self-assessment of health 81, 84
self-care 65, 267, 353, 484, 559, 563
self-care movement 330
self-care programmes 572
self-care record 572
self-care skills 564
self-care techniques 572
self-determination 678
self-health care 559
self-help 378
self-help groups 268
senescence 50, 130, 675
senile dementia 60, 213, 617, 640, 641
senility 211, 329, 373
senior centres 459, 469, 603
senior co-ownership 518
sensory presbyacusis 238
settings for teaching 588
sex differences in aging and longevity 57
sex differentials in mortality 23
sexuality 586
shared housing 519
sheltered housing 5
short-term stay service 395
sight 321
Singapore 355, 356, 357, 617, 643
skills objectives 583
smoking 317, 329
smoking and alcohol consumption 195
social contacts 329
social health maintenance organization 408
social insurance schemes 222, 628
social insurance systems 213
social objectives 582
social policy issues 485
social priorities 647
social security 659
social security measures 663
social support 316, 324, 330, 331, 401, 420,
   436, 474, 477, 480, 485, 541, 569, 619,
   665, 666
sodium fluoride 161
South America 69
southern Europe 22, 27, 213
South Pacific 369
specialists in rehabilitation medicine 444
speech tests 245
speed of population aging 19

sphere of social and vital activity 621
spinal osteoporosis 150
Sri Lanka 369
standard auditory tests 243
status 118
stereotypes 330
strain on the caregiver 86
stress/urge incontinence 283
stroke 28, 56, 59, 60, 63, 94, 101, 172, 173,
   174, 176, 177, 178, 180, 181, 183, 184,
   185, 186, 188, 189, 191, 194, 195, 196,
   200, 216, 217, 235, 245, 247, 267, 298,
   317, 690
   incidence 192
   mortality 176, 192, 193, 197
   prevention 187
   rehabilitation 100
   risk factors 190
   types 187
   units 100
stroke-in-evolution 181
subarachnoid haemorrhage 180
supply of health personnel 611
support groups 330
support services to seniors 465
Sweden 21, 27, 173, 329, 412, 418, 444, 523,
   629
syndrome of dementia 688
Syria 371

teaching 576
   methods 583
   nursing home 589
teamwork 350
technologies for long-term care 539
technology development 528
technology for independent living 620
tenth revision of the International
   Classification of Diseases 683
terminal illness 288, 436
Thailand 368, 369, 376, 617, 640
theory of biological aging 128
   intrinsic aging 54
   mortality and aging 32
   the isolated nuclear family 381
thiazide diuretics 159
third age 19
traditional family 365
training sites 588, 603
transportation 5, 85, 102, 402, 412, 528, 530
Trinidad and Tobago 71
true aging 53
Tunisia 375
Turkey 374

undergarments and padding 281
United Kingdom 22, 53, 58, 60, 112, 185,
    285, 296, 300, 306, 323, 407, 411, 440,
    523, 617, 640, 654, 668
United Nations World Assembly on
    Aging 613
United States 15, 21, 22, 24, 25, 28, 39, 40,
    43, 46, 97, 176, 185, 186, 199, 239, 296,
    323, 327, 329, 398, 418, 436, 464, 476,
    477, 492, 509, 531, 599
United States Congress 528
university of the third age 331
urban or architectural environment 625
urbanization 23, 372, 475, 487, 617, 627,
    665
urge and stress incontinence 284
urge incontinence 285
urinary incontinence 273
use of drugs 211
use of medicaments 329
use of physical and chemical restraints 309
USSR 70
utilitarianism 674

values and attitudes 559
vascular dementia 691
vasodilators 184
Venezuela 71
vestibular disorders 305
vitamin D 150
    metabolites 157

weatherization assistance 513
weight 317, 318, 329
Western Pacific 69, 476
WHO Expert Committee on Aging 1
World Assembly on Aging 368, 378, 475
World Health Organization 223

Year 2000 6
Yugoslavia 70

Zambia 371